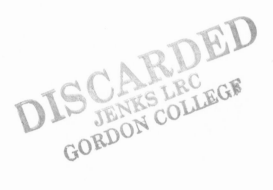

OSLER'S
WEB

OSLER'S WEB

Inside the Labyrinth of the Chronic Fatigue Syndrome Epidemic

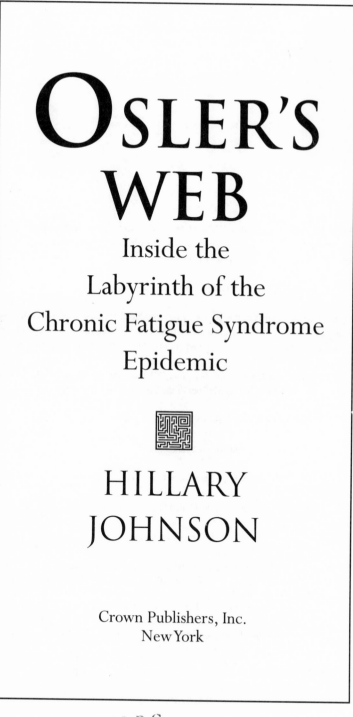

HILLARY JOHNSON

Crown Publishers, Inc.
New York

Grateful acknowledgment is made to Harold Ober Associates for permission to reprint an excerpt from *The Orange Man* by Berton Roueche. Copyright © 1967 by Berton Roueche. Originally published in *The New Yorker*. Reprinted by permission of Harold Ober Associates Incorporated.

Published by Crown Publishers, Inc., 201 East 50th Street, New York, New York 10022. Member of the Crown Publishing Group.

Random House, Inc. New York, Toronto, London, Sydney, Auckland

http://www.randomhouse.com

CROWN is a trademark of Crown Publishers, Inc.

Printed in the United States of America

Design by B. Klein

Library of Congress Cataloging-in-Publication Data
Johnson, Hillary.
Osler's web : inside the labyrinth of the chronic fatigue syndrome
epidemic / by Hillary Johnson. — 1st ed.
Includes index.
1. Chronic fatigue syndrome—Popular works.   I. Title.
RB150.F37J64   1996
616'.047—dc20   95-31149
                                                          CIP

ISBN 0-517-70353-X

10 9 8 7 6 5

For my mother, Ruth Hines Jones (1928–1993)

Contents

Acknowledgments

Osler's Web was forged from the intellectual contributions of a great many clinicians, scientists, patients, and their families who entrusted me with their stories. I am grateful to all of them, particularly the clinicians who, with hardly any time to spare, managed somehow to give me time. Friends and relatives who took my late-night phone calls and supported my effort in countless other ways need to be thanked as well. They are Ann Armbruster, Charles M. Young, Grant Loud, Susan and Bradley Waterman, Elizabeth Andrews, Susan Berman, Barbara Simmons, Chappy Morris, Pam and Summer Rosenberg, Calvin Fentress, Bette Hammel, Liisa Welch, Nanette Dumas, Elizabeth Purdy, Gene Stone, Maria Lenhardt, Don Goodwin, Albert Scardino, John Cantrell, Lionel Horwitz, Ken Sherman, my brother Kimball Johnson, and my cousin Don Wilkin. Ethan Hoffman, a photographer and *Life* magazine colleague who died in an accident while on assignment in 1990, and the late Gilda Radner also helped me in significant ways during the early years of my research. I thank Edward P. Evans, former CEO of Macmillan, for his early interest in this book.

I received financial support in the form of grants from two foundations that saw merit in this project. Their generosity sustained me during critical periods when I otherwise would have been forced to abandon the project. They are the Fund for Investigative Journalism in Washington, D.C., which makes grants to independent writers to enable them to "probe abuses of authority or the malfunctioning of institutions and systems which harm the public," and the CFIDS Foundation of Charlotte, a nonprofit philanthropy that supports biomedical research and educational efforts related to chronic fatigue–immune dysfunction syndrome.

Attorney Quinlan J. Shea Jr., formerly of the National Security Archive in Washington, D.C., and an expert in the Freedom of Information Act, lent his considerable expertise to my efforts to acquire documents from the government through FOIA. On my behalf, he met for long hours with NIH staff to negotiate the release of documents, and vigilantly monitored the government's processing of records, without once abandoning his quick wit. Quin also took an active role in advising me on other crucial First Amendment issues that erupted during the course of reporting this book.

Journalist Spencer Klaw, teacher and friend, offered counsel and support throughout the long, lean years of this project, much as he has done for the last twenty years. I am also indebted to Jann Wenner and Bob Wallace, the publisher and the former executive editor of *Rolling Stone* magazine, who encouraged my first efforts to explore this story and who published my reporting on it in 1987. Charles Ortleb, publisher of the *New York Native,* and *Native* reporter Neenyah Ostrom have been steadily supportive since I began work on this book late in 1987. In addition, their commitment to investigating the nexus between AIDS and CFS in the face of antagonism from many sources is deserving of the greatest respect.

Michael Carlisle of the William Morris Agency exhibited enthusiasm and empathy throughout this project. I am grateful for his help and advice, and for our friendship.

I hold Tom McCormack, CEO at St. Martin's Press, in high esteem and appreciate his myriad suggestions for this book; I employed all of them.

Tina Constable, managing director of Publicity at Crown, demonstrated tremendous energy and a gift for strategic thinking.

Freelance book editor Kitty Ross trimmed five hundred pages from the manuscript with surgical delicacy and offered valuable editorial advice.

My radiant mother, the artist Ruth Jones, who long ago helped me become a journalist, studied this book as it took shape with characteristic insight and concern. She railed against the villains, took umbrage on behalf of the long-suffering, erupted with unprintable witticisms, yet counseled a prose of reportorial calm. Her contributions permeate these pages.

Last, I was extraordinarily fortunate in the winter of 1990 to have landed with my bulky manuscript in the smoke-filled inner office of editor Michael Denneny. He brought an uncommon degree of understanding to the material, was a tireless advocate, and is surely among the most brilliant and dedicated editors in book publishing. Without Michael, there would be no book.

Methods

The following is a work of firsthand reporting. I created no composite characters. All of the people described in this book exist. I conducted the vast majority of the interviews in person and, in most cases, the interviews were tape-recorded. All of the names are real except those of a small number of patients who agreed to be interviewed on the condition that their privacy be protected. In such cases, I used pseudonyms but identified them as such. In the rare cases when I describe someone's thoughts, those thoughts were described directly to me. When I describe private scenes among scientists, patients, or others, I was usually present; in the rare instances when I was not, sources were present who confirmed events, or else dialogue was obtained directly from taped remarks.

I conducted the interviews used in this book over a period of nine years, beginning in the fall of 1986.

I also obtained information through the Freedom of Information Act in the form of memos, letters, and other government documents. The FOIA, in principle, aids citizens seeking to understand the workings of government. The Centers for Disease Control were generally responsive to FOIA requests. The National Institutes of Health were minimally responsive, ignoring repeated entreaties for compliance and even, upon appeal, an order to comply by the assistant secretary of health, James Mason. I circumvented these barriers on occasion when federal employees or third parties provided documents directly to me.

Other sources for this book include scores of scientific papers from the medical literature as well as books written on chronic fatigue syndrome and related subjects by other authors. When I quote or refer to a particular scientific paper or book in the text, the formal citation can be found at the end of the book.

Correspondence between doctors and patients, and between doctors and their colleagues, provided to me by the correspondents, also informed my research process, even though I quoted few of these letters directly.

The edifice of medicine reposes entirely upon facts . . . truth cannot be elicited but from those which have been well and completely observed.

—Sir William Osler, *Counsels and Ideals*

1984
UNUSUAL
OCCURRENCES

Emulating the persistence and care of Darwin, we must collect facts with open-minded watchfulness, unbiased by crotchets or notions; fact on fact, instance on instance, experiment upon experiment; facts which fitly jointed together by some master who grasps the idea of their relationship, may establish a general principle.

—Sir William Osler, *Counsels and Ideals*

1

Clinical Mysteries

San Francisco, California

Her first patient had suggested someone in the initial stages of an autoimmune disease, most probably lupus or multiple sclerosis. By the end of summer 1984, Dr. Carol Jessop counted fifteen such cases in her practice at the Lyon-Martin Health Center, a community clinic for women where she volunteered her time as medical director. The baffling affliction, for which Jessop had no name, was remarkably virulent. In the previous eighteen months, each of her fifteen patients had been leveled by a similar array of symptoms.

Remembering her first patient some time later, Jessop commented, "She had a lot of things going on—abdominal pain, myalgias [muscle pain], headaches. I was really concerned about her. She wouldn't look well; then I would see her again and she would look better. Then—boom! It would hit her again and she would be in bed for sixteen days in a row. She had a family history of connective tissue disorder, so initially I went that route," Jessop continued. "I was looking for lupus or any kind of rheumatological autoimmune disease. I was worried about multiple sclerosis, too, because of some of the neurological symptoms she mentioned. So she got the complete, thorough workup. And I could not make a diagnosis. My comments to her were: 'Listen, I know you've got something, either an autoimmune disorder or maybe a chronic viral thing that we can't diagnose. I'm going to follow you at certain intervals, and we'll check to see if something doesn't show up, because often rheumatological disorders don't really declare themselves for five years.'

"That's what I thought would happen with her," Jessop added. "But then I got a second one. . . . After seeing the second patient I thought, as many physicians would, Gee, I just heard this last week. Then two months later I saw another one, and two months later I saw another. None of these women knew each other. So I was concerned."

Jessop, then thirty-two, was a full-time associate professor in the Department of Internal Medicine at the University of California medical school, an institution housed among several imposing buildings on Parnassus Heights, a windswept bluff in San Francisco's Sunset District. She had served her internship and residency at Massachusetts General Hospital in Boston and been chief resident in the department of medicine at the University of California's medical school for a year

2

before her appointment as associate professor. During eight years of training, the doctor had never heard the constellation of signs and symptoms afflicting her Lyon-Martin clinic patients discussed in any forum. Instinctively she sought the advice of her colleagues at the medical school. "I felt I had the luxury of all those specialty consultants at UCSF," Jessop recalled. After performing complete cardiovascular, gastrointestinal, endocrine, and neurological workups on Jessop's difficult patients, none of her colleagues could put a name to the bizarre disorder. "They found nothing. They told me the patients were depressed," she said. Several male clinicians suggested that Jessop was performing "million-dollar workups on neurotic women."

"Being a woman myself, I took offense to that," Jessop recalled, adding, "I was quite distraught about this disease, but I was even more distraught by the reaction I got from colleagues and peers."

Jessop was stimulated enough by her unusual cases to call Jay Levy, a microbiologist at the university's Cancer Research Institute who was known to be in the business of searching for new agents of disease. Jessop knew Levy was currently looking for the virus that caused the new "gay pneumonia" striking San Francisco men. Perhaps, Jessop mused, she could interest Levy in the affliction she was seeing in her female patients. Levy listened to Jessop's pitch, but declined to help, explaining that he was too busy searching for the cause of the syndrome of immune dysfunction that soon would be called acquired immunodeficiency syndrome.

As the months passed, Jessop's observations about the ailment became more focused. The patients' complaints assumed a familiar pattern "mainly of fatigue," the doctor said, "but fatigue that was profound and made worse upon exertion of any kind and that was associated with low-grade fevers, sore throat, lymphadenopathy [swollen lymph nodes], headaches, myalgias [sore muscles], and, interestingly, a sleep disorder. . . . I did everything I knew how to do," she added, "and I felt like I came from the best of Western medicine. But I was perplexed."

By the fall of 1984 Jessop was uncertain where to turn next, but she felt ominously confident there would be more cases.

Charlotte, North Carolina

The year 1984 marked the fifth year Marc Iverson had gone without a name for the affliction that had upended his career and was threatening to destroy his marriage. Iverson was extraordinarily bright, and he had been extremely lucky. After earning his M.B.A. at the Wharton School of Business, he had returned to Charlotte, his hometown, where he married the love of his young life. There were a multitude of banking institutions in the thriving southern town; he signed on with BarclaysAmerica. Within eighteen months, at twenty-seven, Iverson became the youngest vice president at a Barclays in the United States. Then his luck ran out.

He awoke one morning in 1979 with the disconcerting sensation that his limbs were encased in lead. He did not seem to be hearing or seeing properly; the environment was muted and distant. Iverson also had an excruciating sore throat, which his doctor diagnosed as strep. For the next several weeks the banker's torment continued. A series of brief, apparent recoveries was followed by longer episodes of sore throat and exhaustion. Each time his symptoms abated, Iverson attempted to resume his pace at Barclays, but there was no avoiding the reality of his increasing debilitation.

Iverson's father, president and chief executive officer of Nucor, a steel manufacturer routinely listed in the upper ranges of the Fortune 500, advised his son to search more aggressively for a diagnosis. The senior Iverson encouraged Marc to try the Mayo Clinic. After a week-long stay in the sprawling medical center in southern Minnesota, the younger Iverson returned to Charlotte with assurances that he was perfectly healthy. The Mayo doctors had explained that he was a "type A" who needed to step off the fast track. The banker wanted to believe the Mayo experts. He stunned his employers at Barclays by serving notice and took up gardening in his backyard. For a few idyllic weeks he actually did feel better, but his respite proved fleeting.

Over a period of months Iverson developed puzzling neurological disorders that affected his balance and coordination, his strength, and his thinking. His mind, which he remembered as being "steak-knife sharp," was now, he complained, "a butter knife." He was too weak to walk up stairs or to stand long enough to shower. He could not manipulate his fingers to turn the pages of books or pick up coins. His two toddlers were allowed in his darkened bedroom for only an hour a day. He became practically nocturnal, sleeping during the day, a victim of remorseless insomnia throughout the night. When he finally went to bed, he would wrap a pillow around his head to dim the morning light. "God help me, God help me," he would repeat as he drifted into an uneasy sleep. That state of affairs continued for five years.

In September of 1984 a Charlotte neurologist began to suspect the former banker was suffering from myasthenia gravis, a degenerative nervous system disorder of unknown etiology. He recommended that Iverson seek a definitive diagnosis at the Mayo. Buoyed by the Charlotte doctor's faith in the clinical acumen of the Rochester experts, Iverson undertook his second visit with renewed optimism. As before, his days at the Mayo were consumed by interviews with specialists, who ordered rounds of standard blood and neurological tests. Once more the tests produced results in the normal or near-normal ranges. "They said there was no *clear* sign of neuromuscular disease," Iverson recalled. Ultimately the Mayo doctors asked him to take the Minnesota Multiphasic Personality Inventory (MMPI). When he was finished, they told Iverson that he had scored high on "depressive symptoms." The young man was shuttled through the marble-tiled corridors of the venerable clinic to a psychiatrist. "He told me my symptoms had to do with feeling inadequate to my father and that because I hadn't achieved my father's level of success, it had produced depression," Iverson said.

Another doctor told him, "We could not find any footprints in the sand," a metaphor that assumed increasing irony for the patient as his years of disability wore on. A third pointed out that Iverson had been physically "deconditioned" by inactivity and suggested exercise. Concluding their analysis, the team prescribed a potent antidepressive, which promptly exacerbated Iverson's symptoms. Upon his departure, the thirty-two-year-old was presented with a $7,500 tab.

"I was defeated," he said later. "To feel so sick—to have all these symptoms—and yet to have all these tests come back either normal, or not *significantly* abnormal. I finally thought, I really must be crazy."

Reno, Nevada

Inga Thompson was one of the U.S. Olympic Women's Bicycling Team's best cyclists. Her home was in Reno and she did all her altitude training in Incline Village, a resort town in the Sierras an hour's drive away. Thompson, compact and muscular, had been on the team just six weeks when she fell ill in the summer of 1984. During training, Thompson typically cycled three hundred miles every week. After participating in the 1984 Olympics, she raced in the Coors Classic, a two-week stage race during which cyclists average fifty miles a day. She was unable to finish.

Her Reno doctor tested the athlete for a number of infectious agents, without results. He told Thompson that she had "post-Olympic blues." Even so, the ambitious and dedicated woman remained bedridden. Thompson's father, an orthopedic surgeon, was distressed by his daughter's deterioration and the Reno doctor's diagnosis. He took Thompson to the University of Utah medical center, where she was given a CT brain scan. The scan was abnormal, and the cyclist was treated for a brain abscess. Thompson perceived little improvement after the treatment. She continued to be bedridden.

Raleigh, North Carolina

The North Carolina Symphony was comprised mostly of younger musicians. Their average age was thirty-eight, and they were a close-knit group. The state sponsored them; in return, the orchestra traveled, usually within North Carolina, but occasionally to other states as well. As a result, the musicians spent long stretches of time together. They had their choice of a nonsmoking bus or a smoking bus for the long hours on the road between performances. They doubled up in hotel rooms and dined together. They grew close, formed alliances and cliques. Their informality and friendship was such that they even, on occasion, shared eating utensils or drank from the same glass; more rarely, they had affairs with one another.

In August of 1984 several orchestra members began to experience a strange panoply of symptoms that included exhaustion, sore throat, headaches, insomnia, vision problems, memory loss, and nausea. For many, the severity of the illness seemed to wax and wane and, in a few, the symptoms disappeared after a few months' time. Everyone assumed a particularly virulent flu had visited the orchestra and waited for the siege to end. The malaise persisted well into the fall and winter, however, stealing the vitality of the afflicted and undermining the stability of the orchestra.

Beverly Hills, California

By that same fall, Dr. Herbert Tanney had been logging an influx of exhausted patients into his examining rooms for thirteen months, all of them people he had known for years. "They complained basically of fatigue, and they *looked* very fatigued; depression, and they *looked* very depressed," the doctor recalled. But they listed other complaints: "They also had muscle aching, muscle weakness, recurrent sore throats, trouble concentrating, loss of short-term memory to varying degrees, nightmares, low-grade fevers, an inability to perform simple mathematical computations, insomnia, and," he added after a moment, "*loads* of other symptoms.

"On examination," Tanney said, "frequently I would see small spots on the soft palate just behind the hard palate. Occasionally I would feel [enlarged] lymph glands. Once in a while," he added, "a spleen would be enlarged, but minimally. Basically, nothing else physically was of any great significance." By early 1984 he had collected twenty-two people, all of them "regular, longtime patients," with the same problem.

Tanney had practiced internal medicine in Los Angeles for thirty-two years. His plush offices were high in the dark glass tower of the Century City Medical Plaza in Beverly Hills, and he counted among his patients a number of Hollywood professionals, including filmmakers and actors. Director Blake Edwards was among the first patients Tanney saw with the problem. In June, Tanney had sent Edwards to the infectious disease clinic at Stanford University Medical Center. Thomas Merigan, who was head of the infectious disease department at Stanford and the premier infectious disease specialist on the West Coast, examined the fifty-five-year-old Edwards and drew blood samples.

"I sent Blake to Stanford," Tanney remembered. "And after all the studies were finished, I got a letter from Merigan saying, 'Your patient has mono.' "

The filmmaker, who was profoundly ill, recalled that Merigan tried to downplay the severity of the symptoms he was describing. Merigan, in addition, assured Edwards he would feel better soon.

Atlanta, Georgia

In medical argot, a syndrome is a collection of uniquely presented symptoms and physical signs for which a cause has yet to be found. A disease, in contrast, is a manifestation of illness for which medicine has an explanation—for example, the identity of the bacterium—as well as a scientifically sound explanation of the pathophysiology.[1] In November 1984 a research article in the *Southern Medical Journal* officially dubbed the perplexing new ailment bubbling up in clinical practices around the country a "syndrome," thus establishing it—in the United States, at least—as a specific and tangible problem, even if its cause and natural history remained unknown.

Richard DuBois, an Atlanta infectious disease specialist, was the primary author of the *Southern Medical Journal* article. Prior to publication, his eight coauthors had agreed on virtually everything about their subject except what to name this newfound entity. According to DuBois, that question engendered a heated debate, just as it would in countless other forums throughout the next decade. Because some patients had developed the chronic malady after a case of acute infectious mono, the doctors settled on "chronic mononucleosis syndrome," which then became the title of their paper. Buttressing their decision was the fact that most sufferers demonstrated high levels of antibodies to the Epstein-Barr virus, the cause of mono. As far as the doctors were concerned, in fact, the viral antibodies were the salient laboratory finding in the syndrome.

DuBois had first observed the phenomenon in 1980 in a thirteen-year-old girl who suffered from a seemingly endless case of mono. As the months passed, he identified several more cases of the curious syndrome in his practice. Soon afterward he began his collaboration with his coauthors. The clinicians among them had been seeing in their own practices increasing numbers of patients with identical constellations of signs and symptoms.

DuBois and his collaborators' article appeared that November without fanfare. The authors were disappointed. They had believed that they were describing a new syndrome, one that would have increasing clinical importance and was worthy of national attention, but the publication's readership was small, composed almost exclusively of Southern Medical Association members in Georgia and Florida. In just two months, two more articles on the same subject by other researchers in a larger journal—the *Annals of Internal Medicine*—would garner a vastly larger audience, triggering a response DuBois and his coauthors believed befit the topic. In the meantime, the authors were left with their troubled, and troublesome, patients.

Toulouse, France

Mayhugh Horne lay in a rumpled bed in his hotel room in a state of abject depression. He was in one of the oldest, most delightful cities in France—the "city of restaurants," they called it—and he had been laid low by what the French doctor said was Philippine Type A 2 influenza. An epidemic of the flu had descended on much of western France, the doctor explained. For the muscular, six-foot Horne, whose exceptional health and athleticism had been a source of pride, the imposed helplessness and lethargy were excruciating.

The illness had caused a terrible snag in his training schedule. His employer, Pan Am, had sent the forty-nine-year-old air force veteran to Toulouse to learn how to fly the new airbus. Pilots from Africa, Asia, North America, and Europe were trained there, at the center of the airbus industry, to handle the flying leviathans. Horne had been just four days short of finishing the six-week course when he was forced to take to his bed, although he had been fighting the bug for a week or two before that.

"I'd pop two Panadols," Horne recalled. "I might have been taking away the pain from the headache, but the fever was still there and, as you know, with fever your brain is frying, so you're mentally impaired. I just could not keep up. Pilots don't accept anything below one hundred percent. It's our makeup. There's a lot of friendly competition in the cockpit, and it's really embarrassing—it's the *most* embarrassing thing—to be caught up short in front of your peers."

After three days in his hotel room spent gulping Panadols and cursing the walls, Horne decided to give the training another shot. Once again in the airbus cockpit, Horne found himself struggling more than ever.

"I was not proud of my performance," he said. "Flying *is* concentration, and I could not concentrate."

Two Pan Am engineers had also developed the virulent flu in Toulouse, but they seemed to have recovered. Horne, in contrast, dropped out of the training three days later and returned to Miami, where he was then based. His illness forced him to remain in bed for the next two months. "I couldn't *believe* it—I just couldn't beat it!" Horne recalled.

When he felt he had recovered, he went back to Toulouse and finished the training. He flew the airbus for the next twelve months, but it was a difficult year, unlike any other.

Key West, Florida

By mid-1984 investigators had identified a cluster of at least thirty-seven cases of multiple sclerosis in Key West, the lush tropical island in the Florida Keys that was a holiday destination for more than one million Americans each year. Incredibly, the University of Miami doctor who had spearheaded the research had determined that the rate of multiple sclerosis in Key West was among the highest in the world. William Sheremata, a neurologist and multiple sclerosis expert, was deeply disturbed by his findings. MS, an incurable disease of the central nervous system, was not supposed to occur in epidemic form; it was not generally considered a contagious disease. Additionally, cases of multiple sclerosis were extremely rare in low latitudes; the disease more typically stalked residents of Northern Hemisphere regions such as northern Europe and the northern United States. Finally, the cases themselves were somewhat atypical. Serious questions had been raised by Sheremata and other neurologists as to whether the disease cluster in Key West was multiple sclerosis at all.[2]

Sheremata's involvement with the Key West outbreak had been set into motion with the onset of severe and persistent fatigue in a forty-year-old nursing supervisor at Keys Memorial Hospital on Stock Island, named for its historical role as the site of a cattle slaughterhouse. When the general practitioners who provide medical care in the islands were unable to identify her disorder, the ailing nurse went to Miami, a standard scenario for Keys patients with complicated medical problems. She landed at the University of Miami's department of neurology. The department chairman, suspecting multiple sclerosis, referred her to Sheremata, who was then new to the staff.

"I agreed it was MS," Sheremata recalled several years later. "The patient was having increasing neurological problems—prominent fatigue, heat intolerance, and difficulty walking. Subsequently she returned with additional neurological symptoms—numbness and weakness in one arm."

Soon after, Sheremata was confronted in his examining room with a second apparent multiple sclerosis patient hailing from Stock Island. She too was a nurse at Keys Memorial Hospital. Her illness had begun suddenly with vision problems, but she returned, in time, complaining of chronic exhaustion. "In recent years," Sheremata said, "her major symptom had been fatigue, and this is true for a large proportion of the multiple sclerosis patients I see. It's a prominent, disabling symptom of the disease."

Within weeks Sheremata's Stock Island patients reported to him that another nurse at their institution had fallen victim to the same symptoms. The third patient's most pronounced complaints were the sudden onset of fatigue and visual disturbances. In addition to the nurses, two patients in the Stock Island hospital's forty-bed chronic care wing were suffering from multiple sclerosis, which brought the total cases within the hospital to five.

"The initial patient and the third patient began pushing me," Sheremata continued. "They felt strongly that it was unusual that there were five patients in such a small place. And they had heard of or knew of other people in the Keys who had been diagnosed with multiple sclerosis. Subsequently these other patients were referred to me."

Sheremata responded to his patients' ardent convictions with measured skepticism. "I did not want to be talked into the idea that there was a cluster. It was the patients who thought there was something highly unusual, and they were determined to prove it to me."

In their efforts to persuade Sheremata, the patients undertook their own "barefoot epidemiology," as civilian efforts are frequently termed by professionals, placing ads in local newspapers to locate other multiple sclerosis victims in the region. Interestingly, six respondents turned out to be registered or practical nurses, bringing the total number of nurses with the disease to nine.

By that fall, a surprising new element had entered the debate. According to two microbiologists who had been analyzing blood samples from the Key West patients, the epidemic was now offering a clue to the long-sought cause of multiple sclerosis. Scientists from Philadelphia's Wistar Institute, the nation's oldest independent biomedical research institute situated on the edge of the University of Pennsylvania campus, told Sheremata they had found evidence of an extremely rare virus in the Florida blood samples.

"The question was," Sheremata remembered later, "was this specific for MS patients? Everything had to be repeated and repeated. We asked, 'Is it systematic error? Is it artifact?' It was a very stimulating time," the neurologist remembered later. "But all of us who are interested in reaching the truth had one foot on the brake and one foot on the gas."

Harvard Medical School, Boston, Massachusetts

The malady had a peculiar disconcerting feel, the doctor mused. It was reminiscent of so many other diseases—viral diseases, mostly—but then again, it wasn't really like anything he had ever seen. He was most persuaded by patients he had known for years, people whose lives seemed to deteriorate before his eyes. He found it particularly hard to believe they would fake such bizarre intellectual problems.

Anthony Komaroff, an associate professor of medicine at Harvard, was seeing more and more of these patients in his general medicine clinic at the Brigham and Women's Hospital at 75 Francis Street. He noted that any number of triggers appeared to initiate the syndrome—an influenza-type infection, mononucleosis, even infection with a sexually transmitted disease. Once under way, the symptoms quickly coalesced into the chronic disorder, a condition so engulfing it rendered irrelevant whatever minor disease had launched the slide.

Komaroff was struck not only by the extraordinary quality of the fatigue patients described, but also by the neurologic component of their illness. At first he was skeptical, wondering if there was some ill-defined psychiatric component to the entity. But as anecdote upon anecdote accumulated on his notepads, the doctor grew impressed. He recalled a patient who was deeply disturbed by the fact that he had misplaced his wallet. Komaroff tried to comfort the man, suggesting to him that most people, doctors included, misplaced their wallets on occasion. "You don't understand," the man—a lawyer—said, his frustration evident. "When I found my wallet, it was in the freezer compartment of the refrigerator." Another patient, a real estate saleswoman now virtually bedridden, told Komaroff she had tried to make a pay phone call by slipping a quarter into a parking meter.

Komaroff had noticed the peculiar illness for the first time in 1977 at the Brigham, one of the three major teaching institutions in the Harvard Medical School constellation. Some of these patients were subsumed by exhaustion so severe it prevented them from working or functioning within their families. "I remember two patients in particular," the doctor recalled more than a decade later. "Both of them said, 'It all started with that virus. I've never been the same.' I thought that was very intriguing."

Komaroff was a compact, meticulous man. Unruly black eyebrows shaded his narrow hazel eyes. When patients spoke to him, he met their look empathically. He did not interrupt. The doctor's gift for hearing patients resulted in his becoming acutely aware of the curious intellectual problems described by these unusual sufferers. They complained of an inability to concentrate and demonstrated in their conversations with him pronounced aphasia, or word-finding problems; they reported unusual sleep patterns, including suffering bizarre dreams, waking repeatedly and, in spite of their terrible fatigue, insomnia.

"A strong part of why they were impaired," Komaroff remembered, "was that they couldn't concentrate, they had lost their short-term memory, and so on. But the whole *thing* was outstanding to me," he continued. "The fact that you could get a common virus and still be ill a year later—that was outstanding."

By 1978, the doctor had begun to suspect the existence of a syndrome, but he was stymied in his efforts to investigate further.

"I tried to enlist people to help," he recalled, "but I couldn't find any collaborators who really thought it was a plausible illness or who really wanted to pursue it with me. I was disappointed. I felt it reflected how closed-minded and narrow people could be. But I will say this: in 1978 I didn't vow to go back and study it again someday. It sort of slipped out of my consciousness."

By the spring of 1984, however, a surge of cases had refocused the doctor's attention. Again he was struck not only by the extraordinary quality of the fatigue patients described but by the neurologic component of their illness as well. The symptoms, he mused, bespoke a bona fide organic brain syndrome. To test his hunch, Komaroff began subjecting patients he suspected of having the syndrome to tests of mental integrity that are standard in basic neurological exams. Before beginning the physical exam, the doctor asked the patient to remember three objects—a baseball, an umbrella, and a hat. Five minutes later he asked the patient to name the objects. Rarely could anyone recall them. Komaroff added another time-honored measure of intellectual status to his battery: he asked patients to subtract from one hundred in units of seven. To his surprise, the doctor discovered that even among his patients with advanced degrees the task apparently was impossible; hardly any were able to progress beyond the first reduction to 93.

By the fall of 1984 Komaroff felt certain he was observing the emergence of a discrete entity.

National Institutes of Health, Bethesda, Maryland

Stephen Straus was head of the medical virology section of the National Institute of Allergy and Infectious Diseases, one of the largest, best-funded research arms of the government's premier biomedical research center, the National Institutes of Health. He was viewed by his superiors as a gifted, disciplined investigator. By November of 1984, in his office on the NIH's Bethesda campus, Straus was putting the finishing touches on an article he had prepared for the *Annals of Internal Medicine*. He had satisfied the criticisms raised by the journal's peer reviewers and had only minor changes to make before the January publication date.

When he submitted his article earlier in the year, Straus had limited the number of patients in his study to twenty-three. All were suffering from an apparently identical long-lasting illness that was both incurable and remarkably debilitating. In recent months the young researcher had delivered a few lectures on the malady he described in his paper, and little by little, word of his interest in the phenomenon was spreading. Now calls from doctors seeking to refer additional cases to him were becoming more frequent. Other specialists called simply for advice in evaluating these difficult patients in their own practices. (The previous June, for instance, Stanford University's chief of infectious diseases, Tom Merigan, had called him to consult about the movie director Blake Edwards.) The calls were pouring in from everywhere, in fact. But then, Straus had noticed early on that the disorder seemed to be without geographical boundaries: the twenty-three patients in his study hailed from eleven states.

As the publication date of his study approached and the calls multiplied, Straus realized that he would need to start turning new referrals away. Although he had a medical degree, he was a working scientist, not a practicing clinician, and the NIH was a research institution, not a hospital.

"We do detailed evaluations; we do immunologic studies, virologic studies," Straus would explain some months later when the referrals had reached the level of a dozen each weekday, or about 250 a month. "But we can't do all that for just anyone who walks in. We're here to evaluate medical disorders under specific approved research protocols," he continued, somewhat testily. "We're *not* in a position to crank through patients for the sake of satisfying them."

National Jewish Center for Immunology and Respiratory Medicine, Denver, Colorado

In the fall of 1984, James Jones, a pediatrician and a member of the clinical faculty at the immunology research center in Denver, was anticipating the publication of his own article in the January *Annals*.[3] His would be a companion study to Stephen Straus's investigation. He had first called Straus two years earlier when he heard the government researcher was investigating the same phenomenon of unexplained, devastating chronic illness in previously healthy people.

"The first time we met and described our patients to one another, it was extraordinary," Jones recalled.

Jones had begun to see patients with the baffling illness in 1981. At the time he was performing clinical research in Tucson at the University of Arizona's medical school. His first case, a little boy, was three years old when Jones met him, although the child had been ill since the age of three months. Now the boy was six. Early on, the child's mother had painstakingly documented his monthly fevers, which lasted three to five days. Before Jones entered the diagnostic fray enveloping the tiny patient, assorted pediatricians had labeled the toddler with myriad ailments, including the vague "viral syndrome," aseptic meningitis, and otitis media, a common childhood infection of the middle ear. By the age of three, the boy had begun to suffer a marked pattern of sore throats, swollen glands, and swollen eyelids during his episodic fevers. "Complications," Jones wrote in his account of the child's illness, "included . . . seizures . . . and severe varicella [chicken pox]."

Jones included forty-four patients in his study. Not surprisingly, given the doctor's pediatric specialty, eighteen, or 40 percent, were under the age of fifteen. They had trickled into the university's general medicine clinic over a period of three years.

"The first few came to the clinic without any knowledge or foreknowledge of their confreres, as it were," Jones recalled. "For me, the event that hammered in the concept that these people were all in the same situation was when we got about fifteen of them together in Tucson so they could communicate. It was just amazing how they all recognized their own illness in one another."

Now Jones, like Straus, was beginning to get referrals from every corner of the country. Lurking under Jones's satisfaction at being published was his apprehension that his study's debut, only two months away, would lead to a crush of referrals that might slow the pace of his research.

Incline Village, Nevada

Her neighbors liked to speculate about her financial lineage. A few confused souls were amused by the notion that the heir to the West's largest raisin dynasty lived among them. To those people, she was "Mrs. California Raisin." For most of the citizens of Incline, however, she was just one more rich person who spent her summers in this town on the rim of Lake Tahoe. In truth, she was not the raisin heiress; she was married to a prosperous oilman, and each winter the couple returned to their home in Houston. Her life was one of ease and affluence. When her health began to fail in late August, she went directly to Dan Peterson's medical offices on Alder Street.

A number of such folk residing in the mountain hamlet routinely packed their overnight bags when they wanted to see a doctor, headed for the Reno airport, an hour away, and boarded a flight to San Francisco or Los Angeles. Incline was loaded with wonders of the natural world, but it had for years been short on doctors. Increasingly, however, the rich and the not so rich were skipping the flight to the Bay Area or southern California or wherever they thought they could plug themselves into sophisticated medical care. Where before there had been only family practitioners, there were now, in addition, two AMA board-certified internal medicine specialists, the first such specialists ever to practice in Incline.

Local gossip held that the internists, Daniel Peterson and Paul Cheney, were highly competent. As a result, it was not entirely surprising that when struck by sudden and intense fatigue, the oilman's wife went directly to the medical offices on Alder Street. She asked to see Peterson, a laconic midwesterner with the disarming countenance of a postadolescent Ricky Nelson and the senior man in the practice. Thus it was that the comely young doctor, during the final week of August that year, saw his first patient with the syndrome that had been troubling clinicians in the more densely populated areas of the country for periods of from months to years.

Peterson listened carefully, silently mulling over the possibilities, as the sixty-four-year-old woman described the onset of her profound exhaustion. "I remember going through the whole scenario," the doctor remarked later. "I wondered about diabetes, anemia, hypothyroidism—all of which can cause fatigue." He wondered, too, if she had been pushing her exercise regime too hard or if, despite her outstanding fitness, she was at last beginning to feel the effects of age. "And I considered that she might have a viral illness."

He also considered that her complaint might be related to distress that was psychological rather than organic. "I wondered," Peterson remembered, "if something had changed in her personal life. I went through all of that." But she was convincing in her insistence that her life, were it not for this distressing episode of pain and exhaustion, was placid.

Peterson awaited the results of her blood work, expecting to find his answer when the laboratory reported its findings. Nearly every test he ordered produced results in the normal range. Some of his patient's lymphocytes, or white blood cells, were large or "atypical" in appearance. Lymphocytes are integral components of the immune system. Atypical lymphocytes are a descriptive medium to the extent that they indicate an infection may be simmering: when they encounter a foreign invader, they change their shape in preparation for destroying it. Peterson's second observation was that his patient's white cell count overall had dipped slightly below the normal range. Bacterial infections tend to result in a surge of white blood cells; viral infections more commonly precipitate a crash. However, in the case of this patient, neither finding was dramatic.

Peterson presumed that his patient had been infected with a virus. Her lowered white blood cell count was suggestive, as was her fatigue. He further assumed that, whatever the organism, its effects would be short-lived even without his intervention—in medical parlance, "self-limited"—and quickly forgotten. The doctor was, therefore, surprised when his wealthy patient turned up in his office soon again. This time, she said, she felt "even worse."

Peterson began to suspect cancer. His suspicion was hardly outlandish. In both sexes, cancer reaches its apogee in middle age. A significant symptom, especially when there are no others, is fatigue. In the case of lymphoma and leukemia, cancers of the immune system and blood, it is often *the* symptom. Peterson ordered more-specific blood tests to determine if his dire suspicion had merit. The woman's results were normal. She returned a third time, still talking of extreme, unnatural tiredness.

"I went over and over this," Peterson said, "and I just couldn't figure it out. It bothered me. Every so often you can't handle something as an internist, something comes along that you don't understand because it's not within the limits of your training. You see an abnormal blood test, for instance, and the patient has some rare hematological disease. Then you have to send the patient to a hematologist, who tells you it's hairy cell leukemia—or something like that. But this patient's lab screenings were all *normal.* And I remember thinking, What am I missing? What's deficient in my history taking? Why can't I crack this?"

Late in September the careworn woman departed for Houston as was her custom. Peterson didn't see her again for three and a half years.

Two weeks later a twenty-six-year-old marathon runner who had been his patient for three years came to Peterson's Alder Street clinic. Not only was he unable to run a marathon, the young man told the doctor, he was unable to run at all. His weariness had begun quite suddenly after a sore throat, he said. He complained of low-grade fevers, night sweats, and as the doctor confirmed during an examination, swollen lymph nodes. Peterson, assuming his patient was suffering from a virus, assured the runner his symptoms would abate soon. Two weeks later the runner was in his office again, flattened by exhaustion.

The following week three more of Peterson's patients came to him complaining of upper respiratory infections—sore throats, coldlike symptoms—and crushing fatigue. One of them, Joyce Reynolds, worked as a teller at Placer Savings and Loan in Kings Beach, a woodsy community just across the California-Nevada state line. "I thought it was a flu," the diminutive fifty-five-year-old said three and a half years later, her face a fragile mask of self-control. For the next several weeks Reynolds remained at home, struggling to recover from fevers, a sore throat, headaches, and an exhaustion so profound it seemed actually to pulsate through her limbs with each beat of her heart. Her husband, who repaired power lines for the county, tried to be supportive, but when she had failed to recover after two months, he began to lose patience. Each time Reynolds appeared in Peterson's office, she seemed a little more desperate.

Sonny Dukes was another. Dukes was a thirty-eight-year-old self-described biker, a resident of Kings Beach for seven years. He was six feet three and weighed 260 pounds. The biceps of one of his massive arms was tattooed with the phrase "Live to Ride and Ride to Live." He was bald, with a handlebar mustache, and claimed to have been riding Harley-Davidson motorcycles from the age of nine. "Never was normal," he liked to say. Dukes had seen Peterson once before; the biker had broken his finger, but waited three days before coming to the emergency room at Incline's thirty-bed hospital. Dukes began to feel sick on his way back from a gathering of Harley-Davidson aficionados in Sturgis, South Dakota. The day after he returned home, he lacked the strength to roll his bike from its parking spot next to his small wood-frame house. "Bikers like to pretend they're ten feet tall and bulletproof," Dukes said. A friend drove the demoralized Dukes to the Alder Street clinic.

Sandy Schmidt, an attractive blond woman in her early forties who had run in the San Francisco marathon every year for the last five years, was Peterson's third puzzling case. Schmidt lived in a multilevel A-frame fashioned from brick and pine not far from the center of Incline. Her husband, who was several years her senior, independently wealthy, and a close friend of Nevada's U.S. Senator Harry Reid, ran a financial consulting business from their home. Not long after returning from her fifth Bay Area marathon, Schmidt noticed she was sleeping ten and eleven hours a night instead of her usual seven. She felt "fluish" and noticed she was running a low-grade temperature in the evening. Her reflection in the mirror revealed an ashen-faced woman she barely recognized. After two weeks of rest, the ambitiously athletic Schmidt grew impatient. Telling herself it was merely a problem of mind over matter, she dressed one morning and headed out along her standard eight-mile jogging route, adopting an unusually gentle pace to compensate for her missed training days. Fifteen minutes later she stopped and sat down on the gravel-strewn shoulder of the alpine road. Her hands were shaking and her head was throbbing violently; her feet felt as if they were weighted with granite. She seemed to have lost her peripheral vision, and when she stood, her dizziness made her gasp. It took her an hour to walk back to her house.

Peterson, who typically saw about twenty-five patients a day, might ordinarily have dismissed a connection among these patients. But he noticed they had used nearly identical language in their efforts to describe the severity of their symptoms. The apparent degree of their disablement and the vehemence of their complaints reminded him of the runner he had seen a week earlier.

These new patients were younger than the oilman's wife, although all were well into adulthood. They had swollen lymph nodes under their jaws; two had swollen spleens. In each case, Peterson ordered a round of laboratory tests. By the time the last patient's results came back, he was almost prepared for the absence of remarkable findings. Like the Texan, each had atypical lymphocytes, and white cell counts were down—vague hints of viral infection, but nothing more, certainly nothing to justify the passionate complaints he was hearing. All that linked these people, at first, was the mysterious origin of their infirmities and their failure to recover.

By early December the Alder Street clinician had tested each of his weary patients for anemia, thyroid abnormalities, diabetes and a wide variety of common viruses and bacteria. He sent their thin amber blood serum, centrifuged clean of cell debris, to be analyzed for the presence of antibodies to cytomegalovirus, a member of the herpesvirus family that can cause flu-like symptoms; for toxoplasmosis, a bacterium usually transmitted to humans through cat feces; and for the liver-damaging, exhaustion-inducing hepatitis virus. In every case the results were negative.

One viral offender Peterson mentally toyed with was Epstein-Barr virus, another herpesvirus. Its improbable name, which more convincingly evoked law partnerships or accounting firms than pestilence, derived from the scientist and his lab associate who first isolated the germ in the early 1960s. It was the most ubiquitous known virus in the world, infecting 90 percent of the world's population, even the most insular native cultures, and levied a prodigious toll in suffering. In industrialized nations the virus most commonly caused infectious mononucleosis, the teenage "kissing disease," so named because of its easy transmissibility. Scientists blamed Epstein-Barr virus for certain cancers endemic in parts of Africa and China.

Peterson, who like most practicing clinicians in the United States had missed Richard DuBois's article about the new "chronic mononucleosis syndrome" in the *Southern Medical Journal*, was aware that a number of the symptoms from which his patients were suffering—fatigue, swollen lymph nodes, sore throat—were typical of mononucleosis. But Peterson knew that a number of other viruses could cause the same symptoms. Further, according to the National Institutes of Health's manual on infectious mononucleosis, 80 percent of all documented cases of mono occurred in people between the ages of fifteen and thirty; only one of Peterson's patients was under thirty.[4] If only to reassure himself, Peterson employed the standard test for mono, called the monospot, on his sick adults. Like all the previous laboratory screens, the results were negative.

Another long shot Peterson investigated was human immunodeficiency virus, or HIV, which had been named as the cause of AIDS the previous April. AIDS was rare in Nevada in 1984; state health officials reported less than 1 percent of the nation's total cases. Nevertheless, his patients' signs of chronically swollen lymph nodes and viral-like symptoms correlated with the newly defined AIDS-related complex, or ARC. Again, all test results were negative. The suffering continued unabated.

"They came back—*haunting* me—because they didn't get better," Peterson recalled.

Increasingly the doctor was convinced that his patients were victims of a deft organism capable of sustained warfare with the human immune system. Rather than attempting to sort out what was different about these unfortunate people, Peterson turned his thoughts toward what was the same. "I kept coming back to the fact that they were all well and then had become sick. And I said to myself, This has got to be an infectious disease. And it's got to be a virus."

In late December 1984, five of twelve members of the girls' basketball team at Incline High School were leveled with what at first seemed to be mono. All of the stricken players were teenagers in Peterson's care. Although mono typically resolves itself in four to six weeks, one victim was bedridden for eight months and failed a grade in school. Her teammates remained debilitated for several months. Until the outbreak, the girls had regularly played against other Nevada teams. Now, unable to meet its commitments, the team ended its season.

Neither Peterson nor his partner, internist Paul Cheney, drew any inferences from the cluster—at least not immediately. Clustering of infectious mono is rare, though not unheard of, and the severity of the cases, although unusual, was hardly bizarre.

The winter of 1984–1985 was a superb snow season at Lake Tahoe. Squaw Valley, a forty-five-minute drive from Incline Village, was buried under several feet of base snow and powder; skiers crowded its slopes. The smaller resorts were thriving on the overflow. Incline Village's tourist-based economy boomed with "wall-to-wall skiers," as locals described it. For many residents of the towns around the lake, life that winter had a certain high-spirited buoyancy. When the ski resorts prospered, so did most of the businesses in the region; when the snows were light, the fragile local economies dipped, sometimes disastrously.

The Peterson-Cheney clinic was prospering too. The internists were building what one observer characterized as the "powerhouse" practice in town. The doctors occupied an expensive suite in a new chalet-style medical center opposite the hospital. Mountain light poured into their waiting room through six skylights in a cathedral ceiling, illuminating LeRoy Neiman prints on the walls and warming the ample leather chairs; the piped music was classical. Their offices housed an impressive array of medical technology. The doctors' "Human Performance Laboratory," a trade name for an assemblage of sophisticated diagnostic instruments, was typical. Its components filled a room and included a $60,000 state-of-the-art treadmill to monitor cardiac health; a $40,000 exercise calorimeter which, by measuring oxygen consumption, furnished insight into metabolic states; and a body composition machine, which calibrated fat-to-muscle ratios. In part, the equipment enabled the doctors to work with athletes—skiers, marathoners, Olympic cyclists—who lived in the area. The performance laboratory also satisfied another class of patient, one even more demanding: multimillionaires whose $5 million-and-up life insurance policies remained in effect only so long as they submitted to thorough annual medical exams.

"It was a very busy practice—just thriving," Paul Cheney remembered several years later. "And although you would expect a kind of cross section of patients, like any small town in America, Incline seemed not to be a typical small town. We didn't have a large Medicare population, and we didn't have people in their eighties being shuffled up to us. Most of our patients were in their forties and fifties when we first saw them. They typically were very well educated. Many of them had made lots of money . . . and retired at thirty-five. We were seeing people who had the means to see anyone in the world. So we had a high-tech practice because these people liked that kind of medicine."

Indeed, Incline was no more Small Town U.S.A. than Gstaad was a typical Swiss village. Its residents enjoyed one of the highest per capita incomes in Nevada. A proportion of them lived in multimillion-dollar houses tucked deep into clusters of ponderosa pine on mountainside lots or set like fortified citadels on costly lakefront property. As Cheney had noted, the town was filled with dropout millionaires, retirees who sought the wooded grandeur of the High Sierra after amassing fortunes in their middle years. Many were former Californians lured by the state's low taxes. Rarely did one encounter the native born. Explained a local: "Most of *them* are around ten years old."

As their clinic evolved, Peterson and Cheney came to preside over a health-conscious patient population with a keen interest in preventive medicine. The doctors had the training to practice preventive medicine—a technique that employed frequent high-tech screens for disease, particularly early cancers—and were passionate advocates of it.

"You couldn't deliver sloppy service, because our patients just wouldn't stand for it," Cheney said later of his Incline Village clientele. "You couldn't say, 'Don't worry about it—take this pill and go home. You don't need to know the pathophysiology of this.' You ended up talking pathophysiology with them, because they could understand the pathophysiology and they really wanted to know. They *demanded* to know. And then they would call up their brother-in-law, who was a world-famous cardiologist, and make sure you were right!

"It was actually fun because you got to sit down and talk about these things," the doctor added. "And there was really no subspecialty competition, which made it more challenging. When the passes close in the winter, you are a cardiologist— you are *the* cardiologist. It's like delivering a baby in the woods. *Someone's* got to do it."

Peterson, who had launched the practice in 1981 and recruited Cheney in 1983, shared his partner's enthusiasm. Some years later, his nostalgia nearly palpable, Peterson would remark, "It was a merry practice—made in heaven."

The doctors were, in their own ways, as atypical as their little town. Peterson's decision to start a solo practice in rural Nevada not only broke tradition with his own medical school, the University of Rochester, whose graduates typically set-tled into established, lucrative practices in big eastern cities, it defied a national trend. By the late 1970s and early 1980s, most newly trained doctors were joining multispecialty private clinics or health maintenance organizations. Among those who knew him, Peterson's preference was unsurprising. "Dan was someone who really liked to do things on his own," said a medical school friend, Kansas City cardiologist William Brodine. "He had more of a frontier spirit."

Even before he began his practice at the lake, the doctor's uncompromising ethics nearly upended his career. In return for government sponsorship of his medical training, Peterson opted to serve the poor by joining the Public Health Service in Region Ten, the West. He was dispatched to Burley, Idaho, an insular town near the state's southern border where his mission was to operate a public clinic serving migrant field laborers and vagrants. Observing that the county hos-pital was lax in its handling of laboratory tests for the migrants and indigents from his clinic, Peterson petitioned the Public Health Service to establish a laboratory and employ a technician at his clinic. Reluctantly the government acquiesced. "We then had a full-time technician and a lab," Peterson recalled, "where we were able to do all kinds of tests—and quickly." The establishment of a full-service lab at a one-man clinic was unprecedented within the Public Health Service.

Eventually Peterson faced more intractable dilemmas. When a patient's hand was severed in a conveyor belt accident at a potato factory, for instance, the owner of the factory refused to acknowledge that the person had ever worked there. Peterson began searching, unsuccessfully, for a civil rights–oriented attorney to represent his patient. There were several more incidents in which the doctor's disenfranchised patients appeared to be utterly without advocates, and he took up their cause. Not long before his tour of duty was up, one of his patients was found dead in a ditch. The Burley paper reported the twenty-five-year-old laborer had died of natural causes, but Peterson suspected otherwise. Twenty minutes after be-ing told he would have to file a formal request if he wished to initiate a criminal investigation, he received a call from a well-meaning friend in town. "Dan," he said, "you're not any good to us as the next person who dies of natural causes." Soon afterward Peterson received word from the Public Health Service that he was being transferred to finish the final four months of his tour of duty in Nampa, Idaho, a town west of Burley.

"I was a *terrible* federal employee," Peterson admitted years afterward.

If rural Nevada was an exotic setting for someone with Peterson's training, it was only more so for his partner. It had been, as a friend of Paul Cheney's would later say, merely the "random vagaries of life" that had deposited the sinewy tow-headed doctor in a clinical practice in rural Nevada. By the time he decided to enter medicine, Cheney was a Duke University–educated Ph.D. in nuclear physics. His conversion from physics to medicine occurred when he realized his entrance into provocative research would be through the latter. "The golden age of physics was the first half of the century," Cheney said. "Medicine is the second half." Upon graduation from Emory University's distinguished medical school, the furthest thing from his mind was the practice of general medicine in a private clinic. Instead, he intended to become a research scientist in the prestigious field of immunology.

The twenty-six-year-old physicist and father of a small son was one of two Ph.D.'s in his medical school class of one hundred. To his peers and professors, Cheney seemed cut from a different cloth, and not only because he was older and better educated than most of his classmates. "Medicine is dominated by large numbers of people who are regurgitators of information rather than conceptual types," his Emory classmate, neurologist Chris Gallen, explained. "And Cheney is a conceptualizer."

Dave Gordon, who was then the head of clinical immunology at the Centers for Disease Control, which is next door to Emory, recalled that Cheney approached him for an idea to study the lymphocyte cells in the immune systems of cancer victims. "He was different," Gordon remembered later. "Most medical students see what kind of shoes you should wear to be a doctor, and they climb into them, and they wear them. They listen to all the clues for how you behave. I'm not sure Paul was listening to those clues, which I found very interesting."

Cheney's years at Emory were marked by poverty. "We lived in hovels— garage apartments. Our furniture had holes in it," he remembered. The doctor signed an air force contract that obligated him to three and a half years of service in exchange for an equal period of financial support during medical school. Cheney's chosen subspecialty, immunology, required a five-year postgraduate residency, but because of his air force commitment, he was forced to sign up for a residency in internal medicine, which took only three years. After a grueling internship and residency at Grady Hospital, Atlanta's county hospital, he moved his family to Mountain Home, Idaho, on the Snake River plateau, a treeless stretch of land sixty miles south of Boise. Ten thousand military personnel and their families populated Mountain Home. Cheney was named chief of internal medicine at the base hospital.

As his tour of duty wore on, the doctor's dream of joining the research establishment as a full-time player receded. For Cheney it seemed as if time simply had run out. He was a husband and the father of two rapidly growing children, and had been either a student or in training all of his married life. He found it increasingly difficult to face more years of training.

"I was thirty-five," Cheney said later, "and I had never had a job. And our furniture still had holes in it."

Dan Peterson's gamble that Incline Village would be able to support an internist had paid off—so handsomely, in fact, that he needed a partner. He called a nurse who had worked with him in Burley and who knew the handful of indentured public health and military internists working in the state. She gave him Paul Cheney's name. In early 1983, Cheney became a junior partner, in effect an employee, in the Incline Village clinic, although, at thirty-six, he was the senior man to Peterson, who was thirty-three. And although Cheney's decision to enter into a private practice had been undertaken with bittersweet resignation, he quickly identified aspects of his work that were remarkably well suited to his temperament and training.

"I had never really envisioned myself in a general practice of medicine, especially in a small town," Cheney said later. "And yet there I was in a general practice in a small town—albeit a different kind of small town."

Perhaps predictably, the young doctors had been less than warmly received by the tight-knit band of four general practitioners in town. Peterson had felt the chill long before Cheney joined him. It wasn't merely the obvious symbols of professional success that grated on his colleagues. It was the doctor's "market share" of available patients. Younger, with more sophisticated training, Peterson rapidly became the doctor the emergency room staff at the hospital called.

"Dan was the only one emergency room staff felt comfortable giving a sick patient to," Cheney recalled. "He was getting *all* the patients from the hospital." More often than not, these patients were tourists. "That's where all the sick patients came from," Cheney added. "Heart attacks, strokes, malignant hypertension, decompensated lung disease—people had no business being up in that altitude with their lung problems. All the real hard stuff was seen in the hospital, and they weren't our clinic patients, generally."

As Incline residents began to compare notes about their medical care, people started drifting away from the local family practitioners and into Peterson's clinic. Not infrequently Peterson found himself in the unenviable position of having to correct the misdiagnoses of local practitioners. When he discovered colon cancer in a patient whose family doctor had told him he was too young to require a colonoscopy, for instance, the patient immediately transferred his records to Peterson's clinic; the patient's friends and relatives followed suit. For spurned caregivers, nothing was more galling—or embarrassing. As Cheney expressed it, "Boy, that makes them mad."

Nor did Peterson seem to aspire to the trappings of affluence that doctors frequently covet. His presence in the town where most strivers drove plushly upholstered Range Rovers or late-model Jeep Cherokees could be monitored by sightings of his beat-up bronze-hued Jeep Laredo pickup with a roll bar behind the cab. He typically wore a black leather jacket and running shoes. The house in which he lived with his wife, Mary, and two small children wasn't remotely baronial.

If the family practitioners felt injured by Peterson's success, the young doctor surely added insult by his unambiguous indifference to their society. "Maybe if I had played golf with them or been best buddies, maybe I could have avoided [the hostility]," Peterson once reflected. "But I am just not that kind of a person." And although it was Peterson's way to keep his thoughts to himself, his ideas about the style of doctoring extant in the small town before his arrival had to have seeped out in small ways.

"What was very prevalent here," Peterson said in a contemplative moment years later, "was Band-Aid medicine."

Neither doctor had time to worry about the resentment brewing among members of the tiny medical fraternity in the region that winter. They were occupied seeing patients in their clinic during the week, alternating weekend rotations at the hospital, and spelling each other on emergency duty. Peterson, particularly, was reaching a state of burnout. Shortly before Christmas, however, he found himself faced with an opportunity that for his first three years in Incline had been out of reach: with a partner to cover for him, he could take a vacation. With his wife, he planned a week-long ski holiday in Aspen.

Reno, where Peterson picked up his flight, sits in a pocket of low desert surrounded by mountains; descent or ascent through choppy air created by currents pushing up from the mountains must be swift and steep. To distract himself from the routine white-knuckle takeoff, Peterson opened his January issue of the *Annals of Internal Medicine*. His eye was drawn to the article by National Institutes of Health scientist Stephen Straus in the table of contents: "Persisting Illness and Fatigue in Adults with Evidence of Epstein-Barr Virus Infection."[5] Next, his gaze fell upon the companion study by research clinician James Jones titled "Evidence for Active Epstein-Barr Virus Infection in Patients with Persistent Unexplained Illnesses." Oblivious to the jet's ratcheting and thudding as it careened over the mountains, he began to read. Both articles described a long-lasting flu-like disease with apparent neurological and immunological aspects. As DuBois had done in his article in the *Southern Medical Journal,* Straus and Jones noted the preponderance of high Epstein-Barr virus antibodies among patients; they proposed Epstein-Barr virus as a potential cause of the syndrome.

In the muted, impassive style of scientific literature, Jones's article included the sentence "There were many adverse consequences to the illness." Peterson recognized his patients' distress in the researchers' dry narratives of case histories. Study subjects had lost their jobs or been forced to drop out of school; over time their social support systems had crumbled as friends and family drifted away. Each had received a multitude of medical and psychiatric diagnoses in the years of their illness.

"Most had considerable psychosocial problems," federal researcher Straus wrote of the twenty-three adults he had studied. "Ten could not work at all, and several of these had major conflicts with family and public agencies regarding support. Thirteen of the patients had never married, and two others no longer lived with their spouses. . . . Anger and distrust of traditional medicine was common." In a sentence that had special resonance for Peterson, Straus observed, "Considering the extent of patients' complaints and disability, the results of routine laboratory tests were strikingly normal."

Interestingly, both researchers postulated that the chronic malady might in fact be a form of immune dysfunction. Straus went as far as to suggest that Epstein-Barr virus activation was symptomatic of something more profound. The "apparent persistence of [Epstein-Barr] virus in these patients," Straus wrote, "[may] represent an epiphenomenon . . . of immune impairment of an entirely distinct cause."

Jones, too, theorized that immune function might be compromised in patients with the disorder. He noted that AIDS victims also suffered from "persistent" or chronic Epstein-Barr virus infection and argued that "an abnormality in immune function in [his study subjects]" should not be rejected, "particularly because altered immunity has been seen in other persons with elevated . . . [Epstein-Barr virus] . . . antibody levels."

Peterson was deeply stirred by what he had read. Upon arrival in Aspen, he had to be restrained by his wife from calling his partner at the first opportunity to discuss the articles. Mary Peterson encouraged him to put medicine aside for the week. When he returned to Nevada after New Year's, Peterson pressed the dog-eared medical journal upon his partner and urged him to read the articles.

Paul Cheney complied, but found them anticlimactic. "I wasn't seeing any of these patients, so I didn't know what to think," Cheney remembered. "But Dan was excited."

Peterson immediately sent blood samples from two patients to the Nichols Institute in San Juan Capistrano, California. Nichols was reputedly one of the few laboratories in the country with dependable techniques for determining antibody levels to Epstein-Barr virus. After five months of "soft" or negative lab findings, Peterson was rewarded with positive results. Still, the tests raised more questions. Although most of the world's population is infected with Epstein-Barr virus by age thirty, most people never have symptoms of any kind, and the virus remains latent, or inactive, in the body for life. The laboratory analysis indicated the doctor's patients were suffering from a reactivation of an earlier, formerly latent infection. Why, Peterson wondered, had his patients' immune systems become suddenly incapable of maintaining latency?

It was too late to include the oilman's wife in the sweep, but Peterson decided to send blood samples from his remaining three patients to Nichols for the Epstein-Barr virus antibody panel, a test that measured the level of four different antibodies to the virus. The following week, he learned all three had evidence of reactivation of once-latent Epstein-Barr virus infections.

1985

INVITATION
TO AN
EPIDEMIC

To get an accurate knowledge of any disease it is necessary to study a large series of cases and to go into all the particulars—the conditions under which it is met, the subjects specially liable, the various symptoms, the pathological changes, the effects of drugs ... in the faculty of observation, the old Greeks were our masters, and we must return to their methods if progress [is] to be made.

—Sir William Osler, *Counsels and Ideals*

2

Raggedy Ann Syndrome

Incline Village, Nevada

Paul Cheney's interest in the strange cases of "chronic mono" showing up among his partner's patients began as an academic one until he recognized the pattern in two or three of his own. One of them, Chris Guthrie, was a meter reader from Sierra Power who walked twenty miles a day, five days a week on a route that took her through the rustic terrain of Kings Beach, California, five miles from Incline Village. She wasn't Cheney's first patient to fall prey to the strange malaise. Only later, when his sensitivities to the protean manifestations of the disease were more refined, did the doctor assign Guthrie to the practice's snowballing population of chronically ill patients. But Guthrie was among the early ones that Cheney recollected best.

"I remember her gray uniform," the doctor said. "She came in, sat down, and said, 'Doc, I can't get through the day. You're going to have to give me something.'"

Guthrie, then thirty-two, had translucent skin and long, gently curled brown hair. As a teenager, she had worked as Snow White at Disneyland in her native Anaheim, California. She had been a teacher during her twenties, but Guthrie found her independent outdoor job with Sierra Power more to her liking. A wife and the mother of a toddler, she had established a good attendance record during her first year on the job. Her sterling record began to grow tarnished that winter, however. For most of the summer and fall a seemingly endless succession of strep throats laid her low. She also suffered two miscarriages. Cheney treated her strep throats, but by Christmas, paralyzing exhaustion had emerged as Guthrie's greatest enemy, costing the woman her job. On December 30, 1984, she was unable to complete her route. "I called my boss and told him, 'I can't make it in—I can't finish,'" Guthrie recalled during an interview three years later. Her husband left his workplace in Reno to collect her; he found his wife collapsed on the road shoulder outside Kings Beach.

Following his partner's lead, Cheney had been sending serum samples from patients whose flu-like ailments had endured for suspiciously long periods to the Nichols Institute. He did so now for Guthrie. Her results were impressive. One kind of antibody, which typically becomes elevated during periods of active repli-

24

cation of the virus, was tenfold what the Nichols lab considered normal; another antibody, Epstein-Barr nuclear antigen (EBNA), which was reflective of the body's capacity to sustain Epstein-Barr virus latency, was not detected in Guthrie's blood. In the coming years Guthrie would be hospitalized on several occasions, frequently for pneumonia, dehydration, or dangerously high fever. At various stages of her illness, she would appear to have Legionnaires' disease, multiple sclerosis, and lymphoma; she would never again be able to work. That winter, however, Guthrie's ordeal was only beginning.

By early February 1985, Peterson and Cheney had identified nearly twenty patients who appeared to have the affliction portrayed in the *Annals* articles. All had been active working people; their average age was thirty-seven. Women outnumbered men. Although the phenomenon was not yet a disease the doctors could name, it fit the definition of a syndrome: a constellation of symptoms and objective physical signs, uniquely arrayed, etiology unknown.

As with Chris Guthrie, their most dramatic lab abnormality was low or nonexistent antibodies to EBNA. The doctors' computer search of the medical literature revealed that the condition of low or collapsed EBNA previously had been observed only in patients whose immune systems had been depressed by some radical event such as AIDS, cancer, or the administration of immune suppressant drugs after an organ transplant. In the same patients, antibodies to three other Epstein-Barr viral antigens, which become elevated during periods of Epstein-Barr viral activity, were usually abnormally high. Indeed, it was rapidly apparent to Cheney and Peterson that antibody levels to Epstein-Barr virus had many clues to offer diagnosticians about the status of a person's immune system; the viral antibodies seemed to function as a kind of weather vane of immunological health. Inability to control latency of the virus broadly hinted at immunological dysfunction. The doctors recalled, too, that one of the first infectious agents proposed as the cause of AIDS had been Epstein-Barr virus because, like their Incline Village patients, AIDS sufferers demonstrated reactivation of the virus.

Both doctors read and reread the *Annals* papers describing a syndrome of illness that appeared to be associated with the ubiquitous herpesvirus, but they were disturbed by the nascent theory being advanced by Jones and Straus that Epstein-Barr virus might play a causative role. The Nevada clinicians found another idea, which Stephen Straus had floated with featherweight emphasis, to be far more credible: that Epstein-Barr virus reactivation might be merely an epiphenomenon, or a hallmark, of the syndrome. What if something else, some other virus—call it agent X—was undermining the immune systems of these patients, allowing rampant Epstein-Barr virus replication and other subtle biological disturbances?

Peterson and Cheney began diagnosing the disease that had popped up in their practice as "chronic mono," as the literature suggested. But neither doctor was completely comfortable with that name.

Truckee, California

Truckee, an hour's drive from Incline Village, was nestled in a pine tree–lined valley next to Route 80, the western freeway that dips into California at the Nevada border. A century before, the town had been filled with prosperous loggers and miners. By the mid-1980s its shops catered instead to the après-ski crowd. In stark contrast to the gingerbread-laced hotels and boutiques at one end of town, a lumber mill hunkered at the other, its grounds layered with redwood awaiting processing. Clouds of steam surged from its smokestacks, sometimes mingling with fog in winter, giving the town an eerie cast and rendering travel hazardous.

Thirty-two teachers comprised the faculty of the town's sole high school, Tahoe-Truckee High, when its doors opened for the new academic year. The aging structure was jammed with six hundred students and space was in short supply. Because of the crush of students that year, teachers were obliged to prepare their lessons and eat lunch in a cramped room next to the principal's office on the first floor. Compounding the teachers' discomfort that fall was a newly installed heating system, intended to save money, that recycled the warm air in individual rooms rather than drawing in fresh air and distributing it throughout the building. School administrators instructed employees in resolute terms to keep all windows closed. Reluctantly, the teachers acquiesced to their hermetic existence in the lounge, although many of them found their habitat, polluted by cigarette smoke and fumes from the two bulky copy machines, nearly intolerable at times.

Third and fourth periods, from 9:45 until 11:30 A.M., saw the heaviest traffic in the teachers' lounge. Gerald and Janice Kennedy were among eight teachers who shared the space then. Janice, forty, taught English to students in the top four grades; her husband, then forty-six, taught auto mechanics and drafting. Chuck Pritchard (a pseudonym), a forty-year-old science teacher, shared the room as well. Onorio Antonucci, fifty-two, was the fourth instructor assigned to the third period. A quiet, patrician man known to his friends and students as Andy, he had taught seventh-grade algebra and coached seventh- and eighth-grade girls' basketball for twenty-seven years—twenty-one of them in Truckee. Irene Baker, forty-three, who taught history to eighth graders, was the fifth. A sixth teacher, May Stroud (a pseudonym), taught French. Jack Cooper (a pseudonym) was the seventh and youngest, a man in his early thirties. Lastly, there was Eric Jordan (a pseudonym), who taught math. Jordan, in his fifties, was so put off by the fumes and the meanness of the accommodations that he left school during third period each day, driving his pickup truck with a camper attachment to the lake. There, savoring his view of the largest alpine lake in North America, he perked a pot of coffee and worked in the solitude of his camper.

Chuck Pritchard was the first among this cloistered set to fall ill. For two weeks in January, he stayed home nursing a high fever, swollen glands, and a body-racking cough. Early in February he resumed teaching, but his colleagues observed he was far from recovered. According to Gerald Kennedy, the science instructor spent his ninety-minute prep time lying corpse-like on a tattered couch in the lounge.

Within days of Chuck Pritchard's return to school, another teacher assigned to the lounge during the third and fourth periods became sick: Andy Antonucci. His illness, like Pritchard's, came on suddenly. While teaching his first class of the day, he was nearly overcome by nausea and headache. After school, the algebra instructor drove the ten-mile route that wound around the lake to Incline Village to see Dan Peterson, his doctor of four years. Out of curiosity, Peterson drew a sample of Antonucci's blood for an Epstein-Barr virus antibody test. Antonucci's antibody levels to the virus were in the normal range. Antonucci, meanwhile, deteriorated. He returned to Peterson's office three weeks later, sicker than before. Peterson ordered a second Epstein-Barr virus test. This time the results were positive; the numbers had skyrocketed.

Gerald and Janice Kennedy also found their health flagging in February, though their decline was less abrupt than either Pritchard's or Antonucci's. In Gerald's case, fatigue accompanied by low-grade fevers and headaches began so gradually he was able to discount the problem for some months. Only in retrospect would he realize he had lived those winter months in a netherworld of exhaustion, unable to do anything beyond what was absolutely required of him. He would remember more bizarre problems as well. He found he was unable to bear bright sunlight, for example. For the first time in his life, he began wearing sunglasses, even, on occasion, indoors. Janice, on the other hand, became severely debilitated in a matter of weeks. She awoke in the morning stiff and groggy, as if she were the victim of a monstrous hangover, except that she didn't drink. By mid-March the teacher who loved to go for long hikes in the mountains was unable to walk unaided from her bed to her bathroom. She lacked the strength to raise her arms above shoulder level to shampoo her hair. Janice sought help from her Truckee doctor, who had treated her for a handful of colds and flus over the previous twenty-two years. This time he seemed stone deaf to her words. Gerald Kennedy, too, went to see a local doctor, one who was affiliated with the Truckee hospital. "He spent fifteen minutes with me," the shop teacher recounted, "and then he said, 'I think this is all in your head.' "

By the end of March, three of the eight teachers who shared the lounge in the morning hours were severely ill, as was Chuck Pritchard's wife, Julie (a pseudonym). Julie Pritchard's doctor, also a Truckee practitioner, advised her to get more exercise. Pritchard, who had just finished telling the doctor she was becoming too weak to walk, was flabbergasted, but said nothing.

In April, history teacher Irene Baker grew concerned when her daughter Laurie, a normally ebullient sixteen-year-old, became sick. Later she would note that Laurie had frequently baby-sat with the Pritchards' two-year-old during the winter months. Dan Peterson, the Baker family's internist, tentatively diagnosed Laurie with acute infectious mononucleosis. Three weeks later, just as the girl seemed to be recovering, her mother, Irene, was stricken with a fatiguing viral-like disease. Peterson, assessing Irene Baker's Epstein-Barr test, reluctantly suggested to the teacher that she might be suffering from the chronic malady that had afflicted her colleague, Andy Antonucci.

"I had plans to teach summer school," Baker recalled. "I kept telling the school, 'Just give me another week.' " In mid-July Baker finally conceded that she would have to abandon her summer teaching plans. "Then I thought, Well, surely I'll start school in September, but I wasn't able to walk from the house to the car by September."

Meanwhile, at their friend Antonucci's suggestion, Gerald and Janice Kennedy made appointments with Dan Peterson, becoming the third and fourth Truckee High teachers with the new malady to seek help at the Alder Street clinic in Incline Village. That same month Julie Pritchard made an appointment to see Paul Cheney, bringing the number to five.

Julie Pritchard, who had been ill since February, was suffering increasingly severe medical difficulties. According to Cheney's records, Pritchard had "marked fatigue" and a persistent cough on her first visit in April. Her lymph nodes were swollen, as was her spleen. In addition, she also had a positive monospot test, meaning that she was suffering, at age forty, from acute infectious mononucleosis. Apparently she was one of those medical rarities: a person who had missed becoming infected with Epstein-Barr virus until middle age. Unlike that of many of the chronically ill patients in the doctors' practice, then, Pritchard's Epstein-Barr virus infection was not a *reactivation*—it was a first-time activation.

Two more teachers who shared the lounge during the third and fourth periods came down with a milder form of the malady that spring, bringing the number to six. Jack Cooper, the seventh of the eight teachers sharing the lounge, was not yet ill.

In the end, only one teacher among the eight emerged unscathed: Eric Jordan, the outdoorsman who had chosen to prepare his lessons and grade papers in the stillness of his camper.

"I'll tell you," Gerald Kennedy said years afterward, his voice quavering, "it paid to get out of that room."

Incline Village, Nevada

Until April, Paul Cheney and Dan Peterson had tried to believe they were dealing with sporadic, random cases of the malady described in the *Annals*. The teachers' cluster shattered their fragile equanimity.

"By early March, Dan had fifteen patients, and I had maybe three or four. And there were these girls on the Incline basketball team who had gotten sick—and a few of them really didn't get better," Cheney remembered. "But the thing that made it unusual," he added, "was when the teachers started coming in. You don't see thirty percent of a faculty, whose average age is forty, get hit with mono."

More disturbingly, the Truckee cluster was followed by a sudden prodigious upsurge in the number of adults with the same symptoms. During the first week in May the startled doctors saw what they believed were ten new cases. The next week they saw fifteen, and the third week, fifteen more. Whatever this ailment was, it no longer seemed to be what the literature described.

"It all broke down—began to break down—when the epidemic began to be evident in May," Cheney said. "Because Jones and Straus never talked about an epidemic."

▦

Early in May, Dan Peterson and Paul Cheney identified a cluster of five employees—two casino dealers, an engineer, a hotel maid, and the wife of the general manager—at the Incline Village Hyatt, the largest employer in town. They soon discovered a second cluster of high school teachers at North Tahoe High School in nearby Tahoe City, across the state border in California.

Dan Peterson called Michael Ford, the director of the Washoe County Health District in Reno, to report what he and his partner had been observing in their practice. Incline Village, sixty miles away in the Sierras, lay within the county, and Michael Ford was the area's highest-ranking health officer.

Peterson told Ford that they had more than eighty patients whose symptoms resembled the "chronic Epstein-Barr virus," or "chronic mononucleosis" syndrome, recently described in the literature; most had fallen ill in the previous four months; hardly any of them knew one another. Only recently, with the discovery of time-space clusters of cases in two high schools and at the local Hyatt, had the doctors concluded that the disease was probably infectious.

"There was an eighteen-second silence when I stopped speaking," the doctor recalled.

When Ford, who was then a fifteen-year veteran of the Washoe health department, finally responded, he expressed little interest and offered no help. Soon afterward, in fact, the health official inserted a notice into the county health newsletter, distributed to hospital staffs and doctors in the area; inexplicably, the notice said that mono was most definitely not on the increase in the county.

Peterson was dumbfounded. Ford had missed the point completely.

"I never called him again," the doctor said.

Later, Ford was asked about his response to Peterson's request for help that summer. The stocky dark-haired man, whose medical credentials amounted to a master's degree in public health, grinned and answered, "You really want me to say?" Clearly pleased with the opportunity, he continued, "Through the years, there have been a number of different physicians practicing in the Incline Village area. They kind of come and go. They've all been weird. We had one individual up there who was into vitamin C therapy. . . . There's just always been strange things associated with the clinical practices up there.

"Now, I didn't even know who Dr. Cheney and Dr. Peterson were, to tell you the truth. But when Peterson called, for me it was sort of just another weirdo from Incline Village. It sounded like gobbledygook stuff. It didn't have a lot of credibility."

By early June the doctors realized the number of "chronic mono" patients in their practice had topped ninety, beginning with the three who had consulted Dan Peterson the previous September shortly after the oilman's wife left Tahoe. An epidemic is defined as an unusual occurrence of disease, an unexplained number of cases in a particular time period. Both doctors were convinced that an upsurge of ninety patients with similar symptoms over the course of months in a small-town practice constituted an epidemic, particularly since they had not had a single patient with the same peculiar constellation of signs and symptoms before September. Unfortunately the doctors had no name for the disease they increasingly suspected was spreading across northern Nevada and possibly elsewhere. Had Cheney and Peterson reported an unusual occurrence of, say, bubonic plague, cholera, Rocky Mountain spotted fever, or any exotic-sounding flu, the state's public health officer would have been interested. As it was, lacking a name, the doctors could offer only a confusing litany of symptoms, buttressed in most but not every case with a single laboratory abnormality: aberrant antibody levels to the most ubiquitous known virus in the world.

Paul Cheney's response to Michael Ford's indifference was to burrow further into his own research. His patient load was less crushing than his partner's, and for some weeks already he had been spending hours in his office engaged in telephone conversations with herpesvirus experts and infectious disease specialists all over the country. On a blank eight-by-eleven-inch page that he inserted into a corner of his leather-bound desk blotter, the doctor began noting the names and phone numbers of his contacts in tiny, precise lettering. By December, both sides of the page would be filled.

Werner Henle was the most eminent virologist whose aid Cheney enlisted that spring. With Gertrude Henle, his spouse and scientific collaborator, Werner Henle had done the painstaking research leading to the discovery in 1964 that Epstein-Barr was the cause of infectious mono. The courtly European couple, who had emigrated to the United States from their native Germany in the 1930s, also implicated Epstein-Barr virus in Burkitt's lymphoma, a kind of immune system cancer endemic in the African malarial belt. Gertrude and Werner Henle's brilliant virology established for the first time that, given the right conditions, a common virus could cause cancer. Together they engineered the Epstein-Barr virus antibody test that was in use at Nichols Institute in southern California and at myriad other virological research labs around the world, establishing standards of normality and abnormality for antibody levels to the ubiquitous germ. To a younger generation of herpes virologists, the Henles were known reverentially as the "mother and father" of Epstein-Barr virus; those who had the opportunity to study with the distinguished team universally referred to themselves as children of the Henles.

Cheney had hoped Werner Henle could help him understand why or how this epidemic could be occurring, but the elderly scientist was as confounded as the doctor. Given the pattern of antibody responses Cheney described, however, Henle confirmed that the patients seemed to be suffering a virulent reactivation of a long-latent infection. He also noted that low or absent antibodies to Epstein-Barr nuclear antigen, or EBNA—a common finding among the Tahoe victims—usually was indicative of immune deficiency (in particular, a deficiency of T-cells); the condition was found almost universally in children with AIDS and in a handful of other rare immune-deficient states. The scientist further suggested that Cheney send some blood serum samples from Nevada to the Henle lab in Philadelphia.*

Ten days later Henle phoned Cheney with his news. The virologist had analyzed twenty-nine blood samples from Incline Village; his results were remarkably close to the values being reported by the Nichols lab, although Henle had found consistently higher numbers in one category of antibodies measured. Thus, according to the Henle lab, which was regarded as the gold standard worldwide in Epstein-Barr virus antibody testing, the Nevada doctors actually were undercalling rather than overcalling the degree of the immune system abnormality in their ailing patients.

During the second week in June, spurred by the Henle lab results, Dan Peterson made a decision that has had momentous consequences: with no clear leadership

---

* Since the publication of the Jones and Straus articles linking Epstein-Barr virus to the new syndrome, the Henles' Philadelphia lab had been swamped by serum samples from doctors all over the country whose patients' symptoms mimicked those described in the literature.

coming from Nevada's health department, he opted to notify the Centers for Disease Control in Atlanta about the events under way in Incline Village.

Peterson had never shied away from a cause he believed in, but little in the thirty-five-year-old doctor's experience could have prepared him for the outcome of his appeal that summer. That June, in fact, it could fairly be said that the doctor's political education was just beginning.

Peterson chose to call a former colleague, Mary Guinan, who was doing herpesvirus research at the Atlanta agency. The two had become friends during a shared stint at the University of Utah hospitals in Salt Lake City in 1976. Guinan had been working toward her fellowship in infectious diseases and was a consultant to the internal medicine group; Peterson had been a twenty-six-year-old first-year internal medicine resident with an apparent keen interest in infectious diseases and the rapidly evolving techniques for assessing immune system integrity. Unlike more cocksure residents, Guinan recalled later, Peterson had frequently sought her counsel on difficult infectious disease cases; he had also struck her as a gifted diagnostician.

Historians of the AIDS epidemic remember Guinan, a tall, red-haired Brooklyn native, for her dogged epidemiological forays into the homosexual population of San Francisco during the summer of 1981 to determine what was killing gay men. Her unflinching "shoe-leather epidemiology" earned her high marks at Centers for Disease Control. She was graced, in addition, with the complex social skills required of women to maneuver effectively within a male-dominated bureaucracy. When Dan Peterson, convinced his town was in the throes of a singular medical crisis, resolved to call Guinan in 1985, she was on her way to becoming the highest-ranking woman at the agency; the following year, she was named an assistant director.

Guinan listened as her former colleague described his Tahoe patients, her curiosity aroused by the possibility that this ailment, which three recent medical papers had described, was occurring in epidemic form. Previously, researchers had described it as a sporadic illness. She remembered, too, that Atlanta clinician Richard DuBois had made a presentation to agency staff on the malady early in 1983, even proposing that the new mono-like syndrome might be a second epidemic of immune dysfunction rising concurrently with AIDS.

Guinan was fascinated. Should Peterson's story pan out—if indeed there were nearly one hundred people stricken with it—the event would be a unique opportunity to examine risk factors, transmission modes, and, of course, etiology. She promised to help. If conditions were right, she said, her agency might send epidemiologists to the lake to investigate.* "Just for your information," Guinan told the Nevada clinician, "if we can't get permission from the local health depart-

---

*Each year, doctors, citizens, and state health officers inundate the Atlanta disease center with more than a thousand requests to investigate purported clusters of disease; the agency honors approximately one out of every ten requests for on-site investigation. Guinan's relationship with Peterson was a crucial point in his favor.

ment, we just can't go. They *have* to invite us. The only way we get invited to epidemics is by keeping in good stead with the people who invite us."

True to her word, Guinan moved on Peterson's call the same day. "Dan called as a friend," she said later. "But his call was sufficiently urgent that I felt I had to do something immediately."

Adhering to the then widespread assumption that the disease had something to do with Epstein-Barr virus, a herpes bug, Guinan placed a call to the government epidemiologist who she believed could best assert legitimate claim to the curious phenomenon Peterson described. He was Larry Schonberger, chief of the CDC's Epidemiology Office within the Division of Viral and Rickettsial Diseases and an agency veteran of fourteen years. Schonberger and his staff of epidemiologists had a mandate to monitor and occasionally investigate outbreaks of viral diseases, with the exception of AIDS, which by 1985 had been awarded a separate division and staff and more than half of the federal agency's entire annual research budget.

Among his colleagues Schonberger was known for his affinity for idiopathic diseases—afflictions of unknown etiology. They referred to him jocularly as "our Sherlock Holmes." Like most agency epidemiologists, however, Schonberger was accustomed to diseases with glaringly obvious or sudden onsets and unambiguous outcomes.

"We get these calls all the time," Schonberger, a powerful-looking man with a halo of unruly hair retreating from his hairline, said later. "If someone had said, 'I've got an acute case of paralysis here—it may be polio,' you respond immediately. You go out there—because *that's* a public health crisis. This sounded . . . well . . . strange, not urgent."

The word "chronic" blunted Schonberger's interest in the subject as thoroughly as the word "mono." He opted to proceed in a markedly leisurely fashion before committing his branch to an on-site investigation. His first move was to instruct a young Epidemic Intelligence Service officer to extract better proof from the Nevada clinicians.

Reno, Nevada

Washoe County health officer Michael Ford took the call from the twenty-nine-year-old Epidemic Intelligence Service officer in Atlanta. Gary Holmes, a six-foot-seven-inch native of Denton, Texas, had worked at the Centers for Disease Control for only four months. As his new boss, Larry Schonberger, had instructed him to do, Holmes asked Ford if he was aware of a cluster of "chronic mono" in Incline Village.

Ford had his answer ready. During an interview later he described his response to Holmes: "I gave CDC basically the same response I've given you—that weird things come out of Incline Village. And one tends not to put a great deal of emphasis on them or give them a great deal of credibility. That's just kind of been the general routine in the past."

Ford told Holmes that if the agency should decide to send investigators, he would provide them with assistance from his staff. However, it was Ford's distinct impression, gleaned from his first conversation with the young EIS officer, that the federal agency on the far coast would not be coming. That the agency was interested at all, Ford added in a reference to Peterson and Cheney, was due to "those guys stirring things up."

"*I* didn't see it as being a problem that was unusual or unique," the health officer said, "and, as I recall, at first they weren't interested in taking a look at it."

Incline Village, Nevada

Paul Cheney engaged in so many conversations with Gary Holmes that summer that he grew accustomed to Holmes's rich Texas drawl and his seeming imperturbability.

"He didn't know very much," Cheney recalled. "He *never* knew very much. But what he would do is say, 'Well, let me talk it over with someone.' So he'd go talk to some expert at CDC. And then a couple of days later I would call him back and ask what the expert said. Gary would say"—Cheney paused to laugh— " 'Mono doesn't occur in epidemics. It must be something else.' "

That, of course, was precisely what Cheney and Peterson were trying to convey to the federal investigators.

"I remember telling him what these people were like," the doctor said. "That they seemed to be clustering, that they had swollen spleens and lymph nodes, that they had been sick for months. And he would listen politely and say, 'That's interesting.' I sensed that [Holmes and his superiors] didn't quite fathom what we were saying," Cheney added. "They wondered if we were crazy. But I could understand that," the doctor said after a moment, "because this was beyond their experience."

Clinically, the malady was a hydra-headed monster. As victims increasingly monopolized them in their Alder Street examining rooms, the doctors' sensitivities to the manifold aspects of the syndrome grew. Physical signs and symptoms associated with the malady accrued seemingly without end. Patients described bouts of dizziness, mysterious rashes, abdominal pain and diarrhea, rapid pounding heartbeat and chest pain, shortness of breath, blurred vision. People complained that their hair was falling out. A third of the patients said their joints ached as if they had arthritis. Two-thirds had become highly sensitive to light; some were unable to leave their house or sit near a window without donning sunglasses; others reported they could no longer drive after dark because the headlights from oncoming cars blinded them.

Still other patients complained their peripheral vision was lost to them. More than half described a ringing sensation in their ears, or tinnitus. The worst sufferers kept their sanity by wearing portable stereo headphones to drown out the perpetual whine in their heads. Nearly everyone seemed to lose weight initially, but those who had been ill the longest were now beginning to gain significantly. Another commonly voiced grievance had to do with sex: women talked about their loss of libido; men reported they had become impotent. Marriages and relationships, already strained by one partner's inability to function in the workplace or care for children, were beginning to unravel.

So far, two young women with the disease had suffered miscarriages. Another curious observation was that within one year of the beginning of the epidemic, six sufferers had required gallbladder surgery, including Truckee High's disabled

teachers, Andy Antonucci and Janice Kennedy. "Some were atypical," Cheney remembered later. "Some of these patients had *no* stones." The clinicians were puzzled by this curious outbreak of gallbladder surgery, but even more troubling were
the long and infection-plagued recoveries each of the patients experienced. All of
them took far too long to bounce back from the effects of surgery, and four developed rare bacterial infections after their operations, suggesting that their immune
system was compromised.

There were even more unusual complaints. A number of people said they were
losing sensation in their fingertips or were experiencing numbness in their face.
Victims' ankles, feet, hands, and eyelids swelled. They reported that they became
light-headed—nearly drunk—after one or two swallows of wine or beer. Twenty
percent said they had suddenly developed allergies to substances that had never
triggered an allergic reaction before. A few patients broke out in cold sores or genital herpes, sometimes concurrently, for the first time in their lives. One of
Cheney's most desperately ill patients, a nurse, tested "four plus" positive—or extremely positive—for genital herpes, oral herpes, Epstein-Barr virus, and herpes
zoster, manifested by shingles: in other words, every known human herpesvirus
but cytomegalo was actively replicating in her cells, yet another suggestion of impaired immunity.

Cheney and Peterson were fascinated by the constellation of ailments, unified
by two constants: abnormal Epstein-Barr virus antibody patterns, and a kind of fatigue neither doctor had encountered before in training or in clinical practice. It
was a global disablement, nearly comparable to paralysis. Years later, recounting
the Tahoe experience to a gathering of curious doctors in Albuquerque, Peterson
tried to convey the quality of the pervasive symptom, calling it "absolutely striking—like nothing you have ever heard in taking histories before. This isn't tiredness. This is a carpenter who says, 'I can't raise my arm to hammer,' or a marathon
runner who says, 'I can't make it to the corner.' "

Several patients, too weak to stand, took their showers seated on lawn chairs.
Others reported that their feet seemed encased in invisible tubs of cement or that
their legs felt as weighty as telephone poles. One woman said she needed both
hands to lift a telephone receiver. A patient in his twenties complained that he typically felt "like a POW after a forced march through the jungle." Said another
young patient, an athlete: "I feel as if I'm wearing a suit of armor and there is a
magnet in the floor."

One Incline woman's memorable description inspired a new name for the disease. "I feel like a Raggedy Ann without the stuffing," the once-vigorous fifty-
year-old teacher told a reporter when the epidemic became news fodder several
months later. In time, a magazine article about the Raggedy Ann syndrome that
had "knocked the stuffing out of Incline Village" appeared on newsstands.[1]

San Francisco, California

Nearly a year after meeting her first patient with the malady, Carol Jessop had
identified an additional fifty San Francisco women suffering from the devastating
disease, which seemed to her to be rising in equal proportion to and concurrently
with the city's AIDS epidemic.

"I was really worried about them," she said. "I went from thinking they had everything from ovarian cancer to multiple sclerosis to myasthenia gravis. Ultimately, I kind of thought they had a smoldering autoimmune disease that just hadn't declared itself. But while watching my patients deteriorate to the point where they were unable to work," she recalled, "I continued my search for an understanding of this problem."

Jessop combed the medical literature for clues. In January 1985, she had felt a surge of adrenaline when she opened her copy of the *Annals of Internal Medicine* and saw the articles by James Jones and Stephen Straus.

"I was pretty excited," she said. "I thought, My God! This is exactly what I'm seeing! So I called James Jones. He said, 'By all means, send your patients' serum back to Denver'—where he was then working—'and I'll run it.' And it all turned out positive."

As the winter progressed and Jessop continued monitoring her disabled patients for the Epstein-Barr virus antibody levels, she discovered that a third of them tested in the normal ranges. The statistic suggested to Jessop that the ubiquitous herpesvirus's role in the disease was probably minor. In addition, like her contemporaries in Nevada, she began to wonder if the real problem might be immune system failure.

Beverly Hills, California

In March, internist Herbert Tanney notified Shirley Fannin, an epidemiologist and Los Angeles County health officer, of an unusual occurrence of disease in his Century City practice.

"I told her that I had seen, by then, well over fifty patients with this syndrome and that we were having an epidemic. Fannin said it was interesting, and that she would have loved to send somebody over, but that they were too tied up with AIDS."

Neither Fannin nor anyone else from the L.A. County health department ever spoke with Tanney again. That same month he convened a meeting of his fellow practitioners at Century City Hospital to alert them to what he felt certain was an epidemic. "I gave a presentation on it one day at the doctors' meeting, just to let everyone know what they should be on the lookout for. There were about twelve doctors present. There was, basically, skepticism," he remembered.

Lacking a diagnostic test, Tanney was beginning to develop a sixth sense for the disease. "There are a few key words: fatigue, depression, muscle aching, muscle weakness, nightmares, trouble concentrating, loss of memory. That's usually all you need to start thinking about this seriously." It was the combination of these symptoms and their remarkable duration that distinguished the malady, he continued. Asked if he had ever seen the same constellation of symptoms in his clinical practice before August of 1983, he responded, "Absolutely not."

In the face of his colleagues' rebuff, Tanney pursued his research independently. "After I read all the textbooks on mononucleosis," he said, "I called professors of infectious disease at Stanford, Michigan, Harvard, and Cornell to find out all I could about mono, and they basically recited to me what the textbooks said."

Having satisfied himself that none of the best infectious disease specialists in the country had insights superior to his own, Tanney turned his efforts toward his disabled patients. By spring, he believed the disease to be the most confounding medical problem he had encountered in thirty years of practice.

Glenview, Illinois

Theodore Van Zelst, a soft-spoken civil engineer from Chicago, had first learned of "chronic mono" when his adult daughter, a clinical nutritionist, was diagnosed with it by Denver researcher James Jones in 1984. The woman had been virtually bedridden for three years although doctors in her own hospital judged her a malingerer. The patient's referral to Jones was fortuitous: when an astute nurse overheard Van Zelst's daughter describing her symptoms, she followed the family out of one doctor's office and suggested they call an Albuquerque patients' organization she had read about; it was this contact that eventually led them to Jones.

Twenty-five years earlier Van Zelst had created a charitable foundation, Minann, Inc., to encourage science education in private schools. After his daughter fell ill, he refreshed his foundation's mandate: in future, Minann would furnish seed money to researchers seeking to study his daughter's disease. Harvard's chief of internal medicine, Anthony Komaroff, was the first to approach Van Zelst.

"Komaroff said he felt more and more people were coming into the Harvard hospitals with this," Van Zelst recalled later. "He wanted to study the incidence of the disease at the Brigham's general medicine clinic. He was trying to convince about thirty of his colleagues, but no one would give him any support or encouragement."

Van Zelst funded Komaroff's project, but the Harvard researcher cautioned that results were two years away.

On June 12 the *New York Times* published an article by reporter Jane Brody about the curious new syndrome recently described in medical literature and included Minann's three-digit post office box number in Glenview, Illinois. In a matter of days, Van Zelst said later, his foundation began receiving "trays" of mail. After three weeks the local post office launched an investigation: two postal inspectors made a surprise appearance at the foundation's tiny office to ascertain the nature of its business. Before the mail abated, the foundation had received more than 12,000 pieces of correspondence. Letters poured in from people who claimed to suffer from the disease and from their friends and families; doctors, too, wrote seeking information to help them diagnose the disease.

By summer's end, a volunteer staff of two had created a mailing list. Using these names, Van Zelst planned his own simple demographic survey to establish a statistical base, however small and unscientific, as a preface to a more serious inquiry into the prevalence of the disease.

Raleigh, North Carolina

By the spring of 1985, it had begun to seem as if no one in the North Carolina Symphony orchestra was immune to the depressing malady. In May, however, the first orchestra member to have fallen ill the previous fall was given a definitive diagnosis: infectious mononucleosis, a surprising disorder in a thirty-nine-year-old. Between May 1985 and April 1986, the same local doctor would diagnose another six orchestra members with mononucleosis.

Wistar Institute, Philadelphia

By January, Hilary Koprowski, the director of the Wistar Institute, and his young protégée, immunologist Elaine DeFreitas, had made three trips to the Florida Keys to pursue their investigation of the epidemic of multiple sclerosis there. The scientists spent their days at the Keys Memorial Hospital on Stock Island, where three of the victims had worked as nurses. With Miami neurologist William Sheremata as his host, the Polish-born doctor and microbiologist Koprowski interviewed and examined the patients; DeFreitas worked in the small hospital's laboratory processing the blood and spinal fluid samples.

The Key West patients weren't the first group of multiple sclerosis victims in whom the Wistar team had discovered evidence of a rare lymphotrophic virus, one in the same class of viruses thought to cause AIDS. Similar findings had shown up in a study, undertaken in early 1983, of multiple sclerosis patients in Sweden. What Koprowski and DeFreitas found increasingly puzzling was that the Florida patients had vastly higher antibody counts and had more virus-infected cells than the Swedes.

Although neither DeFreitas nor Koprowski could explain the substantial lab disparities, they believed their discovery of the same rare virus in two geographically distinct populations was important and should be published. With their collaborators, they began preparing their paper for publication in the venerable British scientific journal *Nature*. In their article, published the following November, they took pains to describe the differences between the Key West patients and the Swedish patients.[2] The antibody data in both populations was "suggestive, but not conclusive," of a viral etiology for the disease, they wrote. The pair planned further studies to attempt to isolate the novel virus.

National Cancer Institute, Bethesda, Maryland

Sayed Zaki Salahuddin was annoyed by the large organism that kept lumbering into his line of sight as he stared into the eyepiece of his laboratory's $500,000 electron microscope. Salahuddin was scanning a vastly magnified world of blood tissue from a twenty-nine-year-old man afflicted with AIDS, Kaposi's sarcoma, and B-cell lymphoma. He was looking for anything except what—for all the world—appeared to be an enormous herpesvirus.

The rakish Indian was a lieutenant in the federal government's burgeoning war on AIDS and a top-ranking investigator in Robert Gallo's Laboratory of Tumor Cell Biology at the National Institutes of Health. In 1985 the lab's scientists were basking in the prestige afforded them by their achievement of the previous year: isolating a strain of human immunodeficiency virus. Their boss had promptly hailed the new bug as the cause of AIDS. A year after the Gallo lab was feted for its pioneering science, Salahuddin was busying himself with studies of lymphocyte cells of AIDS sufferers.

"I was looking for something else," Salahuddin remembered much later, "but I found, from time to time, the expression—the very *overt* expression—of a virus that looked like herpes. It kept coming up. So I said to myself, It must be EBV."

Salahuddin had good reasons for his assumption, beginning with the size of the bug. Human immunodeficiency virus is in the retrovirus family, a genus of viruses vastly smaller than herpesviruses. Under an electron microscope, the proportionate difference between the two was comparable to the contrast between a mobile home and an office tower. Further, AIDS patients typically suffered reactivation of latent Epstein-Barr virus infections as their immune system function deteriorated. Additionally, Salahuddin was looking specifically at B-cells, the immune system cells targeted by Epstein-Barr virus.

There was another reason to surmise that the ungainly virus was Epstein-Barr. Cell death is at the core of the disease process in most infectious diseases. Epstein-Barr is unusual because it typically "immortalizes" cells rather than destroying them. However, a number of reports had been appearing in scientific journals about a new variant of Epstein-Barr virus that was exhibiting highly unusual behavior: it was blowing up cells. The virus Salahuddin observed was killing cells like crazy.

Salahuddin tried to ignore the proficient giant for a day or so, but the damn thing kept announcing itself, as well as annihilating the very cells he wanted to study. Had he been looking at serum from a patient with a better-understood disease, he might have been less inquisitive. Hardly anything was known for certain about AIDS, however, and in such a case, the scientist reasoned, everything was of potential significance.

Salahuddin enlisted the expertise of his longtime friend, Dharam Ablashi, who worked in the Laboratory of Cellular and Molecular Biology, a sister laboratory in the National Cancer Institute. Unlike Salahuddin, Ablashi *was* a herpesvirus expert. The latter undertook experiments with the virus-contaminated cell culture Salahuddin gave him. Two weeks later Ablashi reported to Salahuddin: Salahuddin's find was not the new cell-killing strain of Epstein-Barr virus; it was not, in fact, any form of Epstein-Barr.

"My answer to him was," Salahuddin joked later, " 'Dharam, you are making my life more difficult.' "

3

Foot Soldiers from Atlanta

Incline Village, Nevada

While the staff at the Centers for Disease Control pondered the Nevada situation from afar, Cheney and Peterson tried to contain an incipient panic among patients and their families. By the end of July the doctors realized that the number of chronic mono patients in their practice had topped 120.

"We were so bogged down trying to take care of these patients that I remember the time frame of that summer in the context of the patient count rather than the actual dates," Cheney said. "I just kept calling up the CDC and saying, 'Now we're up to one hundred twenty.' And then another week would pass, and I would call and say, 'Now we're up to one hundred thirty-five.' We were horrified," the doctor recalled. "We felt like we were in a nightmare that would not end."

By the end of the summer, the doctors had 150 patients with the syndrome, many of whom had been disabled for months. By early September, however, having heard little from the agency, the clinicians' hopes that the Centers for Disease Control would send its disease detectives to the lake began to fade.

Throughout the summer, knowledge of the drama under way in Incline Village remained confined to a handful of staff at the Centers for Disease Control, the Alder Street clinicians and their patients, and increasingly, the family practice doctors who were Cheney and Peterson's competitors in the town. "No media knew anything about this," Cheney said later, "but other doctors did."

Indeed, the issue was fairly smoldering among the small medical fraternity of lakeside practitioners. Incline's four family practice doctors were seeing patients with the Jones-Straus disease, too, but their view of the malady contrasted starkly with that of the "powerhouse" internal medicine specialists on Alder Street. "Hypochondriacs. Neurotics. Depressives," said one of them, Gerald Cochran, when he was asked some time later to characterize his local patients who complained of exhaustion and a host of other "vague" symptoms that summer. Although there had been a recent marked influx of such patients into his practice, Cochran was confident that these unfortunates represented a species known to physicians for eons. "We used to call it 'poor protoplasm,'" the doctor said. "They tend to be personality types. They're a group that's always looking for answers, looking for diagnoses, and you have to be very careful with the labels you put on them, because they latch on to them."

Cochran avoided words like "hypochondriac" and "neurotic" in his conversations with his weary patients as scrupulously as he avoided words that evinced bona fide medical conditions, but he often jotted his assessment of their problem—"psychoneurotic"—in their charts. "Or else I disguised it better than that," he said.

In case his patient should acquire the chart?

"That's exactly right. You have to be careful what you chart."

The doctor was a large, slow-moving man in his early sixties who had given up a practice in Santa Rosa, California, in 1979 to move to the lake. With the exception of one other, he boasted the longest tenure of any practitioner in Incline Village. By Cochran's estimate, fifteen of his patients had left his practice by the summer of 1985 after he refused to supply them with a label—at least a label he cared to share with them. All fifteen were members of the contingent who had complained of crippling exhaustion. Their defection failed to sadden him. "This is typical of these people," he said. "They will always give histories of having gone through many doctors—that's always a red flag."

Cochran was rattled, however, when all fifteen eventually transferred their records to Drs. Cheney and Peterson. He noticed, too, that the younger doctors were unimpressed with his psychiatric acuity; Cheney and Peterson eventually diagnosed all fifteen defectors with the chronic malady.

Harry Weigel was another local family practitioner with equally fervent beliefs about the disease his younger colleagues were diagnosing with such frequency. That summer he was heard to say in private that the Tahoe malady was a "hoax" perpetrated by the specialists on Alder Street. He himself had seen exactly "zero" such cases in his Incline practice, he explained some time later. "Oh," he amended, "I saw some people who had been diagnosed by Cheney and Peterson and came in for second opinions, and I told them promptly that they didn't have the disease." When asked how he knew the patients were not ill, the doctor answered, "Because the disease didn't exist."

By summer an underground network was flourishing among sufferers and their acquaintances along the north shore of Lake Tahoe. The Alder Street doctors, if they couldn't cure the malady, at least were dealing with it. As a result, the specialists were beginning to feel some "heat," as Cheney described it, from their colleagues.

"There began, in the summer," Cheney recalled later, "a split among the medical communities. The split was between myself and Dan and the subspecialists who were not in primary care, who trusted us because we were the internists and they had no reason—no economic reason, at least—to differ with us. And also, of course, they depended on us for their referrals—you don't cut off your referral source. It was those people on one side. On the other side, you had the general practitioners, the family practitioners, with whom we were in direct competition for patients."

Centers for Disease Control, Atlanta, Georgia

Whether the disease was spreading beyond a tiny resort town in the Sierras or, conversely, had been carried to the mountain hamlet by residents of larger cities were issues less important to Gary Holmes and his boss, Larry Schonberger, than was the reality of the disease itself. Schonberger, in particular, was unconvinced that anything extraordinary had occurred in Nevada. Until he had satisfied himself to the contrary, he could hardly be expected to persuade his agency to undertake a more ambitious investigation. Weeks passed as Holmes negotiated, via telephone, the chasm between his skeptical boss and an unusually bright doctor who was by then up to his elbows in the clinical mysteries of a new disease.

The Nevada clinicians, cloistered in the Sierras, were unable to sense it, but eventually there was movement at the Centers for Disease Control. One steamy morning in mid-August, Federal Express delivered twelve samples of Tahoe blood to the agency's herpes laboratory. It took lab chief John Stewart about ten days to run his tests. Like Werner Henle and the technicians at the Nichols lab in southern California, the government scientist found the same abnormally high Epstein-Barr virus antibody levels when he studied the serum. Thus Larry Schonberger's staff presented him with a major piece of evidence supporting Cheney's claims.

"[This evidence] suggested that it was worthwhile to go ahead with the investigation," Stewart said.

Gary Holmes was less restrained. "We felt, Shoot, we've *got* to go out," he said. "I mean, two hundred patients had been described to us!"

In the second week of September, Holmes called Paul Cheney. They would be coming, Holmes said—he and a senior investigator from the viral epidemiology branch—the following week. The agency had asked for and received permission from George Reynolds, the Nevada state epidemiologist in Carson City.

After weeks of seeming indifference and occasional resistance by the agency, Cheney and his partner were stunned, then pleased. "I thought, My God! They're really coming!" Cheney said. "We were very excited—and actually sort of shocked. We thought, We're really going to get some help now. *Someone's* going to be able to figure this out."

The Centers for Disease Control occupied a jumble of red and yellow brick buildings within walking distance of the marble colonnaded halls of Emory University. Building 1, an eight-story yellow brick structure that fronted on Atlanta's Clifton Road, housed the capacious offices of the agency's administrators as well as the cramped cells of an array of scientists and AIDS labs. The edifice had no doubt looked contemporary when it was dedicated in 1960. Across the street, De Kalb County's Fire Station Number One faced the agency, its red trucks aimed at the agency's front door.

Seven other disparately sized buildings, most of them featureless red brick, fanned out along a slope behind Building 1. Nearly half were connected to the Clifton Road building either by underground tunnels or by caged steel walkways suspended several stories above asphalt alleyways. Irrespective of weather, white-coated agency employees unable to kick the nicotine habit stood outside, singly or in groups, cigarettes glowing, near the doorway of each building and along the catwalks, as the alfresco corridors were called. Inside, a featureless grid of linoleum-floored corridors led to countless crowded labs and to the cubbyhole offices of scientists. Main arteries connecting the buildings pulsed with clerks and secretaries, Ph.D.'s and the rare M.D. Laminated card keys hung from chains draped around their necks, or dangled from clips attached to breast or hip pockets, affording entry to locked buildings. If there was an unofficial uniform among the scientific staff, it was probably jeans and running shoes. The agency was one of the few federal fiefdoms based entirely outside the capital, and its staff was decidedly clannish.

Thirty-nine years earlier, when the Centers for Disease Control was launched as a field station of the Public Health Service, its scientists were charged with coordinating a nationwide assault against an immense array of communicable diseases. The agency's quarry included not only diseases that spread from person to person, but those that spread from animals to people. Its mandate was unique in the annals of American, if not world, medical history. Certainly it was the first government agency created to attempt containment of so many diseases at once.

The agency was, in addition, bound by congressional charter to promptly address requests from the states for epidemic aid. The goal was laudable, but by 1949, agency officials realized that a shortage of epidemiologists was undermining their best intentions. "An intensive recruiting effort yielded the sum total of two young physicians who were genuinely interested but totally untrained," the late Alexander Langmuir, the agency's chief epidemiologist during the 1950s and 1960s, noted in his memoir. Epidemiology—a difficult, even arcane, science that was not easily mastered or taught—was an obscure pursuit at mid-century. It was, as one agency veteran later described it, "the mathematical analysis of health problems," and, some might argue, called for a temperament to match.

Seeking to correct this shortage, Joseph Mountin, an assistant surgeon general and a founder of the Centers for Disease Control, suggested that the agency itself become a training ground. He proposed the establishment of an in-house Epidemic Intelligence Service, its purpose to generate a perpetually refreshed pool of epidemiologists-in-training. These novices could be dispatched under the supervision of more experienced epidemiologists in Atlanta whenever states asked for help. Officials at the National Institutes of Health in Bethesda, threatened by the prospect of competition, vigorously protested Mountin's proposal. Asked by Congress if they would accept responsibility for responding to all requests for epidemic aid, however, the NIH officials replied, "Certainly not. Only the interesting ones." The matter was settled.

The Epidemic Intelligence Service was launched in 1951 and rapidly earned an estimable reputation. Today the agency characterizes the corps as a "cadre of disease detectives." Its officers have played a pivotal role in every agency success of recent decades, most notably the investigations of Legionnaires' disease and toxic shock syndrome in the 1970s and a study of the epidemiology of hepatitis B in the 1980s that enabled researchers to engineer a vaccine.

Approximately twenty-five EIS officers are assigned each year to state health departments for their two-year tour of duty; another twenty-five are assigned to the Atlanta headquarters. Lyle Conrad, who for many years supervised the EIS staff who work outside headquarters, called the corps "one of the smallest, tightest fraternities in the world." A jocular thirty-year government veteran when he was interviewed in 1989, Conrad was unmistakably proud of his troops. "Every year," he said, "we interview about two hundred people who think they want to be EIS officers. We look at dentists, veterinarians, M.D.'s, Ph.D's—Ph.D.'s make terrific epidemiologists! And we look for five characteristics—native intellect, aggressiveness, enthusiasm, energy, and a sincere interest in epidemiology. We pick fifty."

Winning Epidemic Intelligence Service officers, Conrad said, "are willing to go anywhere and look at anything. You can't study epidemiology sitting on your butt in a chair in Atlanta," he added amiably. "By the time you talk to half a dozen of these types, you'll kind of get the idea. . . . Part of the excitement in working at this place is to have a chance to take a bid on something that's weird and wonderful."

For the team of disease detectives about to be dispatched to rural Nevada, the medical dilemma awaiting them in Incline Village held little such appeal. Their early distrust of the two clinicians who were their tour guides was their most serious handicap. The peculiar chemistry that developed between the government team and the Alder Street practitioners precluded illumination. In part, it was a problem of sending epidemiologists, both of whom harbored a disdain for clinical medicine, into a conflagration more deserving of meticulous clinical evaluation. Instead of embracing as an opportunity the "weird and wonderful" nature of a new disease in the High Sierras, the government's investigators quickly came to regard their involvement as a professional liability.

In the introduction to his book about the discovery of DNA, *The Double Helix,* James Watson noted, "Science seldom proceeds in the straightforward, logical manner imagined by outsiders. Instead, its steps forward (and sometimes backward) are often very human events in which personalities and cultural traditions play major roles."[1] Such words might well have been written about the enigmatic disease flourishing in northwestern Nevada and the men who were about to meet there.

Incline Village, Nevada

The disease detectives at the Centers for Disease Control are often described in military terms. The nation's "shock troops" against epidemic diseases and the "front line" in public health emergencies are two metaphors that have found their way into print in recent years. In his 1987 book about the AIDS epidemic, *And the Band Played On,* journalist Randy Shilts characterized the agency staff as "a rapid deployment force [that] could be relied upon to pounce on a crisis and establish a beachhead."[2] The agency's foot soldiers in the war against the Tahoe mystery flu came in the form of two young epidemiologists, Jon Kaplan and Gary Holmes, who were eager to abandon their cubbyhole offices in Atlanta for Lake Tahoe.

"If we had heard about this happening in, you know, Podunk, Nebraska, I wouldn't have been so quick to go," Jon Kaplan said later. "But the fact that it was out *there* made it a little more exciting. I knew it was a nice place. That obviously had something to do with it. I had never been there before, and it *was* spectacular."

Gary Holmes, who was fond of mountain hiking, was equally captivated by the prospect of a trip to the pristine high-altitude lake. "It was beautiful, and I must admit, that was one reason I wanted to go," Holmes remarked afterward. "It was an additional impetus, certainly. Lake Tahoe was magnificent—it really was."

Kaplan, at thirty-seven, was the senior man on the job. A native of Columbus, Ohio, he had completed his postgraduate residency in internal medicine and infectious disease at the University of New Mexico. He had launched his agency career four years earlier as an Epidemic Intelligence Service officer. During his first year, cases of dengue fever, a debilitating mosquito-borne disease, erupted along the Texas-Mexico border. Kaplan and a superior were sent to Texas to plot the course of the disease and gauge its threat. Later, Kaplan traveled to Hawaii to investigate a cluster of Guillain-Barré syndrome cases among children. "We tried to figure out what happened there," Kaplan said. (Only later was it discovered that the Hawaiian Guillain-Barré outbreak was part of a U.S.-wide epidemic of the disease caused by the agency's ill-conceived swine flu vaccination program of 1976.) Kaplan was rewarded with a permanent agency job at the end of his training, landing in Larry Schonberger's viral epidemiology group. From the confines of his office, a room with painted cinder-block walls at the end of a short corridor in Building 6, he performed disease surveillance, monitoring the spread of ailments such as Rocky Mountain spotted fever and typhus.

Kaplan, who spent exactly one week in Incline Village, developed an archly skeptical view of the Incline epidemic that remains unequivocal to this day. The crisis described to him by the Nevada clinicians was less an epidemic worthy of the government's attention than it was a roadside freak show.

"The whole situation was bizarre," Kaplan said. He was thin, with long fingers, their nails bitten short. His brown hair was shaggy, framing a narrow face and large, intelligent eyes. "It was almost like being on another planet out there. I mean, here you have this exceptionally beautiful place with weird people and weird doctors and a weird medical problem—the whole thing was weird. And yet," he continued after a bitter-sounding laugh, "we were happy to be there because it was so pretty." Later, asked if he sensed, like Nevada health officer Michael Ford, that Incline Village was a refuge for medical quacks, Kaplan responded incredulously, "Did I sense that? What have I been telling you for the last forty-five minutes? If I haven't conveyed to you that I thought Peterson and Cheney were a little weird, then I haven't made myself very clear. I hesitate to use the word 'quack,' but . . . the situation was definitely strange."

Kaplan's reputation among his colleagues in Atlanta was excellent. "He's very bright—extremely bright," Mary Guinan would offer almost reflexively when Kaplan's name arose in conversation. Kaplan's boss, Larry Schonberger, too, thought highly of Kaplan. Decidedly, in September of 1985, Kaplan was vastly more experienced than Holmes, who had never worked as an epidemiologist before. Later, Paul Cheney, too, observed that Kaplan was bright—and that Holmes was green: "Gary didn't know anything about epidemiology. Jon knew some things. Jon seemed to be the brighter of the two." But the doctor was disturbed by Kaplan's mien, which seemed to Cheney to have hardened into a worldview that had little room for surprises or even new ideas.

"I don't know that Jon was less eager," Holmes would say eventually of his

Tahoe partner. "But I think he had been around long enough—whereas I hadn't been—to know that there are a lot of so-called epidemics reported that turn out not to be. His concern was that this was going to be another."

Kaplan's wariness of the doctors' interpretation of events had to do with his agency training, which had instilled in him a skepticism toward virtually any unverified report of epidemic illness. Workaday clinicians, in the view of Kaplan and his Atlanta bosses, were prone to confuse statistically *insignificant* increases in disease with statistically *significant* increases. The epidemiologist's skepticism went deeper than issues of biostatistics, however. He was perturbed by the very nature of the illness that Cheney and Peterson had described to the agency, especially by the fact that they had tentatively associated their malady with Epstein-Barr virus. In previous years, physicians had reported clusters of acute Epstein-Barr virus disease, or mononucleosis, to the agency. But as government epidemiologists sifted through the evidence, in most instances by means of telephone calls and letters rather than on-site investigation, the reputed epidemics evaporated under the statisticians' computations.

"Infectious mono—the acute disease—is notorious for having pseudo-epidemics reported," Holmes confirmed. "The previous EIS officer got so sick of hearing about these things that he was overjoyed when I took over." According to Kaplan, the reported epidemics consistently failed to materialize. "I don't think *any* have panned out, so there definitely was skepticism," Kaplan said.

Of course Peterson and Cheney had not reported an epidemic of acute mono. But because Kaplan and his superiors were weary of previous encounters with falsely reported epidemics of the acute ailment, the doctors' case was tainted. Nor did the Atlanta scientists dare to imagine, as the Nevada clinicians clearly had, that a new infectious agent was abroad in the land. As a result, Kaplan arrived in Nevada with more than his usual distrust of the situation. And although he sought to achieve objectivity, his skepticism endured, eventually transmuting to profound disbelief and even anger.

"Early on," Kaplan confessed, "I said, I've got to be open to this. But the doubts were there the whole time I was there. They never disappeared. I never got to the point where I said, I really believe this. I *never* got to that point."

Kaplan's partner, Gary Holmes, was new to the pursuit of epidemiology when he embarked for Tahoe, his first field trip for the CDC. If one is to believe a maxim of EIS supervisor Lyle Conrad—that the agency preferred new EIS officers to wet their feet in shallow ponds before wading into ocean gales—then the agency was disposed to imagine that the Nevada epidemic fell within the limits of a mundane investigation. "We don't send them to the difficult problems right away," Conrad explained. "We try to give them a food-borne disease or a measles—something routine."

Holmes had attended medical school at the University of Texas in San Antonio and then pursued a fellowship in infectious diseases at the University of Kentucky. His ambition, in September of 1985, was to complete his two-year Epidemic Intelligence Service stint, then parlay the credential into an epidemiology post at a university. He hadn't the emotional constitution for clinical practice, and he knew it. "Primary care," he would explain, "is not my bag." The "continuous onslaught," as he phrased it, of patients calling "day and night" horrified him. "You *never* get away from it."

The young officer labored within a cubicle just down the fluorescent-lit hallway from Kaplan's in Building 6. Holmes had a pale moon-shaped face with large features and wiry salt-and-pepper hair that he kept close-cropped. "My impression," he said, "until I got out there, actually, was that this was going to be the ultimate opportunity to find out what's going on with this disease. I had read about it in the *Annals of Internal Medicine*. And those papers looked interesting. Reading them, it seemed that EBV was pretty directly linked, and that was the way I was going to approach it, initially."

Cheney and Peterson had described their patients to the agency as having the appearance of "*chronic* mononucleosis" victims, or as resembling patients Jones and Straus described in their recently elucidated syndrome. But the Nevada internists were astounded by the contagious nature of the Jones-Straus syndrome in their town. And although they considered Epstein-Barr virus abnormalities to be the singular consistent marker in the syndrome, they doubted it was the cause of the disease. The fact that an epidemic had occurred was hearty evidence, in fact, that the ailment's cause was anything *but* Epstein-Barr, since that virus was already endemic in the American population. They assumed the government's disease detectives would arrive at the only possible conclusion: that this was something other than Epstein-Barr virus disease, perhaps even something other than what Jones and Straus had described, and that they would then settle down to the arduous process of elucidating what else it might be.

Kaplan and Holmes, on the other hand, needed first to prove to themselves that an epidemic actually had occurred before they could begin to deal with matters of causation and transmission. Some time later, in 1988, having achieved three years of agency tenure and having absorbed a considerable degree of his more senior colleagues' worldview, Holmes explained forbearingly: "You have to go in with a certain degree of skepticism, because there are many reasons why physicians will report an epidemic. And it's not only just because there's an actual epidemic going on. There's the possibility of getting papers, prestige, and publicity."

Incline Village lies at the northern edge of Lake Tahoe, less than ten miles from the California state line. Gold miners trekked through the region by mule on their way to California in 1849. By the turn of the century, the mountains looming above the town had been stripped bare of trees and scarred by logging roads, their landscape a network of rotting flumes and log chutes. Victorian-era loggers harvested over a million cords of wood here, most of which was used to shore up the subterranean galleries of the Comstock Lode or to fuel the locomotives of the Central Pacific railroad. Today only the deepest logging scars remain; the landscape is rich with pine and manzanita.

There is no easy way to get to Incline unless one is already in the high-altitude vicinity of the lake. From Reno, the nearest airport that accommodates commercial jets, one sets out by automobile, preferably four-wheel drive. The journey begins on the desert floor and advances to the summit of Mount Rose, an 8,000-foot mass indented by a snaking, thin strip of pavement often obscured by fog in winter. On a clear day, the continent's largest alpine lake is starkly visible at the top. The liquid expanse—12 miles wide, 22 miles long, and so pristine a white dinner plate can be seen 120 feet below the surface—straddles the California-Nevada border. Incline Village, invisible from this vantage, clings to the shore, emerging suddenly from verdant stands of pine at the bottom of the slope.

Jon Kaplan and Gary Holmes made their bumpy landing in Reno on Wednesday, September 18. They rented a sedan at the airport and navigated the ninety-minute route over Mount Rose. They were stunned when they reached the summit and saw the lake's expanse for the first time. "To come from Reno, with its flat, desert-looking terrain, and then to go over the mountain to see this—this *thing*—it was like seeing the promised land," Holmes would remark later.

Their parsimonious government per diem obliged the epidemiologists to share a room at the Hyatt. Their view was of the parking lot. Kaplan was put off by the cavernous gaming pit at the Hyatt. The space between the hotel lobby and the guest rooms was occupied by computerized slot machines that gurgled inane melodies into the smoky atmosphere and blackjack tables manned by costumed dealers. "I thought it was rather yucky to have to walk through that casino just to get to our room, which we had to do, obviously, many times. But other than that, it was beautiful. The hotel was right across the street from the lake. We didn't have a view, but that didn't keep us from getting out and seeing the area. Gary and I climbed a mountain one day—Mount Talac. It's at the south end of the lake. It was a long hike. We took a whole day and climbed up there. It was gorgeous."

What Cheney recalled was his frustration at trying, and failing, to convey to the investigators the alarming nature of the problem that had consumed him unlike anything else in his life. He and his partner desperately wanted the federal researchers to grasp the dimensions of the calamity—and not only its epidemic aspect. They hoped to make the young epidemiologists comprehend the magnitude of the affliction itself, to see it as a distinct entity that, once detonated, shattered the health of its victim in myriad ways. "Dan and I were saying, 'Gosh, look at this patient,' and shoving the chart at them. And 'Look at this one . . . and this one.' And, '*This* is an interesting case,' " the doctor said. "We were imparting—*trying* to impart—the *sense* of what we were dealing with.

"As I remember, they weren't excited. They wouldn't *say* anything. It reminded me of many bureaucrats. You know—it was just a job."

From the beginning, the clinicians' incredulity was returned, with disproportionate vehemence, by the investigators.

"Peterson is very quiet and reserved," Holmes remembered. "He didn't really make a big deal of it. I mean, he did verbally, but he wasn't being dramatic about it. Paul Cheney is more open and, I guess, it's a little easier to read what he's thinking by the way he acts. Initially, my feeling was that, Gosh, there's something really *incredible* going on here. That was my initial feeling going into it. It was only when we started digging into it that we just couldn't find anything to support that feeling."

Kaplan, for his part, seemed almost spooked by the panorama he found in Incline Village. Virtually everything and everybody the investigator observed during his short stay made him uneasy. Among other anomalies, the federal epidemiologist was put off by the affluence of Incline's inhabitants.

"Within a day, we saw a number of patients," he recalled. "And I was really struck with just how bizarre a place this was. It seemed like there were some people who were obviously very rich and didn't have to work at all. They were just kind of hanging out there. There were other people—I remember talking to some schoolteachers from Truckee, so there were obviously different levels of society there, but it's an extremely rich community. Gary and I went running a lot on that street right around the lake. There were some incredible houses back there. These are not normal Americans living out there. You can't sit there in that kind of environment and not feel strange," Kaplan said.

"I'll tell you the other thing that fed into this feeling of uneasiness," Kaplan continued. "Dan Peterson took us to lunch. Again, he was just terrific, and he took us up to this real nice place that overlooked the lake—God, it was a gorgeous afternoon. I'll never forget it—bright sun, looking out over the lake, real nice food. And I started asking him about himself. And he had a very unusual history for a doctor in practice.

"He trained in Salt Lake City—nothing wrong with that; it's a good training program. He had gone up to Idaho on the National Health Service bill—again, not terribly unusual. Some docs like to do that; it's an unusual experience, and interesting. But apparently he became a real advocate of migrant workers. Migrant workers are kind of the scum of society up in Idaho. And he sort of became their advocate, and there was, at one point, I think, a death of a migrant worker, and Peterson decided he was going to investigate it. He took things to the extent where his life was apparently threatened and where he was literally thrown out of the state—by a local politician or somebody. And that is definitely beyond where most physicians would go. That is an unusual story. I mean, it is one thing to go to an area like that and kind of get pissed off at what's going on and maybe leave after a year or two with some bitter feelings. But it's another thing to end up with your life being threatened and having some local politician or somebody manage to get you thrown out of a government job. And I was hearing this and thinking, This guy is . . . different. He's *different*. And then he ended up in Incline Village and started that practice.

"Now, Paul Cheney, his partner, was nice. In fact, I remember using his office most of the time we were there. He had an interesting background, too. He had a Ph.D. in physics before he went into medical school. Well, a Ph.D. in physics in *that* position—*that's* really unusual. They both had unusual histories for physicians, and their patients were unusual. But then, the whole community was unusual."

In a letter to Nevada health officials, Holmes wrote in October 1985 that he and his partner had interviewed and examined sixteen patients in the offices of Paul Cheney and Dan Peterson during their Tahoe investigation. A year later, however, in a speech to a small gathering of epidemiologists about his Incline investigation, Holmes reported that he and his partner had seen only ten. When he was interviewed nearly three years later, he used the figure ten once more. "We figured that with ten people we could get a pretty good idea of whether there was something that we really wanted to bite down on and do a thorough investigation," Holmes recalled, "or whether we should back off and kind of take it easy."

Kaplan, reaching back into his memory, estimated that he and Holmes had examined "a dozen—fifteen—something like that. I think we asked to see patients that they thought were most likely to have [the disease]. So *they* picked," Kaplan added, disdain entering his voice. "We didn't pick."

Inevitably, shifting nuances and permutations in human memory begin to haunt events with the passage of time. Sometimes significance emerges more from the passion with which people dedicate themselves to their recollections than from the specifics of their accounts. In the case of the CDC's 1985 investigation of an unusual occurrence of disease in Nevada, it was the clinicians' heartfelt conviction, as well as that of their patients, that Kaplan and Holmes exhibited hardly any interest in meeting or examining victims of the purported epidemic.

Neither Cheney nor Peterson can recall Holmes or Kaplan ever asking to see patients. In fact, according to Cheney, the investigators at first begged off. "We asked them, 'Do you want to see anybody? We'll bring some people into the office.' " The investigators, by Cheney's account, were vastly more interested in studying patient charts than patients. It is Cheney's recollection that Holmes and Kaplan spoke to fewer than ten people with the disease, and all of them virtually by coincidence. "No detailed histories were taken," Cheney said. "We dragged Gary and Jon upstairs and had them feel a spleen here or a lymph node there, but they engaged in no systematic examination of even a subset of these patients."

Truckee High teachers Gerald and Janice Kennedy met Holmes, but Gerald Kennedy confirmed, "It wasn't by his request—it was by ours." Upon arriving for an appointment with Peterson, they learned from the doctor's staff that a federal investigator was on the premises. Gerald Kennedy, by now convinced that he, Janice, and their Truckee High colleagues had been victims of an environmentally transmitted disease, sought a meeting with him. Apparently Holmes was agreeable. "We went into the examining room and asked him some questions," Kennedy said. High among the teachers' concerns was the possibility that fumes from the ditto machine toner—which, after all, was packaged in a can decorated with a skull and crossbones—had made the teachers ill. Another culprit proposed by Kennedy was the encrusted, infrequently changed air filters in the room's heating system. Could they have allowed a viral agent to infect the teachers?

"I remember telling him about the filters," Kennedy said. "You could tell he thought we were a bunch of loonies. That was early into it, and we were still thinking, Well, maybe we *are* crazy. But you would think that we would be *questioned,* at least, and there weren't a lot of questions. He just nodded his head and said, 'Uh-huh, uh-huh.' Very little information was exchanged." By his countenance of indifference, Holmes communicated his bias to the Kennedys: "He seemed to have already made up his mind about us."

Joyce Reynolds, the former Placer Savings and Loan teller, had been bedridden for nine months when her doctor, Dan Peterson, called and asked her to come in to meet the men from CDC. Reynolds remembered that after she described the pain under her rib that had persisted since the onset of her "flu," Holmes examined her, although both he and Kaplan were present in the examining room. Holmes palpated Reynolds's spleen, which, according to Peterson, had been swollen for several months, and her liver, which was painful to the touch; Holmes also felt the enlarged lymph nodes under her jaw. "It was very brief," Reynolds said of the encounter. "They asked me about my symptoms and how long I had been ill, but I don't think they thought this was very much to worry about. I believe they said they didn't see anything remarkably abnormal. I really think they thought that this was pretty much in my head. I wasn't too impressed with them."

It was Peterson's sense that the Atlanta visitors were "somewhat impressed, as everyone has been, by the physical patients—I mean, by the patients sitting there." Cheney was less confident—and closer to the mark. In fact, neither Holmes nor Kaplan was much abashed by the illness in the course of meeting its victims.

"On interviewing them," Holmes recalled, "two or three of them appeared to be quite ill. One of them, in particular, came in looking like she was about to be hospitalized. She was incredibly ill. She could barely talk. I can't describe exactly what it was like, but I've taken care of enough patients to know that this woman was sick. And she was convincing enough that I felt there was *something* going on, even though there were others who did not appear to have anything distinctive. A bunch described themselves as being ill, but did not—I mean, they *walked* in, they didn't *look* like they were especially tired, and their descriptions seemed much more severe than they looked. And we couldn't find any distinct physical findings."

Kaplan was even less compelled by what he saw. Rather than share the clinicians' alarm, he surmised a complicated psychological conspiracy was afoot.

"First of all, I was impressed that all the patients *thought* there was something wrong with them. I mean, you can't minimize that. They all *knew* why they were there. I mean, they knew they were there because they had an illness, and they were there to tell us about it," Kaplan began. "To me, what that suggested was 'A lot of what you're saying I'm hearing from you, but I have a feeling I'm hearing your doctor's voice through you at the same time.' I got the impression," the epidemiologist continued, "that there was a kind of collusion going on between some of these patients and the physicians. Well, this isn't totally fair, because there were definitely some people there who had been feeling well and then all of a sudden they had been feeling lousy. And as a doctor I have to have compassion for that. But at the same time there definitely seemed to be some people who had some kind of emotional overlay. They had some symptoms, and they wanted to make the most of them and were looking for some credibility," the investigator continued. "And all of a sudden here comes these two doctors who not only listen to them but give them credibility. They give a label to their disease. They do a test and say, 'You've got this.' And the doctors like doing it, and the patients like hearing it. And so it's a collusion.

"In a sense, there's always a collusion between patient and doctor," Kaplan added. "And it looked like these doctors had good relationships with their patients. A lot of doctors in private practice tell patients what they want to hear. So it's not unique to Lake Tahoe; it happens everywhere. It's just that what was going on there was a little different. They were perhaps doing it on a level that I hadn't quite imagined before."

Kaplan's cynicism can be attributed in part to his training. In epidemiology, the phenomenon of self-perceived, self-reported illness is considered a danger to the impartiality of any study. A patient who says, "I have cancer," is not tallied as a cancer victim until the radiologist finds the tumor on the X ray, the surgeon biopsies the tumor, and the pathologist determines the tumor to be malignant. The scientific method is undermined when the data are soft, and epidemiologists regard virtually all self-reported illness as soft. To Kaplan and Holmes, who knew little about the clinical manifestations of the ailment when they arrived, the Tahoe data seemed soft indeed. The patients Cheney and Peterson provided, in fact, merely confused them; nothing the investigators heard fit tidily any of the disease models with which they were familiar.

"Their symptoms were really quite different," Kaplan recalled. "With regard to the main thing—fatigue—some people had been laid out for months and months while others hadn't been as severe. That was the main symptom, but the other things that went along with it were incredibly varied. I mean, it wasn't like an epidemic of shigella [dysentery], where everybody comes in and they've got exactly the same thing. These people were coming in with very different stories. It wasn't as if everybody had fatigue, sore throat, and a cough. This patient might have fatigue, sore throat, and itchy feet and scratchy legs. And another patient might have fatigue that's only half as much, and a headache and can't fall asleep. All different things. And yet they were all coming in saying they had the same disease."

Holmes, too, was put off by the varied symptomatology reported by sufferers. "It was pretty apparent early on," he said, "that the illness just wasn't cut and dried. It wasn't simply that you could diagnose it."

"Gary was every bit as skeptical as I was," Kaplan confirmed. "Epidemiologically, I obviously had a few years' experience over him. But we had the same medical training. So I think we looked at those patients the same way."

For Kaplan and his neophyte partner, the Tahoe patients might as well have said, "I have cancer," without offering any hard proof. In fact, from Kaplan's point of view, it was even messier than that. It was as if they were insisting, "I have cancer," but neither they nor their doctors nor the CDC investigators knew for sure what cancer was.

That Kaplan and Holmes quickly lost their spirit for examining these perplexing patients whose symptoms seemed all over the map and whose complaints, to strangers, sounded suspiciously like the anxious ramblings of hypochondriacs or neurotics, is not surprising. Their task was to bring order out of chaos, quickly and without much support from their equally mystified colleagues in faraway Atlanta. One can sympathize with them even if, to Cheney and Peterson, their behavior seemed to evoke the stereotypical comic detective who pleads, "Don't confuse me with the facts."

Charles Darwin, upon hearing a giraffe described for the first time, reportedly said, "There cannot be such an animal." This was the first instance, but certainly not the last, that Cheney and Peterson were faced with similar incredulity. It had been Cheney's heartfelt contention that "all you have to do is talk to these patients to understand that they are different and that what they are describing is real." But he had miscalculated.

For the moment, it was just a rift among four troubled doctors in rural Nevada.

Despite the disappointment and perplexity that swiftly enveloped the investigators, there was no turning back. Somehow they had to come to grips with the spectacle confronting them, whether it was mass hysteria, a real epidemic, or, as Holmes would eventually characterize it, "two doctors isolated in a mountainous area who had worked themselves into a frenzy." Had the ailment been Rocky Mountain spotted fever or typhus or dengue fever or plague, they might have been more certain of their next move. Unfortunately the manual for the Tahoe malady had yet to be written.

As the senior epidemiologist, it fell upon Kaplan's shoulders to devise a means to elucidate the claims of two doctors and scores of patients along the lake's perimeter. "The big thing for me while I was there," Kaplan said, "was figuring out a way to systemize our observations so that we could end up with some kind of systematic conclusion. Eventually what I did was say, 'Let's pick some clinical definition to work with.' That was the trick. And that's what we worked on. What's the common denominator? Everybody says they're tired. Okay. Let's use tiredness as a definition. That was what we did with the case-control study, which ended up being about as nebulous as the whole situation out there to begin with," Kaplan said, sounding a bitter laugh.

Step one of Kaplan's plan was to characterize, by duration and severity, people's tiredness. How long had it lasted? How dramatically had it interfered with their lives? Kaplan decided to limit the inquiry to 149 patients for whom the clinicians had ordered EBV tests since January 1, 1985. The difficulty, again, was the variability of the symptoms even among the most severely tired people. That was where step two came into play: "We decided to try to define a group of severely fatigued patients with as homogeneous an illness as possible," explained Holmes.

After one week, however, and before either step had been initiated, Kaplan returned to Atlanta, leaving Holmes to implement his strategy. Kaplan's departure compelled his partner to abandon the luxurious Hyatt. "I moved into some little ski lodge–looking motel," Holmes said. "A couple of evenings I went to the casinos, just because they were there. There's not a whole lot else to do in that town at night. It was either that or sit in the motel and watch TV or work on the patients' charts." Culling patients who best seemed to fit the fatigue syndrome portrait, Holmes, assisted by Barbara Hunt, a nurse employed by the Washoe County health department, began to make a series of calls, taking phone numbers off the charts.

"It was a very simple questionnaire," Cheney recalled. "They got people to class their fatigue by asking, 'How many weeks were you out of work?' or 'How many weeks were you unable to function?' They devised a system of scoring the length and severity of the fatigue from one to four. And four was the most significant fatigue."

Three-quarters of the patients reported they had been fatigued for more than a month, although there were varying levels of ability to cope with work and responsibilities. Holmes placed thirty-one patients into a fourth class: people who had been fatigued for at least a month and absolutely disabled or bedridden by their fatigue for more than two weeks.

Kaplan's step one, characterizing the tiredness, had been achieved. Step two, culling a "homogeneous" group from among the class fours, was Holmes's next task. "The approach we had to take," he explained, "was that the syndrome was so nonspecific that we had to focus on people who had no other definable potential causes for their illness." Holmes methodically excluded every class four patient who appeared to have other medical problems, such as congestive heart failure, thyroid disease, persistent bacterial infections such as otitis media and sinusitis, unspecified colitis, pneumococcal pneumonia, chronic low back pain, hypertension, and, as Holmes would report later in a letter describing his work to Nevada health officials, "similar diseases that might have explained their fatigue."

The investigator's decision to make such exclusions, prompted by his phone calls to Atlanta, was the second major perceptual breach to occur between the clinicians and the federal agency; it was a rupture that would persist for years. In the view of Doctors Cheney and Peterson, the simultaneous emergence with this chronic syndrome of heart, thyroid, respiratory, gastrointestinal, bacterial, and any number of other kinds of ailments was hardly coincidental. It was their precocious notion, based on their clinical observations and their knowledge of their patients' histories, that these manifestations of disease were features of the multisystem constellation of a single entity. To the investigators, however, whose clinical experience was limited, whose exposure to the Tahoe patients was negligible, and whose acquaintanceship with the entity in question was ephemeral, their exclusionary methods seemed the only reasonable way to yank sense from a bewildering universe of symptoms.

In the end, Holmes winnowed the number of patients who fit his retooled, impromptu case definition of the ailment down to fifteen people, from the clinicians' roster of over 150. The mean age of the now-tiny group was 37.5 years; thirteen were women; all were white. One of them was Julie Pritchard. Neither Kaplan nor Holmes had met or examined even a majority of the fifteen.

Much later Holmes would defend his decision. "What else could we *do*?" he inquired in his liquid Texas dialect, his voice rising. "*They* were wanting us to go out and do this thorough investigation of everybody that *they* thought had the disease. And it would have yielded no useful information whatsoever. Because there was such a mixed bag of stuff going on. That's not the way you do research. That's the old garbage in, garbage out, basically. You can't get good data if you don't have a well-defined group to start with."

Before returning to Atlanta, Holmes, at the suggestion of his superiors, declared he needed thirty controls—two for each of the fifteen cases. In an eleventh-hour effort, he enrolled Alder Street office employees, including lab technicians in the basement, and a number of patients who came through the doctors' offices with minor complaints, into his control group. His only requirement for his controls was that they had never had their Epstein-Barr virus antibody levels tested. His logic was straightforward: if they had so far avoided the test in this hotbed of EBV testing, they were unlikely to have the syndrome. Sadly, as Peterson and Cheney would discover only a year later, the Texan erred, and fatigue patients were unwittingly conscripted into the control group.

Holmes's final moments before departing were devoted to obtaining blood from the people he had deemed to be bona fide cases. "After Kaplan left, they had a phone discussion, and it was decided to bring blood back," Cheney remembered. "This was not something they thought about early or even in the middle of this thing. Gary almost missed his airplane trying to get blood to bring back."

Cheney held in his mind for years a picture of the investigator's frantic moments before leaving Incline. The doctor watched, oddly mesmerized, as the basketball player–sized Holmes struggled with desperate ferocity to cram several plastic tubes of blood drawn from his fifteen cases into a Styrofoam box lined with vaporous dry ice. "Gary was trying to get down the hill to Reno," Cheney said. "I remember the top wouldn't fit, and he was madly pushing it down."

Clearly, the young Epidemic Intelligence Service officer had seen enough of Tahoe.

Key West, Florida

Days after Holmes and Kaplan headed for the High Sierras, a second team of novice epidemiologists left Georgia for an equally exotic setting: the Florida Keys. Chad Helmick and Matthew Zack were luckier than their westward-bound EIS colleagues: the disease their superiors in the Division of Chronic Disease Control had instructed them to track was hardly the mysterious entity without a name that investigators faced in Tahoe. Their mission was to determine whether there had been an epidemic of multiple sclerosis in Key West and nearby islands.

Helmick and Zack arrived at the southernmost point of the continental United States eight years after the surge of multiple sclerosis cases began. The federal government's delay could be attributed, in part, to foot-dragging by the Florida state health department. Like many states, Florida had long ago decreed that federal epidemiologists would be invited to disease outbreaks only after a state investigation had been performed. Although the outbreak was reported to state officials in 1977, the state had refused to investigate until early 1985, when a series of articles about the outbreak ran in the *Miami Herald.* By then, according to Miami neurologist William Sheremata, the multiple sclerosis victims were so angry that not a single one of them authorized their doctors to release their medical records to the state investigators.

One can easily imagine the institutional inertia that might attend a request to investigate an alleged epidemic of multiple sclerosis in one of the country's most popular vacation meccas. Key West in 1985 boasted just 26,000 residents, but the tourist influx each year was more than a million.

The very week Helmick and Zack launched their on-site cluster investigation, Miami neurologist Sheremata's observations about the outbreak were published in a letter to the British medical journal *Lancet.* Sheremata's letter was headlined, rather awkwardly, "Unusual Occurrence on a Tropical Island of Multiple Sclerosis."[3] The doctor reported that the rate of multiple sclerosis in the Keys approached that of the Shetland Islands, where the incidence of multiple sclerosis is among the highest in the world.* The doctor was keenly impressed by the suggestion of contagion manifest by the time-space clustering of the epidemic as well as by the preponderance of nurses among the victims. Nine of the thirty-seven multiple sclerosis patients were nurses. Like doctors, they are exposed to many diseases and, presumably, infectious pathogens in the course of their work. These nurses, Sheremata pointed out, "had worked in the community. This observation," he concluded, "raises the question of exposure to a common infectious agent."

Privately, Sheremata had begun to wonder, in fact, if some of his patients were afflicted with an altogether different ailment, one that might mimic multiple sclerosis but had credentials as a bona fide infectious disease. He was thinking about tropical spastic paraparesis, a central nervous system disorder common to the tropics and the southern islands of Japan that has similarities to multiple sclerosis. Tropical spastic paraparesis was thought to be caused by a retrovirus called human T-cell lymphotrophic virus, type 1, so named because it was the first of three known human retroviruses to be discovered.†

Doctors have always found multiple sclerosis a tough disease to diagnose. There exists no single definitive test. The fact that doctors graduate cases from "possible" to "probable" to "definite" is one measure of the disease's diagnostic intricacies.[4] Multiple sclerosis waxes and wanes, with symptoms submerged during remissions lasting months and years. Many patients must wait for symptoms to worsen to receive a "definite," the AAA rating, as it were, of multiple sclerosis. Contrary to popular perception, symptoms fail to progress in the majority of sufferers, an ambivalent kindness that leaves them adrift in a limbo of medical ambiguity, often for a lifetime.

Exhibiting the singular logic of the modern clinician, Sheremata explained the problem: "I want to emphasize that the diagnostic criteria for MS are really quite clear," he said, "but there are *patients* in whom the diagnosis is not clear." Doctors, in other words, know very well how to diagnose disease; it is patients, with their confusing hodgepodge of symptoms and signs, who fail to cooperate.

Helmick and Zack undertook to graduate their cases in the prevailing fashion of the times: from possible all the way to definite. Over the next two years they would return to the Keys several times. "We tried to find all the possible MS patients," Helmick recalled some time later. "We came up with a list of fifty or sixty people, got their medical records, and decided for ourselves whether they had

---

*Interestingly, epidemics of multiple sclerosis have been reported only on islands. The Orkney Islands, off the northeast tip of Scotland, have the highest prevalence of MS of any island group. For nearly three decades the existence of high MS rates on islands has fueled speculation that the chronic neurological ailment is virally caused. By 1985 at least twelve different viruses had been under suspicion (Peter Newmark, "Multiple Sclerosis and Viruses," *Nature* 318 [Nov. 14, 1985]). The most intensely studied island epidemics have been in the Faroes in the North Atlantic between Scotland and Iceland, and on islands off the coast of Iceland. Both outbreaks were linked to the presence of British troops stationed on the islands during wartime (M. Sosa, A. Font De Mora et al., "Multiple Sclerosis on Islands," *Lancet* 1, no. 8543 May 23, 1987): 1199.

†Scientists had tentatively linked its cousin, human T-cell lymphotrophic virus, type 2, with a rare leukemia, or blood cancer, called hairy cell leukemia after the strange appearance of the blood cells of the victim. The third human retrovirus, formerly known as human T-cell lymphotrophic virus type 3, is HIV.

MS." The team never met any victims of the outbreak. "We didn't have the resources to examine the patients," Helmick said.

The epidemiologists ended up with thirty-three patients they considered to have probable or definite multiple sclerosis. They began making plans to publish their findings.

National Cancer Institute, Bethesda, Maryland

Retroviruses occupied a controversial niche in American science. For decades scientists thought they caused disease only in animals. The first known retrovirus, avian sarcoma virus, was found in a chicken in 1910. Its discoverer, veterinarian and microbiologist Peyton Rous, suffered the ridicule of his peers as a result of his claim that the bug actually caused a disease—a cancer of muscle, bone, and blood vessel tissues. Discouraged, Rous gave up retrovirology, and there was little activity in the field again until the 1950s, when scientists found that retroviruses caused tumors in lab mice and other animals. For some time such retroviruses were thought to be mere lab contaminants. Then, in 1960, a University of Glasgow scientist proved that a retrovirus caused disease in cats—feline leukemia— and that the virus could be transmitted among unrelated cats within households. Not until 1978, however, when scientists in Robert Gallo's government lab discovered the first known human retrovirus and proved that it caused T-cell leukemia, were retroviruses considered a factor in human disease. Gallo and his associates called the virus HTLV, for human T-cell lymphotrophic virus, since it used T-cells as its refuge in the body. In 1982, Gallo reported isolation of a second retrovirus, another T-cell germ he felt certain also caused leukemia, albeit a different kind: hairy-cell leukemia, a rare cancer named for the appearance of the afflicted cells.

"HTLV-two differs subtly in form and function from its viral cousin, and is associated with less aggressive T-cell leukemias," Gallo wrote of the find some years later, adding, "In the most significant ways, however, the two viruses are quite similar. . . . They show the same capacity for transforming cells in culture."[5]

Retroviruses derived their name from their ingenious method of replication. Throughout most of nature, genetic information in cells flows from DNA to RNA. In turn, RNA stimulates cell proteins, in effect telling the protein molecules how to carry out their functions. For decades, scientists believed genetic information flowed in only one direction. This certainty was in fact, as Gallo himself wrote, the "central dogma" of molecular biology.[6] The discovery of retroviruses transfigured that dogma. In a retrovirus, genetic material is harbored in RNA rather than DNA, and the flow of genetic instructions is reversed. The virus is aided in its curious feat by an enzyme, "reverse transcriptase," which uses the virus's RNA as a template to make DNA. The DNA then inserts itself into the host cell's chromosomes, where it begins replicating. It was the virus's ability to lodge itself in the genetic material of the host's cells that resulted in diseases which were, if not terminal, certainly chronic.

In 1987 Japanese researchers proved that HTLV, type 1, was strongly associated with, if not the cause of, tropical spastic paraparesis. In the Caribbean islands, where 3 to 5 percent of all blacks were infected with the virus, the disease was not uncommon.* As Miami neurologist William Sheremata and other brain specialists knew, tropical spastic paraparesis had much in common with multiple sclerosis, a fact that made the Wistar finding of HTLV, type 1, antibodies in multiple sclerosis patients that much more intriguing.

By 1985, Gallo and others had begun to suspect that both HTLVs, type 1 and type 2, caused myriad other neurological and immunological diseases, although they could not yet name them. Writing in *Scientific American* in 1987, Robert Gallo noted that HTLV, type 1, was "the direct cause of T-cell malignancies in adults" and was also associated with tropical spastic paraparesis, "a neurological disease resembling chronic multiple sclerosis." He further proposed that HTLV, type 1–infected T-cells might also contribute to the development of leukemia in another immune system cell: the B-cell. In addition, he continued, "HTLV, type 1, may be an indirect contributing factor in several other pathological conditions. . . . It seems clear that the overall impact of HTLV, type 1, on public health is just beginning to be recognized," he added. "The diseases caused by HTLV, type 1, and HTLV, type 2, are . . . relatively rare. This may not always be the case."[7]

Interestingly, although scientists have long recognized that retrovirus infections among animals are transmitted "casually," current scientific orthodoxy holds that human retroviruses can be transmitted only by means of inheritance, mother's milk, blood, or sexual intercourse.

---

*After discovering that the virus was endemic in parts of southern Japan, the Caribbean, and South America, some scientists hypothesized that HTLV, type 1, had originated in monkeys and been spread from Africa to the Americas via the slave trade. It arrived in Japan, their theory went, via Portuguese traders who stayed in the Caribbean islands on their way to Japan and brought with them slaves *and* monkeys. (Robert C. Gallo, "The First Human Retrovirus," *Scientific American* 225 [6] [Dec. 1986]: 95.

4

Rural Disasters

Yerington, Nevada

Yerington was a lackluster oasis sixty-five miles as the crow flies from Lake Tahoe, an arrangement of ranch-style houses, bungalows, coffee shops, gas stations, and the occasional fast-food enterprise. Lawns were unfenced; cars hunkered down on cinder blocks next to rusting swing sets. At the town's perimeter, desert stretched out in all directions, a lavender and sand-colored landscape interrupted by occasional mountainous outcroppings of rock. In large part, the town was populated by people without any particular occupation seeking a quiet, inexpensive life in the desert. They included California retirees and younger people who had threaded into Yerington over the years, attracted by low taxes, vastly deflated property values, dry, steady weather, and something of which other little towns in the Mason Valley were unable to boast: a hospital. The remote, folksy institution served a spectrum of humanity scattered across a large region. Although the population of Yerington was just under 2,000, with another 1,000 farmers and ranchers inhabiting its outlying regions, the hospital drew its patients from the population base of the valley, which was five times larger.

Until 1979, when the nearby Anaconda Copper Mine closed, mining had been the vital spark of Yerington's economy. Its operators abandoned the mine when the price of copper dropped, and many miners moved to Elko or Eureka where gold was booming. By 1985, the year James and Vicki Dunlap's son, Jimmy, turned twelve, Yerington had been returned to its agrarian underpinnings, specifically the raising of cows and the cultivation of potatoes, alfalfa, garlic, and onions.

The Dunlaps were California natives who had moved to Yerington twelve years earlier, months after their only child was born. James Senior was a core driller; he performed expiration drilling in the desert at the behest of geologists whose calculations suggested there was silver or gold at points beneath the surface. As he grew, Jimmy Dunlap usually begged to go hiking with his father in the mountains outside town on weekends and holidays. During the summer of 1985, however, two months before he was to enter eighth grade, Jimmy's characteristic enthusiasm for mountain hiking suddenly dwindled. He complained of being tired all the time. His mother hoped the boy's malaise would dissipate with the activity and excitement of a new school year, but her hopes were not borne out.

"After school started that fall," Vicki Dunlap said some years afterward, "the school would call me within half an hour just about every day—Jimmy was sick; he had to come home."

After weeks of this routine, Vicki Dunlap became exasperated. She threatened her son, demanding that he stay in school each day to the end of classes. "I didn't understand what was happening," she said. "So he *tried* to stay at school all day. And that was when he got *really* sick."

As the Dunlaps eventually learned from their doctor, family practitioner Judy Hilbisch, one of three such practitioners in town, their son wasn't the only person in Yerington with a chronic health problem that fall. It seemed to Hilbisch that an epidemic of infectious mononucleosis had struck her town, although she knew such an event defied conventional medical wisdom. In the annals of medicine, Hilbisch was aware, bona fide clusters of mono were exceedingly rare; some said nonexistent. Nevertheless, the doctor was unable to squeeze from her medical lexicon anything more apropos to describe the fast-moving illness. At first the problem seemed confined to a group of children attending a nursery school. By the end of the month a number of their parents were bedridden. Soon afterward a sizable portion of the members of a church group, adults and children, became ill. Then the malady spread to students at Yerington's middle school and high school. Two entire classes fell sick in the same two-week period. Over the next two months there were days when more than half the student body was absent. Faculty members were on sick leave as well.

Early that fall, Hilbisch and the other doctors in Yerington, general practitioners Robin Titus and William Mayhew, began to confer on the outbreak. They learned that each of them had scores of patients with similar complaints. In addition to the obvious clusters in the schools and churches, the affliction had spread to bank employees, restaurant workers, and several of the staff of the Lyon County Courthouse. Common to these professions, the doctors observed, was a tendency to interact with the public.

Doctors Hilbisch and Titus began sending blood from their ailing patients to the hospital's diagnostic laboratory for the monospot test. It was a cheap and easy test for mononucleosis, though it lacked the specificity of the more sophisticated Epstein-Barr virus antibody panel. Jim Rathbun, an affable, slight-of-build man in his thirties, was one of the hospital's laboratory technicians. Eventually he was also among the sick. Because Rathbun was responsible for processing the monospot tests local doctors began to request for their patients in early November, he personally handled hundreds of blood samples before he became ill that winter. Before the epidemic subsided the following spring, his lab had processed a total of 487 blood tests for mononucleosis. Nearly all the blood samples came from residents of Yerington; a smaller number were from ranchers and their families in outlying regions. "We were picking up weird stuff. The doctor would order a CBC [complete blood count], and the patient would have these unusual-looking lymphocytes," Rathbun said. "The docs started out making the diagnosis of mono, because that's what the tests showed, but it wasn't mono."

Certainly many symptoms were mono-like, but mono was hardly so contagious, nor was the age group hardest hit—adults—considered susceptible to mono. More significantly, the disease was longer-lasting and was more severe than any form of mono they had ever seen. In the following two months approximately one hundred more Yerington residents came down with the illness. Jimmy Dunlap, among others, was bedridden by Thanksgiving.

"He went numb in his legs, off and on," his mother recalled later. "It was a semi-paralysis. His coordination was *way* off. With that and the numbing in the legs, he would just fall down. And then he couldn't get up. It was scary. First he was up, then he was down. I would have to pick him up. He couldn't really walk anywhere. He also had severe unbearable headaches. And he would forget things really bad. He couldn't remember anything from one minute to the next."

Howard Penney, who taught physical education and wood shop at Yerington Intermediate School, began his eighteenth year as a teacher the fall Jimmy Dunlap fell ill. He also coached football, basketball, and track at Yerington High. During the autumns of 1984 and 1985, Penney had made numerous excursions with his teams to Lake Tahoe to play the school teams in Incline Village. Penney, in fact, had presided over a number of matches between the girls' high school basketball teams the year the outbreak of "mononucleosis" prematurely ended the Incline team's season in 1984.

Of all the children who suffered from the illness that fall, Penney would come to remember Dunlap best. "I had him in my P.E. class [when Dunlap became ill]," Penney said years afterward. "I feel guilty now, because I thought, Mono—it couldn't be *that* bad. Even so, I remember thinking, With my luck, I'll probably get it."

Penney fell sick with the disease a year after Dunlap.

Lyndonville, New York

For decades Orleans County had suffered the unhappy distinction of being, by every index, the poorest county in the state of New York. The region's economy centered around growing apples and raising dairy cattle, two endeavors that, despite their omnipresence, plunged a fair number of locals into bankruptcy each year. The tiny village of Lyndonville, population 1,200, bounded on its northernmost edge by Lake Ontario, was hardly immune to the county's economic vicissitudes. Few of its residents had ever been out of New York State, much less the Northeast; they regarded Buffalo and Rochester, fifty miles west and east of Lyndonville, respectively, as big cities. A great many inhabitants were tradespeople and blue-collar laborers; they worked on assembly lines at Fisher-Price in Medina, or at Eastman Kodak in Rochester, or they toiled in the chemical factories of Niagara Falls and Buffalo. Others were migrants who came up from the South each year to pick fruit; some of them stayed on at the end of the season. A substantial group in town survived on welfare, particularly when they couldn't find work performing day labor in the apple orchards or on the farms.

Virtually anyone in Lyndonville could claim a blood tie to a number of others. Certainly everyone knew everyone else. The poverty that hovered within the ramshackle houses and mobile homes at the edges of town was imperceptible along the village's stately main thoroughfare, however. Handsome brick Victorians graced by generous verandas lined the street, silent testaments to a grander era.

Jean Pollard and her husband Paul lived with their four daughters in a weathered Victorian with white trim and black shutters on Main Street. Their friends, Debbie and David Duncanson, lived around the corner on Maple Avenue. The Duncansons boasted eight children, all of whom seemed to overflow the tall yellow house, topped by a widow's walk, in which they lived. To the delight of both couples, their children had become fast friends over the years.

One Saturday afternoon in October, in the midst of the season's first snowfall, the eleven-year-old Pollard twins, Megan and Libby; their ten-year-old sister, Hannah; and five of the Duncanson children took sleds up to Dates' Hill, a short, steep incline next to the Central Trust bank at the corner of Maple and Main. At the end of an afternoon of sledding, they convened for cocoa with marshmallows in the Duncanson household. Like many in Lyndonville, the Duncansons drank raw goat's milk, a cheaper, local alternative to pasteurized milk and one that was deemed tastier. In the next several months virtually every child in both families fell ill with an inscrutable disease, which at times required their hospitalization and which in some cases resulted in failing one or more grades in school.

Much as a fissure in a dam or smoldering leaves on a forest floor can be overlooked, it was some time before the children, their parents, and their doctor understood the proportions of the calamity. Pediatrician David Bell, who had seen a multitude of sick children in his career, was impressed by the intensity of the affliction from its earliest stages, however.

"It looked like a fairly severe viral illness," the doctor remembered. "Clinically it was not mononucleosis, although some of the symptoms were similar." When tests for mono were uniformly negative, Bell recounted, "I did what every prudent pediatrician does: I tried to ignore it. That worked for about two weeks, but unfortunately these children remained sick. And the illness became, very clearly, something that was unusual."

The Harvard-educated doctor and his wife, Karen, who was the deputy director of health for the Monroe County Health Department in Rochester, lived in a farmhouse on the Lake Ontario shore. In 1976, David, whose pediatric subspecialties were chronic childhood diseases and children's behavioral disorders, had accepted a post as a clinical instructor of pediatrics at the University of Rochester's birth defects clinic. A year later he had quit and opened a small practice in a one-story, postage stamp–sized building with a peaked roof on Main Street in Lyndonville. (Three years later, when the ceiling collapsed on him and a patient whose wounded arm he was stitching, the doctor moved to better quarters around the corner; the doctor's old office became "Bob's Sub and Pizza Shop" after repairs.) "The whole academic environment was bearing down upon me," the doctor said some years later. "I just didn't want to deal with the undercutting and the worries about who's going to steal your research. And I didn't want to spend the rest of my life having ego fights with these cocky residents. So I said to hell with it all."

Of nearly twenty doctors in the vicinity of Lyndonville and Medina, a small upstate town thirty miles away, Bell was the only one willing to accept Medicaid as full payment for his services; his practice eventually also embraced every child in foster care in the region. At least one-third of the school-age population of Lyndonville were his patients, as were most of their parents. "I wanted a nice, quiet practice with very poor, very simple people," David Bell recalled. "And the area that we're in is as poor as it gets."

Karen was an infectious disease specialist who had spent her fellowship year at the University of Chicago; a first-rate clinician, she had diagnosed the first case of toxic shock in western Massachusetts.

Shortly after Thanksgiving, the Bells asked the Pollard and Duncanson families to come to David's clinic. The doctors grilled parents and children about the events of the past year, searching for some lead. Oddly, three of the nine children seemed to have escaped the disease that fall; the remaining siblings in both families were desperately ill.

"I went through a differential of about ten or twenty diseases they might have," Karen Bell remembered. "David and I talked about the possibility of everything from typhus to Rocky Mountain spotted fever."

Ultimately it was the October afternoon sledding party, and what the doctors came to call the "raw milk factor," that riveted their attention. Every child who was ill had consumed cocoa made from the same batch of unpasteurized goat's milk.

Karen began a mental inventory of milk-borne infections. Brucellosis, or undulant fever, was at the top of her long list; in the absence of antibiotics, the disease can persist for years. Brucellosis tests were uniformly negative, however. Two other diseases they investigated were Q fever and yersinia, the latter characterized by—as Karen Bell described it—"the runs." The Q fever postulate was dashed when tests yielded uniformly negative results. The Duncanson patriarch, David, although symptomless, was positive for yersinia, however. For the next month both doctors assumed the outbreak was yersinia.

On December 14, the three sickest children were hospitalized. The admitting diagnosis was yersinia. For two weeks the doctors infused the children with a powerful antibiotic, gentamicin; a second antibiotic, doxycycline, was to be swallowed. On day five all three children began to respond. They were released on Christmas Eve, their ordeal seeming to be over.

Incline Village, Nevada

It was unlikely, of course, that in a town of just under 6,000 a federal investigation of an epidemic should go unnoticed. What was remarkable was how long the Centers for Disease Control's presence on Alder Street had remained submerged. Gary Holmes was instinctively wary of publicity and had identified himself in telephone conversations with patients as an official from the Washoe County health department. "I did not want to make it known that we were doing a CDC investigation," he explained later. "You get the local newspapers and radio stations involved and all this stuff, and you can't get your work done."

Nevertheless, 134 patients had been interviewed by either Holmes or his nurse assistant and the news slipped out. The day before he left Incline Village, a banner headline in the local paper, "CDC Investigates Tahoe Mystery Disease," heralded the story. On October 11, soon after Holmes's return to Atlanta, a reporter for the *Sacramento Bee* picked up the ball with a piece titled "Mysterious Sickness Plagues North Tahoe." Holmes, now back at the "house," as the agency's headquarters were known to its employees, agreed to be interviewed by the *Bee,* and that story was scooped up and sent out on the Associated Press's national wire.

"The symptoms . . . are similar to mononucleosis," wrote its author, reporter Chris Bowman. "But Holmes, who just returned from a three-week study of the situation at Incline Village, said, 'There is little evidence that mono occurs in outbreaks. It is pretty unlikely that this many people had mononucleosis.' "

In his first public criticism of the doctors, Holmes also told the *Bee* reporter that Peterson and Cheney "were making more out of a test than probably should be done. It is such a new test that nobody knows the true value of it." Of course, it was Gary Holmes and his agency colleagues who were uncertain of the Epstein-Barr virus panel's value. Virologists like Gertrude and Werner Henle, the clinicians' scientific consultants, viewed the test as a sensitive measure of both viral activity and immune system health. Holmes also told the *Bee* writer that he had found "no evidence" to indicate the putative mystery disease was "highly contagious" and that the patients he had interviewed had "little or no contact" with other patients. That last was, as Cheney would later complain, "patently untrue."

The following day the *Reno Gazette-Journal* carried the story with an article headlined "Health Officials Dismiss Mystery Disease at Incline." Its lead: "A national public health agency's investigation has turned up no evidence of infectious mononucleosis at Incline Village, despite a rise in the number of reported cases." In the second paragraph, Washoe County's Michael Ford hewed to the opinion he had held for months. "The bottom line is there's no problem as far as we're concerned," he said.

Television reporters, too, interviewed Ford. Filmed in his office at the health department's four-story edifice in downtown Reno, Ford again assured journalists there was "no problem" with mononucleosis or anything else at Incline Village. Ford's comments were broadcast on the six o'clock and eleven o'clock news programs in Reno.

Dismissive comments clearly intended to calm fears had the opposite effect. Cheney and Peterson were deluged with requests for interviews from Bay Area reporters, all of whom were suspicious the Tahoe malady was AIDS. The rumor proved to be pervasive. Canada's Olympic ski team, for example, promptly canceled their two-week Christmas meet in Incline Village. "The ski team is highly active, in more ways than one," said a Canadian doctor who worked for the team. "They didn't want to take any chances."

However much county officials tried to deflate the story, locals swiftly grasped the potential economic downside of revelations that their town was the epicenter of a contagious, disabling illness. As one journalist later observed, word of the baffling outbreak was received in Incline "about as cheerfully as might have been, say, a great white shark attack." Members of the local convention bureau, which financed an 800 number for out-of-towners seeking to reserve rooms, grew edgy as callers tied up the line for hours each day with unanswerable queries about the Tahoe malady. Tourists inquiring about the mystery flu called realtors, too. Just how many Tahoe visitors canceled reservations that winter for fear of catching the mystery flu is a hotly contested issue in Incline Village, even today. When asked, even the most alarmist citizens are unable to provide anything beyond an anecdote or two, usually from secondhand or thirdhand sources, about a realtor who claimed to have lost a condo booking due to fear of contagion. Still, rumors of cancellations reverberated like thunderclaps through the tourist-linked business people in town.

While her boss, Michael Ford, was reassuring locals, Washoe County nurse Barbara Hunt was fending off the inquiries of a multitude of out-of-towners. "Anybody who was the least bit fatigued would call up and say, 'Oh, my God, have I got this disease?' " Hunt said. "People were calling from Los Angeles, even as far away as Connecticut, saying, 'I was in Incline a year and a half ago for two days. Do I have to worry about getting this disease?' Travel agents and people who were running tours would call and ask, 'Are we going to get sued if [clients] get sick?' "

Hunt recalled another class of caller, too. "There were these other people who really *were* sick with something," she continued. "They would say, 'I've been sick for a long time, and I was in Incline a year ago'—or six months ago, or whatever. 'My doc doesn't know what I've got, and he's run a bunch of tests. What tests should he do to see if I have this?' " Having been assured by Holmes that the Epstein-Barr virus test was "too new to be valuable," Hunt could offer little practical advice to such callers. Even so, sick people continued to call Washoe County for some time.

Cheney and Peterson, preoccupied by their ailing patients and their disillusionment with the Centers for Disease Control, were blissfully unaware of the consternation the news coverage was creating among Incline's hoteliers and realtors. But the doctors, too, were disturbed by the coverage. At best, it was uninformed; at worst, by relying on a version of reality proffered by the government's Gary Holmes, it cast them as bumblers and hysterics.

"It was a difficult time, one of the most difficult of all," Cheney said. "Because it was hard for *us* to explain it. And these reporters, who were after a quick story and some headlines that grab you, would somehow always get it wrong. No matter what I said or how carefully I said it, they would *always* get it wrong. And every time they got it wrong, they made me look like, and certainly feel like, an idiot. So the frustrations—I felt very defensive."

Holmes, whose experience had hardly prepared him to be at the center of such intense journalistic inquiry, was feeling equally under siege. But he had clearly acquired, in his short tenure, the federal bureaucrat's knack for soft-pedaling potentially disastrous news: "The newspapers were talking about it being a widespread epidemic. And I said, 'There isn't any evidence that it's a widespread disease.' I was basically telling the truth, as far as I could say it," Holmes recalled later. "The curve of patients that we felt were the best patients [was] in May. This was in September. So the disease appeared to be decreasing, if anything. I never expected it to be such a big to-do in the press," he added. "I never actually considered that I was undermining [Cheney and Peterson]."

Cheney and Peterson soon perceived, worst of all, that rather than clarifying what they believed were pressing public health issues of portent to the entire nation, the federal investigation had merely obfuscated them.

On Monday, October 14, Cheney appealed to his partner to take action. "There were so many misstatements flying around," he remembered. "I said, 'Dan, with all this innuendo being published, we're going to have to do something. We're going to have to set the record straight.' " It was Cheney's idea to hold a news conference. Peterson, who dreaded public speaking and whose faith in the press to be either fair or accurate was scant, reluctantly assented. On October 15, before a gathering of journalists in a conference room at the local Hyatt, the doctors gamely sought to illuminate the medical perplexities with which they had grappled privately for nearly a year.

"I was struggling mightily with how to describe this thing," Cheney remembered. "There were no words, there were no references to point to, except the few we had, such as the Jones and Straus articles and the opinions of some experts, like Werner Henle, who I felt knew *far* more than the CDC."

After the press conference, the doctors believed they had cleared the air at last. But they had seriously miscalculated. As a result of the press conference, the existence and implications of the Tahoe flu ceased to be a subterranean debate among medical intellectuals. The disease entered the public domain and became, to the horror of the town's merchant class, part of the topography of Incline Village. It was a subject upon which everyone might have an opinion, however uninformed, including the board members of the local chamber of commerce, convention bureau, and resort association and any number of private citizens with an economic stake in tourism. If sympathy was evinced in any quarter for citizens who might have been suffering from a severe, apparently incurable illness, it—like room cancellations and lost sales—was difficult to track. One unnamed victim of the disease would tell a journalist in 1987, "Nobody wanted to hear that you were sick. If they believed you, they didn't want to get near you. And if they didn't, they said you were ruining the economy."

For the internists, a long, meandering attack on their clinical acumen by other doctors in the local press was the realization of a long-dreaded scenario: being dragged into public confrontation with their colleagues over medical issues more appropriate to hospital grand rounds and scientific papers. Peterson's wife, Mary, at the end of her patience, told her husband she would leave him if he spoke to the press again; the doctor was more than happy to comply. For years to come, Peterson turned away the vast majority of reporters' requests for interviews, rarely, in fact, returning their phone calls. Cheney, by contrast, struggled patiently at every turn to explain the medical issues to journalists, with only occasional good effect.

Press coverage grew exponentially, bringing news of the Tahoe epidemic to the rest of the nation and, in time, the world. "It sort of crescendoed," Cheney remembered, "and within a number of days, we had phones ringing off the hook [with calls] from all over the place. TV reporters, radio stations—everything went wild."

Wildest of all was a tide of two hundred calls in three days from people claiming to have the disease described in news reports. Emotional pleas for help poured into the Alder Street switchboard from as far away as Florida, New York, and Canada. For those who had been suffering in isolation, particularly those who had been written off by their doctors and families as hypochondriacs or malingerers or lunatics, news of the Nevada outbreak crystallized the nature of their problem. An uncounted population of sufferers experienced the news as a powerful epiphany: they weren't crazy.

Centers for Disease Control, Atlanta, Georgia

One month after his return to Atlanta, Holmes drafted a three-page, single-spaced letter to George Reynolds, the epidemiologist for the state of Nevada. With his letter to Reynolds, the young Epidemic Intelligence Service officer laid the first brick in the foundation of what would become an intractable federal policy on the Nevada epidemic and, in turn, the disease. The investigator wrote Reynolds that there was no way the government could conclude whether or not there had been an epidemic of disabling fatigue at Tahoe. Holmes reported that since there had been no Epstein-Barr virus tests performed on patients in the Peterson-Cheney practice until 1985, it was impossible to know if there had been an upsurge in cases of the debilitating illness. After all, what if the problem had always existed, but the doctors simply failed to test for it? Hence, Holmes wrote, "We do not think we will be able to conclude whether an outbreak of excessive fatigue, or of chronic EBV infection, occurred in Incline in 1985."

He acknowledged that there appeared to have been a definite upsurge of cases in May compared to other months of that year, but "some patients," he wrote, "may have referred themselves to these physicians on the recommendations of friends who had similar symptoms, inducing a referral bias which might explain the peak."

That Cheney and Peterson likely would have noticed an upsurge of fatigue cases among their patients in 1984 as easily as in 1985, whether or not the technology to measure Epstein-Barr virus antibodies was available to them, seemed to be irrelevant to the agency. Without incontrovertible proof, or the "baseline data" the agency was now demanding, little the Nevada doctors said any longer carried weight.

If anything untoward had occurred in Nevada, Holmes cynically postulated to George Reynolds in a theory that would become deeply entrenched at the federal agency in Atlanta in the years ahead, it had been an epidemic of a *diagnosis*.

National Cancer Institute, Bethesda, Maryland

Having established that the mystery microbe in the cells of AIDS patients wasn't Epstein-Barr virus, Zaki Salahuddin knew his next step: to determine whether the virus was a variant of some other known herpesvirus or an entirely new organism. If it was the first, that would be interesting; if it was the second, that would be historic.

Salahuddin enlisted the molecular biologists at the National Cancer Institute to undertake a genetic mapping. They would look for genetic similarity, or homology, between Salahuddin's find and the rest of the herpes family members. If any part of the new organism's DNA strand "recognized" any part of another herpesvirus DNA strand, it was probable that Salahuddin's agent was a variant of that virus. To the astonishment of everyone involved, none of the known human herpesviruses recognized the new virus.

Dharam Ablashi and the other cellular biologists continued to play a crucial role even after the molecular scientists joined the investigation. Ablashi exposed Salahuddin's bug to antibodies from other herpesviruses. If the antibodies responded to it, there remained a high probability that the organism was a known quantity—or closely related to one. However, antibodies from each human herpesvirus failed to react to the novel virus.

When both groups had ruled out human herpesviruses, they turned to the animal kingdom. Perhaps an animal herpesvirus had jumped species. The virulence of the new agent in human cell cultures certainly hinted at that possibility, since, when viruses change host species, the resulting disease is far more severe in the aberrant host than in the traditional one; after all, the customary host population has enjoyed the benefit of thousands of years in which to adapt to the parasite.

It was logical to look to apes and monkeys first, since viruses, when they jump species, rarely go far; herpesviruses tend to be not only species-specific but even organ- and system-specific. With the lavish resources of the National Cancer Institute at their command, the scientists obtained blood from five chimpanzees, three gorillas, two orangutans, three baboons, two stump-tailed monkeys, nine rhesus monkeys, ten African green monkeys, ten squirrel monkeys, six owl monkeys, six common marmosets, and three cottontail marmosets. Antibodies from all fifty-nine animals failed to recognize their virus.

The team labored on, testing their virus against herpes antibodies from cattle, pigs, horses, cats, dogs, mice, rabbits, chickens, turkeys—even deer. They drew the line at frogs.

"We have tested every damn thing—every animal herpesvirus," Ablashi said some time later. "Even deer sera—the deer herpesvirus—we tested that one too!"

"We went from the exotic to the ridiculous," Salahuddin confirmed, adding, "We did the sublime first. The process, as you very well know, is that of elimination. As you do it, the virus gets newer and newer. You understand? It's not new to begin with. It only becomes new when you eliminate everything else, and then you say, 'Okay, there's a chance. And the chance of it being new is, say, two percent now.' You go in little stages, and things accumulate. Then you look at it and you say, 'All right, if there's nothing else that I can do with it, then it's a new thing, and now it's my responsibility to describe it'—which is a heck of a responsibility. That's a very disturbing part of science. As long as it is already done by someone else, it's an easy thing to do."

Eventually, Salahuddin recalled, "There came this day when we decided it was something new."

San Francisco, California

In July, Carol Jessop helped found a clinic dedicated to women's health problems in San Francisco. Healthworks for Women was located at the busy intersection of Post and Divisadero Streets and drew more than 500 patients weekly. Jessop contributed twenty hours of her time each week. Within a year, another 70 patients in

Jessop's new practice presented de novo with the syndrome she had identified in patients from her old clinic, bringing the total of people under her care with the ailment to 136.

Like Dan Peterson and Paul Cheney in Nevada, Jessop was increasingly persuaded there was a new infectious disease abroad. Unfortunately, her effort to interest the local scientist who was perhaps best qualified to undertake an investigation into the chronic malady had failed. Eighteen months before, after meeting a handful of such patients, Jessop had taken her medical mystery to Jay Levy, a microbiologist at the Cancer Research Institute of her university's medical school. Levy was reputed to be in the business of searching for new agents of disease. The scientist had been cordial, but he made it clear to the internist that he was on the trail of the agent of immune dysfunction causing the plague sweeping through gay men in San Francisco and could spare none of his time.

In the interim, however, government investigator Robert Gallo had announced his discovery of the human immunodeficiency virus. Levy, too, isolated HIV late in 1983, just months after the French team at the Pasteur Institute did so, though he received hardly any public kudos for his work. In order to accumulate proof that the virus was the true cause of AIDS rather than another opportunistic agent, Levy postponed publishing his find. As sometimes happens in scientific competitions, his caution went unrewarded: he was subsequently scooped by the French and by Robert Gallo's team in Bethesda.

That fall, a sympathetic colleague proposed to Jessop that Levy's disappointment might be turned to her advantage. Suggesting a meeting with the microbiologist, Jessop's colleague predicted Levy's recent ill fortune would predispose the microbe hunter to tackle something altogether new. The professor's intuition proved correct. A few days later Jessop arranged a meeting with Levy, an elfin, dapper man with an authoritative manner.

Levy's lab in the medical sciences building on Parnassus Hill was small, with a closet-sized office for Levy. In this private space, the scientist kept a portrait of Werner and Gertrude Henle, with whom Levy had trained as a young scientist. His working style was one of resolute independence if not autocracy. At any given time he rarely had more than one technician or postdoctoral fellow on the premises. Even so, by 1985 he was widely viewed as a major player in the AIDS research drama. Yet, in contrast to Robert Gallo, who had assumed an executive post as the administrator of a large team of federal researchers, Levy remained a solitary figure in his little lab with a loose cadre of outside collaborators, his intimate link with wet lab, or bench, research wholly intact. "Jay doesn't have very much patience for administration," one of his collaborators confirmed.

Levy found Jessop's description of her patients compelling. Further, he knew she was regarded as a rising star at the medical school, irrespective of her fascination with a disease most of her colleagues considered bogus; she taught several popular classes and was a favorite of the dean of medicine. Levy was most impressed, however, by her theory that the malady was a new infectious disease that hobbled the immune system in some way distinct from the immune disruption seen in AIDS. The promise of an unknown, possibly new infectious agent, in fact, was the glue that cemented Levy's commitment to the project. Ancillary issues relating to the disease, issues such as the gamut of its clinical manifestations or its social toll, bored him.

"I really don't care if it affects one person or a million," Levy admitted later. "The fact that there is a brand-new infectious disease is terribly exciting for someone who spends their life looking at infectious diseases . . . and I have been, from the very beginning, interested in attempting to find the virus that causes this disease. . . .

"Now, Carol said she had more women than men, and it seemed strange that AIDS was affecting mostly men, and we had chronic fatigue affecting mostly women. That seemed a queer, strange quirk of nature. But that was just an initial observation. Then I began realizing that what I had learned from the Henles about Epstein-Barr virus was probably true with this disease—that it wasn't just hitting women. The women were showing the symptoms, but *everyone* was being infected. Well, one of my interests is viruses and autoimmune diseases, and autoimmune disease primarily hits women. So I started putting it together and said, 'This could be a new virus.' "

Jessop agreed to send ten patients to Levy's lab. There he would draw their blood and begin his search for viruses new and old. To her dismay, however, Levy began to show signs of disgruntlement immediately upon meeting patients.

"When I started seeing [Jessop's] patients, I could understand why other doctors wouldn't believe it," Levy recalled. "People would say they were tired. Later they would say the fatigue had gone away, and even later they would be tired all over again. I said to Carol, 'I've got to find a way to separate the wheat from the chaff.' I was worried I was working up *normal* people, and that was simply too much effort."

The scientist's creeping incredulity graphically illustrated to Jessop the barriers to understanding the disease among researchers whose clinical skills were either poorly tuned or hampered by sexism. "Sexism," Jessop frequently said, "is the worst malpractice there is." She decided to send Levy a male patient who she believed had the syndrome.

"Jay saw ten women," the doctor recalled later. "And he thought they were all hysterical. Then he saw a man, whose complaints he took seriously."

Having met a male sufferer, the virologist persevered. He conscripted Evelyne Lennette, a herpes virologist in Berkeley who was one of Levy's AIDS collaborators. For the next several months, Levy and Lennette looked for a multitude of known viruses, as well as for cell death in cell cultures grown from patients' blood serum. (Cell death would suggest viral infection.) They financed the project with a few thousand dollars cribbed from Levy's AIDS grants from the state of California and the National Institutes of Health.

Wistar Institute, Philadelphia, Pennsylvania

Elaine DeFreitas felt under siege that November. On the first of the month, her paper—written in collaboration with Hilary Kaprowski and others—relating multiple sclerosis to a retrovirus had appeared in the British medical journal *Nature*.[1] It seemed as if all of the MS patients in the nation suddenly wanted her to test their blood for the microbe. Her desktop was papered with scores of pink telephone messages; her secretary stacked the scientist's mail each day in rows on DeFreitas's office floor.

DeFreitas was an immunologist by training. Her field was among the most erudite branches of biomedical investigation. For all the immune "boosting" schemes available in bookstores, the human immune system continued to so perplex researchers that it was widely viewed as the black box of medicine. DeFreitas was comfortable inside the Zen-like complexity of her work. "I am *not* a clinician," she took pains to emphasize. She spent her days scrutinizing cells rather than people, and like many bench researchers, she felt her preference deeply. In the sanctity of the lab, one held the emotional chaos of illness at bay; the wrenching, often tragic quandaries of the sick became intellectual puzzles requiring solutions. Now DeFreitas's delicate contract with disease was torn asunder.

Amid the deluge that November, one voice penetrated DeFreitas's defenses: that of Jake Lindsay (a pseudonym). A cardiologist–turned–medical investigator, Lindsay had been diagnosed with chronic mono by Denver researcher James Jones three years before. Lindsay's illness had left his busy group practice in the Pacific Northwest in shambles and forced his retirement. Just thirty-four at the time, the doctor provided neither his astonished colleagues nor his patients with an explanation; he had none to offer.

Since falling ill, he had developed an insatiable appetite for medical literature. Ensconced in his study, a comfortable room with floor-to-ceiling windows overlooking a wooded vista in suburban Indiana, Lindsay sat before his computer several hours every week. He was wired into the major medical literature search services via modem; without leaving this sanctum, he could call up citations for scientific articles on any topic, however obscure, from virtually any journal. With a keystroke, he was able to fill his screen with the text of any published study whose title caught his interest.

The ailing doctor proposed to DeFreitas that she explore the possibility that a retrovirus might also be at the heart of the new syndrome under investigation in Nevada.

"Jake started calling me and sending me all sorts of material," DeFreitas recalled. "I was overloaded just opening my mail, and his call came in the midst of this. He was very serious about us looking at this problem. But . . . it was a whole new disease! I remember I kept saying to the people in my lab, 'I can only take one disease at a time!'"

The immunologist was in possession of only the most rudimentary information about the affliction Lindsay described. "I knew that the research hadn't gone very far," DeFreitas recalled. "But I knew of about fifty other diseases, too, and that didn't mean I could work on them. I already had two people working for me on MS. And that was it—I was maxed out."

Nonetheless, Lindsay—and the ideas he proposed to DeFreitas about the possible relationship between retroviruses and this new malady—left an impression.

"I could see, just based on his letters, that he really knew the literature. I absolutely respected him," she said. "He would write, 'There are twenty-two articles about the possible role of a DNA virus reactivating a retrovirus,' for instance—and he would enclose all twenty-two reprints. This man had done his homework."

Ironically, Lindsay had learned of DeFreitas's multiple sclerosis findings not through his computer searches but through the mail. A former colleague had sent him the *Nature* report suggesting human T-cell retroviruses might play a causative role in MS.

Lindsay often had ruminated upon what he felt were striking similarities between the disease Jones and Straus were calling "chronic mono" and the vastly more familiar brain disorder. Many symptoms were comparable, among them extreme fatigue, muscle weakness, and vision and balance disorders. Another multiple sclerosis symptom, rarely discussed, was a variable degree of cognitive dysfunction, which seemed to draw the two ailments even closer together. Antibodies to Epstein-Barr virus frequently were elevated in multiple sclerosis patients, too. There were differences, however. Symptoms like aching muscles, painful joints, and migrating tingling sensations in limbs that were common in the Tahoe malady weren't typical of multiple sclerosis. Remissions, common in MS, were rare in chronic mono. Still, it seemed to Lindsay that the two ailments were kindred, not only symptomatically but epidemiologically: multiple sclerosis seemed to favor adults in their prime, usually from the middle and upper classes. The doctor pondered a third ironic affinity: although multiple sclerosis garners respect as a potentially fearsome, crippling ailment today, it was dubbed the "faker's disease" at the century's start when first described in medical journals. The disease gained credibility only in later decades when better tests hastened interpretation of its frequently confusing and inconclusive signs.

After reading the Wistar study, Lindsay began to wonder if the agent X in his own debilitating disease might be a retrovirus.

When DeFreitas indicated to him that she would be unable to follow up on his research suggestions, however, Lindsay put his retrovirus theory aside temporarily.

Incline Village, Nevada

When Cheney and Peterson scanned their patient files that fall, they discerned that approximately 20 percent of their patients claimed to have recovered from the disease. Another 50 percent were improving but had failed to recover entirely. The 20 to 30 percent who remained were, according to Cheney, "significantly impaired."

The social ramifications of the disease overwhelmed many patients in the latter categories. "It was ripping up people's jobs and relationships," recalled Chris Guthrie, who had been unemployed and nearly bedridden, unable to care for her child, for over a year. Somehow Guthrie's family remained intact, but she watched as the families of other victims disintegrated.

Apparently the disease was not fatal, since, so far, no one had actually expired, but that observation failed to cheer anyone. In their efforts to describe the actual sensation of the illness, patients frequently said they felt as if they had been poisoned or were experiencing something akin to radiation sickness. A perverse "good news–bad news" joke about the Tahoe malady began circulating. "The good news is, you're not going to die," it began. "The bad news is, you're not going to die." Behind the humor, pathos reigned. For many, the disease was so severe its impact was a kind of half-death, a paradoxical "dying but not dying," as

Cheney described it. Sufferers invoked the specter of death so regularly, in fact, it seemed to be an integral part of the sign-symptom complex.

"It was a theme I kept hearing: 'I think I'm dying.' So many patients said that—again and again," Cheney recalled.

Stephen Beale, an Episcopalian priest from Paradise, California, had been diagnosed with the disease that fall. Beale had been a lively participant in his community; in his adolescence he had been the state chairman of Teenage Youth for Reagan; his family knew Nelson Rockefeller and Barry Goldwater. In Paradise, he had a young thriving congregation. But when stricken at thirty-six, the man was physically devastated. The day Beale arrived in the Alder Street waiting room, the priest of Incline Village's Episcopalian church was waiting to see Cheney as well; the two men prayed together before their appointments.

Two years later Beale was still sick, frequently bedridden, and had been forced to cut down on the number of services he offered. During a phone conversation that fall from his California parsonage, a severely depressed Beale pondered the strange, ersatz lethality of the disease with a gloominess typical of most patients.

"We *apparently* don't have a life-threatening disease," he said, adding, "although I'm not sure. I'm reasonably certain that it may turn out to be far worse than it looks. But at least in the short term it doesn't look like it's a life-threatening disease—unless you think losing your job and your home and your family isn't too bad. Some people would rather die."

The Centers for Disease Control's visit polarized the tiny medical community and raised the ire of locals, but it did nothing at all to elucidate the mysteries of the disease. Cheney and Peterson were alone again, only now their adversaries were mobilized and vocal.

"It was in the midst of all this," Cheney said much later, "that some really important things began happening among the patients we were seeing. That fall, increasingly, the neurologic component of this illness began. I think some of it was always there, but somehow we just started seeing it in more striking examples. We started hearing more and more of 'I can't read,' 'I can't add,' 'I can't teach,' and 'I can't think.' Those were certainly the most common complaints. But on top of that, we had these very dramatic neurologic impairments."

Chris Guthrie had developed focal paresis—a weakness or numbness—in her left arm. In a drift test, during which both arms are raised in front of the torso to shoulder level, Guthrie's neuropathic arm slowly dropped from shoulder height until it hung at her side; the right arm held steady. This symptom, combined with other complaints such as blurred vision and a mild dementia, in which Guthrie's powers of memory and cognition seemed impaired, caused Cheney to wonder if the former meter reader had suffered a stroke. Balance problems and migraine headaches plagued Guthrie as well.

Dizziness was extremely common, as were depth-perception problems. Patients fell victim to what is described in neurology texts as the Alice in Wonderland syndrome, a disorder common to people with temporal lobe epilepsy. Spatial distortions characterize this syndrome; sufferers see objects as either smaller and farther away or larger and closer than they really are. Given these unusual symptoms, the doctors began to question the origin of the fatigue. Was it in the muscles, or was it central fatigue, originating in the neurotransmitters of the brain? Fatigue played a powerful role in multiple sclerosis, they knew; MS experts believed the symptom was rooted in the brain.

They wondered, too, about the significance of the phenomenon that algebra teacher Andy Antonucci called "brain rot." Initially, random complaints of confusion and intellectual debilitation had sounded immaterial in contrast to the general devastation of the disease. After all, what was absentmindedness compared to being suddenly too weak to stand or walk? As the illness ground on, however, its intellectual infirmities were becoming more problematic for patients.

Paul Thompson (a pseudonym), a patient of Cheney's, was a computer programmer who had made a fortune in that burgeoning industry after writing a best-selling software program. Soon afterward, the forty-three-year-old had moved to Incline Village and started his own business. Thompson acquired the Tahoe malady in May, at the epidemic's peak. He became excessively sensitive to cold and complained of visual disturbances. For months his temperature had hovered between one and two degrees below normal, and his EBNA (Epstein-Barr nuclear antigen) level was depressed enough to indicate that his immune system had lost its ability to control Epstein-Barr virus latency. His most startling symptoms weren't so much malaise and fatigue as they were alarming changes in his thinking ability. Thompson had always been proud of his 800 math score on the SATs. One day in early November, however, he drove from his house on Lakeshore Drive to the 7-Eleven on Tahoe Boulevard, the main thoroughfare, a near-straight shot of less than a mile. Once inside, he forgot why he had come; he returned to his car empty-handed. Nothing to get upset about, Thompson told himself. His composure ebbed, however, when he realized he was lost in the center of a town with two traffic lights. The computer prodigy sat for several minutes gripping the steering wheel, trying to remember where he lived and how to get there. Eventually he returned to the store and asked the clerk for directions. On another occasion he took his family camping in the desert. When a friendly camper asked him where he was from, Thompson drew a blank. He tried mentally re-creating the map he had followed to the campsite, hoping that if he could retrace his path he would arrive at the name of his town on the map. Before he could work it out, Thompson's young children, incredulous at their dad's inexplicable silence, blurted, "Incline Village!"

"My logic skills had been outstanding," Thompson said later. "But now everything was getting zapped."

Neurologists called such episodes "jamais vu," translated from the French as "never seen"; they were the opposite of the more universal phenomenon known as déjà vu.

Stories like Thompson's were increasingly common within the Alder Street examining rooms. Parents forgot their children's names; secretaries were unable to commit seven-digit numbers to memory long enough to dial; certified public accountants could no longer add columns of figures. Driving on the wrong side of the road was not unusual. Many patients experienced frequent periods of transient amnesia, losing track of their surroundings and thoughts for several minutes. The doctors speculated that the blackouts might be the result of petit mal seizures. Yet while memory problems were legion, there were other, stranger symptoms.

"Some people were not so much severely affected as unusually affected," Cheney remembered. "They had problems with processing sensory information . . . they might come up to a green light and not know whether it meant stop or go. We heard some very interesting stories," he continued, "such as people trying to read a book, and rather than, as is normal, focusing on one line and reading across while x-ing out the other lines in the periphery, these people would instead see *all* lines. It was as if they could not process visual information. They couldn't calm down and process what they needed to process, and avoid processing what they didn't need to process."

Patients were experiencing dyslexia as well: they transposed letters when they wrote; they misread words on the page; they even transposed words when they spoke. Nor could they always find words appropriate to their sentence. The word-finding problem noted by the doctors was hardly the simple aphasia that claims everyone on occasion. Peterson described a typical patient: "They will say, 'I went skiing and I hit a—hit a—you know—that thing that grows by the side of the slope?' I say, 'Tree?' They say, 'Yeah, a tree.' "

It was becoming evident that the disease's ability to befuddle and bewilder was among its most devastating properties. One patient who had been fired from her job and divorced by her husband during the course of her illness wrote Cheney, "Of all the things I've lost, I miss my mind the most."

Another striking aspect of the disease was the periodically suicidal depressions patients experienced. This seemed to be fundamental to the illness. In fact, the doctors found it difficult to sort out depression that was biochemical and linked inextricably to the disease process from that caused by the disastrous social consequences of the illness. An emergency room physician in Reno killed himself that fall with a shotgun. Throughout the two years of his illness, his colleagues in Reno had accused him of malingering. It was the first suicide the doctors had heard of, but there would be many, many more in the years ahead.

Depression is a frequent companion of many chronic neurological diseases, including multiple sclerosis, Alzheimer's, and Parkinsonism. Neurologists believe this symptom derives at least in part from brain damage that occurs as those diseases progress. Patients recovering from head trauma also experience profound depression. For decades, doctors had assumed the depression was the patients' emotional response to the trauma. More recently, doctors have come to believe it is the brain injuries themselves that give rise to depression. There are a number of infectious and chronic diseases, too, without any outstanding brain linkage, that are known to cause depression. Liver disease is one; pancreatic cancer is frequently preceded by approximately six months of mild to severe psychiatric disturbances, including depression. On the other hand, virtually any illness is marked by a "psychological overlay," to borrow from the medical idiom, of depression, anxiety, and other emotional states having to do entirely with the patients' response to their condition.

A final layer of complexity facing the clinicians was the fact that depression, no matter what its source, typically induces a dulling of intellectual capabilities, including impaired concentration. Somehow they needed to find tools to help them distinguish between cognitive impairment due to depression and that due to brain damage. As with many of the most significant discoveries in science, a clue to all of these perplexities presented itself serendipitously—in the form of a coltish blue-eyed twelve-year-old with a passion for ballet.

Shortly after Thanksgiving, Cheney received a call from Mary Hawkins, a wealthy born-again Christian whose daughter, Katie, was in seventh grade in Incline Middle School. Hawkins sounded desperate. As Cheney listened, she described the previous several days in her daughter's life.

Two weeks earlier, on the drive over the mountains to Reno, Katie had experienced what her mother suspected was "some sort of an inner-ear or equilibrium problem." Consequently Hawkins had taken her daughter to see an ear, nose, and throat specialist in Reno. The doctor dismissed the child's complaints as "nothing," according to Hawkins. Assuming the doctor was correct, Hawkins took her daughter home.

For the next three days Katie stayed home from school with severe headaches and an intensely painful sore throat. The child, a lissome girl with chestnut hair, could still remember the torment of those headaches three years later when she was interviewed. "I felt like a hammer was smashing in my head," she said. A day or two after the headaches and sore throat began, she developed a new symptom: "I got dizzy, and my speech got blurred." Most frighteningly, when she tried to stand, she fell over.

After five days of these symptoms, Katie awoke on a Saturday morning and insisted she was well enough to attend her dance class. She was a bright, sweet-tempered student, but she lived for ballet. Her devotion to dance had won her the prima ballerina role in her dance school's Christmas recital. She told her mother she could not afford to miss a rehearsal so close to her star performance.

Katie's sore throat and headache were gone by that Saturday, Hawkins told Cheney, but it was soon apparent something else was terribly wrong. Not long after depositing her daughter at dance class, Hawkins got a call from Katie's ballet master. He told her Katie was unable to stand on one foot without toppling over. By Sunday the child was unable to keep her balance even on two feet.

Embarrassment entered Hawkins's voice as she told Cheney her next move, which was to take her child to a chiropractor.

"It was just on my mind that there was something out of *balance* with her," Hawkins said.

Katie had attributed her inability to walk to dizziness, but her mother noticed that one side of the girl's body had become ungainly and uncoordinated whereas the other side seemed unaffected. The child's speech was slurred again, too. On closer examination, Hawkins realized in a moment of suppressed horror that the slurring was a result of what appeared to be paralysis on the right side of her daughter's face. After examining Katie, the chiropractor told her mother that the child's problem was "out of his realm." The following day Hawkins returned her daughter to the Reno ear, nose, and throat specialist. The specialist proposed that Katie be seen by a neurologist immediately.

Within an hour the seventh grader underwent her second exam of the day, this time in a neurologist's office. "I'm afraid there might be a tumor," the neurologist told Mary Hawkins when they were out of Katie's hearing range. No doubt confused by Hawkins's beatific expression, the specialist struggled to impress upon Hawkins the fact that her daughter's entire right side had failed to respond to stimulus. "She's a gift from God," Hawkins remembered telling the doctor. "She's in the Lord's hands." The neurologist conveyed his admiration for the depth of Hawkins's faith, after which he made arrangements for her daughter to undergo a CT brain scan. The next morning, Hawkins learned that her daughter's brain was tumor-free. The tentative diagnosis was encephalitis, a brain inflammation that can occur as a result of viral or bacterial infection.

The neurologist sought permission to perform a spinal tap to determine the extent of the brain swelling, but Hawkins refused. She was against invasive procedures, particularly since the doctor had explained there was no treatment available for Katie's condition. She signed her daughter out of the hospital and took her back to their luxurious house on Country Club Drive in Incline Village, where she put Katie to bed.

Hawkins was aware that Paul Cheney and Dan Peterson had been investigating some kind of viral outbreak in town. But, she recalled years later, "there was this criticism of Dr. Cheney that once he gets hold of you, he'll find the [Epstein-Barr] virus. I thought, I don't *want* to find the virus."

In the end, Hawkins's impulse to consult Cheney won out.

"Would you mind if I examined her?" Cheney asked when Hawkins came to the end of her story.

The doctor was impressed by the child's degree of mental deterioration. She was suffering from pronounced neurological abnormalities, including cerebellar ataxia, a clumsiness of deliberate movements, including walking and talking. The doctor hospitalized her that night under quarantine in the intensive care unit at Lakeside Hospital. He ordered an electroencephalogram, which indicated the child was in danger of suffering seizures. Late that night Mary Hawkins finally sanctioned a spinal tap on her daughter. There was significant pressure upon opening, indicating a substantial degree of brain swelling.

For months the doctor and his partner had been central witnesses to an epidemic of an apparent viral disease striking adults and, more rarely, adolescents. They noted that once the most acute flu-like symptoms subsided, more disturbing complaints arose—an inability to see properly, to speak normally, to remember, to comprehend. There had to be a neurological component to the illness, Cheney reasoned; there had to be brain involvement. Could this child be another victim of the epidemic, albeit in more acute form?

After performing the spinal tap, Cheney drew a small tube of Katie's blood for an Epstein-Barr virus antibody profile. He arranged for a third diagnostic test to be performed at the University of California medical center in San Francisco: a magnetic resonance imaging (MRI) scan of Katie's brain.

MRI scanning was then in its infancy; the technology had become available only the year before with Food and Drug Administration approval. Nevertheless, MRI was the most sensitive imaging technology available, light-years ahead of CT scanning, which in turn had been light-years ahead of the X ray. The machine was capable of creating a magnetic field 60,000 times more powerful than the earth's. During the test, the magnetic field was switched on and off, agitating the nuclei of hydrogen atoms in the body. The scanner's computer noted the tiny electrical pulses in these atoms and used them to create a picture. Different water densities in organs allowed the machine to distinguish shapes and structures with startling clarity. MRI's earliest contribution came in the field of multiple sclerosis. The machines revealed for the first time lesions, or plaques, in the brain that today are synonymous with the disease. One multiple sclerosis patient had spent eighteen years in a mental institution with a diagnosis of schizophrenia until an MRI scan of her brain clarified her problem. MRI's pictures of the brain were exquisite, and the technology was rapidly becoming the modality of choice for central nervous system imaging. Unfortunately the machine's $2 million price tag in 1985 ensured that only the largest medical centers in the country could afford one.

Early on Wednesday the Hawkinses made the four-hour drive to San Francisco. The university's lone MRI scanner was housed in the former Fireman's Fund building on California Street. Katie was asked to don a shower cap before being fitted into the cavity of the machine. She was told to lie stock-still. Forty minutes later, having survived the nearly deafening clanging sounds emitted by the coils of supercooled electromagnets inside the unit—the technicians had forgotten to supply her with the earplugs that are customarily mandated—she was liberated.

The pictures arrived in Cheney's office several days later. Katie's left temporal lobe was dotted with several white, pencil-point–sized perforations. Cheney was puzzled, but he quickly learned that the experts in San Francisco were equally perplexed. The neuroradiologist described them alternately in his report as "T2-weighted high-intensity lesions" and "punctate lesions"; the word "punctate" denoting their pencil-point size. In conversation with Cheney, he used the colloquial term UBOs, for "unidentified bright objects." No one knew, apparently, whether UBOs were related to an infectious agent or even a disease process. They had never been seen before the advent of MRI scanning. Since the new technology had been in use, UBOs had been observed almost exclusively in the brains of sixty- and seventy-year-olds and then only rarely, in 2 to 3 percent of all scans. Some people speculated that UBOs might be associated with aging, the neuroradiologist said; perhaps they accounted for memory loss among the elderly. Without question, their appearance in a twelve-year-old was unusual.

Cheney asked Katie's parents to come to his office. There he showed them an array of six-inch negatives—images of their daughter's brain. He aimed the pictures near the ceiling lights and, with his forefinger, directed the Hawkinses' gaze to the small white spots. Damage on the left side made sense, Cheney told the stunned couple, since it was Katie's right side that had been affected. What else was implied by these lesions, the doctor continued, he was unable to say with any authority.

The following day, Cheney obtained the results of Katie's Epstein-Barr virus panel. The pattern of antibodies, in general, indicated she was experiencing a reactivation of the virus rather than a first-time infection. She had, in other words, the curious antibody profile unique to the practice's epidemic patients and other victims of immune dysfunction.

The second finding set off a bomb in Cheney's consciousness. Although he was uncertain precisely what Katie Hawkins's illness represented, he found the drift sinister. His own daughter, another twelve-year-old named Kate, was a student at Incline Middle School, too. What if the epidemic was spreading to a younger population in which the symptoms would be acute neurological damage?

While he was discussing the lesions in Katie Hawkins's brain with his partner, Cheney received a call from Inez Kates, the mother of yet another twelve-year-old who was Katie Hawkins's classmate at Incline Middle School. The child, Mimi, had been diagnosed in Reno with cerebellar ataxia two weeks earlier and had been hospitalized for several days. She had lost her equilibrium and was unable to walk; her speech was slurred. The Kateses agreed to bring Mimi to see Cheney. The doctor confirmed the child's cerebellar ataxia diagnosis, drew a blood sample, and ordered an MRI scan. The child's blood revealed the curious viral antibody profile with which the doctor was by now all too familiar. Against expectations, however, Mimi's scan was clean. There were two possibilities, Cheney realized: either the child's brain had been spared by her illness or the damage was so deep within the cerebellum that the MRI scan was unlikely to pick it up.

On a hunch, Cheney sent two adults in his practice with the chronic disease to San Francisco for brain scans. Both of the adults were positive for several small T2-weighted high-intensity lesions, or UBOs.

Reno, Nevada

The opening of Reno Diagnostics, a medical radiology business on Eureka Avenue just blocks from the Circus Circus hotel and casino, coincided with Cheney and Peterson's heightening curiosity about the integrity of their patients' brains. As it happened, Reno Diagnostics was home to Nevada's only magnetic resonance imaging scanner, which was enclosed in a sparkling white geodesic dome adjacent to the one-story medical firm. The dome was an architectural conceit inspired by the unusual specifications for housing such machines; its walls and floor were lined with copper to prevent radio waves from penetrating the multimillion-dollar contraption. As one Reno Diagnostics technician explained, "You don't want the local top forty rock station beaming their radio waves in to ruin your magnet or your scans." The business drew patients from all over the Washoe Valley and from communities in eastern California, southern Oregon and Idaho, and even Colorado; the cutting-edge scanner was a substantial part of the allure.

Royce Biddle was a young neuroradiologist hired by Reno Diagnostics to read MRI scans of the brain and spinal cord. The doctor was a subspecialist, trained not only in radiology but in diseases of the brain and spine. But like most Reno doctors in the winter of 1985, regardless of specialty, Biddle was ignorant of the disease Cheney and Peterson were attempting to characterize a mountain range away. He was drawn inexorably into the web, however, when he began reading the MRI brain scans ordered on patients in the Peterson-Cheney practice. In conversation some time later, Biddle couldn't recall the first such scan he analyzed, but he did remember that Reno Diagnostics began performing MRI scans on several adults Peterson and Cheney referred to the center that December, and he read all of them. "A high percentage of those scans—approximately fifty percent—were abnormal," Biddle said.

More problematically, the neuroradiologist had never before seen abnormalities like the ones he saw in the Incline Village patients' brains. More than anything, they resembled the brain lesions seen in multiple sclerosis, but there were significant differences. In multiple sclerosis, the lesions—or plaques, as they were known—were anywhere from three to four millimeters up to a centimeter in size. There were far fewer of them, and they were located in the central white matter areas of the brain next to the ventricles or brain cavities. In contrast, the Tahoe patients' lesions were tiny pinpoint, or punctate, spots; there was nearly always a multitude of them and they appeared in a different part of the brain.

"In my mind, I just didn't think these could easily be confused with the MR scan abnormalities that you see in multiple sclerosis," the doctor said. "They were new—located near the top of the brain near the white matter tracks, some distance from the ventricles. To be perfectly honest with you," he continued, "we weren't sure what they were or what they meant. Even now we are not one hundred percent sure what they mean. But they were there. And the patients were sick."

Among the first patients Biddle scanned that winter were Onorio Antonucci, Chris Guthrie, Julie Pritchard, and Gerald and Janice Kennedy. Antonucci, the former algebra teacher who now found simple addition and subtraction beyond his ken and had been bedridden in his mobile home in Truckee for several months, was profoundly afflicted with multiple lesions, but Guthrie, Pritchard and the Kennedys had positive scans too.

Because medicine was exploiting the scanners chiefly to image the brain and spine, neuroradiologists like Biddle were rapidly dominating the MRI field. These specialists often found themselves trying to analyze an interior topography of which they knew frustratingly little. At issue was the question of what was *normal* among the myriad structural details revealed by the new scanners. Neurologists, too, were puzzled. Said one, "We can see abnormalities we never saw before. The sensitivity of the tests is so high that they're picking up *everything,* and we're not really able to tell whether any of it has any bearing."[2] For Biddle, the touchy issue of normalcy and its converse was about to explode.

In his first two years at Reno Diagnostics, the doctor read between 5,000 and 6,000 brain scans, but it is fair to say he was enthralled from the very beginning with the wide window that magnetic resonance imaging opened on diagnostic dilemmas. "MRI scanning has basically left CT scanning of the brain in the dust," Biddle said. One of the first patients he scanned was an eighteen-year-old who had undergone seven CT scans of her brain since developing acute hydrocephalus in early adolescence. Biddle's first magnetic resonance imaging scan revealed a 2 1/2-centimeter-size tumor in the young woman's brain that had been missed on every successive CT scan. (Surgeons removed the tumor and the patient recovered fully.) The doctor's enthusiasm was such that he began compiling for his colleagues a teaching file of medical cases in which the new scanner had picked up significant brain disease missed by CT scans.

Although his observations of multiple punctate lesions among the patients from Lake Tahoe were original and obviously important, the cases were hardly ready-made for the teaching file. There were no diagnostic triumphs, no happy endings—only perplexity. The doctor was confounded by the "tiny areas of abnormal signal in the white matter," as he characterized them, in the brains of so many adults in their prime years.

"When we first started seeing these things," Biddle remembered, "my initial reaction was uncertainty, because MR scanning is so sensitive it can pick up things the significance of which you don't even know. That's part of the excitement of working with a new modality, but it's also part of the mystery of dealing with this disease."

Nevertheless, it was Biddle's unabashed respect for the new technology that led him to his heartfelt conclusions about the Tahoe patients: the multiple bright spots in these brains weren't normal; they were not supposed to be there. Several years later, Paul Cheney would remark, "People who really understand MRI scanning— and not many people do—know that there is never anything that is not significant on an MRI scan. There is much that is not understood, but nothing that is not significant." Biddle agreed. He would argue passionately and in the face of chilling skepticism from his peers that although the meaning of the lesions was uncertain, their presence and importance could not be discounted.

"I just don't—I just *do not believe,*" Biddle would avow two years after studying his first Tahoe brain scan, "that one can dismiss these tiny punctate lesions as being normal or variants of normal. Exactly what they mean we just don't know at this point. I wish we did, but we don't. But I do not believe these findings are normal."

That winter, however, Biddle was just beginning to feel his way along the learning curve of the disease. He had only his simple equation: the UBOs were there, and the patients were sick.

5

Folie à Deux?

Yerington, Nevada

Late in November, Judy Hilbisch made a series of phone calls to Cheney and Peterson. "We started hearing from Judy that fall," Cheney recalled later. "Her outbreak began six months after ours. She said, 'I read about your problem up in Tahoe in the newspaper, and I wanted to tell you what I've been seeing in Yerington.' "

The Yerington doctor's description of the disease spinning out of control in the Nevada desert was remarkably similar to what Peterson and Cheney had been observing in the high-altitude region of the lake. Cheney listened carefully to Hilbisch's description of the monospot test results, most of which were positive, although, Hilbisch explained, the illness seemed more severe than classic mononucleosis. In addition to the profound exhaustion her patients suffered, Hilbisch said, there were a number of schoolchildren who appeared to have cerebellar ataxia. Several were so severely affected by a balance disorder that they were unable to walk without stumbling or falling. Adults complained they were having problems thinking and remembering. When the Yerington doctor began describing some of the neurological events occurring in patients, Cheney was almost certain they were talking about the same disease. Hilbisch was inclined to agree.

In late December, Hilbisch told a reporter from the *Sacramento Bee,* "This is possibly something trickling down from Lake Tahoe. The timing is right." Unfortunately there was little Hilbisch or her Yerington colleagues, Doctors Titus and Mayhew, could do to investigate that possibility, because most of their patients were too poor to pursue elaborate diagnostic testing. Yerington was, in Cheney's words, "just a poor farm town on the desert, the farthest thing from a yuppie place you could ever imagine." Most inhabitants weren't even subsistence landowners. "People don't come here to pursue a career; they come to pursue a rural lifestyle," said Russ Colletta, Yerington's high school principal. "When they enroll their kids in the schools and you ask their profession, they're unemployed."

Certainly, few Yerington residents carried health insurance that would cover $800 brain scans and esoteric, labor-intensive laboratory assays, particularly for an ill-defined mystery disease. An even larger portion lacked health insurance of any kind and were able to afford only the most basic and inexpensive care. Even the Epstein-Barr virus antibody panel Cheney and Peterson routinely ordered, a $57 test, was too costly for a majority of the afflicted in Yerington. In many cases, however, the impediment to investigating the disease wasn't simply a matter of cash. In Yerington, as in most Nevada desert settlements, a passionate sense of independence and self-reliance ruled the communal temperament. Ultimately, that peculiarly western ethos defined people's response to illness. According to Colletta, many of the sick failed to seek medical care of any kind.*

"A lot of people came here three generations ago and literally carved a life out of the desert, and they're very proud of it. They are very provincial," Colletta said. "There are people who lived here their whole lifetime without seeing a doctor. They don't want anyone to tell them what to do." When the disease began its spread, Colletta continued, it was accompanied by a sense of shame in many of its victims. "The people who were sick were neither articulate nor vocal, unlike people in Incline Village," he said. "They felt it was their fault that they were sick, and they just sort of hung their heads. There's no virtue in being sick if you're tough and independent and macho."

As a result of all these things, then, schoolchildren with apparent cerebellar ataxia and encephalopathy simply were sent to bed for several days; adults with unusual, if less acute, neurologic symptoms and extreme fatigue drifted off their jobs for weeks and months at a time, abashedly returning to work with no vocabulary to explain what had happened to them—that is, if they still had jobs.

Yet, Yerington's epidemic was a powerful signal to Cheney and Peterson that what they were seeing in their own town was real. "Yerington was an important issue to us," Cheney said later, "because it was such a different population from ours. Incline Village was the most affluent town in Nevada. And there was this feeling at the Centers for Disease Control that there was selection bias going on there, with the bias toward rich people. But Yerington was insular, populated by farmers and the lower middle class—people who could barely afford to pay for a doctor's visit. And there was enough lab work done there to *suggest* this disease," he continued. "The peripheral [blood] smears showed atypical lymphocytes."

On December 26, Judy Hilbisch reported the outbreak to the Nevada State Health Department. Nevada officials responded much as they had to the crisis in Incline Village—that is, with the merest modicum of interest. Certainly no one from the state health department ever came to Yerington to investigate the outbreak Hilbisch reported, nor did state officials notify the federal agency responsible for identifying and tracking epidemics, the Centers for Disease Control.

Unlike state health officials, Cheney believed the events in Yerington were deserving of the federal government's notice. He called Gary Holmes to tell him about Yerington two days after Hilbisch called the state, but the CDC never investigated the possibility that there had been an unusual occurrence of disease in Yerington.

"All they had to do was go in there," Dan Peterson would comment bitterly some years later on the subject of Yerington. "It was all there."

---

*Colletta himself was diagnosed with the malady during the winter of 1985–1986, but after six weeks, he seemed to have recovered to a great extent.

On the final day of 1985, an article by *Sacramento Bee* journalist Chris Bowman about the events in Yerington appeared under the headline "Mysterious Illness Strikes Another Town." The *Bee* story indicated that 105 Yerington residents were ill.

Incline Village, Nevada

By late November, the local epidemic had come to an end. In the next few months the doctors identified an additional fifty people with the disorder, but nearly all of them had been sick for some time; their diagnosis was new, in other words, but their disease was not. "We seemed to be seeing some sporadic cases," Cheney recalled. "But most had become sick within the time frame of the epidemic, which peaked in May and June, and so were really part of the epidemic. We were just seeing them late."

The objective diminution of cases only fueled the doctors' conviction that an epidemic had occurred. A surge of cases followed by a dropping off was compatible with the pattern of an infectious agent: pathogens sweep through populations, causing disease in all who are vulnerable, leaving those who are not unscathed; as immunity develops, the ravagement subsides.

The total number of cases by that fall was 160 from a population base the doctors determined was approximately 30,000. The clinicians included in their calculations not only the population of Incline Village but also residents of the north shore of Lake Tahoe, the region from which most of their epidemic patients hailed, including Truckee, Kings Beach, and Tahoe City, California. Based on those numbers, the attack rate was one out of every 188 people, a startlingly high rate compared to the attack rates of other chronic diseases, particularly those that strike in the prime of life. An estimated quarter-million people in the United States are afflicted with multiple sclerosis, for example; the attack rate of that disease turns out to be one in every 960 people. By 1990, five years after the Tahoe epidemic, doctors had reported 124,984 cases of AIDS to the Centers for Disease Control, with the result that the AIDS attack rate was one in every 1,920 people. The infectious disease with which Cheney and Peterson were struggling in 1985, then, was already ten times more common in northern Nevada than AIDS would be nationally five years *deeper* into the AIDS epidemic.

The doctors realized the attack rate might be higher if, as was probable, some percentage of north shore victims had eluded their detection. If Cheney and Peterson were seeing just half of the afflicted, for example, the attack rate was actually one in 93 people, or slightly more than 1 percent of the population of Lake Tahoe's north shore. It was an awesome rate for an infectious disease of the severity of the Tahoe malady. Unknown variables, particularly the length of the incubation period, added another dimension.

As a result of news coverage, a new chronically sick population was infusing the doctors' Alder Street practice. Like pilgrims journeying to Lourdes, ailing patients from every state were flying to Reno. Upon landing, the gamblers on board these flights hailed complimentary limousines to Bally's Grand or Circus Circus; the human wrecks launched themselves in Hertz and Avis four-wheel-drive vehicles and navigated the snow-dusted road over Mount Rose to Incline, their destination the sleek Peterson-Cheney clinic. There they hoped to find relief—or at least medical validation; if Cheney and Peterson could not alleviate their symptoms, the young internists might at least certify their sanity. One patient from Louisiana had already seen twenty-eight doctors, but everyone who came had seen at least a handful of practitioners in an effort to be accurately diagnosed. They brought with them medical records labeling them victims of a multitude of ailments. Their diagnoses included atypical multiple sclerosis, mitral valve prolapse syndrome, Lyme disease, atypical lupus, and any number of psychiatric disorders. Some of them had been incarcerated by relatives in mental institutions at points in their ordeal. Cheney and Peterson were utterly absorbed by their descriptions of their illnesses, not because the progressive symptomatology these people recounted was so variable but because, once the doctors stripped the stories of personal minutiae, it was the same. From the high school basketball player to the postal worker with teenage children to the middle-aged retiree, the tale rarely varied: a sudden onset of flu-like symptoms accompanied by an engulfing, life-altering exhaustion and neurological deterioration affecting vision, balance, coordination, and thinking.

The doctors also had letters, hundreds of them, from patients from all over, tremulous with an agony reminiscent of their local epidemic patients. Their authors had typed them on embossed stationery, scrawled them in pencil on notepaper, or spun long-winded epics in ballpoint pen on pages torn from legal pads. The missives were laden with the dyslexic spelling errors and jumbled syntax that typified the composition style of the doctors' local patients. Invariably they concluded with a plea for help.

A waitress from Big Pine, California, wrote, "My symptoms wax and wane. . . . I have strange dreams, memory problems, depression and I just do the most idiotic things you can imagine." A former editor at a national magazine in New York City typed pitifully on her magazine's letterhead stationery, "I am forty-three, single, chronically fatigued, and sick to a point where sometimes brushing my teeth is all I have the energy for in a day. On good days, I am able to work for an hour or two." An art history major from Sarasota, Florida, complained, "I cannot concentrate or see clearly. Confusion, depression, anxiety, and loneliness are my constant companions. I am unable to support myself." There were letters from a psychiatrist in Winston-Salem, North Carolina, who had been disabled by fatigue and poor cognition since 1983; from a former director of public information for a Manhattan arts council, with degrees from Radcliffe and Columbia, now living on disability from the Social Security Administration; from a nun in Chicago. A single thirty-seven-year-old wrote, "A little piece of me has died every day for the last fourteen years. . . . The sense of loss of control over my life hurts so deeply, I cannot find words to describe it."

Some of the letters were dictated or written by someone else on the patient's behalf. One came from the father of a concert cellist whose debilitating illness had forced her to drop out of Oberlin College. "She was a brilliant student," the man wrote. "Whatever the cause, my daughter's life has been wrecked." The parents of another young woman, who recently had married and "begun a promising career as an electronics engineer," wrote, "Our sad experience has been to watch our youngest daughter suddenly lose all energy to the point of incapacitation. She saw more than thirty doctors, including physicians in some of the major diagnostic centers in the Boston area . . . they all failed to identify the root cause. Some wrote her off as a hypochondriac."

The disease posed the greatest intellectual challenge of Paul Cheney's life. It was vastly more intricate and pressing than anything he had encountered in physics. By some remarkable turn of fate, he had abandoned his research dream and reluctantly retired to a life of small-town doctoring only to have, as he ingenuously phrased it, "the most exciting research project of my life" drop with a resounding thud in his lap. By the fall of 1985, the Tahoe malady had acquired a transcendent significance for him.

"There's this thing that's joked about in internal medicine: you're bored with ninety-eight percent of your patients, and the other two percent keep you stimulated and thinking," Dan Peterson said when conversation turned to the subject of his partner some years later. "So if you don't get the two percent, you get burned out—or out to lunch. Well, Paul lived for that two percent. And when this thing came along, Paul just took up the gauntlet, because he had been tweaked where he operates best."

For Cheney, in fact, the 2 percent had become 100 percent. He was performing fewer physicals, attending to fewer colds and flus, opting to see fewer new patients. Half of the doctor's long days were spent examining and interviewing a handful of chronically ill patients. His consultations often consumed more than two hours, a radical departure from the national average of seven minutes harried internal medicine specialists were devoting to individual patients in the late 1980s. Rather than attempting to examine a large aggregate of patients in whom he suspected the disease, he was looking tenaciously at a few, searching for the disease in its purest, or least ambiguous, form to allow him to define it with precision.

He was impressed that the patients from out of state complained of the same unusual symptoms suffered by locals. These included numbness in their faces and limbs, pronounced sensitivity to light, weight gains of thirty and forty pounds, hair loss, intolerance to alcohol, heart palpitations, loss of libido, and a sleep pattern characterized by unpleasant dreams alternating with insomnia. Their anecdotes about their self-confessed "off-the-wall" behavior raised the doctor's suspicion index, too. People described finding objects like gloves or car keys in their microwave ovens and dinner leftovers in their china cabinets, and being unable to find their way home from familiar landmarks. A number of them had lost their jobs as their illness progressed, an event they more frequently blamed on their intellectual deterioration than on their exhaustion. One thirty-year-old woman, a system programmer for Apple Computer, reported she began to experience thinking problems soon after the onset of her disease. Eventually she was fired. In high school, she told Cheney, her IQ was 132. A year after her illness began, she was tested again: her IQ was 98.

The other half of the doctor's days were spent on the phone. Ensconced in his office one floor below his partner's, with Lake Tahoe's glistening surface visible between the stands of ponderosa pine outside his window, he called scientists. His curiosity was boundless. Could a mutant Epstein-Barr virus have caused the Incline cluster? Was EBV prone to infect the brain? Could EBV cause brain lesions? Were any diseases besides leukemia and childhood AIDS associated with collapsed Epstein-Barr nuclear antigen? His inquiries were costing the practice $2,000 a month in long-distance telephone charges.

Dan Peterson was no less compelled by the problem than his partner, but his patient load was significantly greater than Cheney's. Having been in practice three years longer, he had approximately three times as many patients, in fact. As a result, the clinician was spending very little time on the phone and a great deal of time in the Alder Street examining rooms. He had always run an efficient office, and he was loath to allow the epidemic to endanger the practice he had built so painstakingly. Even so, he was nearly overwhelmed by the epidemic patients, whose health problems dwarfed those of other patients in his practice. In all his experience, in fact, he had never seen people who were so ill. Peterson's perception of the problem was shared, on occasion, even by those who were wholly unfamiliar with the disease. His nursing staff grew accustomed to healthy patients tapping on the glass partition between the waiting room and their office to alert them to a patient slumped over in his chair in what appeared to be an unconscious state. Inevitably, the gray-complexioned, corpse-like subject in question was a "fatigue patient," as the nurses would calmly explain.

Until the epidemic hit, chronic disabling diseases in Peterson's practice had tended to be those, like multiple sclerosis or lupus, that resulted in referral to another specialist. Unhappily, there were no specialists to whom Peterson could refer patients with this new affliction.

"There would be bright spots," Peterson recalled. "Paul would talk to someone, and he would come up—he would come *running* up the stairs; he had just tremendous energy—and he would say, 'Well, we've got to pursue this, because I talked to so-and-so today.' Stuff like that. Once I had him hooked, there were times when he was more hooked than I was. And then we just fed each other. . . . But [the patients] weren't getting better. They were bitching and moaning and complaining, and there seemed to be more and more of them. What was I going to do? I just seemed immersed in the middle of a mess that I couldn't get out of and that I didn't fully understand myself. And it just kind of went on, day after day."

The clinicians had heard nothing from the Centers for Disease Control since Holmes and Kaplan's departure, but on October 24, Truckee's *Sierra Sun* quoted Gary Holmes in a story about the Incline epidemic. "Our feeling," Holmes said, "is we just don't have an outbreak."

During that fall, Cheney and Peterson gathered in the senior partner's office each day at dusk. "I don't think Paul and I ever differed once in a major sense on the way that we would manage a particular case, which is just incredible," Peterson would remember. "But we were trained the same way, we thought the same way, and we did the same things, which subsequently became very important in this whole issue. Because there were many, many times when one or the other of us would get discouraged or at a dead end in our thought processes, and I swear if it hadn't been for the other, it all would have been gone."

Despite their daily exchange of observations and hunches, by November a sense of exile was beginning to settle on both men. During these twilight moments they occasionally found themselves wondering if the Tahoe malady was indeed a folie à deux. "I remember sitting down at the end of the day and looking at Paul and saying, 'Am I nuts? Have I now made *you* crazy?' " Peterson said. "We used to try to keep ourselves honest. We'd say, 'Is the lab sending us fake results?' We would always go back to the stuff we could measure. You know, I would feel a big spleen, and then I would do a CT scan. I would spend *five hundred dollars* to measure the size of the spleen. And the report would come back, 'Spleen enlarged.' "

Cheney, too, frequently looked to his partner for a reality check: "I'd say to Dan, 'Can we both be deluded at the same time? Are we seeing this in so many people simply because we're attuned to it?' If enough people tell you your diagnosis is garbage, you start to believe it. The thing that kept pulling us back, though, was our patients."

That month, the clinic's office manager, who was Peterson's older sister, had a grand mal seizure while driving her car and plowed into a snowbank. The woman had no history of a seizure disorder, but like a growing majority of the practice's fatigue patients, with whom she had daily contact, her magnetic resonance brain scan revealed multiple small lesions in the temporal lobes. Her antibody levels to Epstein-Barr virus were elevated in the familiar pattern as well. Like Chris Guthrie, she developed a temporary weakness, or paresis, in her left arm. Two weeks later a male nurse in the practice suffered a grand mal seizure in the office, hitting his head on the exam table with an impact that shattered his glasses. The nurse had been ill for several days with an upper respiratory ailment, but like the office manager, he had no history of seizures. His MRI brain scan was positive, and his antibody levels to Epstein-Barr virus were "sky high," Peterson recalled. The office manager recovered in a matter of days, seemingly unfazed by her experience; the male nurse did not.

"For the next few months," Cheney remembered, "he was encephalopathic. He was confused, disoriented, disarthric—had trouble forming words, and he had ataxia—equilibrium problems." Eventually the nurse filed suit to obtain workers' compensation disability from Nevada for industrial related contact. His was one of the few successful disability lawsuits that would be filed with various state agencies by victims of the Tahoe flu in the years to come. He remains disabled at this writing.

The loss of his nurse was a point of demarcation for Peterson. "After that," the doctor said, "there was just absolutely, categorically no question in my mind about [the disease] being infectious and about it being real. From that point onward, I didn't care who I argued with. You couldn't convince me otherwise. There was such a marked change in people—a *marked* personality change. And the more people said, 'Oh, it's just craziness,' the more adamant I got."

During the same period, Cheney underwent a curious change in his health. For several months, off and on, he experienced disequilibrium, but no loss of vitality. Eventually the balance problem went away, only to recur in a milder form a year later. Soon afterward the symptom disappeared completely and never returned. The athletic doctor enjoyed robust health in the future, never again experiencing symptoms reminiscent of the disease. (Peterson has never developed symptoms of the disease.)

Cheney, like his partner, was persuaded that the disease was contagious, though he remained uncertain by what route. An apprehension that had simmered for months loomed larger that fall as the breadth of the epidemic became manifest: the prospect that unwitting blood donors were contaminating the nation's blood supply with whatever unnamed pathogen caused the disease. A plethora of letters from patients who said they had contracted their disease after blood transfusions fired Cheney's concern.

Sexual transmission, too, seemed possible. Peterson discovered that five of his male patients had had sex with the same prostitute the previous year; the prostitute was one of Cheney's sickest fatigue patients. The prostitute's weight had fallen by fifty pounds; she ran a low-grade temperature intermittently and was suffering from chronic lymphadenopathy. Cheney had ruled out AIDS, leukemia, and Hodgkin's lymphoma in the patient, but she had the classic Epstein-Barr virus antibody reactivation pattern as well as numerous other clinical signs and symptoms of the new disease.

By this evidence, anyway, the Tahoe malady would seem to be, like AIDS and a number of other viral diseases such as hepatitis and mononucleosis, transmitted sexually. On the other hand, with the exception of the Pritchards and the Kennedys, who seemed to be victims of an environmental rather than a sexual exposure, neither doctor could think of another incidence of two spouses falling ill. In time, that perception would change, however.

Saliva might be yet a third route of contagion. One of Cheney's patients, a sixty-two-year-old anesthesiologist who practiced in Reno, became ill soon after cutting his hand on the incisor tooth of a woman undergoing elective surgery. The woman had been ill with a vague, undiagnosed illness for months prior to her operation. After several months of disability, the Reno doctor opted for early retirement.

Until the agent was identified, the doctors knew, the mode of transmission would remain inscrutable.

Raleigh, North Carolina

Normally, Seymour Grufferman would have dismissed the call that autumn. The Duke University cancer epidemiologist, whose expertise lay in the complex and controversial field of virally caused cancer, had little patience with cranks. The caller was living in northern California about fifty miles from Truckee, she explained, and she was worried that her recent move to the northern Sierras had launched the epidemic of chronic Epstein-Barr virus disease in the region. She told Grufferman that the outbreak began soon after her arrival in mid-1984. She and her husband had discovered they enjoyed casino gambling, she continued, and, after their move to the area, the couple had made several day trips to Incline Village to gamble. She promised to send Grufferman an article from the *Sacramento Bee* that she said would buttress her theory. A few days later the clipping arrived: it was a chronology of the Incline Village epidemic.

Far from rebuffing the caller and her far-fetched-sounding theory, Grufferman was cordial and respectful. He was thoroughly engrossed in her story, in fact. She was well known to him personally as a member of an upper-middle-class family of Danish descent that had suffered, as one journalist would later describe it, "a singular catastrophe." Within months of each other, one family member in each of four households in different corners of the country had come down with rare but related cancers. Each was diagnosed with non-Hodgkin's lymphoma, a category of immune system cancers encompassing several B-cell lymphomas, including Burkitt's lymphoma, a cancer that is exceedingly rare in the United States but endemic in the African malarial belt. One of the four, a fifty-eight-year-old man, was diagnosed with Burkitt's.

Though trained at Harvard to be a pediatrician, Grufferman had been "waylaid," as he once described it, by cancer research, a turn of events that eventually led to his interest in cancer epidemiology and the possibility that some cancers were infectious. His most pressing professional interest for some years had been the relationship between viruses and cancer. Until the early 1970s the notion that cancer could assume an infectious form, like measles or the common cold, was widely disavowed. But Grufferman, in common with a number of his peers, was unconvinced: there were enough apparent clusters of some kinds of cancer to suggest that a transmissible agent had played some role. Nevertheless, for most forms of the disease, unassailable proof eluded researchers. Anecdotal reports of cancer clusters abounded, but Burkitt's lymphoma was, so far, the only *human* cancer for which there existed unequivocal evidence of time and space clustering.

Grufferman had first learned of the family in 1983 when the caller's sister-in-law, a bright, enterprising person who had undertaken considerable medical research in an effort to comprehend her family's bizarre ordeal, came upon Grufferman's name in the course of her studies. The epidemiologist, who had an unreserved passion for studying cancer clusters, agreed to investigate. Immediately he ruled out genetic predisposition as a risk factor, since only two of the afflicted were blood relatives. But one common thread rapidly emerged: during a six-week period in the summer of 1982, each of the four households had been visited by a South African relative.

A recently widowed sixty-three-year-old, the South African had planned a happy reunion with her American relatives in California, Georgia, and Washington State. Just before leaving South Africa, however, she was beset by a severe sore throat and fatigue; these mono-like symptoms had tormented her, in fact, off and on, for years, although she had never actually had bona fide mono. Early in her American tour, the South African woman required antibiotic treatment for chills and a worsening of her sore throat, and her relatives recalled that good health eluded their aunt for virtually the entire duration of her excursion. The woman returned to South Africa in late August, leaving in her wake an outbreak of cancer that would doom four people in the next seven years.

Grufferman had studied the family's misfortune exhaustively. His report in the *New England Journal of Medicine,* "Burkitt's and Other Non-Hodgkin's Lymphomas in Adults Exposed to a Visitor from Africa," appeared in December.[1] By that time one of the four cancer victims was already dead; two more died in the ensuing three years, and the fourth, Grufferman's astute caller from Nevada, died of lymphoma in 1990 at age sixty.

The average period between exposure to the South African woman and the onset of cancer symptoms in her relatives, Grufferman determined, was 198 days, a remarkably brief latency period compared to most cancers, which are thought to have latencies of from ten to twenty years. Two patients, a sixty-seven-year-old woman and a fifty-seven-year-old man, were diagnosed within three days of each other in March 1983. The last victim received her diagnosis of non-Hodgkin's lymphoma in late July, exactly a year after her South African relative had been a guest in her home.

Grufferman established, too, that at least three and probably four of the lymphomas originated in the patients' B-cells, vital components, along with T-cells, of the immune system. The B-cell finding prompted the researcher to look for Epstein-Barr activity in the cancer victims' blood. As it turned out, only one of the three surviving patients had antibodies to the virus, indicating that the other two had escaped infection altogether. Whatever agent had caused the wave of cancer, then, it was not Epstein-Barr virus. Several other family members without symptoms of either cancer or fatigue were discovered to have elevated antibodies to the virus in a pattern that suggested reactivation of a latent infection, however. These apparently well family members had been exposed to some unknown pathogen that had harmed their immunity.

"It is possible that the Epstein-Barr virus was involved in some way," Grufferman concluded in his *New England Journal* article. "The symptoms of the visitor's illness suggested infectious mononucleosis, and her [blood] contained early antigen antibodies, thereby suggesting a recent or reactivated EBV infection. Secondly, several of the persons exposed had very high antibody titers to EBV." But because two of the three surviving patients had no evidence of exposure to the virus, Grufferman continued, "the data are most consistent with an unidentified transmissible agent, *with the findings of antibodies to EBV representing secondary activation responses*" (italics added).

In other words, a mystery virus, spread unwittingly by the South African to her hosts in America, had resulted in four cases of immune system cancer; the same bug simultaneously caused an immune system disturbance that allowed Epstein-Barr to be reactivated in other family members.

In a report to scientists at the National Institutes of Health many years later, Grufferman wrote that he and his collaborators initially dismissed the curious outbreak at Lake Tahoe as having nothing at all to do with the tragic events that had befallen the South African's American relatives. "We thought [the Tahoe epidemic] was part of the emerging picture of chronic fatigue syndrome," as the disease had then been named by federal scientists. But four months later the caller sent Grufferman a second clipping from the *Sacramento Bee* about a new outbreak of presumed Epstein-Barr virus associated disease in Placerville, California. Like Incline Village, Placerville was a community from which the caller lived a negligible distance and which she had visited.

"We then began to wonder whether she didn't have a point," Grufferman continued in his report, "and that her presence in the area might have been related in some way to the epidemics."

Incline Village, Nevada

Starting that fall, Peterson and Cheney began to observe an outbreak of rare immune system cancers not only among people who were ill with the epidemic disease but among other previously well residents of Lake Tahoe's north shore.

During the first week in November a fifty-four-year-old attorney who was Peterson's patient showed up in the clinic with a tumor at his jawline. The man had retired from an active law practice and now dwelt in the evocatively named Zephyr Cove, a community a few miles south along the lakeshore from Incline Village. Peterson sent the attorney to Stanford University's medical center for surgery. Following routine procedure, Stanford's pathology lab biopsied the tumor. Soon afterward, the surgeon who had performed the surgery called Peterson to inform him of the biopsy results. The mass was indeed malignant and the diagnosis most unusual: according to the pathologist who studied the cells, the attorney was suffering from Burkitt's lymphoma.

By the time an astonished Peterson called Stanford's pathology lab to discuss the finding, however, a second, more senior pathologist had studied the lawyer's tumor cells and changed the diagnosis to "undifferentiated B-cell lymphoma." The tumor cell's "architecture," the senior pathologist explained to Cheney some time later, did not display the regular, "brick-like" construction of a Burkitt's tumor. The tumor, in fact, failed to fit into any single category of B-cell cancer.

Buried in the parotid, or salivary, gland, a standard site for Burkitt's, the tumor had completely destroyed the tissues around it. "It was so distorted," the doctor remembered. "We asked to have it probed for Epstein-Barr virus, but they didn't have much to look at because it was such a destructive necrotic mass."

The lawyer's diagnosis prompted a flurry of speculation between Peterson and Cheney over whether his cancer might be related to the epidemic. The lawyer had not complained of severe fatigue, Peterson remembered, though there were hints of a problem during the year before his tumor appeared. "He had nothing that was marked," Cheney said. "On closer questioning," however, the doctor learned that "he had not been completely normal in the year leading up to this development. But he would not have said, 'I am very tired.' He would say, 'I don't have all the energy I used to.' It was that kind of thing. Nothing marked."

Acting on a hunch, Cheney ordered a magnetic resonance imaging brain scan on the attorney; the resulting image was one of the most pockmarked the doctor had yet seen. In the following months the attorney developed the chronic syndrome.

A week later a second previously healthy patient walked into the Alder Street clinic with a tumor on his neck. This thirty-eight-year-old plumber and handyman in a local casino had been a patient of Cheney's for two years. The plumber's tumor was also in the parotid, or salivary, gland, although it was a benign growth, characterized at Stanford as a "mixed salivary adenoma." (Adenomas are, by definition, benign, although they may become malignant.) Nevertheless, the Stanford lab probed the tumor tissue for Epstein-Barr virus at Cheney and Peterson's request and found it to be infused with the herpesvirus.

The plumber's diagnosis jogged Peterson's memory; one of his fatigue patients, a woman from San Francisco, had undergone surgery for the removal of a tumor in the parotid gland early in the course of her illness, which had begun two years before. That tumor too had been described as a mixed salivary adenoma. At the time, Peterson had thought little of the incident.

The implication of these uncommon immune system tumors arising spontaneously in the context of an epidemic characterized by immune dysfunction was ominous. What if, as was sometimes the case in AIDS, lymphomas and other cancers were the inevitable culmination of this so far untreatable disease?*

The doctors were engaged in discussions about this possibility when the lawyer, who was recovering at home in Zephyr Cove, telephoned them with an alarming story. The attorney was calling to report the death from lymphoma of a six-year-old Los Angeles boy, the grandchild of a couple who lived in Zephyr Cove. The child had spent his Christmas season the previous year with his grandparents in Zephyr Cove. While in Nevada he had become debilitated by an illness for which none of the doctors his parents consulted in Los Angeles could find a name. The boy's lymphoma diagnosis came three months after his illness began. His older sister had spent Christmas in Zephyr Cove with her brother that year as well. She too became ill. Hers was a lengthy flu-like illness, much like her brother's; unlike her brother, however, the little girl had recovered.

Was it possible, the clinicians asked each other, that the siblings had picked up the bug that was just beginning its rampage through the north Tahoe area during the winter of 1984–1985 and had acquired the fatigue syndrome, except that in the boy's case, his immune system response was inadequate?

Then one of Cheney's favorite patients, a retired seventy-year-old engineer, complained to the doctor of a sudden onset of exhaustion that was keeping him housebound. On examination, Cheney found that the man had swollen lymph glands and low-grade fever. His Epstein-Barr virus antibodies were extremely elevated, and he was suffering from focal myocarditis, an inflammation of the heart muscle resulting in arrhythmias and heart murmurs. The principal causes of myocarditis are viral infections and rheumatic fever; Cheney was able to rule out the latter. Not surprisingly, the doctor suspected that yet another of his patients had contracted the Tahoe malady. The news was hardly welcome, but it was not astonishing. Six months later, however, the engineer's sixty-nine-year-old wife developed a malignant tumor mass on her jaw, which was diagnosed in Los Angeles as an "infiltrating, necrotizing B-cell lymphoma" of the parotid gland. Unlike her husband, the woman had no history of fatigue.

"I would say that to see—within one year—two B-cell lymphomas of the parotid gland was just unthinkable," Cheney said later. "I haven't seen that before or since. And I think the mixed salivary adenomas were unusual too."

The doctors were deeply alarmed.

Faced with the extraordinary possibility that the disease which had struck the north shore might be an epidemic of cancer, Cheney, in particular, began to mull the likelihood of spotting lymphomas at a presymptomatic stage. Was there a window of time, he wondered, when ominous changes at the cellular level could be detected, even interrupted? "I wondered if there was a test that could tell us what was going on in these people microscopically," the doctor said.

*In 1982 doctors in San Francisco had diagnosed nine gay men with Burkitt's lymphoma, a disease so rare that statisticians for the California Tumor Registry expect to find only two or three cases of the disease in the entire state every two years. The surge among gay men in San Francisco so impressed that city's infectious disease specialist, Selma Dritz, that she instructed the Centers for Disease Control to assume in the future that "Burkitt's lymphoma is a form of AIDS."

His queries led him to Susan Wormsley, a biochemist and flow cytometry expert at Cytometrics Laboratory in San Diego. Flow cytometry is an expensive, rarefied technology for quantifying and qualifying immune system cells; this technology is used to diagnose and stage the severity of lymphomas.

"Its value," Wormsley explained some time later in her sun-drenched office at Cytometrics, "is that it enables you to detect very small numbers of circulating abnormal cells whose presence, under a microscope, would be impossible to appreciate. What we do," she added, "you just couldn't do working under a microscope. You couldn't see enough. Flow cytometry is highly quantitative, very reproducible, and very sensitive," she continued. "The measurements are done on a single-cell basis—a *per cell* basis. That's really its strength."

Not long after establishing Cytometrics, Wormsley had begun to take advantage of one of the technology's most significant applications: monitoring the progression of B-cell lymphomas. In 1976 three Harvard scientists had developed the test, which was a highly sensitive method of finding monoclonal, or cancerous, B-cells in the blood. Called the kappa/lambda clonal excess assay, the test was able to detect lymphoma cells even when they were present in extremely low numbers.

"Say, for instance, a person normally had ten percent B-cells," Wormsley said. "If only one percent were abnormal, you wouldn't be able to find them using standard technology. But this test allows you to identify that one percent."

As helpful as it would seem to be, the kappa/lambda test was, for nearly a decade, a tool used almost exclusively by researchers rather than clinical oncologists. That was because, in late 1985, Cytometrics was the sole commercial lab in the country with the technical skill and equipment to perform it. Once Wormsley's expertise became known, there was a terrific surge of interest among oncologists in the region. Curiously, Wormsley found that the test's original function, which was to stage B-cell lymphomas, or determine how far the disease had advanced, was less frequently utilized by oncologists than was its secondary function, which was to identify microscopic changes that presaged the disease's onset. She devoted the lion's share of her time to evaluating very early B-cell lymphomas.

The biochemist thought she had seen every unusual result or combination of results one could see in a flow cytometer. Then, in December 1985, Paul Cheney called.

"Paul said he had this group of patients," Wormsley remembered. "And it seemed that, within that initial group, two or three went on to develop lymphoma. At that early stage, the worry was, 'My gosh, is this disease going to cause lymphoma in a *lot* of patients?' "

Wormsley asked Cheney to send her a handful of green tops, tubes capped with green rubber tops signifying that the anticoagulant heparin had been used to preserve the fresh blood. The clinician eagerly complied.

"We did a few samples," Wormsley continued, "and . . . there *were* abnormalities. But the abnormalities and the patterns we saw weren't really that similar to what you see in a patient who has lymphoma. These were very *strange* patterns. But they have been consistent over a long period of time for those given patients. The only problem is, we *still* don't know how to interpret what's going on."

One disparity between cancer patients and the Tahoe patients had to do with quantitative differences among the several categories of B-cells that circulate in the immune system. In the cancer patients, the differences were "very subtle," Wormsley said. "In Paul's patients," she added, "we saw very large differences."

"When I first saw some of these abnormalities," Wormsley continued, "I said, 'Wow! Send another tube of blood!' And they did, and, *boy,* they were just *exactly* the same abnormalities! And now we've followed some of these patients out two and a half years, and they remain identical. They haven't changed. It is a very worrisome finding."

Cheney and Peterson began drawing blood from all of their epidemic patients and sending it to Wormsley.

"In the early stages we were getting three or four a week," Wormsley recalled. "We also did some serially." In most cases, the abnormalities remained stable in the same patients over periods of months and eventually years.

For Peterson and Cheney there was one problem: the kappa/lambda test cost $400. On the frequent occasions when their patients' insurance companies refused to reimburse them for the test or when an indigent patient was unable to pay, the doctors drew cash from the practice to cover the Cytometrics bill every month. Within two years Peterson's personal debt to the lab was $200,000.

After studying samples from approximately fifty patients, Wormsley estimated that the rate of clonal excess abnormality in the fatigue patients from Nevada was at least 25 percent. But that wasn't the only aberration Wormsley found.

"Actually there were several abnormalities that we saw in these patients," she continued. One was a voluminous amount of cell debris. "Right from the time we separated and stained the cells, we saw a lot of debris," she said. "Just broken-apart cells, *pieces* of cells and platelets. And we don't see that in anything else that gets sent to us. Now, naturally, with everything that is sent to us, the people are sick, and most of them have cancer—leukemia, lymphoma—but we didn't see this kind of debris except in these patients."

Obviously something—a virus or some kind of toxin—was killing cells in the Tahoe sufferers.

Wormsley was struck by another phenomenon. In order to successfully perform the kappa/lambda test, she needed a sizable population of B-cells in her samples.

"Right from the beginning," she said, "these people seemed to have extremely low percentages [of B-cells], sometimes only one percent or two percent of their white blood cell population instead of the eight to twelve percent that we normally see. I noticed it because with a normal person, ten milliliters of blood gives you plenty of cells to do the entire assay. But I wasn't able to get enough B-cells to feel comfortable with Paul's patients. The background-noise level was almost at the same level as the positive cells. Again, we just didn't see that in a lot of our other patients, and certainly not in our normals."

Wormsley was perplexed. Here was a so-called Epstein-Barr virus disease, but the sufferers had lost their B-cells. One would expect the opposite, a profusion of B-cells, since EBV "immortalizes" B-cells. (In acute-phase mononucleosis, B-cell counts explode.) Yet three of the first five Tahoe patients tested had no B-cells at all, a finding that was repeated on additional tests. "It *was* curious," Wormsley said.

She discovered another immune system disorder that was possibly related to the B-cell deficiency that Cheney's patients suffered. Several Tahoe victims had abnormally low levels of several classes of immunoglobulins, immune system proteins produced by B-cells that act as antibodies.

"If you add that into all of the other abnormalities," Wormsley said, "then the number or percentage of the abnormalities goes up even higher than twenty-five percent."

One of the most striking immunological aberrations Wormsley observed, however, was abnormal ratios of T-cell subsets. T-cells are a major category of immune system cell; they regulate production of disease-fighting antibodies. Two primary T-cell subsets are "helper" and "suppressor" T-cells, which boost and suppress antibody production, respectively. In AIDS the normal ratio tends to be dramatically skewed in favor of suppressors. Since this finding is virtually diagnostic of AIDS, Cheney and Peterson were curious to know the T-cell subset profile in the Tahoe malady.

Wormsley's results showed that four of five Tahoe patients did have abnormal helper-suppressor ratios. But, unlike the ratios in AIDS sufferers, they were low in the numbers of suppressor cells. Instead of one-to-two or one-to-three, which are typical of healthy people, the Incline patients had helper-suppressor ratios of five-to-one, ten-to-one, and higher. It was the mirror image of AIDS.

Cheney and Peterson decided to run all five samples again; the results were identical. Then they expanded the test to include more people. Approximately half of the twenty additional patients were found to have abnormally low ratios of suppressor cells to helper cells. When they searched the medical literature for other diseases that produced similar inverse ratios of T-cells, they discovered that the finding had not been reported before. Researchers had observed elevated ratios in certain autoimmune diseases such as multiple sclerosis and lupus, but always the elevation was due to an increase in the helper cell population, as in AIDS, rather than a decrease in suppressors.

The finding continued to be unique to the disease as the years passed. Said one virologist, some time later, "There is not another disease that mimics this, except perhaps some relatively rare T-cell lymphomas. But you could practice your whole life and never see a T-cell lymphoma."

Peterson and Cheney began using the curious helper-suppressor ratio as yet another laboratory abnormality—in addition to the abnormal Epstein-Barr virus antibody profile—to support their diagnosis of the disease. It was a fragile strand, they knew, and they were uncertain of its significance. Yet it was real, and it was not normal.

During one late-November after-hours session, Cheney and Peterson tried to extract a manageable hypothesis from the immensely complex events under way in their region of Nevada. Something—agent X—was being transmitted from person to person within their community, and perhaps in many communities, if the letters in their overstuffed correspondence files were to be believed. Agent X appeared to target the human immune system, in rare cases undermining the body's ability to ward off cancers but more frequently fomenting a relentless illness characterized by the classic symptoms of a viral infection. To these scenarios the doctors added the wild card: the neurological complications that seemed to afflict, to some degree, virtually everyone who got sick. If agent X wasn't Epstein-Barr virus, as it clearly was not, then what, precisely, was it?

"We had collected increasing evidence that there was an immunologic problem going on," Cheney recalled. "And so we were trying to figure out what causes immune system problems, makes people sick for a long time, is probably new, and could cause an epidemic? Well, we came up with a retrovirus."

In the fall of 1985, the most famous retrovirus was human immunodeficiency virus, for which all of the Tahoe patients had tested negative. With the discovery of HIV, the bulk of scientific muscle and money had been redirected from the first two retroviruses; a commercial test for human T-cell lymphotrophic virus, type 2, did not yet exist. A test existed for HTLV1, however, and that was the virus for which Cheney and Peterson decided to test five of their patients.

Cheney sent five tubes of serum by overnight mail to Jim Peters, the head of Specialty Labs in Los Angeles, which performed a wide range of esoteric high-tech diagnostic tests. "[The five patients] weren't the sickest, and they weren't the mildest," Cheney recalled. "Two of them were teachers. They were what we considered classic cases, and they were part of the epidemic."

Three days later a Specialty Labs technician phoned Peterson with the results: four out of the five were positive for the first human retrovirus. The doctors were stunned.

"I had to find a chair to sit down," Cheney remembered. The predicted rate of HTLV1 infection in the American population was .031 percent.

Soon after the Nevada doctors learned of the positive HTLV1 results, Jim Peters, head of Specialty Labs in Los Angeles, called them to express his astonishment. He suggested that they have the samples retested at Biotech Research Laboratories in Rockville, Maryland, the manufacturers of the HTLV1 test kit used by Specialty Labs.

Cheney and Peterson agreed. In the meantime Cheney composed a letter, in which he described the retrovirus finding, to the British journal *Lancet,* a century-old weekly publication widely devoured by American medical practitioners. The *Lancet* was famous for its newsy letters section where an international sweep of biomedical findings was discussed in short takes. Cheney's goal was to rapidly disseminate the finding, then let the world-class virologists in the university laboratories confirm or disprove it.

He heard from *Lancet*'s editor first. The letter would be published, the editor said, pending verification from a second lab. Soon after that, a Biotech employee called Cheney. On the second test, all five samples had been negative for HTLV1. Cheney immediately called a Biotech laboratory technician who had worked on the company's HTLV1 test kit development. "She had done two different tests for the virus and reported that they were both negative," Cheney said. "She was very defensive about this, and her nuance seemed to be that perhaps they hadn't done the test correctly at Specialty."

Because the original results were so incredible in the first place, Cheney and Peterson were easily persuaded that the Los Angeles laboratory's findings had been a flukish series of false positives. For the moment, the doctors put aside their retrovirus theory.

On December 4 a frustrated Dan Peterson wrote to Gary Holmes in an effort to spark the Centers for Disease Control's apparent dwindling interest in the Tahoe epidemic.

"Dear Gary," he wrote. "It has been some time since we have heard from you. We continue to find out some interesting things about the phenomenon that we have observed." Peterson went on to describe the influx of new patients into their practice "with primary complaints of severe fatigue and/or chronic cough." He gave a case history of one patient with enlarged lymph nodes, extreme fatigue, atypical lymphocytes and, in the beginning of the illness, low levels of antibody to Epstein-Barr virus. As the patient's illness progressed, "with a significant increase in disability," Peterson added, the EBV antibody levels increased fivefold. "We have had other, similar cases," the doctor said, "and continue to be concerned about exactly what these scenarios represent, particularly due to the long disability and lack of prior history of significant illness in these patients. We continue to look to you for guidance in terms of additional evaluation of these patients. . . . Additionally, we continue to have patients from the original group who demonstrate ongoing lymphadenopathy, positive [EBV] serologies, and no clinical signs of improvement since the time that you visited," Peterson wrote.

Jon Kaplan, rather than Holmes, responded to Peterson's letter on December 18. With his one-paragraph letter he enclosed a copy of a short summary of his own and his partner's observations about the Tahoe outbreak. He and Holmes planned to present the summary, or abstract, at the agency's annual Epidemic Intelligence Service conference the following April, Kaplan wrote. "This is an in-house conference at which EIS officers give oral and poster presentations of the work they have done at CDC. As you can see," Kaplan continued, "preliminary analysis of the data suggests that the diagnosis of chronic EBV infections in persons [who are ill] less than one year is practically impossible given the nondescript nature of the symptoms. . . . It might be easier to diagnose chronic EBV in persons who have been ill one year or longer, at least according to the literature, but I think this also will take some time to sort out. Gary is continuing to work with the data to write a final report, but in the meantime, I would suggest that you make the diagnosis of chronic EBV in your patients only with great caution, and perhaps not at all."

Kaplan ended his note with the wistful comment "I wish I were out there skiing."

Peterson examined the abstract Kaplan had stapled to his letter. Its cumulative effect was spirit-sapping. The "data" Kaplan referred to had to do with the variables in Epstein-Barr virus laboratory testing. The abstract seemed to imply that the test was a meaningless diagnostic tool, since it had an element of subjectivity and different labs achieved different results. Additionally, the investigators were hewing to their original impression, based on their examination of a handful of patients and a hasty chart review, that just fifteen Nevada patients actually had the infamous Tahoe malady or, as the federal investigators were now calling it, CEBV, for chronic Epstein-Barr virus. All of the other patients, the abstract seemed to imply, had symptoms that could be attributed to other health problems.

Kaplan and Holmes's impression of the degree of illness in Incline, Peterson believed, was indicative of their clinical inexperience with the disease. Its victims, Peterson knew, were hugely vulnerable to misdiagnoses. But the illness was hardly the "nondescript" entity Kaplan had dubbed it in his letter. Almost as disheartening to Peterson was the realization that the crises of the last eighteen months would amount to little more than fodder for a young Epidemic Intelligence Service officer wishing to ingratiate himself at the agency's annual epidemiology conference. Most unsettling, however, was the investigators' continued intractable, even simpleminded approach to the problem. Cheney and Peterson were well acquainted with the variables in Epstein-Barr virus laboratory testing. These variables hardly meant that people weren't sick or that the unusual clustering of illness at the lake was a product of two doctors' fantasies. Vastly more than fifteen patients in the Alder Street practice had been disabled for periods longer than two months, as the government maintained. Yet Kaplan seemed to find in these variables a reason to ignore the crux of the matter: the epidemic nature of the syndrome. The government's first official words on Incline avoided any indication that something out of the ordinary had occurred there.

Jake Lindsay had first called Paul Cheney in the summer of 1985, a period during which Cheney and his partner were diagnosing an average of fifteen new patients a week with the chronic malady.

"I didn't know at first who he was," Cheney recalled later. "And his call came in with a jumble of calls from people far less knowledgeable. But I kind of gradually began to get a sense of his power and his interest."

By the end of that year, the relationship among Peterson, Cheney, and Lindsay was cemented by mutual esteem and a shared passion for the medical conundrum consuming their lives. Lindsay was an invaluable resource. The ailing cardiologist was creating an international network of bench researchers and clinical investigators, who were inching toward discovery in this ponderous medical dilemma; he was the linchpin at its center.

"His letters are marvelous," Cheney recalled some years later. "What he'll do is he'll start out by saying, 'The following things have been observed.' And then he'll indent into microprint from his computer and give you an abstract paragraph from an article. Then he'll go back into big print and develop ideas. Then he'll sweep back into microprint and then sweep out into his own ideas. It's a very powerful, persuasive technique to researchers, because he's not just a guy giving his ideas; he's going into peer review material, extracting that, making his point, coming back. He's continuously connecting himself with valid scientific information. He comes across as kind of a scientist, which he is. Because he is committed to the scientific method—he's not a crazy who wants to proselytize a pet idea."

It was not until late in December that Cheney happened to mention to Lindsay the false-positive results on the five Nevada patients sampled for HTLV1.

When Lindsay proposed offhandedly that the results produced by Biotech might actually have been false *negatives,* it was quickly apparent to him that Cheney's enthusiasm for the retrovirus theory had never really died. Lindsay then described the Key West epidemic to Cheney and the Wistar Institute's preliminary evidence for retrovirus infection in multiple sclerosis. The two men shared their suspicion that the disease being diagnosed as multiple sclerosis in the Keys might actually be something else—something akin, if not identical, to the disabling neurologic disease prevalent in Tahoe.

"That's when Lindsay suggested I send the samples to Elaine DeFreitas," Cheney recalled.

Cheney had heard of neither the scientist nor her institution, but he trusted Lindsay's recommendation. By outward appearances, the Centers for Disease Control was remaining inert, and he knew commercial laboratories like Specialty Labs lacked the resources and expertise to settle a problem of such magnitude. The doctor was impatient. Perhaps, he reasoned, the enigma would be resolved only within the confines of a high-powered independent research institution, as Lindsay portrayed the Wistar to him.

Philadelphia, Pennsylvania

"Paul started calling me," Elaine DeFreitas remembered later. "In the beginning I had the same response to him as to [Lindsay]. I would listen. What he was telling me about these patients was fascinating, and his theories and experiments were very interesting. And he seemed absolutely convinced that there was a retrovirus involved in this. And I would tell him, 'I'm [working] on multiple sclerosis. I can only handle one disease at a time.' But he was *so* persistent. Finally I decided that the quickest way of shutting him up was to take five or six patients, to run the samples—to do what we could do with them here. And they were all going to be negative—I was absolutely convinced of it. And then I could tell him they were negative, and then he would stop calling me."

Cheney sent DeFreitas samples from each of the four patients whose sera had been tested first at Specialty Labs, then at Biotech, for HTLV1. The doctor hoped for a rapid answer, but days, then weeks, passed without word from DeFreitas.

Incline Village, Nevada

By early December, the acrimony seemed to be spreading from Cheney and Peterson's competitors to the population at large. Together the clinicians agonized about whether to continue on the course on which the epidemic had launched them. Some of their distress revolved around finances. "The epidemic cost the practice money because we paid for—and Dan is still paying for—tests that insurance companies would not cover, such as the immunologic studies, which were new technologies," Cheney recalled some years later. "A lot of the insurance companies began balking and saying, 'We don't even have a code for this disease, so we're not going to pay you.'. . . We had this negative cash drain, having to pay for people's tests we felt obligated to order.

"But I think we felt trapped. I mean, what were we going to do with these people? Tell them we weren't going to see them anymore, or only see the ones who could pay? Obviously there came a point when we had to decide whether we were going to get into this or avoid it like the plague," Cheney added. "We decided to get into it. And I think one statement . . . says something about Dan," Cheney continued, laughing as he spoke. "He said, 'Paul, we're going to have to get ours in heaven, 'cause we're sure as hell not going to get it here.' "

As winter settled upon the lake and the towns along its shoreline, a number of those afflicted with the Tahoe flu were marking their one-year anniversaries. Sandy Schmidt, the marathon runner, Sonny Dukes, the biker, and Joyce Reynolds, the bank teller, were virtual shut-ins. Reynolds's son, a registered nurse who lived in San Francisco, had ceased visiting his mother with his children for fear that she might infect them; Reynolds's relationship with her husband was growing increasingly brittle.

Andy Antonucci, whose health had been deteriorating since midsummer, was unable to return to teaching that fall. The headache Antonucci had experienced every waking moment for the last several months was now so painful it was nearly blinding. Perhaps the most remarkable aspect of Antonucci's decline was his progressive inability to do algebra. He "was beginning to suffer from a sort of dementia," Cheney recalled. "He couldn't manipulate numbers anymore, which was very strange for a math teacher. The more complex the problem, the more dysfunctional he became."

Gerald Kennedy, the auto mechanics and drafting teacher, had recovered from a case of bacterial pneumonia that resulted in his hospitalization in September. But while antibiotics had cured his pneumonia, nothing ameliorated the other symptoms that were now hard upon him; they included paralyzing weakness, migraine headaches, irregular heartbeats, dizziness, and an inability to think straight. There was little question of his returning to school. Instead, Kennedy remained housebound, watching the days slip by on the calendar. Like his wife of twenty-eight years, herself bedridden for six months, the normally sanguine man was sliding into a depression that occasionally veered into the realm of suicide.

Julie Pritchard, who, like the Kennedys, had been conscripted as a bona fide "case" by Gary Holmes, was becoming more disabled as well, after a short spell during which she thought she might be recovering. She had missed most of the first month of school that year and was extremely distraught. Her brief remission had been a cruelly frustrating experience. She dreaded another winter of illness.

Irene Baker was yet another Truckee High teacher who remained disabled.

Biker Sonny Dukes was exhibiting a kind of despair typical of most sufferers. "I'm a fighter," he said during a conversation late one afternoon in his small house near the lake. "But there are days when I can't even get out of bed. I don't remember what it feels like to feel good." While his collie idly licked Dukes's tattooed hands and leather-banded wrists, the biker described his head-on collision with a Kenworth semitrailer truck in Powell, Idaho, while riding his Harley back to Lake Tahoe the year before. The 260-pound man had flown 40 feet over the nose of the truck and rolled 300 feet down an embankment. He wasn't wearing a helmet. "A Kenworth can't kill me," Dukes said, "but this virus might. I've been through a lot of shit in my life," he added. "I've done things normal people just fantasize about. I would take on a Kenworth again, but this thing scares me, because you've got no way to fight it. You keep hoping there's going to be good news tomorrow—" Unable to continue, Dukes hung his head and cried.

Harvard Medical School, Boston, Massachusetts

Of all those whose names Cheney jotted on his list of experts that fall, Anthony Komaroff was the most captivated by the epidemic as it was presented to him by the clinician.

"We had received a number of calls from around the country by the time Tony called us," Cheney remembered later. "He was just a Harvard doctor who had some interest in this, and so we gave him the litany of stuff—the brain scans, the lymphomas, Yerington. And of course all he could say was 'Let me think about it, and I'll get back to you.' "

It isn't difficult to imagine the excitement Komaroff must have felt as he listened to Cheney's eventful story. Komaroff had been tracking the same entity in his New England patients for some time, albeit without the support or confirmation of his Harvard colleagues. Even more compelling to the doctor was the fact that just one year had elapsed between the upsurge of victims at the Brigham and the Tahoe outbreak. Komaroff would say much later that he had no proof that his patients were part of an epidemic. "When you're a doctor in a big city," he explained, "it's nearly impossible to spot an outbreak of something unless it's like the influenza epidemic, which is *so* big that it's obvious." Tahoe was another matter. "What [Cheney] was describing was nearly identical to what I had been seeing in Boston for two years. What was different was that Tahoe was a small community where apparently a reasonably large number of people had become ill in a pretty limited time period. That's what intrigued me—that a very similar-sounding illness had happened in what sounded like an outbreak."

Komaroff, in short, glimpsed in tiny Incline Village, Nevada, what the Centers for Disease Control's young epidemiologists and their superiors had missed: a chance to probe the etiology, routes of contagion, and risk factors of a new disease. A similar undertaking would be vastly more difficult in a metropolis like Boston.

Shortly after Christmas, Komaroff called Cheney again. "I've got an idea," he said.

The Harvard doctor proposed that he come west and, with Cheney and Peterson's aid, undertake the scientific inquiry that the government had failed to perform. It would be a classic epidemiological study, Komaroff promised. He would provide detailed questionnaires; he would collect blood samples from every patient as well as from controls. Statistical analysis of the data would be performed at Harvard. He indicated he would enlist, in addition, a network of collaborators in Boston and at the National Institutes of Health, the federal agency that had provided grants to him to pursue other areas of research in the past. In addition, he continued, the team would have the luxury of comparing two geographically distinct populations of patients, those from Nevada and northern California, and those from New England.

The doctors were elated. At the very least, they imagined, the collaboration would serve to rehabilitate their decimated reputations. More important, a study such as Komaroff described was likely to see publication in a major medical journal. The involvement of a well-connected Harvard researcher would help make the subject matter palatable to medical journal editors.

"What I wanted, I guess," Peterson remembered later, his features conveying an ironic awareness of his naïveté, "was to impress somebody like the National Institutes of Health or Harvard, who would then say, 'Thanks for tipping us off to this. We're going to take it from here. We're going to bail you out of debt. We're going to set up a ten-year study. All you have to do is fill out our forms.' "

1986
AIDS MINOR

No men among us need refreshment and renovating more frequently than those who occupy positions in our schools of learning. Upon none does intellectual staleness more readily steal "with velvet step, unheeded, softly," but nonetheless relentlessly. . . . These unrefreshed, unregenerate teachers are often powerful instruments of harm, and time and again have spread the blight of blind conservatism in the profession. Safely enthroned in assured positions, men of strong and ardent convictions, with faithful friends and still more faithful students, they too often come within the scathing condemnation of the blind leaders of the blind, of those who would neither themselves enter into the profession of new knowledge nor suffer those who would enter.

—Sir William Osler, *Counsels and Ideals*

6

The Prepared Mind

Miami, Florida

After finishing his airbus training in Toulouse, Mayhugh Horne had returned to Miami and begun flying the planes.

"I had good days and bad days," the pilot remembered. "I was always using an awful lot of headache remedies. And I went from being a person who would jump out of bed at six A.M. to someone who could barely wake up. Among pilots, the ability to be very sharp upon waking is something you're proud of.

"At first I noticed I was having difficulties with numbers," he continued. "We have a navigational system, and it requires precise insertion of numbers. I found I was making more mistakes than I normally would have made. Someone always does a full double check, but you don't like to be wrong."

Horne assumed that his intellectual problems were a transient effect of his headaches. He presumed the headaches and fatigue were temporary, as well. Coasting on a surge of optimism about his future, Horne put in a bid at Pan Am for training on the 747. Like any ardent pilot, he was eager to fly the highly rated planes, and piloting the bigger equipment commanded a bigger salary. The airline accepted Horne's bid. Much of the training took place in a newly constructed climatized Pan Am building in Miami.

"I got *real* sick during the training," Horne remembered.

The symptoms that had leveled him in Toulouse returned full force. The headaches grew worse. Some days he wondered if he had a brain tumor. He was able to numb the pain somewhat with Panadol, but he couldn't control the mental spaciness that was afflicting him. Frequently Horne sat alone in the simulator cockpit provided by the FAA to test his piloting skills. Occasionally, when his symptoms were mild, he performed well. During a period when he felt ill, he was able to lift the plane from the runway and establish his flight pattern on four successive attempts, but on each of the four landings, Horne crashed the plane. What should have been a three-week training session turned into a five-month ordeal. Horne's training was interrupted countless times when he succumbed to his symptoms and returned to South Carolina, where he and his family were now living, to recoup his strength.

Horne had been flying for twenty-eight years, since he was twenty-one. He was what the air force called a triple-rated monster: a certified jet pilot, navigator, and radar observer. During the Vietnam War, Horne flew cargo and supplies into the war zone. In the early 1960s, as part of the United Nations peacekeeping force during the Congo War, he flew missions into Zaire that few pilots would have dared to undertake. A career officer, Horne was about to be promoted to captain when he left the air force in 1966. "The airlines were hiring," he said. "I knew the job market was going to be saturated by 1975, when I would have retired from the air force." He joined Pan Am, then the biggest and most glamorous of the international airlines. For the next two decades, based in Berlin for a significant portion of them, he flew passenger jets to Australia, Pago Pago, Tahiti, Singapore, Bali, Hong Kong, London, Paris, Frankfurt, and Buenos Aires.

Horne's robust physique and sterling flight record likely made it hard for his colleagues and superiors at Pan Am to believe anything could be seriously wrong with him that year. Horne, in contrast, was certain something had gone haywire in his brain. He decided to seek an opinion at Duke University's medical center in Durham, North Carolina. "I didn't want to go up for my line check on the 747 until I found out what was wrong with me," Horne said. "So I went to Duke for three days. They did a CAT scan. There were no problems—they could not come up with anything. The only thing I had was an allergy to smoke and dust."

Horne passed the FAA line check. He began flying 747s from Miami to London, Paris, and South American cities. He found himself humiliated near the end of the long flights when his computations were corrected by junior pilots and engineers. "Say you started at midnight out of Miami and you're flying down to Rio or Buenos Aires," he said. "You're supposed to be at your best at the landing phase. And when you're doing a landing by controls, an instrument landing, and you've flown all night—well, I noticed it was requiring much more effort than it normally did. It was apparent to me and to the other pilots." Afterward Horne would collapse in his Buenos Aires hotel room and lie motionless for hours, bone-weary but unable to sleep. The flights back were even rougher: "If I started a trip, I finished it. But after a while I was just holding on with my fingernails."

Truckee, California

Andy Antonucci, thinking he might be able to teach again, had made a tepid reentry into the working world earlier that year. He returned to Truckee High to teach two periods of algebra in the morning. "It was all I could do to get through these two periods," he recalled later. "I would come home and totally collapse." Although his primary symptoms were extraordinary fatigue and chronic head pain, his intellectual infirmities interfered most dramatically with his work. "I remember once I was standing at the blackboard," Antonucci recalled. "I was about to demonstrate a math problem to my students. All of a sudden my mind went completely blank. For few seconds I forgot what I was doing. When I remembered what I was doing, I could not remember what I should be doing *next*. I didn't know how to solve the problem."

When school ended in June, Antonucci decided to wait until the summer was over before deciding whether or not to return to school in September. "I knew by August that I wouldn't be able to go back for the new semester," Antonucci said.

"I was really very depressed over the fact that I would not be teaching that fall and that perhaps, as far as I knew, I might not ever be able to go back."

Yerington, Nevada

During the remaining winter months and the early spring, approximately one hundred more Yerington residents came down with the lingering illness. In some cases, several members of the same family were afflicted. Martha James (a pseudonym), a forty-six-year-old bank employee, and her two adult children were all diagnosed with the disease by Yerington clinician Judy Hilbisch. James's twenty-two-year-old daughter, who lived next door to James with her husband and two young children, and James's son, who lived in another part of town entirely, fell ill on the same day. Their mother fell ill not long afterward. Of the three, James's daughter, Sally Bentson (a pseudonym), was the most severely afflicted, bedridden by weakness, headaches, and extreme pain in the muscles and joints of her upper body. After two months Bentson began to feel better. At one point, in fact, she believed she had almost recovered. But just as she seemed to be over the disease, she relapsed. The second bout, Bentson said, "was much more devastating, physically and emotionally. I really did not want to go on." The young woman slept for long hours, often round the clock. Her mother would come next door periodically to wake Bentson in order to feed her. "This is just an incredible, *different* kind of sickness," Bentson said years afterward. "I remember saying to myself, 'I don't care if I never wake up, because I just cannot do this anymore.' "

Incline Village, Nevada

Julie Pritchard's attempt to resume teaching in the fall served only to exacerbate her symptoms. It was as if the disease were wired to a rheostat under the control of a malevolent hand; any effort to transcend it was met with another cruel twist of the dial. A month into the school year, subdued again by the malaise that had defined her life for ten months, she abandoned her grade-school class. Her husband, the first of the Tahoe-Truckee High teachers to fall ill, had returned to work, though he continued to complain of exhaustion and a kind of persistent absent-mindedness.

On January 10, 1986, Pritchard underwent her eighth office consultation with Paul Cheney in as many months. She reported that her headaches were unceasing. Her eyesight was increasingly affected; blurred vision and "floaters," specks of black in the visual periphery, were an everyday occurrence. She haltingly described to Cheney a new frustration: her inability to keep her mind on one thought long enough to act upon it. Her concentration problems alone, she said, guaranteed she would be unable to teach anytime in the foreseeable future. By her own account, she was experiencing dramatic mood shifts as well. She would weep, but in the middle of wrenching sobs she would begin to laugh; moments later the crying would begin anew.

Cheney and Peterson already had observed that a number of their epidemic patients were emotionally labile, or mercurial. Both James Jones and Stephen Straus had included emotional lability in their descriptions of patients in the *Annals* the year before. Straus favored a psychiatric basis for the symptom, theorizing that such distress "may reflect [patients'] poor adaptation to a debilitating illness that can be considered psychosomatic to the casual observer." The Alder Street clinicians, however, were loath to ascribe the epic mood swings in patients like Pritchard to vagaries of "poor adaptation." Based on the mounting number of abnormal brain scans, the Nevada clinicians wondered if the condition was related to a larger problem of organic brain dysfunction. On February 11, Cheney asked Pritchard to submit to a magnetic resonance imaging brain scan. The news from Reno was bad: the forty-year-old had numerous small lesions in the white matter of her occipital lobe.

Pritchard was, Cheney had begun to suspect, a classic case. Her particular constellation of signs and symptoms might even be the pure form of the disease that he and his partner had been seeking: virtually every test of the teacher's immune system and neurologic integrity had revealed disturbing abnormalities. She was especially compelling to him, in addition, because she had been a part of a discrete outbreak: the Truckee teachers.

Raleigh, North Carolina

In January, seven members of the North Carolina orchestra were still disabled by "mono." Their ages ranged from thirty-three to forty-four. That month an eighth player fell suddenly and severely ill. Initially the thirty-two-year-old woman was diagnosed with viral meningitis, a sometimes deadly brain infection. Later, when she survived, the local doctor changed her diagnosis to mononucleosis. In all, eight musicians in the fifty-eight-member orchestra—or 12 percent of the orchestra—now had the chronic illness.

Lyndonville, New York

By late spring, David Bell had determined that, in the four months between September 1985 and January 1986, about twenty-five people in his practice, sixteen of them children, had become ill with the strange ailment that had afflicted the sledding party. The children ranged in age from seven to eighteen; the adults were as young as twenty-eight and as old as fifty-two. For months, these patients had suffered intermittently from sore throats, low-grade fevers, swollen lymph nodes, crushing fatigue, and, occasionally, swollen spleens and livers. Their more curious symptoms—rashes, eye pain and extreme sensitivity to light, migraine headaches, tinnitus, and earaches, numbness, joint pain, chest pain, nausea—endowed the entity with its conspicuous, if peculiar, signature.

The doctor was startled when he identified another entire family among the new score of patients. He had painstakingly itemized its members' symptoms and the conspicuous pattern had emerged the way a photographic image materializes on the blank paper. Bell's observation raised the number of family clusters in his practice to three, and it crystallized a thought that had been, until then, just a suspicion. "This was obviously a disease in families," the doctor said.

Two percent of the population of Lyndonville was now suffering from the disorder.

Incline Village, Nevada

Harvard researcher Anthony Komaroff arrived in Incline Village on February 23, accompanied by two Harvard Medical School fellows. One of them, internal medicine specialist Dedra Buchwald, was helping Komaroff determine the frequency of the disease among patients in his general medicine clinic at the Brigham. The third member of the team, Nicholas Fiebach, had no particular stake in the malady but had been encouraged by Buchwald to "more or less volunteer," as Buchwald phrased it, for the Incline trip.

"Their attitude and perception of this problem was far different from CDC's," Cheney later remarked. "These people had a gleam in their eye. They abstracted twice as many charts as the CDC in a third of the time. So that means they were almost six times faster. I think the CDC looked at ninety charts," Cheney added. "Komaroff looked at one hundred and seventy, one hundred and eighty. Komaroff was abstracting charts for four days. Holmes and crew were there for three weeks."

A month before his arrival, Komaroff had sent a batch of questionnaires to the Alder Street clinic, which the Nevada doctors distributed to their patients. It was a hybrid version of the questionnaire the Harvard team was using to ferret out bona fide cases of the disease in the Brigham clinic and a questionnaire that Cheney and Peterson had devised for their own use. Upon arrival, Komaroff and his fellows studied patients' charts along with their recently completed questionnaires. (The Boston trio did not go mountain hiking, nor did they sample the casinos.) Unlike their government predecessors, either Komaroff or Buchwald met nearly all of the patients, each of whom was invited to the Alder Street clinic to provide a blood sample. In four days they enrolled 178 patients in their study. Fiebach's job was to draw blood from each one, which he did day after day until the team's departure.

"We got chart abstracts, questionnaires, blood—the whole epidemiological kit and caboodle—in four days," Dedra Buchwald said later. "It was pretty wild."

If the Harvard investigators made the Centers for Disease Control look inept, one could argue in the agency's defense that Komaroff had an advantage over Gary Holmes and Jon Kaplan. The federal researchers were like hunters assigned to bring down a mythical beast they had never seen and weren't convinced existed. Komaroff had not only tracked the beast longer, he had made numerous sightings and had been close enough on many occasions to actually feel and smell it. Further, the Harvard doctor had a powerful intuition about the authenticity of the Nevada epidemic. Any doubts he might have entertained were dispelled on the second day of his stay, when he abandoned his research fellows on Alder Street and, in a late-model rental car, sped through the desert along the flat, monotonous route to Yerington. The doctor turned right at the green interstate sign announcing the town and drove directly to the medical office occupying the front rooms of the narrow shingled house where Judy Hilbisch practiced.

"It was my intention when we came out," Komaroff said some time later, "to include Yerington in a serious study."

The doctor's ambition withered soon after his arrival. He rapidly deemed the Yerington outbreak far too elusive for study: too little investigation at the height of the outbreak had resulted in a dearth of medical records. Now, it seemed to Komaroff, reconstruction of the breadth and natural history of the Yerington outbreak would be impossible. The epidemic on the north shore of Lake Tahoe was different. Cheney and Peterson's sweeping inquiries into their patients' immunologic and neurologic status, as well as the doctors' documentation of each twist and turn in their patients' medical histories, had generated not only insights into the pathophysiology of the disease but also a database from which to launch a retrospective study. Swallowing his disappointment, Komaroff met and examined approximately twenty Yerington patients that day. In doing so, he made an important discovery, one that would cement his fascination for the disease even more solidly.

"Between November of 1985 and March of 1986," Komaroff recalled some time later, "there appeared to be a sudden increase in that community of an illness that was very much like the illness we saw in Tahoe, that probably involved from one hundred to two hundred people, of whom I was only able to meet about twenty, and study fewer because the medical data were not complete. The impressions that I had were, first, that this was a world apart from Incline Village and the surrounding communities," the doctor continued. "It was demographically and socioeconomically a completely different situation. And, second, as it was described, it sounded like the same illness. The fact that it was such a different population of people was important in that regard, because many of them, for example, were and are farmers and had no disability insurance. [They had] nothing to gain and everything to lose from being ill."

Jimmy Dunlap, the junior high student who had been disabled for several months, was among the patients Komaroff met that day. The boy's brain problems were then so severe that he was unable to stand without tipping over; his parents supported him on either side as he entered the examining room. During one test, a measure of brain integrity known as Romberg's sign, the doctor asked Dunlap to stand with arms outstretched and eyes closed. When the boy began to sway, Komaroff leaped from his chair to support him. Komaroff experienced a frisson of recognition. He had observed a similar result in a minority of his New England patients with the chronic malady, although they appeared to be less debilitated than the Dunlap boy. The doctor also met Russ Colletta, the Yerington high school principal, and several patients who worked at the Lyon County Courthouse.

Cheney recalled that the Harvard doctor was exhilarated upon his return to Incline. "Tony was very excited that night," Cheney said, "because this had been increasingly characterized as a yuppie disease. And unfortunately Incline *is* a yuppie place. Well, Tony found out that it wasn't a yuppie disease when he went to Yerington."

Komaroff's harried presence in Nevada made the front page of the *North Lake Tahoe Bonanza*. The doctor and his support team were photographed at work in Cheney's office; the photograph and accompanying story ran just below the paper's logo. In addition, ninety-five locals, most of them victims of the Tahoe malady or their relatives, attended a community meeting convened by Cheney, Peterson, and Komaroff, during which Komaroff answered questions about his research.

The Harvard cachet failed to mend the credibility gap created by the federal investigators. Skepticism about the validity of the disease abounded outside the Alder Street clinic. The hospital's nursing staff, formerly respectful of the internists and eager to please them, had become increasingly uncooperative. Not only were doctors in Incline Village maligning them, but doctors in Truckee and Reno were beginning to scoff at the phenomenon, too. Charles Goodman, a radiologist at the Tahoe Forest Hospital in Truckee, was typical. Goodman attended a medical staff meeting at his hospital where Paul Cheney discussed the disease during the winter of 1986. Before Cheney was finished speaking, an agitated Goodman stood and, in a raised voice, disputed Cheney on the matter of the magnetic resonance imaging findings. "There are no doctors that I know of on this staff," he said later, "who would render that diagnosis. We haven't seen any good evidence that it exists. My feeling is that people are going to get bored with this disease and eventually it's going to disappear."

By the end of February, Cheney and Peterson were beginning to feel a pressing need to settle the matter of their patients' sanity. Royce Biddle's findings of multiple brain lesions added fuel to their growing conviction that their patients were the luckless victims of an infectious organic process that injured the brain. It was manifestly obvious, however, that they would need even harder evidence to convince the rest of the world.

Berkeley, California

Sheila Bastien was captivated when the Nevada internist called that winter. She had heard of the syndrome Paul Cheney was describing, but mostly as it was discussed in the lay press and, she would later confess, at dinner parties in the expensive Berkeley Hills neighborhood where she lived. She had no idea it was so sweeping in its impact, nor had she realized it was such a frankly neurological disease.

Bastien was a Jungian psychotherapist, but her second, more consuming discipline was the little-known field of neuropsychology, a specialty that throughout the previous decade had propelled her into the curious, often tragic world of the brain-injured. Her patients were referred to her by doctors seeking to understand the source of their patients' complaints, and by courts and lawyers who sought objective documentation of head injuries, including those caused by medical malpractice. Sometimes the problem was congenital, like arterial malformations in the brain. Far more frequently, the harm occurred after birth. Included among her many hundreds of cases were people who had suffered traumatic injuries to the head or been exposed to intolerable levels of toxic chemicals. An even larger portion of those sent to her for neuropsychological evaluation were victims of diseases that forcefully undermine brain integrity, like Alzheimer's, Addison's, myasthenia gravis, brain tumors, and multiple sclerosis.

"And of course I saw patients who just had depression—and every other psychiatric disorder, too," Bastien said during an interview some years later.

Cheney and Peterson became aware of Bastien and her specialty when one of Peterson's patients, a San Francisco resident in her twenties, showed the doctor a report Bastien had written about her condition. The woman had been ill with an undetermined illness since 1978, but in 1985 she was accidentally exposed to formaldehyde on her job in a print shop. The woman's long-standing fatigue and "mental spaciness" became completely disabling after the chemical exposure. Her San Francisco doctor had referred her to Bastien for further evaluation. Cheney and Peterson were particularly impressed by the apparent sensitivity of Bastien's tests, which measured not just general IQ, for example, but also a multitude of cognitive functions, including abstract and concrete reasoning abilities, judgment and logic, visual-spatial relationships, and several categories of memory skills. Cheney called her immediately.

"He described a neurological syndrome to me," Bastien recalled. "He talked about discalculia [inability to perform math problems], gait disturbances, balance problems, memory disturbances, word-finding problems, severe headaches, and increased cranial pressure on spinal taps. He even told me about a small portion of people who had had seizures. And he described some of the biological markers, like the Epstein-Barr antibodies and the T-cell helper-suppressor ratios. He said a lot of [body] systems were involved, but that he and his partner thought it was probably a neurological problem."

In March, Cheney arranged for one of his patients, a Nevada postal worker, to go to Berkeley for testing. The woman, who had one of the worst magnetic resonance imaging scans of all of the Tahoe patients and who seemed to be among the most mentally impaired, was eager for help from any quarter. Bastien made the woman's test scores available to Cheney soon afterward. "She was grossly abnormal," Cheney remembered.

Bastien, a diminutive, bright-eyed woman in her mid-fifties, described neuropsychologists as "gatekeepers" who patrol the ragged, war-torn boundaries between medical and psychiatric diagnoses. "Many medical disorders present as psychological disturbances," she said. "Pancreatic cancer can cause visual hallucinations. Adrenal tumors will cause behavior that can seem psychotic. So you have to be very careful not to accept psychiatric diagnoses at face value. One in ten of my patients who is referred to me for depression, for instance, turns out to have hypothyroidism. Recently," she continued, "a patient was sent to me labeled 'depressed.' She had a master's degree from Berkeley and she's a working professional. When I asked her to draw a person, she did a drawing that was at the level of a two- to three-year-old child. She's not just depressed; I think it's early dementia. It's not that I don't respect and understand that some problems are psychological," Bastien added. "But I have an ax to grind, as it were, in seeing psychologists clean up their act and physicians clean up theirs so there aren't so many false negatives."

In the next several weeks Peterson and Cheney referred a handful of patients to Bastien. Her curiosity was piqued by the visibly distressed people who made their shaky way from the Sierras to the redwood-sided house in Berkeley where she had her office. While they *appeared* to be normal, she noted, they often had difficulty performing the simplest tasks, beginning with untying the latch on a wooden gate to gain entry to her front yard. More than once she had to send her adolescent son to meet the fumbling patient at the sidewalk. She noted that, unlike Alzheimer's patients, a majority of whom expressed puzzlement about the necessity of being tested, the Nevada patients were excruciatingly aware of their disabilities.

"I was very stimulated by trying to identify the pattern of impairment in these patients," Bastien remembered. "You go into any of these psychological testing sessions like a detective. You know, What is it we have here? What is the pattern? And I remember thinking that if I were testing nothing but Alzheimer's patients, then I would say, 'This group isn't very impaired.' But they were *more* impaired than the head concussion cases that I've tested that have been in litigation. And they were more impaired than the average chemical-injury patient. It was also worse than hypothyroid conditions I've tested for and, in some cases, worse than brain tumors. And it looked worse than most of your average depressions. This ain't no little thing. In a normal, healthy person, we would not expect to have results in the severe range. A little anxiety might put someone into the mild range— but not the severe. I was concerned about these people."

Incline Village, Nevada

Before Christmas, during one of his frequent literature searches for clues to the confounding Tahoe malady, Cheney had come upon Seymour Grufferman's *New England Journal* paper about an outbreak of apparently contagious lymphomas in an American family. Cheney called the epidemiologist and, sensing his interest, invited him to Incline. The overture served as the final impetus for Grufferman, whose curiosity about events in Nevada had been escalating as a result of press reports and correspondence with the family member who worried she had carried the cancer pathogen to Nevada and launched the epidemic. He promised to come west that winter. Although Grufferman eventually would report that his experience in the High Sierras was "fascinating," his efforts there ended in frustration.

The investigator was a small, studious figure typically attired in tweeds and suspenders. In the course of his career, Grufferman had acquired three doctorates in epidemiology, an achievement that led him to boast on more than one occasion that, among that fraternity, he was best qualified to undertake epidemiology on the new disease. Although his claim was likely true, Grufferman's eventual contributions had less to do with his credentials than with his mind-set. "Chance favors the prepared mind," he often said in homage to Louis Pasteur.

Few among his brethren in epidemiology focused Grufferman's wrath around this philosophical sticking point like the Centers for Disease Control's epidemic intelligence team assigned to investigate the Nevada outbreak. Grufferman was confounded by the frank disbelief with which Gary Holmes and Jon Kaplan had approached the epidemic, particularly given their opportunity to immerse themselves in territory unsullied by other investigators.

"I don't understand it," Grufferman said. "Maybe it's because I don't have an infectious disease background. But I think I've had pretty rigorous scientific training, which really trains you to be open-minded and to consider all possibilities. And I think unusual distributions of new diseases offer potential clues for gaining new knowledge. And to close your mind and dismiss it out of hand is, to me, absurd and very nonscientific. Holmes and Kaplan came in with preconceived notions and just missed an extremely interesting situation. Those guys *weren't* prepared."

In Grufferman's opinion, the government's investigators were further taxed by an inbred arrogance pervading agency staff. "The CDC has this notion," he said. "It's sort of the Peace Corps mentality that any one of ours can do better than the best of yours. And so they send out these inexperienced investigators. Very often they find nice things because it's so obvious. But they also botch things up."

Unlike the CDC's youthful epidemiologists, unlike even Komaroff, each of whom came to Tahoe with a bias either against or in favor of the disease, Grufferman had no bias at all; he was merely curious. "I was just approaching this as an investigator who'd done lots of field investigations to see if I could piece together some ideas as to what might be done," he said. "And I was curious to learn more about the disease."

The investigator stayed in Nevada for three days. He spent his nights at the lakeside Hyatt, his days at the Alder Street clinic. He met several patients and, with Paul Cheney's help, took blood samples from them. As Grufferman began to interview patients, he quickly concluded that too much probing had already occurred; it was the old problem of suggestibility in a population that had been scrutinized and examined by multiple investigators over time. By the end of his second day, Grufferman had begun to view Tahoe as a horribly squandered opportunity.

"The major evidence was a footprint in the mud," he said, "and a herd of elephants had gone through and trampled it." The elephant herd he referred to was, of course, the government's foot soldiers, Gary Holmes and Jon Kaplan, followed by the team from Boston. But Grufferman included even Paul Cheney in his turbulent imagery. "Paul meant well," Grufferman said, "but he was so puzzled by the epidemic and so desperate to get help that he got too much help. Basically," he continued, "there was no way that I could do anything systematic that would be unbiased given the numerous investigators who had already been there asking questions. You really want to ask the questions once, and ask them well."

The scientist departed Nevada under a cloud of melancholy.

Children's Hospital of Philadelphia, Philadelphia, Pennsylvania

Complementing the avid interest of the Harvard investigators, international Epstein-Barr virus expert Werner Henle continued to provide the intellectual foundation for Cheney and Peterson's ideas that winter. The Henles, like the Alder Street clinicians, believed that the world's most ubiquitous known virus, Epstein-Barr, was blameless in the drama at Tahoe. "In my opinion, and I believe you share it," Henle wrote to Cheney on December 10, "the evidence does not implicate EBV as the cause of the Lake Tahoe epidemic." Additionally, given the time-space clustering described to them by Cheney, the Henles were persuaded that the high levels of Epstein-Barr virus antibodies observed in sufferers suggested immunological damage from an altogether different source, likely an infectious agent which, Henle wrote, "activated . . . latent EBV infections."

In December, Cheney had sent twenty-nine blood samples to the Henle lab to make sure that the Sierra Nevada Laboratories in Reno, which by then were processing most of the blood from the Tahoe patients, were meeting the gold standard of the Henle lab. Cheney had begun staging the disease, categorizing patients simply as "sick or recently sick," and "not so sick or improving."

On January 10, Henle, calling the affliction under investigation the "Lake Tahoe disease," reported his results: "I am pleased to inform you that we were able to confirm in principle the EBV-specific serological results recorded by the Sierra Nevada Laboratories. The 'sick or recently sick' patients had a geometric mean [Epstein-Barr Virus] antibody titer about 2.5-fold higher than controls. . . . The 'not so sick or improving patients' had overall lower [titers] but their [geometric mean titer] was still 1.5 times above that of the controls."

Cheney had also told the elderly virologist about the Wistar Institute project to investigate five Tahoe cases for retroviral infection. In response, Henle exhibited a temperament for which great scientists are remembered. "It would be most surprising if HTLV1 would turn out to be the cause," he wrote, "but right now we have to have an open mind and await confirmation. . . . I shall be interested to learn the final disposition of this very puzzling situation."

Wistar Institute, Philadelphia, Pennsylvania

Paul Cheney's hope for the rapid identification of the mystery agent causing the disease in Nevada and elsewhere was crushed that month upon hearing from Elaine DeFreitas. Although she had found some suggestions of retroviral infection in the five tissue samples from Nevada, ultimately DeFreitas could not call her results positive.

The immunologist and her assistants had been using several techniques for finding evidence of HTLV1, all of them more sensitive than the Biotech test kit used at Specialty Labs in Los Angeles. Initially she had detected antibody known as the P24 core protein, which was known to be a product of a number of retroviruses, in three samples. "They weren't *dramatically* positive. . . . But it looked like *something*," DeFreitas said later. She called Cheney with her results: "Elaine could not explain why [the patients] had an antibody to P24," Cheney remembered. "And I had the feeling we were at an impasse, except that she agreed to do two more things. First, she agreed to take whole blood and attempt to assay for reverse transcriptase." Reverse transcriptase, an enzyme manufactured by retroviruses as they replicate in cells, is a telltale footprint of retrovirus infection and easier to detect than the virus itself. A standard technique for finding reverse transcriptase called for the scientist to grow patients' cells in test tubes for about one week, then search for the substance in the supernatant, a fluid that floats above the cells' surface.

"I was intrigued enough," DeFreitas confirmed, "that I said, 'Okay, we'll look for reverse transcriptase activity.' We could have done a lot of things," she continued, "but at the moment that's what we had up and running for the multiple sclerosis studies. Again, we saw either one or two, as I remember, that were above background level for reverse transcriptase. It looked like there was *something* there," DeFreitas continued, "so we thought we should repeat the tests." DeFreitas and her staff launched a second week of cell-growing, with poor results. "We couldn't get those samples to repeat. We grew the cells a second time, we took off the supernatants again—and now *all* of them are negative."

DeFreitas consented to a final task: she promised Cheney she would sort into categories and count the white cells, or lymphocytes, in his four patients. "Eventually," Cheney said later, "she called and said, 'This is very strange—there is a complete loss of T4 helper cells. Under normal circumstances this should not have happened.' So," Cheney continued, "we had this antibody [to P24] we couldn't explain, and there was an unusual loss of T4 cells." Neither the doctor nor the immunologist knew precisely what the T4 helper cell loss augured for these patients or why it occurred.

With little more at hand to hold DeFreitas's interest, Cheney realized to his immense disappointment that the tantalizing collaboration would end.

DeFreitas, by contrast, was relieved. "I said, 'That's it. It's finished.' I called Paul and told him exactly that. And that kept him quiet—for a while."

Harvard Medical School, Boston, Massachusetts

In the two months since his first call to Cheney, Komaroff had assembled an array of collaborators in Boston and at the National Institutes of Health in Bethesda, Maryland. "Enter the grand old men, the guiding lights in the east," was how Cheney, his tongue gently lodged in his cheek, later characterized the progressive involvement that winter of Komaroff and his network of medical bright lights. Komaroff's recruits were bench researchers who relied on the Harvard doctor to shepherd their efforts; they had little sense of the unique entity Komaroff was so methodically tracking. He characterized their relationships with him as "feel-the-goods collaborations."

At the top of Komaroff's research agenda was an idea Peterson and Cheney had been mulling for more than a year: could the disease be caused by a new, mutant strain of Epstein-Barr virus to which the race lacked immunity? Reports of a "wild-type" isolate of Epstein-Barr in some patients* had been appearing with increasing regularity in the scientific press.[1] Cheney and Peterson, searching for some way to explain the multiple brain lesions in their patients, had been particularly taken with the idea of a wild "lytic," or cell-destroying, strain; something, after all, had to be destroying brain tissue; Epstein-Barr virus was known to immortalize or transform cells rather than destroy them. Months before Komaroff's arrival, on a hunch, Cheney and Peterson had sent Tahoe blood samples to Duke University's Joseph Pagano, an Epstein-Barr virus expert. Pagano earlier had identified a wild strain of the virus that was both lytic *and* transforming, but he reported to the clinicians that he saw nothing unique about the Tahoe strain. In spite of Pagano's negative findings, Komaroff felt the matter of a wild strain remained an open question. He engaged John Sullivan, a University of

---

*Two years earlier, for instance, a Canadian medical journal had reported the case of an eight-year-old child with "chronic, active EBV infection." Researchers had discovered a wild-type isolate of Epstein-Barr virus in her tissues. The most remarkable aspect of the new strain was its cytolytic, or cell-killing, ability. Most Epstein-Barr viruses immortalized rather than destroyed cells. The Canadian researchers claimed theirs was the first documentation of a wild-type strain of the virus that killed cells.

Massachusetts herpes virologist, to look again for a cell-destroying wild-type—or any other unusual isolate—of Epstein-Barr virus in the Nevada patients' blood.

The resurrection of one hypothesis failed to sink another. Komaroff had been as impressed as Peterson and Cheney by the immune system abnormalities that flow cytometrist Susan Wormsley was observing in Tahoe patients, and he was as willing as the Nevada clinicians to entertain the idea of a retroviral cause for the disease. Few pathogens, Komaroff reasoned, seemed guaranteed to hamstring an immune system with greater efficiency than a retrovirus, since it infected the very cells that constituted the immune system. The chronicity of the disease was suggestive, too: the fact that retroviruses integrated themselves into the genetic substances of those cells, thereby avoiding detection and sustaining themselves over periods of years, lifetimes, even generations, hinted at their role in any number of puzzling chronic diseases. Komaroff engaged a retrovirologist at the National Institute of Allergy and Infectious Diseases, Tom Folks, to look for telltale reverse transcriptase in twenty Tahoe samples. Folks was principally an AIDS researcher working in a satellite of Robert Gallo's larger laboratory at the National Cancer Institute. Folks's expertise lay in culturing cells, a scientific discipline better described as an art form; coaxing viruses through their life cycles outside the human body was a task fraught with variables and pitfalls. Finding suitable culture media to support not only cells but the viruses infecting them was the crux of the problem: each new virus represented a cache of unknowns that might be revealed only by painstaking trial and error.

Folks committed himself to a thirty-day experiment with two objectives. First, as Elaine DeFreitas had done, he sought to identify reverse transcriptase in the samples, thereby establishing retroviral activity. Second, he planned to observe the cultures for large or bizarrely shaped cells that would indicate infection with either of the first two retroviruses, HTLV1 or HTLV2. After receiving blood samples from ten Nevada patients, Folks prepared his test-tube cultures. Every three days he studied the supernatant for evidence of reverse transcriptase. The results were always negative. A second, more difficult chore was observing the cultures for signs of unusual cell shapes or cell death. "We looked for changes all the thirty days," Folks remembered, "but the Tahoe blood never looked any different from our control cultures."

By his own admission, Folks's effort, however well intentioned and elegantly performed, nonetheless fell into the quick-and-dirty order of scientific endeavor. "The assay we were using for the reverse transcriptase was made for HIV, so we would likely have missed an oncogenic virus like HTLV," he said. "Our experiment was not done in enough detail to completely rule out the presence of a retrovirus, but that would have taken me six months, and this was a short collaboration. There are many other things that could have been done, but I guess anytime you find negative results based on your philosophy of what you think might be there, you halt your work to preserve assets."

Komaroff engaged a third collaborator at Harvard's Dana-Farber Cancer Institute. Michael Caligiuri, a young immunologist, was an expert in a second nascent realm: natural killer cells, a newly identified class of white blood cells. Natural killer cells were primitive immune system components able to target cancerous or virus-infected cells and promptly destroy them without needing first to develop specific antibodies to them. (Sharks, prehistoric animals, have no other kind of immune cell.) Scientists had been studying the unusual lymphocytes since the early 1970s. Only recently, with the aid of electron microscopy, researchers had revealed the life cycle of natural killer cells to be a remarkable, if infinitesimal, drama. They stalk their target cell, bind to it, then punch the cell's outer membrane full of holes with a "killer protein" called perforin. The virus-infected or cancerous cell sprouts leaks, takes on water, and disintegrates.[2] If the Tahoe disease was initiated by a virus, as Komaroff suspected, then perhaps the illness was perpetuated by an upset in the natural killer cell surveillance system. Reports in the medical literature suggested that viral illness prompted changes in natural killer cell function. During an acute viral infection such as a cold in an otherwise healthy person, natural killer cells increased; in immunodeficient people with severe viral infections, natural killer cell competency was depressed. "Profound depression" of natural killer cell activity had been documented in people suffering from X-linked immunodeficiency syndrome, a genetic disease in which 40 to 50 percent of all patients die from Epstein-Barr virus infection.[3] Komaroff asked Caligiuri to measure not only the numbers of natural killer cells in patients and matched controls, but the cytotoxic, or cell-killing, ability of the cells. Potency might be as crucial as quantity.

Los Angeles, California

In contrast to the small-scale, if high-tech, investigations being conducted in the East, an army of medical quacks and charlatans was conducting its own experiments upon the rising tide of victims in the West. Their efforts were vastly better funded than those of Komaroff, whose collaborators were supporting their investigations with, as Komaroff described it, "midnight oil." These New Age and old-fashioned theorists—herbalists, homeopaths, hypnotists, aroma and massage therapists, psychics, faith healers, even purveyors of snake venom—rushed to fill the void left by mainstream medicine's helplessness and outright neglect, capitalizing on their patients' desperation. Typically, they supplemented their methods with an endless bounty of expensive nonprescription pills and potions.

Flush with their own literature and bywords, these practitioners, once on society's fringes, had come into their own with the AIDS epidemic. By the time the new chronic malady began its ascent in the mid-1980s, this community was firmly in place, ready to embrace an equally desperate constituency of victims of "Epstein-Barr," as the chronic malady increasingly was known. In fact, unlike AIDS, the new ailment lacked established clinical or therapeutic protocols of any kind. As a result, vulnerable sufferers were eased by the gurus of "wellness" into a maelstrom of absurd and costly practices.

Beginning in mid-1986, Epstein-Barr clinics began to emerge in southern California, their existence announced in newspaper and magazine ads. Inevitably the ads promised a cure. Treatment frequently consisted of exercise regimes, massive injections of vitamins or minerals, and possibly stimulants such as amphetamine-based diet pills—all of it prescribed in complex combinations and justified by pseudoscientific rationales. Putatively curative substances either ingested or injected by victims ranged from the relatively benign-sounding bee pollen to the powdered adrenal glands of baby pigs. Exotic physical therapies abounded, including steam baths, acupuncture, acupressure, and colonic irrigation. New Age "healers" promoted biofeedback, relaxation tapes, Zen meditation, visualization, and so on, typified by meditation sessions in which sufferers were instructed to tap their thymus gland at the base of their throat—"the seat of the immune system," claimed the wellness gurus—and to utter statements such as "I profoundly and deeply accept myself just as I am," or to visualize the cells of their immune system vanquishing toxic invaders. The cost of such programs tended to be extravagant, rarely less than several hundred dollars, and occasionally in the thousands. When such regimes failed, as they inevitably did, promoters suggested that ailing consumers look within themselves to discover why they preferred illness to health.

Seductive ads for Epstein-Barr clinics appeared routinely in the *Hollywood Reporter* and *Variety,* the daily bibles of the film and television industries. The ads did not escape the notice of trend-spotters on the opposite coast. Later that year *New York* magazine reported on a disease its editors dubbed "the Hollywood blahs." "A mysterious epidemic is sweeping Hollywood," L.A.-based reporter Steve Pond wrote. "Screenwriters, actors, producers, and studio executives alike are coming down with Epstein-Barr, a nonfatal viral disease that causes deep fatigue and has no known cure." Pond interviewed sufferers, including a screenwriter named Lyn Hemmerdinger.

"It's rampant in the film industry," Hemmerdinger said. "It's hitting cameramen, technicians. Every week I hear about a friend who's got it."

Doctors who had been trained in and adhered to the methods of mainstream medicine were at an ethical crossroads with such patients. Their choice was either to dismiss their complaints, thus encouraging the patients to seek care elsewhere, or to attempt to help them feel better in the absence of any information as to how such a goal might be achieved. Some clinicians chose to treat the disease globally—that is, to level an assault at what they deemed to be the primary source of the symptoms: a dysfunctional immune system. Atlanta infectious disease specialist Richard DuBois, the lead author of the 1984 paper about the disease in the *Southern Medical Journal,* and others infused patients with gamma globulin, a substance made of the pooled blood serum of thousands of donors and rich in antibodies to any number of infectious pathogens, particularly Epstein-Barr virus. Other doctors tried a less sophisticated approach—treating the symptoms. They prescribed anti-inflammatory agents, more typically used in rheumatoid arthritis, for joint and muscle pain; antidepressants for the severe depression that seemed to be universal among victims; and drugs to promote sleep. Common to all of these therapies was an apparent improvement early on, but one that seemed unsustainable over time. Hovering in the atmosphere above these private dramas between patient and doctor was the possibility of the placebo response, a well-established tendency of people to feel better, for a while at least, after treatment even with inert substances. That the disease's severity waxed and waned added another layer of complexity to efforts to learn what might ameliorate its symptoms.

Los Angeles internist Herb Tanney had approximately 150 sufferers in his practice by that spring, all of whom had been his patients for some years. Typically, they had been ill for a few months before seeking his help. "They usually waited anywhere from three to four months before seeing me—just waiting for it to go away," Tanney recalled. "They would come in and say, 'I've had this flu-like illness, and I don't know if I'm cracking up or I've got a brain tumor.' " Given the rise of cases in his own practice, Tanney was absolutely persuaded the disease was infectious. "I don't know *how* highly contagious," he said, "but in order to have an epidemic so that one doctor—me—would see well over one hundred and fifty patients in a two-year period, it had to be an enormous epidemic and therefore had to be highly contagious."

Betty Agee, head of Los Angeles County's Acute Communicable Disease Control Unit in 1986, confirmed that a number of doctors concerned by the growing phenomenon in their practices had called her offices that year. "I've had doctors call to say they really think we should be studying this, but we're a small unit and this is a huge county," Agee said. "It's better undertaken by the Centers for Disease Control."

In addition, Agee said that her staff took numerous calls each month from people claiming to have been diagnosed by their doctors with a long-term debilitating form of mononucleosis and showing high levels of antibodies to Epstein-Barr virus. Months later, however, they remained sick. Agee was clearly puzzled by the curious phenomenon and she was suspicious of the mono diagnosis offered to so many of her callers.

"Eighty percent of the calls are from women," she continued, "most of them in their thirties; I haven't heard from anyone over the age of forty-two. Perhaps the only men, in fact, have been doctors calling to see what we're doing about it." She also noted that the callers were single, married, some with many sexual partners, others with few or none. "They're all exhausted," she added. "Before it hit, many say they were running four or five miles a day. Now they can't walk to the corner."

Since neither L.A. County nor federal health officials took action to determine the breadth of the crisis, the rate of spread in that city is unknown. Yet by spring of that year, the rise in the number of cases of the chronic disease in Los Angeles was becoming conspicuous. Writing in the now defunct *Herald Examiner,* conservative columnist Ben Stein asked flatly, "Is *everyone* in Los Angeles sick?" Stein's column, published on March 26, was titled "The Spread of 'Non-Stop Flu' Is Cause for Concern." "Can anyone help?" he asked. "Isn't this worthy of national attention?"

San Francisco, California

Although media pundits and phrasemakers had spotted the disease in Hollywood, by 1986 an increasingly significant portion of Peterson and Cheney's patients hailed from San Francisco and its suburbs, a densely populated zone 500 miles north of L.A. but just 170 miles by car from Incline Village. In San Francisco that year, Carol Jessop was following slightly more than three hundred patients with the disease in her busy clinic on Divisadero Street. Many had been ill for some time and had learned of her growing expertise by word of mouth. But others presented de novo—that is, they came down with the disease while under Jessop's care.

"It is my opinion," the doctor said that year, "that there's a new virus—and people are getting it. We don't know how it's transmitted. We don't know who's likely to get it. But I see too many people who have been totally healthy, who get struck with a definitive onset and then have these characteristic stories. And I can't believe that these same people," the doctor continued in reference to a theory then being propagated by academic clinicians within her own institution, "have nothing better to do than to read what's in the newspaper and come in and complain of this disease."

Jan Montgomery began to read about the Incline Village epidemic in the San Francisco newspapers that year. News of the Nevada epidemic was a revelation to the tall auburn-haired woman who had been mostly bedridden for two years with what a doctor had called "chronic Epstein-Barr syndrome." In 1985 the former bank vice president had begun to notice ads in the *San Francisco Bay Guardian* for support-group gatherings of people suffering from EBV. Montgomery went to some of the meetings out of curiosity; she found it difficult to believe so many others might be suffering from the same malady. She went, too, out of her need to make a connection with people with whom she could share the burden of her despair. To Montgomery's amazement, the people at these meetings described bouts of illness identical to her own: "It became clear to me quite quickly that it wasn't just me in the Bay Area who was sick with this."

By early 1986, Montgomery, who had been an energetic participant in San Francisco's progressive politics, decided to marshal her remaining energy to forge a patient coalition to petition the city's year-old health commission for a hearing. The Tahoe epidemic provided enough evidence, she believed, to characterize the affliction to the health commissioners as a public health menace. In addition, she said later, "We had people in support groups whose partners were showing signs of the disease." In the spring of 1986, Montgomery petitioned the commission for a hearing on the grounds that the malady appeared to be contagious.

The health commission, whose eight members, half of them doctors, were appointed by Mayor Dianne Feinstein, had been born of pressure from citizens who believed that the health department's initial response to the AIDS outbreak had been inadequate; the commission was the health department's governing body.

"We had been in touch with Paul Cheney and followed that epidemic," Montgomery said, "believing that we were having a similar epidemic going on down here. And it was mostly because of Paul's findings that we were able to convince the health commission to have a hearing on the subject."

On the afternoon of April 14 the commission convened a public hearing at 101 Grove Street, health department headquarters. Fifty citizens attended; a handful were doctors, including Carol Jessop and Paul Cheney. Those remaining were patients whose lives had been engulfed by the disease for months or years; several testified that their spouses had developed symptoms of the disease. Florence

Stroud, the health department's deputy director, reported on the new disease, beginning with a pedestrian account of Epstein-Barr virus and its widespread distribution among the world's population as well as its role in mononucleosis, Burkitt's lymphoma and other B-cell lymphomas. She noted that one of Carol Jessop's patients had developed B-cell lymphoma, but she reported Gary Holmes's view that there was "no evidence of transmission."

"Physicians seeing patients with this symptom complex in the Bay Area," Stroud concluded, "state that physical findings are sparse and that they do not believe that the syndrome is passed from person to person. Most authorities state that there is no solid evidence for transmissibility of the syndrome and that, to the extent that clustering occurs, it is random."

Montgomery was struck by the disparate versions of reality generated in the course of the hearing. "What was interesting was the juxtaposition of about fifty people standing up and saying, 'I'm sick,' and the written report that the health department presented saying, number one, 'This disease has been around forever and it's just lately that people are becoming aware of it' and, number two, 'It's impossible to transmit it.' The testimony totally contradicted the report, but that didn't bother them at all."

At least one commission member was bothered, however. Philip Lee, a doctor who had been assistant secretary of health in the Johnson administration, had a friend who had fallen suddenly ill with the disease while visiting San Francisco months before. On May 2, Lee sent a letter to James Mason, the director of the CDC, prodding him to release his agency's data on the Tahoe investigation and urging that the agency "reconsider its priorities" and spend more money on the disease. Lee told Mason about the hearing. "There was compelling testimony from various physicians who stated that they were concerned about the lack of scientific research conducted on this syndrome," Lee wrote. "Many patients testified that they were transferred from physician to physician for years prior to receiving a diagnosis of chronic EBVS [Epstein-Barr virus syndrome]. . . . A recent investigation of an outbreak of EBVS at Incline Village by CDC personnel was not given wide distribution in spite of the many cases reported by local physicians. The Health Commission urges that Disease Control reconsider its priorities on infectious diseases research and investigation," Lee concluded, "and place financial resources in the area of EBVS research, because it is a nationwide phenomenon."

Incline Village, Nevada

Clearly, Incline Village was not the epicenter of chronic Epstein-Barr virus disease, in spite of its frequent portrayal as such; Herb Tanney had recognized an epidemic of the same disease in Los Angeles a full year before the Tahoe epidemic began, and it was apparent to Cheney, after his visit to San Francisco, that Bay Area residents were at risk as well. "Since we are a resort area," Cheney remarked that spring, "we are umbilically connected to all the major metropolitan areas on the West Coast. We *are* San Francisco. We *are* L.A.—are, or will be. And looking at how long this disease complex has been in the Bay Area or Los Angeles versus how long we've been observing it here, it may be a little older in the Bay Area and L.A. So rather than [L.A.] getting it from us, we got it from them."

But was the rate of spread in Los Angeles and San Francisco as volatile as it had appeared to be in Incline Village?

"We may have the net too wide, pulling in people who don't belong," Cheney postulated. "And in Los Angeles and San Francisco, the net's too small, pulling in too few people because the recognition of the disease is so poor. But if you applied our 1.5 percent to the greater Los Angeles basin, for example, there would be 105,000 cases there [assuming a population base of 7 million]. If you were to take those cases and spread them over, say, eight thousand doctors, there would be thirteen cases in each doctor's practice. Some doctors might only have one. And they may think that person has a viral disease they just can't recognize. Or has lupus. Or has multiple sclerosis. Or is a hypochondriac. Or is crazy."

Like Carol Jessop, Anthony Komaroff, and other doctors with large constituencies of such patients, Cheney and Peterson continued to be struck by the degree of disability and suffering in their epidemic population and frustrated by their inability to help. The best any compassionate doctor could do was treat the disease symptom by symptom. Typical therapy might include medications to induce better-quality sleep, anti-inflammatory drugs to ease joint and muscle pain, painkillers for the severe head pain many if not most patients described, antidepressant medications for depression, and cautionary words against imbibing either alcohol and caffeine, two drugs that seemed to have a decidedly deleterious effect on sufferers. (A decade later, these therapies remained the most commonly employed by doctors treating such patients.) Early that spring, however, Cheney came upon an article in the medical literature that described the successful use of a drug called acyclovir in cases of severe Epstein-Barr virus reactivation in renal transplant patients whose immune systems had been suppressed. Manufactured by the British pharmaceuticals firm Burroughs Wellcome, the expensive new drug was one of the few antiviral therapies on the market and the only drug with proven efficacy against herpesviruses in their active state. The doctors had heard as well that federal scientist Stephen Straus was experimenting with acyclovir on a group of people suffering from the chronic disease.

Cheney and Peterson decided to try intravenous acyclovir infusions on a small group of patients who were totally or partially incapacitated by their disease and had been among the third of patients whose immune system status, as evaluated by flow cytometrist Susan Wormsley, had suggested they might be vulnerable to lymphoma. During their conversations with Burroughs Wellcome staff, the clinicians were warned to administer large amounts of fluid to their patients; Straus, according to Burroughs Wellcome, had inadvertently caused temporary kidney failure in some of his subjects by failing to ensure that they took sufficient fluids with the drug.

The doctors chose twenty patients—eighteen women, two men—ranging in age from twenty-eight to sixty-five. All the patients lived in a thirty-mile radius of the Peterson-Cheney clinic and had become ill within the time frame of the epidemic. Sixteen of the twenty were completely bedridden when they began taking the drug. The patients were infused with acyclovir in amounts of up to 800 milligrams each day for seven to ten days. None of the patients experienced ill effects from the infusions and by the end of the infusion period a bare majority—eleven—felt dramatically better. The doctors noticed that among all of those who felt better, antibodies to Epstein-Barr virus early antigens—the antibodies that rise when the virus is actively replicating—dropped. In three people, however, there was no change, and the same antibodies actually rose in two patients. Neither doctor was ready to call the drug a cure. But they were encouraged, and they remained intent upon following the progress of the patients who had received the drug.

Ten weeks into their acyclovir experiment, Cheney and Peterson continued to be ambivalent about the drug's effectiveness. Although most patients had responded to the drug, all but one had begun a slow descent into the disease once again when the infusions ended. Still, the doctors speculated, for those patients in the severe, nonfunctional state, maintenance on the drug might be the answer until a cure was found.

The doctors began to offer the expensive therapy to a small number of their worst-afflicted patients, including Andy Antonucci, Sandy Schmidt, Sonny Dukes, and Gerald and Janice Kennedy. In cases where insurance companies refused to reimburse for an experimental therapy, Dan Peterson bore the cost of the drug. It was soon apparent that the longer the patient was on the drug, the longer the remission. "We were mostly experimenting with the length of treatment," Cheney recalled some years later. "The dose was fairly stable."

Naturally the doctors wondered to what extent acyclovir therapy might have generated a placebo response. Their question was answered by Reno neuroradiologist Royce Biddle. As the months passed, Biddle observed that the brain scans of a majority of acyclovir-treated patients became negative for the multiple small, or punctate, lesions known colloquially as unidentified bright objects, or UBOs. Unfortunately, when the same patients were removed from the drug, the UBOs returned, although in new places in the brain.

7

Not Normal Americans

Palo Alto, California

On March 18, Julie Pritchard, the fourth-grade teacher from Truckee who had
been sick for fourteen months, appeared more ill than Cheney had ever seen her.
She had to be helped into his office by a nurse. Two weeks later, she reappeared
with cognition problems, headaches, disabling fatigue, and an upper-respiratory-
tract infection. A week later she returned again. Shortly after that visit, Pritchard
requested copies of her medical records from the Alder Street clinic in anticipation of an appointment at Stanford. "Where else would anybody go?" she asked
some time later. "You wouldn't try any other local doctors. It was the obvious
thing to do. I wasn't getting well through [Cheney and Peterson], and I was getting desperate. I *had* to find somebody else to help me."

In mid-April, Pritchard arrived at the medical complex at 300 Pasteur Drive on the
stately palm-lined Stanford University campus. She carried a taped manila envelope, heavy with her Alder Street medical records. One piece of evidence had
been sent from Reno Diagnostics ahead of her: magnetic resonance imaging
scans, which were positive for UBOs in the right occipital lobe of her brain. The
teacher had secured an appointment with Lucy Thompkins, a former medical
school classmate of Anthony Komaroff's and now an associate professor in the infectious disease department at Stanford. But when she arrived, Pritchard learned
that she would be seeing the head of the infectious disease department, Thomas
Merigan, instead.

Merigan was a short, brawny man with small hands. In his office, crammed
with medical texts from floor to ceiling, he kept a wooden plaque on a wall above
a file cabinet. It read, "If you can't dazzle 'em with brilliance, baffle 'em with
bullshit." At fifty-two, he was, by reputation, the most powerful man in his field
on the West Coast. His lab specialized in the study of chronic viral infections. In
September of that year, in fact, Merigan and several of his colleagues at Stanford
would receive a $2.5-million grant from the National Institute of Allergy and In-
fectious Diseases in Bethesda to launch the first clinical trial of AZT drug therapy

in AIDS.* Nearly two years after meeting Pritchard, Merigan remembered her. She was the first of two Tahoe victims who came to Stanford.

"We saw two," the department head confirmed, "and one of them I particularly remember was a woman who was very concerned about an abnormal MRI scan. We didn't have any sign of progressive disease in her, and yet she was very worried. And as I view it," he continued, "she had been kind of overstudied. She had anxiety as a triggering factor to refer her to a physician. I concluded that she had a lot of anxiety, and I didn't believe there was any evidence for a chronic virus infection going on in her."

Merigan reported that he examined Pritchard, then asked one of his colleagues, associate professor of neurology Leslie Dorfman, to examine her as well. Although Merigan assured this reporter that both he and Dorfman examined the patient, Pritchard herself was adamant that they did not. "Let me just be brief," Pritchard said later. "I went to Stanford, and they never, ever—they never touched me, basically. Neither one of them. They never examined me. *I was not physically touched by either of them.* They spent fifteen minutes with me—combined—and drew the conclusion that I was a neurotic middle-aged broad who had mental problems. Then they told me to go away. There wasn't anything real subtle about what was going on."

Pritchard held her medical records from Nevada on her lap during her brief dialogue with the doctors; when she left Stanford, the envelope's seal was intact; neither man expressed the slightest interest in its contents, according to her. Had they done so, they would have seen vivid documentation of a life-altering illness of fifteen months' duration, including highly abnormal immune status test results. One piece of medical evidence did pierce the Stanford specialists' alleged indifference, however: the magnetic resonance imaging scan of the teacher's brain. Before Pritchard's arrival, Merigan had asked Leslie Dorfman to evaluate the scan; neurologist Dorfman was unimpressed by Reno neuroradiologist Royce Biddle's conclusion that the scan was abnormal.

In a letter to Cheney penned after Pritchard's departure, Merigan wrote that he agreed with his neurologist colleague that the lesion or "demyelination" in the right occipital lobe of Pritchard's brain was "within normal limits." Given that, Merigan told Cheney, he had informed Pritchard that further demyelination was "unlikely."

"With all the new procedures introduced in clinical medicine," Merigan said much later, "we can't define right away the anatomical variances, the things that aren't in all people but are in a few people and yet are not really associated with disease. They're just variations on the normal, like someone who has a sixth finger or a bald head. They're the small things that don't signify the site of true disease. Now, some of those kinds of things were being called disease," he continued in a reference to the Tahoe epidemic, "and the patients were becoming worried about it. They were anxious patients who were caused to be even more anxious— patients in whom grave fears were being generated."

---

*By 1995 the trial had been in progress for nine years and Merigan et al. had received a total of $8 million from NIAID to study the drug's efficacy.

Long after Pritchard's visit to Stanford, Dan Peterson was apprised of Merigan's "sixth finger" postulate. The Nevada clinician by then had ordered sequential magnetic resonance imaging brain scans on several hundred patients and discovered that, over time, the number and position of the brain lesions changed. "I have MRI scans where the lesions are there, where they go away, and where they come back," the doctor said. "Sixth fingers don't do that."

Stanford neurologist Leslie Dorfman also wrote a letter to Cheney after Pritchard's departure. Dorfman implied that he had performed a physical exam and that he was familiar with Pritchard's medical history, which Cheney knew to be untrue. "He didn't even do a mental status exam," Cheney complained, "which is part of a good neurologic exam. What you're doing is looking for organic dysfunction. Tony Komaroff likes to use serial seven subtractions. And when you have this disease, you can't do it—or you get it wrong. And Dorfman didn't do that. There are other variations of the mental status exam, but Dorfman never did them."

In his letter, Dorfman also stated in chastening, unequivocal language that, although Pritchard was physically healthy, she suffered from "considerable psychiatric disability," a problem he blamed on Cheney. Dorfman rebuked the Nevada internist for failing to appropriately diagnose Pritchard with what the neurologist believed was anxiety, depression, and somatization disorder—physical symptoms generated by emotional stress. The neurologist stated categorically that Pritchard's symptoms stemmed from her belief in the unlikely scenario, inculcated in her by Cheney, that she was suffering from a viral disease of the brain. After ostentatiously reprimanding Cheney for causing Pritchard's woes, Dorfman concluded with the comment that, in all probability, Pritchard would need "intensive psychotherapy to put her life back together again."

Dorfman's next action suggests that he was considerably affected by his encounter with the Nevada schoolteacher. In a letter to the widely read *Science* magazine the following February, Dorfman embroidered upon the ideas he had expressed in his letter to Cheney about Pritchard nearly a year earlier, giving Cheney a public slap in the process. Postulating that the symptoms of the "Lake Tahoe mystery disease" are typical of "the chronic stress syndrome so prevalent in our society," Dorfman added, "These symptoms may be expected to persist and increase when the sufferer is told they indicate brain damage from a mysterious viral infection." He further proposed that "chronic mono" was a "dubious diagnosis" of "questionable validity."[1] Like most of his counterparts in other academic and federal research institutions, Dorfman focused exclusively on complaints of fatigue, depression, anxiety, insomnia, and the other so-called subjective symptoms, as if they were the only hallmarks of the disease. He ignored the objective findings, such as lymphadenopathy, aberrant T4–T8 ratios, and chronically reactivated Epstein-Barr virus.

Cheney agreed that Pritchard was an anxious patient. "But," he insisted, "she wasn't crazy. Her objective database, her lab work, was one of the strongest to suggest an organic etiology. There were a lot of things in there that just can't be ignored. Now, Merigan sat down with her, saw this was an anxious woman, and immediately made a snap judgment," Cheney continued. "He didn't even examine her. He sent a neurologist in to sort of cover his tracks, to make sure she really *was* normal. I can see it now: 'Go in there. She's okay; just get it over with.' You know," Cheney said after a moment, "it's almost as if you sort of see what you're looking for. They were trying to see an anxious, neurotic woman, and so that's what they saw. And I have to ask myself, was I looking for a disease and couldn't see an anxious, neurotic woman? I saw elements of anxiety in this woman, but that wasn't what I was focusing on. I was focusing on the things that were *not* normal. I also saw this within the context of a third of a teaching faculty, of which she was a member, becoming sick. And none of *them* had an anxiety problem."

Cheney's partner was equally nettled by the Stanford doctors' misreading of the illness. Dan Peterson generously ascribed it to their inexperience with the multi-faceted disease. "We learn a template—a model that fits, okay?" he said. "If the critical features are there, then it doesn't matter to me how depressed they are or anxious they are or crazy they are or whatever, if they have the other features of the disease. But I think for an outsider, that's impossible to do. Now, I'm not here to argue with Merigan, but I think he was very gutsy to claim that we were crazy and the patient was crazy."

Thirty-year-old Stephen Ciatti (a pseudonym) was the second Alder Street patient to turn to the Stanford experts. Like Pritchard, he wanted a second opinion. According to Peterson, Ciatti was awarded only slightly more credibility than Pritchard by Stanford's experts. "The difference is that with [Stephen]," Peterson remembered, "Stanford didn't tell him that he had not been sick. They told him, 'You had a little virus that people made way too much of.' After all, how could they tell him he was an hysterical middle-aged woman?"

Ciatti was one of the few patients in the Alder Street practice to eventually recover. Pritchard never joined that privileged circle. In 1988 she and her husband moved from Truckee to a small town in Washington State, where her husband got a teaching job; she abandoned her teaching career. She had contempt for the Stanford specialists, neither of them psychiatrists, who had labeled her a woman of "considerable psychiatric disability."

"They said things that I absolutely don't believe are true, but other than suing them, what's the point? I wanted to get well." Now, Pritchard said, although the virulence of her disease had eased, "I have symptoms. I get a lot tireder than most people. I have memory lapses. So does my husband. We try not to think about it."

Unknown to Cheney and Peterson, Merigan and his colleagues in Stanford's infectious disease clinic were hardly innocent of the medical phenomenon represented by Pritchard. Far from being an isolated incident, Pritchard's treatment by Merigan and Dorfman was to a great degree pro forma. By Merigan's own estimate, the infectious disease clinic at Stanford had been, since 1985, the destination of 100 to possibly 250 people every year with a chronic disease resembling Pritchard's. Los Angeles filmmaker Blake Edwards had been among them.

"We saw at least four or five people with this a week for fifty weeks a year for a couple of years," Merigan admitted during an interview in 1987. "I would say we saw at *least* one hundred patients with this a year—easily," he added. However, the infectious disease specialist explained, he and his staff had decided that year to begin discouraging private clinicians in their referrals of patients with the illness because "we look for certain underlying disease that is serious and that might explain reactivation of herpesviruses in these people, and we've not seen it very frequently."

🔢

Enmity, subtle or not, traditionally has informed relationships between clinicians in private and academic medicine. In the 1925 Pulitzer Prize–winning novel *Arrowsmith,* Sinclair Lewis's searing examination of a young doctor's rise from private practice into the realm of academic research, Dr. Coughlin of tiny Leopolis, Dakota, vents the great frustration of his career to the novice Arrowsmith. "I tell you," the loutish Coughlin complains in a rare moment of acuity, "a plug G.P. may not have a lot of letters after his name, but he sees a slew of mysterious things that he can't explain, and I swear I believe most of these damn' alleged scientists could learn a whale of a lot from the plain country practitioners, let me tell you!"

The action in *Arrowsmith* begins at the century's turn and moves to its middle. During the decades covered by Lewis's story, clinical medicine was ascending in importance and prestige, due in great part to the Canadian clinician Sir William Osler, who lived from 1849 to 1919 and who taught medicine to students in Canada, the United States, and at the time of his death, England.* Osler's international eminence derived from his descriptive and diagnostic gifts. He defined the sign and symptom complexes of many of the most perplexing, obscure diseases of his era, favoring the substitution of observation and method for speculation and theory. In short, Osler believed in listening to the patient. In the course of his luminous career, he became a prolific lecturer and essayist, frequently extolling the virtues of meticulous clinical observation. He knew that the conservative nature of his profession often blinded it to the obvious. And he exhorted his medical students to be on guard against lockstep thinking.

In the decades after his death, Osler's diagnostic ideals began to be supplanted by the rise of medical technology. Like a shifting of the stony plates beneath the earth's surface, technology's force transformed the clinical landscape. Cognitive medicine, the art of divining and interpreting the nature and source of illness, lost ground to the laboratory bench. One bug, and one bug alone, caused each disease, according to the microbe hunters, and scientists seemed to be closing in rapidly on ways of identifying every bug. In time, blood tests emerged for several of the major infectious diseases, including syphilis, tuberculosis, gonorrhea, rabies, and typhoid. These developments were an undeniable boon, ending untold cycles of suffering, but they began subtly to erode the tradition of "well and complete" observation extolled by Osler. Once the spirochete at its source could be isolated, the degree of clinical skill required to recognize syphilis, for instance, a disease with mutable, elusive signs and symptoms ranging from lesions to lunacy, receded.

For an ailment like the one afflicting people in northern Nevada, California, and elsewhere—an ill-defined disease lacking a single, indisputable marker—technology alone offered ambivalent relief; technology needed to be harnessed, much in the manner of Paul Cheney and Dan Peterson, by clearheaded clinicians who favored Osler's style of scrupulous clinical observation. Cheney, in addition,

---

*Lewis was himself the son of a country doctor.

brought a physicist's ebullient creativity to the dilemma, a contribution, it might be added, his conservative critics in medicine distrusted profoundly.

By the early 1980s, half a century after Osler's death, the breach between doctors in private practice and clinician-researchers in academia was gaping. Michael Gottlieb, an assistant professor at UCLA from 1980 to 1987 and the first research clinician to describe AIDS as a coherent disease entity, elaborated on the phenomenon during a conversation in Santa Monica in 1988.

"A misconception that clinical observation does not lead to new knowledge prevails widely in academic medicine today," Gottlieb said. "There is a widespread view that the age of seminal clinical observation is over and that the only progress now will be through the laboratory. Certainly I will be among the first to point to the successes of laboratory investigation since the early part of this century. There has been dramatic progress. However, occasionally something very important of a clinical nature is observed and can lead to further breakthroughs," Gottlieb continued. "That was the case with AIDS. It could be the case with other conditions."

Gottlieb was thirty-two and a freshly trained immunologist when he began his UCLA career. In 1982, using the government's *Morbidity and Mortality Weekly Report* as his vehicle, he filed the first scientific report on AIDS, describing five cases of young, previously healthy men who had T-cell deficiencies and had died of an extremely rare disease: *Pneumocystis carinii* pneumonia.[2] Gottlieb's colleagues at UCLA failed to reward him for his effort. Many, in fact, advised him to turn his energies toward a more "legitimate" area of medical research. By 1987, Gottlieb had been denied tenure three times, even though his research ultimately had secured his university a $10.2 million AIDS research grant. There was gossip that the academicians who had prevented his tenure would blackball him at other university labs. In 1987, Gottlieb, who had foreseen for himself a research career in academia, opened a private clinical practice of immunology in Santa Monica. He placed much of the blame for his loss of favor among the UCLA faculty on the overtly clinical orientation of his research.

"The moral of the story is, I suppose, if you're going to make brilliant observations, be sure that they're in the laboratory," he continued. "And do steady, inconspicuous work until you have tenure. Academia breeds small minds," he added. "It's rare that the truly brilliant, insightful person survives. The system selects for mediocrity."

Incline Village, Nevada

In mid-April, neuropsychologist Sheila Bastien and a colleague, Berkeley psychologist Bob Thomas, undertook the four-hour drive from the Bay Area to Incline Village. They set up shop in an examining room in the Alder Street suite. On that first visit, Cheney and Peterson funneled fifteen patients to them over three days. All fifteen had positive brain scans and had complained of cognitive changes with the onset of their disease. Otherwise, the selection was not particularly scientific; they tended to be patients the doctors were most concerned about. One of them was Peterson's nurse, who had suffered a seizure and had been,

Cheney said, "encephalopathic" for some months; another was Truckee algebra teacher Andy Antonucci.

Bastien's earliest and most startling observations had to do with IQs. She was baffled by the patients' low scores given their educational backgrounds and their professions, which included not only nursing and teaching, but heading a high-technology business. The legal periphery of mental retardation in many states was 69; 100 was considered average. It was unusual, Bastien said, to find average or near-average scores in a group of people with college degrees and relatively high levels of professional achievement. In the months ahead, as she continued to test more patients, she documented post-morbid IQ losses of up to 40 points in patients who, for the purposes of applying for government jobs and for other reasons, had taken an IQ test before their illness began. Even with so small a sampling, the psychologist and her associate quickly concluded that the depressed IQ levels were due mostly to a remarkably poor showing in tests of nonverbal, right-hemisphere skills. Full-scale IQ, after all, is a synthesis of a multitude of intellectual skills that are rooted in different areas of the brain. In the Tahoe patients, the right side of the brain was causing the average of combined measures of intelligence to plunge.

Gross disparity between hemispheres is indicative of brain damage. Neuropsychologists generously allow for a fifteen-point spread between verbal and performance, or nonverbal, IQ before introducing the specter of brain dysfunction. In the Tahoe patients, performance IQs frequently were 20 to 25 points below verbal IQs. (Two years later, after having tested three hundred people with the disease, Bastien had measured verbal and performance IQ disparities as great as 45 points, with many patients' performance IQs at or below the legal level of retardation.) A few performance IQs were startlingly close to the legal definition of idiocy.

A gap between verbal and performance intelligence was Bastien's first hint that Cheney and Peterson's patients were, as the doctors had suspected, suffering from an organic brain disease. Whatever injury had occurred, however, it was focal—that is, it was hitting some regions of the brain and sparing others. Intellectual torpor induced by depression, in contrast, is global: verbal and performance skills are equally dulled.

Initially, the patients seemed quite bright, Bastien remembered. They were able to define most of the words on the vocabulary list she read to them and were able to articulate in some detail their medical histories. It was when tasks edged into the nonverbal, the visual and the abstract, that they unraveled. Among her tests to gauge visual acuity, for example, was a series of simple drawings of common objects with one vital feature missing; the patient's task was to name the missing object. An intellectually normal seven-year-old could be expected to perform the task successfully. The Tahoe patients typically stared at the pictures for long minutes until, with obvious embarrassment and frustration, they admitted defeat. When asked to assemble a four-piece jigsaw puzzle of an elephant, they toyed with the pieces, shuffling them around on the table before them as if they were blind. Although Bastien chose not to impose a time limit on the test, it was apparent that all the time in the world would have been inadequate to allow these patients to assemble the puzzle. On several similar tests, the patients were handicapped in the extreme, exhibiting severe visual-discrimination deficits.

The intellectual resources for visual discrimination rest in the visual cortex of the occipital lobes at the rear of the skull. For a while Bastien wondered whether the dysfunction was rooted there. But several even more bizarre anomalies existed in the realm of memory, the mechanisms for which are moored in both the right and the left temporal lobes at the sides of the brain.

Bastien discovered that although patients were only mildly impaired in their ability to remember written words and images, a left brain skill, they were severely impaired in their ability to recall the import of spoken words, a right brain skill. There were other findings. Not a single patient was able to count backward from 100 in decrements of seven. Sufferers had, in addition, what Bastien described as "spatial perceptual" difficulties, manifested by an inability to draw a correctly proportioned human being. Patients' grip strength was abnormally weak, about half as powerful as what would be considered normal for their sex and age; frequently, the left hand, controlled by the right side of the brain, was weakest.

As Bastien pursued her investigations, right brain deficits arose again and again, making the patients' left brain problems seem minor by comparison. The psychologist was struck, too, by the remarkable range in each patient's scores on different tests, which she termed "intellectual scatter." "What that suggests," she said, "is that there are pockets of dysfunction in the brain. It would be like if I were a ninety-word-per-minute typist but I had trouble dialing the phone."

Of course, it was premature to draw any conclusions after testing only fifteen people. That winter, Bastien was able to surmise only that something rather startling was occurring in the right brain hemispheres of fifteen people, something that could neither be faked nor be the result of even the most severe depression. "I was very aware of their profound depression and anxiety," the psychologist said of her original Tahoe subjects. "But because of the laterality and the focality, it turned out not to be the pattern you find in depression and anxiety."

Bastien was particularly impressed by her first subject, the Nevada postal worker who was Paul Cheney's patient. "This woman is now completely demented," Bastien said later. "But when I first saw her, she was well groomed, well spoken. She tried very hard to hide her deficits, although she looked tearful. She was forty-seven or so and had worked as a civil servant in Nevada. She had a terrible time with numbers, counting both forward and backward. Her math was terrible, and her job was partially dependent upon calculation. She also had terrible short-term memory loss. She was out of work as a result. Emotionally, she was very distressed. And her drawing was poor. She drew a person—and it was very bad. That tips you off to parietal lobe dysfunction. The parietal lobes are at the top of the brain, and they process spatial relations and perceptual construction ability. She continued, over the next year, to deteriorate to the point where I recommended she not be let out alone. She was found one day sitting on the curb in front of her house not knowing where she lived."

Although the postal worker seemed to be the worst afflicted, Bastien was struck by the poor performances of all the patients. She and her partner, Bob Thomas, felt they had stumbled onto something altogether frightening.

"My impression was, My God! This is a lot of damage to be seeing in a group of people who have these flu-like symptoms," Bastien recalled. "I was horrified that what seemed like a ubiquitous virus was so dangerous to so many people. Whatever the virus was doing, it was clearly neurotropic. I wondered, Is this progressive or just temporary? And I wondered how damn contagious it was."

During one of their visits to Incline Village that spring Bastien and Thomas went to Reno Diagnostics at neuroradiologist Royce Biddle's invitation to see the magnetic resonance imaging brain scans of the Tahoe patients as well as the scans of patients suffering from multiple sclerosis. Although Bastien had been testing multiple sclerosis patients for two decades, she had never seen the visual evidence of the disease. "The lesions were bigger in the MS patients," she recalled, "but there were *more* lesions in the Tahoe patients." Of course, multiple sclerosis was a well-established clinical entity known to cause brain damage; the other disorder wasn't even on the map. Both psychologists were shaken by the Tahoe scans. "I thought, What is *causing* this?" Bastien said.

The clinicians were buoyed by the addition of Bastien's tools to their arsenal of investigative techniques. They were increasingly confident that they had marshaled incontrovertible evidence to prove the disease was real and that neither they nor their patients were crazy.

"Parallel with trying to figure out what caused this, we had worked on trying to define it better," Dan Peterson remembered later. "And it seemed that we had a clinical description that we could make: Acute onset. *Some* degree of contagion by *some* route. Cognitive function abnormalities that we could measure by psychometric testing and the shadows of which we could visualize through MRI scanning. Impaired immune systems. A group of complaints that people gave us over and over and *over* again. And while they were vague, they all fit together, in that everybody said the same thing. So," Peterson said after inhaling deeply, "it seemed clear."

Unfortunately "it" was clear to almost no one except Dan Peterson, Paul Cheney, their patients, and the handful of specialists who had gamely entered the fray, some of them lured by the tantalizing array of unusual test results, others compelled by the heartbreaking predicaments of the victims.

San Diego, California

That spring, Cheney decided to seek the opinion of his medical school friend and soul mate, neurologist Chris Gallen, who was then a member of the neurology department at the University of California at San Diego. "I had just a *slew* of brain scans by then," Cheney remembered. The doctor's decision to consult a friend was one measure of his developing political consciousness. News of the Centers for Disease Control's apparent unconcern about the "purported"—as it was increasingly characterized by skeptics—Tahoe epidemic was quickly making its way through the corridors of American medicine. Cheney needed to find a neurologist who could either confirm or dismiss Royce Biddle's observations; but it had to be someone he could trust. Chris Gallen was unusually bright and well trained, Cheney believed. Moreover, he knew Gallen would listen to him. "Chris was my best friend in medical school," Cheney said. "I thought, Here's a friend of mine who knows I'm not crazy." Best of all, Gallen confessed to knowing virtually nothing about the Nevada epidemic or the disease.

Gallen was fascinated by his former classmate's story of an enfeebling pestilence moving through the High Sierras. But he was even more interested in the brain scans Cheney carried under one arm when he visited Gallen at the university. Gallen invited Cheney into the medical center's MRI unit where, in a darkened viewing room, the latter began slotting scans against panes of backlit glass. On each scan, the tiny white lesions emerged in contrast to the gray sections of the brain that surrounded them. Gallen was surprised by the number of lesions in every brain. He had seen such things before, but only rarely, only in the elderly, and only in far lower numbers. He was gripped, too, by Cheney's clinical histories. "This woman is unable to count backwards," Cheney said as the two stared at the image of one pockmarked brain. "She was a postal worker. . . . This man was an accountant," Cheney continued. "He can no longer add or subtract."

Gallen invited a colleague, neuroradiologist Mark Healy, to join the animated colloquy. Healy examined the scans and, after a moment of study, said, "Very interesting. Let me show you some of mine." He reached over to his own sizable stack of negatives and slotted several of them against the backlit glass; with a floor pedal, he began to rotate the display around the sides of the room. The scans were identical in every way to those Cheney had brought. They were images of the brains of AIDS sufferers. Cheney knew, as did most clinicians by 1985, that AIDS patients sometimes developed dementia in the final stages of their disease. Healy, who studied the brain scans of such patients routinely, told Gallen and Cheney they frequently were notable for evidence of multiple punctate lesions in the white matter. Sometimes the lesions were slightly larger, Healy added.*

Later Gallen invited Cheney to accompany him and a senior professor of neurology on hospital rounds. "After we rounded, I presented a case of this syndrome to Chris's professor," Cheney recalled. "His comment was 'Sounds like AIDS minor.' He just coined the term. He said, 'We should call it AIDS minor.' "

Chris Gallen recalled Cheney's visit and the Nevada brain scans with some clarity afterward. By then the neurologist had left the University of California and was practicing at the Scripps Clinic in La Jolla.

"The bottom line is that no one knows *what* the hell they mean," Gallen said of the unidentified bright objects Cheney had displayed for him. But, he added, "There's a tendency in medicine to dismiss data because it doesn't fit with your understanding of a problem. As a neurologist, I've had docs explain that they wanted me to see a patient who they thought was probably a crock because the patient had this or that odd set of symptoms. But by the time I finished listening to *their* history of what I'm going to see the patient about, I knew what the disease

---

*Multiple punctate lesions, or UBOs, were increasingly understood to be a frequent finding in AIDS sufferers, particularly in those suffering from dementia, but it wasn't until 1992 that a report appeared in the medical literature documenting the same finding in 85 percent of all victims of chronic fatigue syndrome. (Dedra Buchwald et al., "A Chronic Illness Characterized by Fatigue, Neurologic and Immunologic Disorders, and Active Human Herpesvirus Type 6 Infection," *Annals of Internal Medicine,* 116, no. 2 [Jan. 15, 1992]: 103–113).

was because those symptoms that seemed like odd, quirky symptoms to the doc added up to a classic neurologic syndrome that they just happened to not know about.

"When you see that happen enough," Gallen continued, "it begins to make you realize—if you're open-minded about it and if you can live with the fact that you don't know everything—it makes you realize that most of the time when patients are giving you a history, they're giving you the right history. It's really a question of Can I figure out what this history means? Rather than What can I throw out from his history to make it fit into my existing slot?"

Incline Village, Nevada

That spring, nearly two years after the epidemic began, the clinicians were more dispirited than ever. The heady anticipation that had attended the launch of their collaboration with Anthony Komaroff in February had worn thin as weeks passed without news from the Harvard researcher. In mid-May they learned from Komaroff that Tom Folks, at the National Institute of Allergy and Infectious Diseases, and John Sullivan in Boston had failed, so far, to discover anything unusual in the blood of Tahoe patients. Sullivan, in particular, had been unable to identify the long-sought wild-type strain of Epstein-Barr; Folks had seen no indication of either retroviral activity or cell destruction. Both researchers deemed their investigations to be concluded. Michael Caligiuri, the natural killer cell expert in Boston, so far had nothing substantial to report, according to Komaroff, although Caligiuri's work was destined to be more time-consuming than either Sullivan's or Folks's.

Cheney's brusque reception at Stanford, followed by Julie Pritchard's psychiatric diagnosis, had been especially chilling to the Nevada internists. The doctors found it hard to comprehend the flip skepticism displayed toward such a calamitous medical problem by professionals of Merigan and Dorfman's stature. They were increasingly demoralized, too, by the Centers for Disease Control's apparent indifference to the epidemic.

During the long months since Holmes and Kaplan's departure, the clinicians had sought, by written word and telephone, to keep the government abreast of new developments that might have broadened its view of the Nevada disease cluster. Independently of each other, Peterson and Cheney had continued to send Gary Holmes letters that included individual case histories they considered illustrative of significant aspects of the disease. And as they struggled to characterize the malady and comprehend its pathways and etiology, the doctors passed their discoveries on to the agency.

For both doctors, the road ahead had begun to seem longer and lonelier than ever before. "I guess it's like the Big Lie," Cheney said. "You know, you hear all those criticisms from enough people who are supposed to be experts, and you begin to wonder if they're right. And then as soon as you get feeling low about that and thinking maybe they are right, all of a sudden some patient walks in with a big tumor on their jaw or some other just *incredible* thing. It was almost as if nature was saying something and wouldn't let it go. The gibberish that should have been coming out of this if it was nothing was not coming. Rather, coherency seemed to be coming out of this."

Centers for Disease Control, Atlanta, Georgia

A startlingly different coherency emanated from the CDC at the end of May when the agency released its first public report on the Tahoe epidemic. Jon Kaplan and Gary Holmes's failure to share the Nevada internists' vision had never been more explicit. The agency's analysis implied what local critics had been saying all along: two small-town doctors had engaged in a frenzy of elaborate misdiagnoses.

The federal agency chose to disseminate Kaplan and Holmes's Tahoe findings in its *Morbidity and Mortality Weekly Report.* The slim, pocket-sized journal, known colloquially as the *MMWR,* was mailed free to approximately 100,000 public health agencies, medical libraries, and medical schools worldwide every Friday.* Its articles and reports lacked the prestige of peer-reviewed medical journal articles, but the lead time between manuscript submission and publication in the *MMWR* was a matter of days.

On May 30, 1986, the *MMWR* began with a summary of a Saint Louis encephalitis outbreak in Grand Junction, Colorado. The article went on to describe three other isolated cases of the disease in Dawson County, Texas, and Riverside County, Los Angeles, and reported on the case of a "sentinel chicken" placed near the Sepulveda Reservoir that became infected with the mosquito-borne disease. Health officials who might have been concerned about the spread of another disease likely were reassured by the Holmes-Kaplan report on Incline Village that followed. The seven-paragraph monograph was titled "Chronic Fatigue Possibly Related to Epstein-Barr Virus—Nevada."

"From November 1984 through August 1985," the young epidemiologists wrote in their eagerly awaited analysis of the notorious outbreak, "approximately ninety patients evaluated for persistent fatigue were diagnosed as having chronic Epstein-Barr virus (CEBV) disease by a two-physician community medical practice near Lake Tahoe, Nevada." Holmes and Kaplan eschewed any discussion of the malady's clinical presentation, nor did they engage in debate about whether or not an epidemic had occurred. Instead, they arrived at the somewhat extraneous conclusion that because Epstein-Barr virus test results varied from laboratory to laboratory, and because "there is a great deal of overlap in the antibody [levels] of case patients and the general population," the diagnosis of chronic Epstein-Barr virus, or "CEBV," should be made only in exclusion of numerous other diseases, "such as endocrine and autoimmune diseases; malignancies, chronic heart, liver, kidney and pulmonary disease; anxiety and depression; and chronic infectious diseases, such as CMV [cytomegalovirus] and tuberculosis."

Not long after the agency released its report, Ottawa clinician Byron Hyde, whose practice was then dominated by CEBV cases—among them his college-age daughter—would retort that the disease was "simple to diagnose—there is no disease even *vaguely* like it."[3] Another researcher, this one an Australian immu-

---

*By 1995 the *MMWR* was available on the Internet, vastly expanding its readership.

nologist, Denis Wakefield, would insist that "[the disease] should be able to be diagnosed at bedside, without doing thousands of dollars' worth of investigation."[4] Nevertheless, a belief among many in medicine that the disease was both rare and exceedingly difficult to diagnose, requiring masses of exclusionary tests, would persist for years.

In addition, by casting Epstein-Barr virus testing in disrepute, the CDC effectively wiped out the most creditable diagnostic tool of the day. Correctly interpreted, the EBV test offered a window into the integrity of the patient's immune system and remained one of the cheapest and most straightforward laboratory markers with an ability to flag a potential case of the disease.

The publication of Holmes and Kaplan's brief monograph was a milestone of sorts because it unveiled the federal government's public face on the Tahoe epidemic for all to see. The federal institution telegraphed to the lay press and, in turn, to citizens, a message that might best be paraphrased as follows: chronic Epstein-Barr Virus Syndrome is a minor illness, both in severity and in the number of people affected, if indeed it is an illness at all. Predictably the report unleashed a spate of lay coverage, some of which reflected the agency's own befuddlement. The Associated Press, for example, carried a lead that likely left its readers scratching their heads: "Federal health officials said there is not yet sufficient proof that a new disease which supposedly ravaged the Incline Village area last year actually exists." The *Atlanta Journal* published an article that purveyed a similar message in somewhat clearer language: "In a controversial report issued by the national Centers for Disease Control," medical reporter Charles Seabrook wrote, "researchers said there is no conclusive scientific evidence that CEBV actually exists, and a diagnosis of the disease is 'unreliable.' "

Not surprisingly, the government report was heralded by Cheney and Peterson's critics in Nevada. Washoe County health officer Michael Ford's remark was typical. "The epidemic didn't have a lot of credibility to begin with," Ford told one reporter. "And the CDC certainly did not find anything to get excited about. . . . I would defer to and seek direction from the CDC with respect to this particular disease entity." Practitioners at higher levels of medicine, too, considered the agency's analysis of the Tahoe epidemic definitive. Stanford infectious disease chief Tom Merigan, for example, made use of the government's investigation to buttress his own convictions. "The CDC looked at the Incline Village patients, and they couldn't find this epidemic that's been cited," Merigan remarked later. "They have the best facilities for epidemiology in the country. And, to me, if they can't find anything worthwhile there, why should anybody else look at it?"

Peterson and Cheney were incredulous at the agency's wholesale dismissal of a health threat they considered potentially catastrophic. But they were also humiliated. Neither doctor was emotionally prepared for the CDC's strangely off-base assessment of the epidemic.

"I was kind of naive about this," Peterson recalled much later. "I think Paul was better attuned. When Kaplan and Holmes were here, I wasn't terribly impressed by their research methodology—I was kind of upset that they *insisted* on putting two patients in the control group. But they were, it seemed to me, impressed by the patients. What I thought is they would take this back, they would research it, they would tell me it was an unusual strain of EBV, and that would kind of be it. I wasn't looking for a paper, a news report, or anything else. I was just trying to make things fit, so I could say to folks, 'Well, the CDC says you're sick. They say it's a virus. It should blow over, and that's all we can do.' "

Cheney maintained his characteristic composure when he talked about Holmes's report, but his language was fervent: "One of the things that upset me the most was not the fact that they had preconceived ideas—why shouldn't they have preconceived ideas? Or that they were not brilliant. They sent third and fourth stringers out here, but why should I expect they wouldn't?" he asked. "The thing that really bothered me was that between the time they left and when they sort of suddenly decided to publish the *MMWR* in the spring of 1986, I kept feeding them all this information. I said, 'Now I've got ten positive MRI scans. Now we have these two tumors, and one of them was read out initially as Burkitt's.' I told them that two people in the office whom they had met had had seizures. I fed them the flow-cytometry data. I fed them the psychoneurological problems from Sheila Bastien. And the more I fed them," Cheney continued, "and particularly the more powerful stuff, it seemed to cause them to suddenly write an article, the general theme of which was that 'nothing's wrong.' And *that* really bothered me. Because it seemed that the opposite should have happened. I would have understood the article if it had been written right after they came, but not after they had been fed all this other information."

Cheney began to suspect a kind of covert pressure had been exerted upon the young epidemiologists to "crush" the reality of the epidemic. "All of a sudden, the interest that hadn't been there for months just erupted—as if someone said, 'We have to crush this—how can we crush this?' To this day," Cheney added, "I don't believe that Holmes and Kaplan were the principal drivers of that botched attempt. I really do think that they wanted to do more, but someone above them was calling the shots during the critical stages when they were in the decision mode of whether to commit more resources to this or whether to cut bait and publish their piss-poor study. I got the feeling they were told to cut bait and publish this view."

Internal agency documents bear out some but not all of Cheney's suspicions. The decision to report on Tahoe in the first *MMWR* of June was, if nothing else, hasty. On May 28, 1986, two days before the report's publication, John Bennett, the CDC's assistant director for medical science, sent a copy of the Tahoe draft to Kenneth Herrmann, then the chief of the Viral Exanthems and Herpesvirus Branch. Bennett attached a memo: "Ken, please review and clear this last minute article for the newest *MMWR*. Looks OK to me, but this appears to be a highly controversial diagnosis." The report itself had been through numerous transmogrifications. Gary Holmes, with oversight from Jon Kaplan and Larry Schonberger, had penned a total of at least ten drafts, the ninth of which culminated with the words "it remains to be proved whether the entity of chronic EBV disease actually exists as a distinct disease."

Cheney was mistaken in his suspicion that Jon Kaplan wanted "to do more" in the way of researching the Tahoe outbreak. In a 1988 interview, the senior investigator indicated he was anxious to drop the disease upon his return from Nevada. He clearly considered the subject a deep, dry hole with the potential to entomb his career.

"I've never had any contact with Cheney and Peterson since that week I spent there," Kaplan said. "I didn't put that much effort into it. I spent one week in Lake Tahoe. You know—great," he added, shrugging. "I don't regard that as any price to pay. I haven't really sacrificed that much for this. . . . It's no secret there aren't that many people working on this," he continued. "Good scientists like to see their work going in a direction where it's going to benefit themselves or their institution or society. . . . So, by definition, the good people are going to drift away from this. On the other hand, you could end up being real famous if you find out what causes it. It's like a high-risk investment. I'd rather plan conservatively. I'm more interested in retroviruses. It's more concrete—more to my liking. And, you know, you want to put your effort in a place where you can see some things develop in a few years. And with retroviruses, there's no question. It's hot. You know they're going to be important. Whereas with this, you could work on this thing for a decade and end up with a total dud."

The fastest and surest way for Kaplan to get out from under the onerous controversy, of course, was to portray the Tahoe epidemic to his superiors as a bogus disease, a non-issue, and above all a waste of agency resources. Nor was Kaplan much moved by most of the observations Cheney and Peterson were relaying to Atlanta in the months before the agency's analysis of Tahoe was published. Some time later Kaplan grew riled at the mention of the more sophisticated tests the Nevada doctors employed in the months after his departure. "When I heard about *that,* I just couldn't believe it," he said. Apprised of Cheney and Peterson's view that magnetic resonance imaging brain scans, neuropsychological testing, and flow cytometry tests could be used to delineate objective signs of the disease, the senior epidemiologist rejoined: "*Bullshit!* What makes them so special? *We're* the scientists, and *we* go out and *we* do the work and *we* find the tests aren't diagnostic and they're not particularly of value in diagnosing this illness—or *whatever* this thing is."

Despite his explosive anger on the subject, Kaplan admitted he was wholly unfamiliar with the technology of either flow cytometry or neuropsychology. On the other hand, he conceded, word of Reno Diagnostics' magnetic resonance imaging scans, which had illuminated the presence of brain lesions, and the Nevada internists' reports of seizures among their epidemic population, had seemed "interesting" initially.

Gary Holmes, in contrast, admitted that he had been "tantalized" by the medical information the Nevada doctor was relaying to him that spring. "I was sitting around," he recalled, "and Paul kept calling me up with all this tantalizing stuff about the tumors. And I would have liked to have gone back out. But the problem was, it took a long time to get our lab results. It took three months before I got enough controls. So we didn't have any results—we didn't have our data back— and I wouldn't have known what to do out there, basically." Not surprisingly, it was Kaplan, according to Holmes, who put a clamp on the younger investigator's early impulse to return to Nevada. "I was updating Jon Kaplan on these developments," Holmes remembered. "But he, by this time, had pretty much decided that we should leave it alone. I don't know if that was definitive, but that was the opinion I got. If there was really something going on, I could have gone back out," he continued, adding after a beat, "I think."

Holmes's latent desire to return to Tahoe dissolved after his report was published in the *MMWR*. The resulting press blitz overwhelmed the young Texan. "I had made some comment about the fact that there was a question whether the disease exists. Well, there *was* and there still *is*," Holmes recalled much later. "So the newspapers picked up on this as saying that we thought it didn't exist, and then they started interviewing all these poor people who had been sick with this, and here we are saying that they're not ill. . . . We were publishing something that we thought was going to be of use to people. Instead, it was completely reversed on us. But I mean, here was my first major investigation. It was not the way I had hoped it would be. It was not a description of a huge outbreak of a newly described disease. But it was still the best that we could do under the circumstances. And to have it just continually lambasted by everyone . . . I mean, it gets on you after a while."

As time passed, those who were doing the lambasting were not only patients but at least one doctor: Paul Cheney. The Nevada clinician's move was unusual, given the unwritten code among doctors that discourages public criticism of one another. A few months after the report's release, Cheney expressed his contempt, inspired more by the agency's myopia than by its conclusion, when he told a reporter, "The design of their study was insufficient for the complexity of this problem. Therefore it is not surprising that the conclusions derived from that study are not very learned, or very surprising. That anyone would think that a week invested here in a simple case-control study of Epstein-Barr virus serologies would solve this puzzle is remarkable. This is far too complex."

"Here I am at CDC," Holmes complained. "We're the ivory tower. It's not appropriate behavior to attack somebody in print because of something like this, and that was what made it all the more irritating. I had no way of responding. If we turn around and say, 'These guys are lying,' how's that going to look? We're attacking these poor country doctors who are trying to help their patients. . . . I was interested in going back," Holmes reiterated, "but here I am being smeared all over the place by these physicians. How am I going to personally deal with somebody who feels I've done a bad job and a disservice? It was just, on a personal basis, I didn't want to go back at that point. It had nothing to do with CDC."

The government's equivocation about the existence of the disease was the initial volley in what would become routine federal policy as the years passed. This policy served to keep panic at bay but it also isolated sufferers in a Kafkaesque universe where what they knew to be real was reported by authorities to be patently false and where their testimony carried no weight at all, disputed as it was by the nation's premier disease detectives. Those who were ill conveniently became, in Jon Kaplan's words, "not normal Americans," but rather people strangely wedded to a mass fantasy of suffering and disability. Eventually, one cynical author who invested heavily in the government's view of the disease would characterize its victims and their support organizations as a "subculture of invalidism" in a withering book on the subject.[5]

Perhaps the most tragic effect of the *MMWR* report was the breach it created between the agency and the two people in the country who were best equipped to lead the agency staff through the labyrinth of the disease. Feeling as if they had hit a brick wall, Cheney and Peterson were suddenly as loath to continue their lobbying efforts with the agency as the Epidemic Intelligence Service officers were to pursue their Tahoe investigation.

An anticipation that the disease might not even exist, that it was a psychiatric disorder thriving among suggestible women, ensured a profoundly lethargic pace of research at the federal agency. And as the months and then years of inaction passed, the agency staff worked to portray Cheney and Peterson to colleagues in the American medical arena as "two doctors . . . who had worked themselves into a frenzy," in Holmes's words. Sotto voce they portrayed the internists as quacks.*

---

*The comments of one agency scientist, John Stewart, to this reporter were typical. "I heard some of the story from Gary," Stewart said several years after the Nevada investigation. "There obviously [was] a bunch of sick people out there. There obviously were a number of other people. I really don't know *what* they had. It seemed like somebody was just running their medical practice by lab test. It obviously was a situation that was out of control. . . . I heard about a bunch of patients who were out of control and a couple of doctors who were out of control."

8

"Dear Sirs, I Am *Sick* . . ."

Incline Village, Nevada

Try as they might, Jon Kaplan and his colleagues could not alter the hard reality: thousands of Americans believed they were ill. By 1986 a patient league calling itself the National CEBV Association emerged in Portland, Oregon; in less than eighteen months it had mushroomed from a living room support group to a staffed organization with national aspirations claiming 10,000 members, each of whom received a bimonthly newsletter, the *National CEBV Reporter.* In addition, although it did not advertise in any venue, the Portland group was soon receiving 100 to 300 letters a day from people who had been diagnosed with the disorder or who suspected they had acquired it.[1] Thirty states as well as Guam and the District of Columbia, had at least one support group. Alaska had three such organizations, two in the state's southeast region at Juneau and Auke Bay, and one in the interior at Fairbanks. California had twenty, organized by area codes from San Diego to the Mojave Desert to Sacramento. Incline Village had its own association, composed of patients from the small towns along the north shore of Lake Tahoe and funded by several multimillionaire members. Incline patients launched a free national hot line; within a year its volunteers were taking 250 calls a day around the clock.

During the first week in June, a front-page story appeared in the *Los Angeles Times* headlined "160 Victims at Lake Tahoe, Chronic Flu-Like Illness a Medical Mystery Story." *Times* reporter Robert Steinbrook described in colorful detail the plague of exhaustion and intellectual deterioration that had visited the mountain resort; then he summarized the government's conclusions and Anthony Komaroff's rebuttal. The *Times* article was sold through syndication to a multitude of smaller newspapers around the country, generating hundreds of inquiries to the hot line and to the Alder Street medical offices.

That summer, Peterson and Cheney began sending a questionnaire to every patient who called or wrote their office. A simple document, the questionnaire asked the date of the patient's onset of illness, the outstanding symptoms, age at onset, and sex. "We mailed out hundreds of these questionnaires," Cheney recalled, "and got most of them back." Over several weekends that summer, Cheney loaded the information from four hundred questionnaires into his Macintosh computer. "I entered it by the date they got ill," Cheney recalled. "And when I was done, you could see this almost perfect exponential curve rising out of the late 1970s—exactly in sync with AIDS." In fact, in the 1980s, the arc looked more like a bell curve, shooting up at a near–90-degree angle between 1983 and 1984, peaking in 1985, then plummeting in 1986. Cheney was struck by the extremely small but steady appearance of cases going back to 1953. "Most of these people had gotten ill in the 1980s," Cheney noted, "but some formed a flat line into the distant past—one or two cases a year, every year. The line remained flat up to the mid to late 1970s. Then, in 1977, this thing starts moving, and by 1984 and 1985 it's going right up to the roof."

Cheney also attempted to analyze the responses by the patients' age at the onset of their illness. He discovered a surprising parity between the epidemic patients in northern Nevada and those who responded to the questionnaire; among the first group, the average age at onset was thirty-seven and a half; among the second, it was thirty-eight. The northern Nevada sex ratio of approximately two women to every man held true among the national group as well.

Finally, the doctor analyzed the questionnaires by geography. "I made a plot to see if there were more patients in one region or sector of the country than another," Cheney recalled. "There was no trend. They were from all over the place."

On the basis of the doctor's graph, one might conclude the epidemic had ended abruptly in 1986, but Cheney wasn't so sure. He knew his survey was hardly scientific; for one thing, he had never examined these people. But in successive years he continued to enter the same simple statistics into his computer's database—date of onset was always the crucial question—for patients he had physically examined and studied in his practice. As the patient base grew, he gained confidence in his data. What he saw gave him little comfort. Each year, the rising arc moved along. When he performed the analysis in 1987, for instance, the arc of new cases continued its steady, dramatic rise well into 1986, but fell sharply in 1987. Similarly, when Cheney performed his calculations in 1988, the arc continued up in 1987 but crashed in 1988. By 1987 the doctor thought he knew the reason for this apparent anomaly.

"People who first become ill with this disease don't know they have it, usually, for at least a year, because it takes about a year to get a diagnosis," Cheney said. "So, on a graph, it *looks* like a bell curve, but it's not. The peak of the thing keeps moving along in time. The numbers are holding steady; it's just that there's a delay in diagnosis. In '82, '83, and '84," the doctor added, "it would have looked the same for AIDS, because [in the absence of a diagnostic test] it took a while for those people to get diagnosed, too."

"Something happened in the late 1970s," Cheney reflected soon after he fashioned his first admittedly crude analysis of the epidemic outside Nevada. "There's a new dynamic afoot."

Washington, D.C.

Cheney and Peterson weren't the only people struggling to measure the breadth of the new disease. Ted Van Zelst, the Chicago philanthropist whose daughter had been bedridden for four years, reported that spring that the survey he commissioned in

1985 was finished. He had mailed 2,200 questionnaires; 1,200 patients had responded with detailed replies—"a phenomenal return rate," Van Zelst noted. Of these, 702 had had at least one positive test for abnormal levels of Epstein-Barr virus antibodies, a requirement for inclusion in the study. Van Zelst's advisers, doctors in the Chicago area, opted to increase the survey's confidence level by further limiting the study to people who had been ill for at least two years. (Slightly less than half of the respondents had been ill for *less* than two years, a fact that correlated with Cheney's graph showing a dramatic rise in cases in 1984 and 1985.) Ultimately, 438 patients were included in the final cut. Among the survey's findings were the following:

- Half of the correspondents had been ill for less than five years, a fact that seemed to support Cheney's theory of a "new dynamic afoot" in the late 1970s.
- Seventy-one percent of the patients were between twenty-four and forty-five years old, with the largest number of patients—close to 40 percent—between the ages of thirty-five and forty-four. The second-largest number were twenty-five to thirty-four years old.
- Women suffering from the illness outnumbered men by approximately three to one.
- Health care workers and teachers were disproportionately victims of the disease.
- Forty percent were completely disabled by their disease; nearly all of the disabled group reported they had been denied Social Security disability benefits.
- Nearly half of the victims knew other people with the same disease; slightly more than one-fifth of all sufferers reported that other members of their family had the same illness.

Van Zelst's questionnaire also explored the nature of the symptoms from which this group suffered, asking whether or not they experienced any of thirty-seven symptoms. Ninety-nine percent reported extreme exhaustion, but the second most common complaints were in the neurologic realm. They included "difficulty concentrating" (88 percent), persistent headaches (81 percent), depression, anxiety and mood swings (80 percent), "dizziness and disorientation" (75 percent), hypersensitivity to light (75 percent), and memory loss (72 percent). Significantly, in light of the seizures that occurred among the Tahoe population, 16 percent of the Chicago survey respondents also reported suffering seizures or "seizure-like attacks." And although the CDC advocated testing for an enormous range of other diseases before conferring a diagnosis of CEBV upon a patient, *93 percent* of the respondents in the Chicago survey had been tested for other diseases, including anemia, tuberculosis, lupus, multiple sclerosis, hepatitis, rheumatoid arthritis, scleroderma, and Sjögren's disease (the last two are autoimmune diseases) with negative results.

During his manufacturing career, Van Zelst had testified on issues of international trade and land use, and he knew a number of senators' aides. Two years earlier, in

1984, he had met little resistance when he requested an opportunity to testify on behalf of the new disease. His suggestion then that House and Senate members "designate funds for specific research," and particularly his proposal that the NIH be directed to focus manpower on the problem, had been less warmly received: "[I]t is not the role of Congress . . . to advocate on behalf of any one disease," John Porter, an Illinois Republican whose district incorporated the Chicago suburb where the Van Zelsts lived, wrote to the engineer. "That would politicize decision-making which should be scientific in nature."

Van Zelst knew there were precedents for political activity around diseases, the most obvious being Richard Nixon's "war on cancer," but he realized that in order to generate interest, he required better proof of the pervasiveness of this disease. "The feeling was," Van Zelst recalled several years later, " 'if it's only your daughter and a few other people with this, then we can't get the government involved.' We had to have something to back up our claims."

Van Zelst now believed himself well armed. He presented testimony on April 28 and May 1 before the House and Senate subcommittees that control the purse strings at the NIH and the CDC. His foundation, the Chicagoan told legislators, had "been in contact with more than seven hundred doctors as a result of their inquiries for information about this disease. . . . New concerns about this disease have developed."

Van Zelst described the Lake Tahoe outbreak and noted that he had been alerted to smaller outbreaks around the country by Anthony Komaroff of Harvard. "Doctors have recently become aware of a fairly large number of patients in San Francisco," he added. Van Zelst told the legislators about the burgeoning network of local support groups and the 12,000 letters his foundation had received after the 1985 *New York Times* story on the disease; nearly a thousand of these letter writers had described their case histories in some detail. "These letters are from extremely articulate individuals," Van Zelst said. "Many are physicians, nurses, professors, and lawyers who have been searching for a diagnosis for years."

Using the survey findings, Van Zelst strove to provide committee members with a sense of the disease and its victims, though he acknowledged that his survey was less than scientific. But, he explained, "the question of 'how many are afflicted?' will not be properly answered as long as the patients themselves must seek ways of finding out this information. There must be a definite medical protocol set up at National Institutes of Health and/or Centers for Disease Control so that physicians will scientifically report the incidence of [the disease] in their [practices]."

Van Zelst's survey was remarkable for one other statistic, which emerged incidentally. All of the respondents were asked to name their doctor and the laboratory where their blood tests had been performed. Nineteen of the 438 people who had been ill longer than two years, or nearly 5 percent, indicated their doctor had been on the staff of the Mayo Clinic and that their tests had been performed there. In a departure from the typical Mayo clientele, which is 80 percent midwestern, these patients had come from all regions of the country, including Ellsworth, Maine; Norfolk, Virginia; McAdoo, Pennsylvania; and San Diego, New Orleans, Honolulu, and New York City.

Of course, if American medicine were Islam, then Rochester, Minnesota, would be Mecca and the Mayo Clinic would be the Mosque of Muhammad. Each year more than a quarter of a million people, arriving at the rate of a thousand each working day, registered at this somber palace of medicine. Here, they imagined, their body's mysteries and betrayals would be fathomed. For many, the Mayo was, as one of its doctors acknowledged, "the last resort." It was hardly surprising, then, that large numbers of people suffering from so-called CEBV sought help at the Mayo in the 1980s, all of them seeking an explanation for their catastrophic illness that had eluded their own doctors. It would be difficult to chart with certainty the number of people suffering from the singular constellation of symptoms established in the Minann survey who sought help at the Mayo Clinic in the 1980s. By any estimate, however, patients with the malady constituted a not insignificant portion of the clinic's five thousand patients a week.

Patients entering the famous clinic were assigned to a primary, or coordinating, doctor in a particular division based on the nature of their symptoms and complaints. People with general, nonspecific complaints were assigned to the department of internal medicine and might never see an infectious disease specialist. The clinic's departments of rheumatology and neurology were processing patients with the disease, as well, and it is likely that hematology, endocrinology, gynecology, and perhaps other departments, too, were playing host to people with the disease.

As early as January 1984 the Mayo had taken a public stand on the disease in its *Health Letter,* an eight-page newsletter mailed to 400,000 health-conscious members of the lay public. In a short article titled "On Chronic Fatigue" the editors noted that:

Occasionally, chronic fatigue is a symptom of a disorder such as chronic infection, cancer, hormone deficiency, or heart, lung, or kidney disease. . . .

Still, in many people who experience chronic fatigue, results of all examinations and tests are normal. The fatigue may even be severe. These people often will state to their physician: "I feel totally exhausted. At times I am too tired to eat or even talk. A sound sleep or extra rest during the day does me no good. I feel more tired when I get up in the morning than when I go to bed.". . .

What is wrong with these people?

Some have an emotional problem (anxiety or depression related ailments are common). In others, the problem is caused by a prolonged reaction to stress. What can be done to help?

In its concluding paragraph, the article outlined what was, in effect, the Mayo's standard recommended protocol for such patients: "Individuals with anxiety or depressive disorders often benefit from psychiatric treatment. In some instances, [antidepressant] medications are helpful."

Although the clinic's senior doctors had clearly cast their lot with the psychoneurotic theorists—those who felt the disease was a disorder of the psyche rather than the body—as an institution the Mayo had much to gain from the epidemic and its victims. Assumptions about the origin of a patient's symptoms might be made within hours of his or her entry through the imposing marble portals of the vast institution, but it was the clinic's practice to send these patients on a round of specialist consultations. As the days passed, the patient's bill burgeoned. Despite the expense, victims of the disease were unlikely to be afforded even compassion.

Typically, after completing their round of medical specialists, suffers were shuttled to the department of psychiatry, the Mayo's elephant graveyard for those presumed to be psychosomatically ill. There they were administered the Minnesota Multiphasic Personality Interview and questioned by a psychiatrist.

One patient who had been bedridden with CFS for several years spent a small inheritance left to her by her mother to pay for a visit to the Rochester clinic in 1985. Although she was wheelchair-bound, she was told by Mayo specialists that she suffered from an imaginary pain syndrome, and she was offered psychiatric counseling. A young man, John Boren of Albuquerque, New Mexico, had fallen acutely ill while on vacation in Paris, and had been bedridden for two years. After costly examinations by numerous clinic doctors in 1987, the Mayo's chief of psychiatry, Gordon Moore, suggested to Boren that he had emotional problems. Another patient with CFS, a disabled dental hygienist, sold her car to pay for her Mayo evaluation in 1988. She was also sent home with a psychiatric diagnosis. Most commonly, the final prescription was exercise, a potentially dangerous recommendation for such patients.*

In 1988, a series of Mayo doctors was interviewed over a two-day period about CFS and their methods of evaluating people suffering from the disease. All of the interviews were taped. In return for permission to conduct the interviews, the clinic's legal department demanded that all information derived from those interviews, as well as quotes, be submitted to the interviewed doctors prior to publication. When this was done in 1995, all of the doctors declined to allow their names or their quotes to be used.

For people suffering from the disease, the Mayo experience was little more than a "wallet biopsy," according to Paul Cheney. For Marc Iverson, however, scion of a wealthy steel manufacturer, the arrogance of the Mayo specialists was vastly more devastating than their fees. "Everything is black or white for them," Iverson said some years after his second and last visit to Rochester. "There can't be anything in the world they don't understand—because they understand everything! They don't believe in their patients—they believe in their orthodoxy. They read their printouts, but they never really listen to what you're saying. It's the worst of modern medicine."

---

*In coming years it was discovered that little was guaranteed to exacerbate chronic fatigue syndrome more rapidly or more profoundly than exercise, particularly rigorous exercise. During aerobic exercise, CFS victims were found to experience a sudden drop in body temperature and a decrease in oxygen flow to the brain—the opposite of what occurs in normal people. The oxygen deficit in the brain persisted for several days after even brief activity (Ismael Mena, "Study of Cerebral Perfusion by NeuroSPECT in Patients with Chronic Fatigue Syndrome," presented at the Cambridge Symposium on Myalgic Encephalomyelitis [M.E.], Cambridge University, England, April 12, 1990).

Reno, Nevada

By the summer of 1986, Olympic cyclist Inga Thompson had been ill for two years. She had spent most of that time in bed. "I was just useless," Thompson recalled much later.

Because Thompson had had an abnormal result on a CT brain scan the year before, her Reno doctor now ordered an MRI brain scan for the cyclist at Reno Diagnostics. The MRI brain scan was abnormal as well. Her father, an orthopedic surgeon, took Thompson back to the University of Utah, where doctors gave a tentative diagnosis of multiple sclerosis. When Thompson insisted that her symptoms were unlike those of MS and requested further evaluation, the Utah doctors told her she was "in denial."

Los Angeles, California

That summer, another elite women's cyclist fell ill. Jill Koval was twenty-four when the disease hit. A 225- to 275-miles-per-week cyclist, she, too, was now bedridden. The first day, her most bizarre symptom was a remarkable weakness in her arms, but her legs, too, tingled as if she had just performed a major workout. She had trouble focusing her eyes.

Although she was not a member of the U.S. Olympic team, Koval was a member of the U.S. National Cycling Team and, the summer before, like Thompson, she had trained at the Olympic training center. Only recently, she had signed a lucrative contract with 7-Eleven, the biggest corporate sponsor in cycling; now the company canceled the contract. She remained severely debilitated for the next two years.

"The worst part about the whole thing," Koval would remember some years later, "is that no one believed me. I started to think I was a mental case."

Washington, D.C.

On July 24 the House Appropriations Committee, as a result of Ted Van Zelst's testimony, encouraged both the NIH and the CDC to address the matter of the new disease. Unfortunately it failed to earmark money for research at either agency. Nevertheless, the report's language acknowledged the problem, noting "an increasing incidence nationwide of a physically and psychologically disabling illness, chronic Epstein-Barr virus infection (CEBV)." Language in the House bill encouraged the NIH "to expand research studies on CEBV to improve diagnostic techniques, develop treatment, and search for an eventual cure of this debilitating disease which is affecting thousands of Americans." In their message to the CDC, the bill's authors were more specific: "The incidence appears to be much higher than was previously indicated. There have been apparent small epidemics of this disease in various parts of the country and reports of thousands of individual cases." The subcommittee asked the CDC to determine the prevalence of the disease by setting up a system whereby doctors could report cases of the disease to the agency.

In August the Senate appropriations subcommittee with oversight over the NIH issued its report on the fiscal year 1987 budget for the Department of Health and

Human Services. The committee urged the National Institute of Allergy and Infectious Diseases "to continue and expand recent studies of victims of [the new chronic disease] and to increase grant support for extramural research." The committee also asked the agency to submit a report before the next fiscal year budget submission, "clarifying the controversy amongst the scientific community and submitting a plan to resolve this controversy through continuing research and public education."

These were the first in a series of congressional requests that the health agencies in Atlanta and Bethesda would ignore in coming years.

Incline Village, Nevada

To Cheney's surprise, Wistar scientist Elaine DeFreitas called him early that spring. She'd had a conversation with Robert Gallo, she told the doctor, and Gallo had expressed interest in the Tahoe blood samples still in her freezer. Would Cheney mind if she sent samples to the federal researcher? Cheney paused, torn between impulses. "You know I'm collaborating on this with some other people," he told her. With regret, he declined DeFreitas's request. For the moment he was unwilling to jeopardize his relationship with Komaroff and the team Komaroff had assembled by second-guessing a member of that team—in this case, government retrovirologist Tom Folks. To do so, Cheney felt, would be particularly grievous since Folks was at the National Institute of Allergy and Infectious Diseases and so was to some extent in competition with Gallo's team at the National Cancer Institute. "If you're dealing with one retrovirologist, to turn around and send blood to a competitor virologist is like stabbing him in the back," Cheney said.

By early June, however, both Cheney and his partner, Dan Peterson, had become discouraged with the pace of the research being choreographed by Komaroff at Harvard. "We were getting no indication from Tom Folks that there was any evidence of retrovirus," Cheney said. "And as time went on, I got increasingly frustrated with the lack of progress in the face of some obvious things that needed to be tracked down—like why was Gallo interested? And why was DeFreitas getting a P24 core protein [a product of retroviruses]? And yet, no evidence . . ."

In early June, Cheney entered into an auspicious series of conversations with Howard Streicher, a researcher in the Gallo lab. A gruff former emergency room doctor from Hawaii who had entered Robert Gallo's inner circle, Streicher pressed Cheney for information about the Tahoe epidemic and the clinical status of his patients. The federal scientists' curiosity, Cheney believed, carried an obvious implication: they too suspected that a retrovirus was causing disease in Tahoe. After all, they were retrovirologists—what else would they be looking for? Streicher, like most in the Gallo orbit, was fiercely protective of the laboratory's scientific secrets. In the course of conversations about the phenomena Cheney and Peterson were observing in Nevada, Streicher did not disabuse Cheney of his assumption that the government lab's interest in the epidemic malady was related to its retroviral potential. As it would for years to come, information flowed mostly in one direction: from Nevada to Bethesda.

"Eventually," Cheney recalled, "Streicher invited me to send some blood, and I did."

The doctor chose not to inform his primary collaborator, Anthony Komaroff. "I knew he would object," Cheney explained. "I guess I felt I had a higher purpose," the doctor continued. "The patients were more important than the ego of a researcher and the etiquette of research. Tom Folks wasn't having to sit there and see these people every other week and listen to their stories and to their frustration like I was. He wasn't in my shoes."

Cheney shipped twelve blood samples by Federal Express to Bethesda. When a month passed without word from Streicher, Cheney presumed the blood had been negative for retrovirus and that the Gallo lab had dropped the inquiry.

National Cancer Institute, Bethesda, Maryland

Gallo and his scientists had been doing anything but searching for retroviruses in the Tahoe blood. They were hunting instead for evidence of their newly discovered herpesvirus; ultimately, they were seeking a disease with which to pair it. By the time Cheney sent them blood from the Nevada epidemic victims, the researchers already knew a great deal about their new bug, even if they knew very little about the Tahoe malady. Those struggling to unshroud the unique properties of the sixth human herpesvirus agreed that it was remarkable in all respects. Initially it appeared that this bug, unlike any other herpesvirus, could flourish only in an environment of fresh human B-cells.* The federal scientists dubbed the germ human B-cell lymphotrophic virus, or HBLV.† Two to four days after infection with HBLV, the B-cells inflated into watery, balloon-like configurations, a growth pattern that mimicked some kinds of laboratory-grown cancer cells; within two weeks they exploded, dumping thousands of virus particles into the cell culture, each particle capable of infecting a new cell.

The Gallo team considered the virus's cytopathic, or cell-killing, ability exceptional: it reduced flourishing B-cell cultures to debris in approximately ten days. The devastation was so extreme, in fact, that the scientists had difficulty keeping the virus alive; it crunched through cells like a plague of locusts, but when it had exhausted its supply, the virus had nowhere to go and promptly died. Finally, unlike any other herpesvirus known to the scientists, this new virus did not appear to have a latent stage. It required little imagination to fathom the implications for human health posed by an organism that targeted immune system cells and expeditiously destroyed them. Theoretically, the disease it caused must be severe—but where or what, exactly, was that disease?

So far, every herpesvirus discovered had been shown to cause a specific "primary" disease, be it chicken pox, mono, or genital herpes. All six patients in

*Even Epstein-Barr virus, notable for infecting B-cells, occasionally can be found in the epithelial cells lining the mouth and throat.

†Herpesviruses are named for the primary disease they cause, not for the cells they target; if the organism's pathology is unknown, it is assigned a number based on the order in which it was discovered. By this orthodoxy, the correct name for the new virus is human herpesvirus six, or HHV6, the name adopted by the National Cancer Institute's rivals at the CDC six months later.

whom the scientists had first spotted the new virus had lymphoproliferative, or immune system, disorders, though not necessarily the same disorders, which left the matter of a single, or primary, disease open to speculation.* The team began testing blood sera from large numbers of healthy people for the presence of antibodies to the virus. They pulled most of their specimens from the massive collection of banked sera in the National Cancer Institute's −70°F. freezers, some of it dating back two decades. Other, fresh samples came from their own staff. The team's earliest test, later refined, picked up antibodies in fewer than 2 percent of all samples, a finding that bolstered the possibility that the researchers had stumbled onto a brand-new virus in humans. Among the National Cancer Institute scientists and lab techs who were tested, the positivity rate was zero. So far, then, infection with human B-cell lymphotrophic virus appeared to be an uncommon occurrence.

When the scientists performed their assay on the samples from Tahoe, a new pattern emerged, however: nearly every sample was positive for antibodies to the new herpesvirus. Thus, after months of investigation, the Tahoe malady, a disease that mystified them, was so far the only candidate for their virus.

Incline Village, Nevada

Just when he had decided the Gallo lab had dropped its inquiry, Paul Cheney received a call from Jake Lindsay, the disabled cardiologist who was increasingly at the center of an information loop that wound its way through the federal health agencies and academia. "Lindsay told me he had heard that Gallo had found something in our blood," Cheney recalled. "He said there was a rumor circulating that the lab had found evidence of a virus." Soon after this conversation, Cheney received another call from his former collaborator in Philadelphia, Wistar scientist Elaine DeFreitas. Robert Gallo had approached her at his annual summer lab meeting in Washington, D.C., to which he invited dozens of outside scientists, to discuss the Tahoe epidemic with her. Gallo had found something in the Tahoe blood, DeFreitas told Cheney.

When Cheney heard that Gallo had "hinted to [DeFreitas] that he knew what might be causing the Tahoe problem," the doctor recalled, "my natural thought was [that] he [had] found a retrovirus. I mean, he's a retrovirologist. If he's found something, then it is a retrovirus." Unable to contain his curiosity, Cheney called Howard Streicher. "Without actually bringing up the rumor, I said, 'Have you found anything?' "

Streicher, characteristically, was enigmatic. In fact, he told Cheney that the retrovirology team had been unable so far to find anything unusual, but he promised, "We will get back to you." Nevertheless, the conversation with Strei-

---

*Although the virus had been isolated from two AIDS patients, it was initially thought to be less than critical to the development of that disease. The scientists looked for evidence of the virus in the blood of twelve AIDS patients who were lymphoma-free; all twelve turned out to be seronegative. By 1993, however, the Gallo group had fine-tuned its HBLV assay, and government scientists changed their original opinion: the herpesvirus was found to be so prevalent among AIDS sufferers that Gallo himself postulated that HBLV worked in tandem with HIV, or was perhaps the trigger mechanism that launched the series of immunological events leading to death.

cher left Cheney feeling frustrated. At last, he phoned his Boston collaborator, Anthony Komaroff, to confess his breach of scientific decorum. "I said, 'Tony, I sent twelve sera to Gallo.' And he said—and I remember I had to hold the phone way out to here," Cheney said, gesturing to a space three feet from his ear. "He said, *'You did what?'* After about a minute, during which he ventilated, Tony said, 'So—what was the rumor?' I said, 'Rumor was that he found something, but I called them and they're not admitting anything to me.' "

"There are three people in the world Gallo won't stonewall," Komaroff told the Nevada doctor, "and I know one of them.' "

Komaroff's friend was Robert A. Weinberg, an oncogene expert working at the Massachusetts Institute of Technology's Whitehead Institute of Biomedical Research, and a friend of Robert Gallo's. Three days later Komaroff called Cheney with stunning news: Gallo had turned positively garrulous in his conversation with Weinberg. Months earlier scientists in the Gallo lab had indeed discovered antibodies to a new virus in a handful of patients with several different illnesses. Apparently, until they began testing blood from Nevadans suffering from the curious Tahoe malady, the federal researchers had been mystified as to what primary ailment this new virus might cause. In the Tahoe patients they had hit upon the first group of people all of whom seemed to be consistently infected—in fact, *royally* infected, based on antibody tests—with the new germ, and all of whom suffered from the same disease. So far, however, only Gallo and his lab associates knew that the newly discovered virus was a member of the herpes family and not a retrovirus.

Bethesda, Maryland

Sixteen thousand people worked at the NIH, making the agency the world's largest institution devoted to biomedical research. With three times more money at its disposal than was allotted to the CDC—more than $10 billion a year—it was also the richest. In the half century since philanthropists Helen and Luke Wilson deeded the agency 45 rustic acres in suburban Maryland, it had prospered and grown larger, in recent years consuming another 250 acres of public land, and its directors had won ever-larger sums from congressional appropriations committees. At last count, the agency comprised seventeen institutes, their offices and laboratories scattered among sixty-three buildings. At the center of the campus, small Georgian-style structures with graceful white columns housed the administrators' offices as well as some of the agency's oldest institutes. Less distinguished edifices of varying sizes, connected by roads and footpaths, fanned out onto the manicured grounds and surrounding neighborhoods. Slow-moving white jitneys shuttled employees among the conglomerate's buildings.

Robert Gallo and his associates worked at the western perimeter of the campus on the sixth floor of Building 37, a glass-and-steel structure that was part of the National Cancer Institute. By 1986 the lab chief was a superstar of the medical world, and his Laboratory of Tumor Cell Biology—formerly just another among a number of overcrowded, grubby immunology labs in the institute—was at the top of the agency's prestige pyramid. The lab's fame accrued entirely from its association with the isolation of human immunodeficiency virus. Irrespective of the shadow that was soon to fall on its HIV claim, the Gallo lab was at the axis of American retroviral research in 1986, its researchers the fair-haired boys of the government's research establishment, scientific superheroes who could do no wrong.

It was into this charged milieu that Robert Gallo invited Paul Cheney and Anthony Komaroff one week after Cheney learned that Gallo had discovered a new virus in patients from the Nevada epidemic. Gallo and the other government scientists working on human B-cell lymphotrophic virus wanted to learn more about the Tahoe malady.

That afternoon, Cheney met Komaroff and the two walked together to Building 37. In his briefcase Cheney carried magnetic resonance imaging brain scans, the results of Berkeley neuropsychologist Sheila Bastien's mental status tests, and documents giving evidence of the array of immunological problems he and his partner had discovered. Inside a large conference room, Cheney stood before Gallo's core research group, approximately ten people, and described the events of the previous two years in Tahoe. Not surprisingly, little he said riveted the federal scientists like his descriptions of non-Hodgkin's lymphomas in Nevada, particularly the apparent cases of Burkitt's.

When Cheney finished, Gallo's lieutenant, Zaki Salahuddin, reciprocated. Using a slide projector with a light beam that spread images over an entire wall, he projected electron micrographs of human B-cell lymphotrophic virus particles erupting from B-cells. Cheney and Komaroff were struck by the destructive force of the virus. What hit the clinicians more powerfully, however, was that the Gallo group, a world-famous retrovirology team, had discovered a new herpesvirus.

"Here we are, sitting in the offices of the nation's premier retrovirologist, looking at a herpesvirus," Cheney recalled. "And then I thought, 'Well, my God, we've solved the case!' "

The fascination and fervor were returned in equal measure by the government scientists. Komaroff later recalled, "I remember vividly the day in July of 1986 when we first went to Bob's lab and—all of the leadership of the lab was there— and Bob says something like 'We're all going to stop working on AIDS for the next three months and work on *this*.' "

Before leaving the campus, Cheney presented his clinical findings from Tahoe to another group. In his audience this time was medical virologist Stephen Straus of the National Institute of Allergy and Infectious Diseases, author of the 1985 *Annals* article on the chronic syndrome. One of Straus's research fellows was also present, as were six or seven fourth-year medical students. The meeting took place in a classroom inside Building 10, the NIH clinical center. In the give-and-take after the doctor's presentation, Cheney noted that Straus was satirical in his references to the discovery in the Gallo lab. Straus called the bug "herpes Gallo." In Cheney's memory, however, the red-haired, impeccably groomed scientist seemed sincerely interested in his clinical observations and laboratory findings. "He was kind of fascinated," Cheney recalled, "and not at all hostile. But amused. I felt like I was a medical student giving a talk and he was the teacher. The venom was against Gallo. He knew what I had with Gallo might be an important lead."

Cheney left the NIH campus assuming Straus was an ally in the effort to elucidate the epidemic disease.

Before the summer's end, Cheney made four trips to Washington at his own expense to meet with the federal scientists in an effort to clarify the clinical manifestations of the syndrome to them. In addition, he and his partner, at the request of the scientists in the Gallo lab, continued to send samples from their patients. By September the clinicians had sent seventy-two blood samples overnight to Bethesda via Federal Express. Komaroff, too, was sending samples to the Gallo group from his New England population. The government scientists were also getting blood from clinicians in private practice in New York City, Houston, Fort Lauderdale, and Miami who were seeing large numbers of patients with the disease.

Although the Peterson-Cheney clinic was falling under increasing financial stress from the high costs of the doctors' own research and their unremunerated collaboration with Gallo, Cheney had developed a strange immunity to worry that summer. He was in high gear, thoroughly enmeshed in the drama of the scientific mystery that had wound its way from a rural town in Nevada to the most prestigious research laboratory in the nation in less than a year.

"By the summer of 1986, during the Gallo thing," Cheney said later, "the medical economics of the practice began to lurch into the red increasingly. Like, four flights to Washington, D.C., from the West Coast. The two-thousand-dollar-a-month phone bills. The mounting bills for patient blood tests that patients were not paying for. Although," the doctor added, "I didn't care—I just didn't care. I mean, I guess I felt like I was young enough that if everything crashed, what the hell? This was a great ride! I mean, you cannot *buy* an experience like this."

Centers for Disease Control, Atlanta, Georgia

As the government's cancer researchers' interest in the Tahoe epidemic quietly escalated, investigators at the CDC were struggling to divest themselves of—or at least to distance themselves from—the entire affair. Nine months after their Nevada adventure, Jon Kaplan and Gary Holmes had achieved a tenuous stasis: with the publication of their report in the *Morbidity and Mortality Weekly Report,* Kaplan had managed to ease himself off the Nevada study and was educating himself about retroviruses. Thus Holmes, who was Kaplan's junior and an agency employee of only fourteen months, came to be the U.S. government's principal investigator into the new disease. The young Texan was now saddled with the task of interpreting, with an eye toward publication in a medical journal, the data he and Kaplan had obtained in Nevada.

In the months since the team's return from Nevada, the infamous entity—few at the agency felt comfortable calling it a disease—had become a dependable source of humor among the epidemiologists in the Viral Exanthems and Herpesvirus Branch. Jokes about it were rife along the branch's corridor in Building 6, where anyone who happened to mention he was tired or feeling stress was barraged with derisive comments suggesting he was falling victim to the bogus affliction. Holmes, who had hoped to carve out a respectable career at the agency, was chagrined. Perhaps in an effort to sustain his dignity among his colleagues, nearly all of whom were relatively young males like him, the EIS officer began decorating his cubbyhole office with cartoons, memos, and posters poking fun either at the disease or at the people he was supposed to be studying. On a large poster of the Statue of Liberty, for instance, he scrawled, "Give me your tired, your weak, your EBV-positive, yearning to be diagnosed." On another wall, he hung a placard that said, "Mono Man." On his door's exterior was another placard: "Just because I'm paranoid doesn't mean they're not after me."

This merriment reached out into the division's public spaces, as well. For some period of time, Holmes's office door was home to a letter composed by the agency's staff lampooning the chronic disease and its sufferers. "Dear Sirs," it began, "I am *sick.* . . . I am so tired, it took me six days to dictate this letter to my secretary." The text of the letter evoked a grotesque portrait of a hypochondriac. It read, in part: "I would like a list of recommended treatments . . . in descending order of trendiness, including acyclovir, gamma globulin, WXYZ-2, 3DOG, Vitamins A, B-1 through 12, C, D, E, F, G, H, I, J, K, L, M, N, O, P, and Q, Zinc, Cadmium, Cobalt, Neodymium, Ytterbium, lecithin, morithin, lessismorithin, sensory deprivation, walking on hot coals, alternating sensory deprivation and walking on hot coals, purified fruit-bat guano injections, and bedrest. I have already tried Valium, Lithium, Haldol, and thorazine, but they only work when I take them." And it ended, "Please inform me about how to get social security and workman's compensation benefits for the above diseases. I have had them for over forty years now, and I am only twenty-nine years old." The letter was signed "I. M. Zappode, 2431 Western Blot, Wornout, California."

The document was widely disseminated and enjoyed throughout the agency, and remained on the division's bulletin board for the next two and a half years until a staffer noticed a reporter copying its text into a notebook. Soon afterward, the staffer urged viral epidemiology chief Larry Schonberger to remove it. When Schonberger demurred, the staffer warned his boss, "This will come back to haunt us." Only then did Schonberger reluctantly remove the letter from public display.

That summer Gary Holmes and his superiors at the CDC first began to indicate that money constraints were impeding their progress in unraveling the elusive mysteries of chronic Epstein-Barr virus syndrome. If only they had more money, the scientists suggested, they could get down to the business of elucidating the true prevalence and the cause of the disease. The agency's response to the letter from San Francisco Health Commission president Philip Lee was typical. Lee had urged James Mason, the agency's chief, to release the Tahoe findings and to direct more agency resources toward illuminating the disease, which Lee characterized as a "nationwide phenomenon." Mason forwarded Lee's missive to principal investigator Holmes for a response. The latter wrote that he received "numerous calls each week" from sufferers and from doctors. "It is quite apparent that there is a great deal of interest in this entity throughout the country," he said. Unfortunately, Holmes continued, given the diagnostic vagaries of the disease, it was impossible to know either how many people actually were suffering from it or if those who had been so diagnosed actually had the disease. Holmes said he and his colleagues "agree a greater research effort into this syndrome is warranted." The problem, he added, was that "recent budget cutbacks make expanding efforts into this disease syndrome very difficult. . . . If additional funding becomes available," he added, "our branch would be interested in initiating studies dealing with the etiology, epidemiology and immunology of this syndrome."

Incline Village, Nevada

On July 31 thirteen million households tuned in to ABC's *20/20* broadcast about the Lake Tahoe epidemic. They were transported into former meter reader Chris Guthrie's living room in Kings Beach, California, where the thirty-four-year-old, who had been largely bedridden for a year, described her experience. The show overwhelmingly focused on the emotional trauma of the disease rather than scientific issues. Guthrie described the sorrow she felt when friends pleaded with her not to touch their new baby for fear of contagion. James Jones's patients in Denver described social ostracism as well. One of them, real estate consultant Darrell Anderson, a fifty-four-year-old father of four, talked about the suicidal fantasies that had beset him after two years of life-altering illness that few among his friends and relatives believed was real. "I got in my car, and I drove up the highway, headed up to the mountains, and I was going to drive off a cliff. Now, that's absurd, but that's really the way I felt. It wasn't a matter of trying to get back at anyone. I just wanted to end it all." Nomi Antelman of Tucson, Arizona, said, "I couldn't face another doctor saying, 'You're doing this to yourself,' 'Think positively,' 'You're crazy,' 'You're neurotic'—whatever they had to say. And one day I simply decided that I had to be released from the pain, and the only release that I could see was suicide." When James Jones diagnosed Antelman, she was stunned. "There's a *name* for what I have?" she asked. "Then I said to him, 'You've saved my life.' And at that time I don't think he really understood what I meant: *You have saved my life.*"

Nearly a decade later, Roger Sergel, the segment's producer, recalled that the show generated an overwhelming response. The deluge of calls and letters was so great that ABC ultimately prepared a form letter to respond to inquiries from the public; the number of requests for transcripts was phenomenal, Sergel remembered. Hundreds of calls poured into the offices of Cheney and Peterson as well; within eighteen hours Chris Guthrie had her telephone number unlisted. Within two days letters began arriving at the Alder Street practice at the rate of one hundred a day.

CDC staff were conspicuously absent from the show. The network sought an interview with James Mason or a Mason-designated spokesperson, without success. Interestingly, although ABC never got its interview, a document obtained under the Freedom of Information Act revealed that someone at the CDC prepared a three-page backgrounder for Mason in the *event* of an interview with *20/20*. After a cursory description of what was known about the disease and the agency's conclusions about the Tahoe outbreak, the backgrounder primed Mason with the following:

Negative for CDC:
   Many people diagnosed with this illness finally thought they had found the etiology and thus the disease was "not in their heads." The CDC study says that EBV may not be the cause, and that serology tests prove nothing. Many are sick and desperate and will be upset that their disease may still be unknown.

Positive for CDC:
   We have helped to identify the major problems facing the study of this illness. . . .

▥

Cheney and Peterson began to feel the disapprobation of their fellow citizens in more overt ways after the *20/20* story. "By the summer of '86, the perception began in earnest that we were harming the economy," Cheney said. "Now, it was not just an intellectual dispute among professionals, it was, 'This summer, business is down, and it's got to be because of this publicity.' " Cheney's children were taunted at school; he and his wife were denied service at a local restaurant. Mary Peterson's shopping cart was overturned in the supermarket parking lot; obscene notes were attached to her car, warning her and her husband to leave Incline Village. Peterson's toddler was nearly banned from his day-care center at another mother's request; the mother happened to be the wife of a local GP. Peterson himself was openly accused by strangers of trying to buy up lakeshore property with the profits from "the virus."
   The business community of Incline Village had struggled to derail the broadcast, at least for a while. Before it aired, chamber of commerce president Jeffrey Quinn penned a letter to *20/20* producer Sergel pleading for a postponement until fall, after the summer tourist season had ended and before the ski season began. "It is our perception that a lot of good would flow from such an action," Quinn wrote, "to the benefit of a small community which survives on tourist dollars."
   The network broadcast was a watershed for Cheney. "After the *20/20* thing," he recalled, "I realized that if I really wanted to pursue this, I could not be living in Tahoe. It just would never work. I mean, you don't do research on a viral disease like this in a tourist area. You do not go to Vail, Colorado, and study an infectious AIDS-like virus. No one in their right mind would do that."
   For Peterson, too, the *20/20* broadcast was a point of demarcation, but unlike his partner it served to cement his commitment to stay in Incline to fight for his patients and for an understanding of their disease. "I was *not* going to be driven out of town by these idiots—by these people who knew *nothing* about viruses, *nothing* about medicine," he said.

Los Angeles, California

With the publication of the government's Tahoe report, the odds had diminished that doctors who, like Peterson, labored in the trenches rather than in the halls of academe, would prevail anytime soon. Influential faculty members grew only more hardened in their views that year, even as the number of sufferers seeking help in university settings burgeoned. Attempting to explain the phenomenon to themselves and others, they attributed the surfeit of victims in their clinic anterooms to the spread of publicity rather than a pathogen. The patients, they implied, were either hypochondriacs—crocks or gomers, in medical slang, the latter an acronym for "get out of my emergency room"—or neurotics seeking undue attention. In at least one such institution, the University of California at Los Angeles, the city's premier medical institution, the degree of cynicism on the subject was profound. That fall, UCLA's infectious disease senior faculty issued a memo on the subject to all doctors and residents working or rotating through the medical center's infectious disease clinic. The memo's harsh skepticism was bound to deaden any impulse on the part of even the most open-minded UCLA doctors to make the diagnosis, no matter how persuasive the patient's symptoms.

Dated September 1986, the notice from UCLA's Division of Infectious Diseases was sent to all "Physicians participating in the UCLA Infectious Diseases Clinic." "The syndrome of chronic EBV infection has become a popular explanation given to patients with fatigue of uncertain cause," it read in part. "This perhaps nonexistent syndrome has been popularized by the media and fueled by physicians in the community who have not reviewed the data critically, as well as by commercial laboratories who make their money doing poorly standardized serologic tests. Consequently," the memo continued, *"we are seeing several patients every week with suspected chronic EBV"* (italics added). Stressing that "the current clinical and laboratory criteria [for CEBV] are unreliable," the memo advised doctors to look instead for anxiety and depression as well as tuberculosis, chronic heart and liver disease, and AIDS.

On October 12, William Hewitt, then the university's chief of infectious diseases, and two members of his staff, David Haake and Steven Blander, made the disease the subject of a public letter to the editor of the *Los Angeles Times.* The trio sounded almost angry. "The bottom line is that since the symptoms and signs are nonspecific, and the currently available laboratory tests are unreliable," they wrote, "the diagnosis of 'chronic Epstein-Barr virus syndrome' means nothing; it is a non-diagnosis." The doctors also cautioned that providing a patient with the chronic EBV syndrome diagnosis would make the patient feel "hopeless," since there was "no effective treatment" for the ailment. This hopelessness, the UCLA experts concluded, "may dissuade these patients from returning to their prior lifestyle and activities." The possibility that patients had abandoned their "prior lifestyle and activities" as a result of disabling illness rather than by free choice was not entertained.

A few weeks later Beverly Hills internal medicine specialist Herb Tanney, striving to give his UCLA brethren the benefit of the doubt, sent his patient Blake Edwards to Hewitt for an evaluation. At the time, Edwards was extremely ill. The film director recalled that Hewitt was deferential in his approach. "He didn't want to come right out and say I was crazy, because I have a high profile—I'm well known—but he as much as told me I had a psychological illness," Edwards said later. "My feeling afterward was very simplistic and perhaps very typical. I wanted to say, 'I just wish *you* had it!' It outrages one. And it makes you terribly insecure. Absolutely *no one* believes you, and you begin to doubt yourself."

Miami, Florida

Researchers like those at UCLA, who were convinced the disease was a psychiatric problem, were usually rewarded with either no clear clinical findings or with findings that reinforced their bias: the patients were anxious and depressed. Researchers looking for ways to elucidate the organic nature of the disease considered the UCLA approach futile. "I'm convinced the majority of patients really become depressed," Anthony Komaroff remarked that year. "But what does that matter? I mean, who wouldn't be? If you were to test a group of patients with multiple sclerosis or lupus, and find that seventy percent of them were depressed, would you say, 'Well, since you're depressed, you don't have a physical illness'? I would think it would be unnatural *not* to get depressed. *I* would be depressed."

Conversely, on occasion researchers who otherwise had no interest in the subject were drawn powerfully into the web when faced with laboratory results providing evidence of organic disease. That was the case with Nancy Klimas, an immunologist who ran the only clinic at the University of Miami where patients with immunodeficiency states other than AIDS could be evaluated. Klimas was, in fact, the only immunologist on the university faculty who actually saw patients. Typically, her clinic was packed with people suffering from congenital and acquired immunodeficiencies. Klimas also ran the AIDS clinic at the Miami Veterans Administration hospital.

An unadorned and plainspoken woman who wore jeans under her white lab coat, Klimas became aware of an unusual and, she later admitted, bothersome group of people in her university clinic that year. All of them had seen numerous doctors before coming to her; all of them insisted there was something wrong with their immune systems. Klimas was highly skeptical of their self-diagnoses. "I was trying to do what we call 'turf,' " Klimas remembered. "I would try to turf them off to a rheumatologist because they also complained of fatigue and joint pain. And they kept saying, 'No, no, please just look at my immune system before you do anything like that.' "

Klimas was lavishly funded with government money to study AIDS. She had used some of that money to standardize several sophisticated measures of immune function in the disease. Frequently she liked to use her new tests to compare AIDS patients to people suffering from other kinds of immune deficiency states. Now she decided to compare her AIDS patients with a few of the university patients she had tried to turf. The doctor was amply rewarded for her efforts. "What was fascinating was the *levels* of immune dysfunction in this population," Klimas remembered. "That's when I really started getting interested.

"These patients kept trickling in with this chronic fatigue syndrome thing just as I was becoming better and better funded in AIDS and was doing a lot of basic immunologic research in AIDS," she continued. "Like every other skeptical clinician, I tried hard not to believe in it. But I kept doing my weird immunologic panels on these patients and saying, 'Well, it looks like there's a viral infection in these folks.' "

Klimas wasn't looking for viruses—virology wasn't her field—but she was struck by changes in white blood cell ratios and other immune system parameters that suggested a body fighting infection. "The immunology is not your run-of-the-mill immunology," she recalled, "nor is it depression immunology, another area I was rather interested in. I had a fairly good idea of what depression did to the immune system. In fact, I was an investigator in the Center for Psychoneuroimmunologic Research in HIV infections, so I had a good background in the literature on immunologic and neuropsychiatric connections. That's *really* what got me into it, actually. I said, 'Boy, this is *different*.' "

Klimas also was increasingly impressed by the clinical severity of the disease. "A lot of my colleagues told me, 'Oh, *everyone's* tired!' Oh *no*. These guys were *profoundly* tired. These aren't normal folks," Klimas said.

When she ran a series of immune function tests on several patients at once, the results convinced her that the psychoneurotic proponents of the disease were one hundred percent wrong. She also gave one presumed-AIDS patient in her VA hospital AIDS clinic who was negative for human immunodeficiency virus a new diagnosis: chronic Epstein-Barr syndrome. "It didn't take long—not more than three months after I became a believer—to have word of mouth spread around that I was a chronic fatigue clinician," she continued. "After that, I was just overwhelmed with patients from the south Florida area and from far away, too."

9

Jerry's Poster Kids

Incline Village, Nevada

On September 12, Jean Lamming, a young journalist for the *North Lake Tahoe Bonanza,* broke one of the biggest science stories of the year, even if the rest of the world failed to notice. "A prestigious medical research center is expected to announce its discovery of a new virus that has been found in blood samples from many of the North Lake Tahoe's chronic fatigue patients," Lamming wrote. The reporter quoted Cheney, who she said had just returned from a meeting with researchers on the East Coast: "They had a virus looking for a disease, and we had a disease looking for a virus and we met up in June of 1986," Cheney said.

Cheney had indeed just returned from the National Cancer Institute with a list of patients proven by the Gallo team to be actively infected with human B-cell lymphotrophic virus. He sat down at his desk and methodically called each patient with the news. Perhaps, Cheney told them, an explanation for the source of their devastation was at hand.

Bethesda, Maryland

By September, the Gallo team had determined that close to 75 percent of the Tahoe samples sent to them by Peterson and Cheney over the summer were highly positive for their virus. So far, fewer than 2 percent of normal healthy people tested had evidence of exposure to it. The federal scientists were aware of only one other group of blood donors with a positivity rate rivaling that of the patients from Nevada: Burkitt's lymphoma patients being monitored by the NCI's Burkitt's Tumor Project in Ghana, Africa.

Not surprisingly, news of the positivity rates in Tahoe was percolating through the offices of the cancer institute's epidemiologists. That month two investigators in the Environmental Epidemiology Branch, Robert Biggar and Paul Levine, decided to head west with the intent of tracking the disease Paul Cheney had described to them with such quiet intensity three months earlier in Bethesda. The federal investigators' interest in the Nevada epidemic was driven exclusively by the mysterious new herpesvirus and by Cheney's report of a cancer cluster. They were unconcerned that teams of researchers already had made expeditions to the

High Sierras before them, thereby potentially biasing the population. Unlike Holmes and Kaplan, who had struggled with elemental problems like defining cases and determining whether or not an epidemic had occurred, Biggar and Levine were armed with something more tangible: laboratory results that pointed toward infection with an apparently new agent that might cause cancer.

Levine was markedly more willing than Biggar to believe a new disease was afoot; his imagination had been stirred by the story of the Tahoe epidemic and by news of the new herpesvirus's prevalence among victims. "A very fundamental question that we're always trying to address," Levine said later, "is what causes different outcomes if a person's infected by a virus. Why is it that some people get cancer, some people get, perhaps, neurologic disease, and some people don't get disease at all?"

Biggar's commitment was less fixed. "When Zaki Salahuddin discovered HBLV as the latest in a group of herpesviruses, the obvious connection was to say, 'Well, let's see if there's something going on related to an oncologic event,' " Biggar recalled later. "And Paul Cheney had reported that there were these lymphomas out there. Although from the very beginning we were—or certainly *I* was—very suspect that herpesviruses don't have explosive outbreaks of the type that Cheney was describing.

"Now, I did not go out there to discredit Cheney; I can absolutely assure you on that," Biggar continued. "We went out there with, if anything, a pro-Cheney bias. The problem was that Cheney was will-o'-the-wisp, which means that as soon as you track something down, there wasn't any evidence. It all disappeared like a mist before our eyes. We couldn't ever get our hands on anything that was truly abnormal. And that was very discouraging. The first time it happens, you think, Eh, that's annoying. The second time it happens, you think, Darn it. And the third time it happens, you think, Wait a minute—is *any* of this right?"

Levine and Biggar arrived in Reno on September 29, one year after Gary Holmes's hasty departure. Cheney spent the day with the federal researchers. In his office the investigators reviewed the doctor's records and interviewed patients Cheney believed might be interesting to them.

That evening Cheney arranged for Levine and Biggar to meet a group of six patients at the Incline hospital. "These were patients Cheney felt were classic cases," Levine said. "And I think that the ones he emphasized were the ones who turned out to be the key ones to look at. I mean, in retrospect I would have to say that it's from those cases that we actually developed what our feeling was of the classic case." Among the patients present that evening were former meter reader Chris Guthrie, former marathoner Sandy Schmidt, former teachers Janice and Gerald Kennedy, and the former postal worker who had been the first patient tested by neuropsychologist Sheila Bastien.

On the second day, the Bethesda researchers crossed the Sierra Nevada to Placerville, California, where an outbreak of the Tahoe malady had been reported in the summer of 1985. They met with ten patients, a group organized by the editor of the local newspaper. One of the patients was also the chief administrator of the local hospital. All ten claimed to be suffering from the disease, but a majority of the diagnoses were complicated by a second disease. As it happened, Placerville had been the site of a large giardiasis outbreak during the summer of 1985; nine of the ten people suffering from the Tahoe flu told the researchers they had become ill after first acquiring giardiasis, a mild gastrointestinal disease. The infusion of a second disease into an already complicated medical puzzle put Biggar and Levine on the defensive. In the end they selected just two of the Placerville patients as bona fide Tahoe malady sufferers, one of whom had become sick *before* the giardiasis outbreak and who had made numerous trips to Incline Village prior to falling ill. The investigators' criteria for their selection was the fact that the two had "features resembling those observed in Dr. Cheney's patients." Even the eight Placerville residents whom Biggar and Levine dismissed as non-cases, however, complained of what Levine described as "neurologic symptoms—dizziness, numbness, tingling of the extremities and impairment of intellect," which, he noted in his official trip report, "are generally not seen with giardiasis."

On the morning of the third day, Cheney accompanied the epidemiologists to Yerington. There clinician Judy Hilbisch introduced Biggar and Levine to a number of her patients, including the teenage Jimmy Dunlap, who had so impressed Anthony Komaroff. (By that fall, Dunlap's parents, at Hilbisch's urging, had arranged for their son to have an MRI brain scan; the boy was found to be positive for multiple punctate lesions, or UBOs.) Levine undertook the interviews with patients while Biggar worked in another room drawing blood samples. Like Komaroff, both researchers were persuaded by the patients in the desert town.

"The Yerington experience was probably the cleanest," Biggar said afterward, "because evidently the community was not at all aware of what was going on elsewhere. I don't know if you've been to Yerington, but it's not a town that casual visitors would idle through. It's a small farm town, and they're not in touch with the Incline Village–Truckee crowd at all. So Yerington was the most interesting and the most plausible case that there might really be something that swept through that community."

Both investigators were sufficiently impressed with Yerington that they chose three patients to send—all expenses paid—to Stephen Straus at the NIH's clinical center for further study; eighth grader Jimmy Dunlap was among them. In his trip report, Levine noted that Dunlap "had primarily been an A and B student who suddenly developed fatigue, syncopal [fainting] episodes (seizures?), mood changes, depressions, and severe fatigue. He developed problems of concentration and began to fall asleep in class, which teachers reported to be entirely out of character. . . . MRI lesions compatible with those observed in the Incline Village patient population were observed." Levine and Biggar also chose to send the mother-daughter team of Martha James and Sally Bentson to Straus. Bentson was described by Levine in his trip report as "an active twenty-two-year-old homemaker with several part-time jobs. . . . Fatigue and depression have been the primary manifestations of her illness. Her depression has been quite severe and uncharacteristic of her personality. . . . This vivacious young woman has intermittently considered suicide in recent months." James, who had become abruptly ill soon after her daughter, told Levine she felt "spacey" and that, although she had returned to work, "concentration was difficult."

That same evening, Cheney, Levine, and Biggar gathered with seven high school teachers in Gerald and Janice Kennedy's Truckee living room. Paul Levine took notes while the teachers described their medical histories. Biggar was highly skeptical. "I remember that group very well," he said later. "They felt that their lives had been totally disrupted and changed by this. But the Truckee people had a support group. And one of the problems you get into with this kind of group activity is that they reinforce each other. This collective myth of 'Oh, yes, I had that *too*,' gets reinforced. They've been talking with each other and arguing their case for long enough that you see this monolithic entity come out that everybody had the same thing. Whether that's true or not is very hard to determine because you've had this sort of inadvertent collusion." Levine, too, was unimpressed. "Many of the teachers were trying to say that their disease was work-related and were trying to get compensation. So the idea of compensation and health-related benefits entered into the evaluation and made it . . . well . . . difficult," he said.

Before leaving Nevada, Bob Bigger called Reno Diagnostics to discuss the magnetic resonance imaging scans the firm had been performing on Tahoe malady victims. Biggar did not speak to neuroradiologist Royce Biddle, whose job it was to read scans of the brain and spinal cord. Instead, he spoke to one of the firm's administrators. In a conversation about the call some time later, Biggar was unable to remember the administrator's name, but he recalled the substance of their exchange: "I said, 'Well, now listen, I understand you've been seeing patients and they have these abnormalities.' And he stopped me immediately and said, 'We never said these were abnormalities. They may be *variants* of normal. We don't have enough information on it.' I said, 'Well, have you seen these before?' And he said, 'We have a brand-new machine. It's about three or four times as powerful as anything we've ever had before. We just set it up. I have no idea if these are really abnormal or normal. We haven't seen them before, but we *wouldn't* see them before because we didn't have the resolution to see them before.' " Biggar was less than satisfied. He next phoned General Electric, the manufacturer of the most powerful grade magnetic resonance imaging machine. "I said, 'What do you think?' " Biggar recalled. " 'I mean, you're the guys who make the machine.' And he said, 'Yeah, we get reports of these things all the time. We have no idea if it's normal or abnormal.' "

By the time he left Nevada, Biggar's skepticism had turned to red-hot disbelief. "When you add that all up and you start seeing this pattern repeated," he said, "you get an impression. And I guess the point I'm coming to is not so much whether I am in a position to evaluate it, but that every time you try to reach out and find a tangible piece of evidence that there really were abnormalities that you could hang your hat on, it evaporates. And in the end, my own conclusion is that there was no objective evidence of any uniform thing going on in this community. Which is not to say that these people were not ill. They may have had a dozen different illnesses."

Levine, on the other hand, returned to Bethesda in an entirely different frame of mind: "I thought that there really was an outbreak of something infectious."

Incline Village, Nevada

On October 10, Incline Village journalist Jean Lamming of the *North Lake Tahoe Bonanza* nailed down her story. She was still way ahead of the national press. Lamming reported that researchers from the National Cancer Institute had found a new virus. She wrote that National Cancer Institute scientists had in their possession seventy-two blood samples from locals afflicted by the Tahoe malady. Better than half of those samples, Lamming claimed, were positive for the new virus. She further reported that federal researchers had been to Incline Village in recent weeks, interviewing patients and drawing more blood samples for analysis in Bethesda.

Bethesda, Maryland

Gallo's team chose to debut their virus in *Science*'s October 31 issue.[1] The discovery of the sixth human herpesvirus had an especially appealing angle for government public relations specialists eager to advertise the news: its discoverer of record, Robert Gallo, was the American scientist then credited with isolating HIV as the cause of AIDS. National Cancer Institute publicists sent word of the breakthrough to hundreds of journalists; stories were carried on the wire services and published in the *New York Times,* the *Washington Post,* the *Wall Street Journal,* the *Los Angeles Times,* the *Sacramento Bee,* the *San Francisco Herald-Examiner,* and *USA Today* during the week of October 24.

"The finding is considered important because it is the first human herpes-like virus to be discovered and characterized in twenty years since an earlier herpes family member, Epstein-Barr virus, or EBV, was identified as the cause of infectious mononucleosis," wrote Marilyn Chase in the *Wall Street Journal.* Harold Schmeck reported in the *New York Times* that Gallo had suggested "there are hints that the virus may attack the human brain and central nervous system, and this possibility is being pursued 'aggressively now' " at the NIH. Most of the coverage indicated that the government researchers thought the virus might play a role in an ill-defined chronic disease occurring in Nevada and elsewhere. "Of particular interest," wrote *San Francisco Examiner* reporter Lisa Krieger, "is a possible link of the virus to a mysterious, bone-weary fatigue reported by thousands of San Franciscans. . . . The scientists are testing specimens of this disease—also found in pockets of Lake Tahoe, Houston, Cleveland and Los Angeles—to determine whether there is a connection." Gallo himself told the *Washington Post,* "All of the known human herpesviruses cause disease, and we expect that will be true" for the new one as well.

Aside from demonstrating the uniqueness of their virus, perhaps the most dramatic revelation Gallo and his colleagues, headed by Zaki Salahuddin, made in their article was that of 220 healthy blood donors, just four were positive for the virus. In a veiled reference to the Tahoe epidemic, the authors added that "sero-epidemiological analysis has recently shown HBLV antibodies in a patient population clearly dissociated from [human immunodeficiency virus] infection." Although they implied that their new virus might cause cancers and other diseases, Gallo and his colleagues left it to *Science* readers to guess which ones. "These results focus our attention," they concluded, "on the possible role of HBLV in some lymphoproliferative and immune abnormalities of man."

An article about the Lake Tahoe outbreak in the same journal, "Mystery Disease at Lake Tahoe Challenges Virologists and Clinicians," complemented the Gallo study. Its author, Deborah Barnes, pointed out that the effort to link the "chronic mononucleosis syndrome" to a virus had been "complicated by the fact that the disease has not . . . been described in any major review. Its symptoms vary greatly," she continued, "although the most striking are chronic, severe fatigue lasting more than a year and neurological problems . . . which in many respects resemble those seen in some AIDS patients. Paul Levine of NCI recently interviewed more than seventy people from Nevada and California who complain of the chronic syndrome and was struck by the fact that many patients are unable to perform mental tasks that were once routine for them. Perhaps different herpeslike viruses, including HBLV, act in concert to produce nervous system damage as well as B-lymphocyte abnormalities." The Tahoe malady, Barnes added, exhibited a pattern of casual transmission similar to that of Epstein-Barr virus, which "can be spread by kissing, sharing food, dishes, or bathrooms, or coming in contact with someone who is sneezing or coughing." She concluded her report with the observation that although this was not a lethal disease, "like mononucleosis it seems to be highly infectious."

In the weeks following the *Science* article's publication, Cheney sensed that Gallo and his associates were growing skittish over speculation in the media about the relationship between human B-cell lymphotrophic virus and the Lake Tahoe disease. "After the association of their virus with the Tahoe outbreak emerged," Cheney recalled, "they were accosted by reporters. They were really uncomfortable about necessarily associating the two." Cheney eventually learned, too, that the government's cancer scientists were increasingly displeased with him. For one thing, the doctor had told his patients whether or not they had tested positive for the new virus. "They objected to that greatly. It put them in a very awkward position," Cheney said. After all, what if more refined tests later on revealed that their original test had generated false positives and false negatives? In fact, that had occurred in the early days of the AIDS epidemic when the Gallo lab was performing much of the testing for the disease nationwide, creating, Cheney said, "a lot of bitterness—bitterness of patients to clinicians, bitterness of clinicians to Gallo."

Cheney, in addition, was apparently far too garrulous for the government scientists' comfort. On the heels of the *Science* articles, Richard Knox, the medical writer for the *Boston Globe,* flew to Nevada to interview Cheney; Knox had just come from Bethesda, where he had seen Gallo. "Knox told me that Gallo had said I was 'out of control,' " Cheney recalled. "But it was a difficult time for everybody. Gallo was in a hot seat not of his making. Dan Peterson and I were in hot seats not of our making. Tony Komaroff was in a hot seat. And the media pressure was enormous. Tony, except for a few slips, pretty much toed the line, saying, 'Well, we really don't know . . .' and 'All the data's not in,' and all the things you say to cover your tracks. But there is this structure with the National Science Foundation and the National Institutes of Health with strings out there passing money to all the researchers. Well, I wasn't on any string. I wasn't getting any money. So I think I was kind of viewed as a leaky sieve—which I was."

Charlotte, North Carolina

In the third week of October, Marc Iverson experienced a spectacular if temporary respite from the despair of the previous seven years. While leafing through an issue of *Newsweek,* he came upon an article in the magazine's Lifestyle section about an illness called chronic Epstein-Barr virus infection. "Malaise of the Eighties" was *Newsweek*'s prophetic headline. The lead enumerated a few of the hallmarks of the disease: "They are plagued by low-grade fevers, aching joints and sometimes a sore throat—but they don't have the flu. They're overwhelmingly exhausted, weak and debilitated—but they don't have AIDS. They're often confused and forgetful—but it isn't Alzheimer's. Many patients feel suicidal, but it isn't clinical depression. They shuttle from doctor to doctor with a variety of vague symptoms—but it isn't hypochondria."

The poignant comments of one Houston doctor, pathologist William Hermann, resonated in Iverson's thoughts for days. "We don't have a word in the English language to describe the tiredness and fatigue these people have," Hermann said. He also noted that "there's reticence among the medical leadership because they're not the ones who introduced this. They should be embarrassed, because it's been staring them in the face for years."

Newsweek described the CDC's inconclusive investigation at Incline, juxtaposed with a comment from Cheney that the inquiry was too narrow and was performed over too short a period of time. The magazine estimated that as many as 10,000 Americans suffered from the disease, although by that fall, the membership claimed by the Portland-based patient organization had grown to 12,000. *Newsweek* noted the Portland figure, even though the number suggested that the magazine's own estimate of the breadth of the problem was far too low.

In the nearly three years since his last visit to the Mayo Clinic, Iverson had seen a total of seventy-five doctors, taken a dozen trips to other major medical institutions, and spent $250,000. One trip to Duke University's prestigious medical center landed Iverson in the center's psychiatric ward. The former banker was too exhausted to care, he said later. He spent a week sleeping virtually around the clock, his respite interrupted only by a daily psychiatric interview. The *Newsweek* article was his first indication that someone, somewhere, might be able to help. "First, I felt elated," Iverson said. "I *knew* I had this." He took the article to the neurologist he was seeing in Charlotte and asked to have his Epstein-Barr virus antibodies tested. His antibody levels, he soon learned, were nearly four times above the normal range. "Later, as it sunk in, I felt angry and bitter," Iverson continued. "No doctor, in seven years, had ever mentioned this disease to me. My neurologist just brushed off the EBV finding, saying, 'What does it matter? We can't do anything for it.' But after a while I was elated again. I thought, God *damn!* I don't have the Marc Iverson disease. Other people have this, too!" Iverson called the Portland organization and began to meet, via telephone, other sufferers for the first time.

Days after the *Newsweek* article appeared, Cheney received a letter from an executive headhunting firm in Virginia looking for a general internist to join a large multispecialty group practicing in a "dynamic, thriving town in North Carolina." The town turned out to be Charlotte.

"I was getting burned out," Cheney remembered. "We had this heavy emergency room operation, and I was on call every other weekend. Plus I was trying to see all these patients. Plus I was trying to do research. I had begun looking for a way out. And then this letter came, and I thought, Gosh, I won't have to be on call very often. And maybe I'll have something I never had in Incline, namely a large group of physicians who are on my side, rather than me and Dan and maybe a surgeon or two against everyone else—and in a town that isn't a resort town.' "

In the months prior to the publication of their paper on human B-cell lymphotrophic virus, according to Paul Cheney, scientists in the Gallo lab were concerned that their competitor in San Francisco, Jay Levy, might have isolated the new herpesvirus as well and might beat them to publication. Such concern was hardly unfounded; Levy, after all, unlike Robert Gallo and Zaki Salahuddin, was a herpes virologist by lifelong training. In addition, the federal scientists knew Levy was researching the new chronic disease currently under investigation in the Gallo lab. Levy had proven that, working virtually alone in his tiny lab, he could nail down the answers to formidable scientific questions: he had discovered HIV concurrently with the Gallo lab, but Gallo had won the race to publication, thus reaping the glory.*

The federal scientists' anxiety, while legitimate, was needless. Seven months into his research, Jay Levy and his Berkeley collaborator, Evelyne Lennette, found themselves empty-handed. The two had studied blood samples from fifty-seven patients referred to them by San Francisco clinician Carol Jessop. Lennette, who, like Levy, was a self-described child of the Henles, had initially looked for evidence of active Epstein-Barr virus as well as other herpesviruses. She discovered that one particular Epstein-Barr virus antigen, according to Levy, "was quite different from what you see in the control population"—that is, it was significantly elevated. But like most knowledgeable researchers before them, Levy and Lennette attributed the finding to immune dysfunction; neither believed the virus had caused the disease.

Levy's working hypothesis was that, as in AIDS, a new agent was infecting the immune systems of people suffering from the disease.

Lennette and Levy isolated the B-cells from patients' white blood cells and put them in test tubes to grow. Periodically they studied the cells, looking for changes, particularly cell destruction or cell death, a telltale sign of viral activity scientists call the cytopathic effect, or CPE.

"There were a couple patients in whom we saw CPE," Levy said, "but we couldn't identify any active virus."

Levy was impatient that fall. Unable to find a virus or even much evidence of one, he felt his doubts about the reality of the disease creeping back. The specter of funneling precious money and time into a bogus ailment returned. He put the collaboration on hold and returned to his AIDS research.

---

* Most scientists are more fearful of being wrong than of being last or even second, Levy among them. Before publishing, Levy took the time to be certain the new virus could be transmitted, thereby assuring himself that it was not merely another opportunistic pathogen afflicting AIDS sufferers. As Levy himself diplomatically described events, "The Gallo announcement eclipsed our ability to be the first to report the virus in the United States."

Raleigh, North Carolina

In September, one of the North Carolina Symphony members suffering from the fatigue syndrome was diagnosed with B-cell non-Hodgkin's lymphoma. The woman had become ill with the ailment that had afflicted seven of her colleagues—or 12 percent of the orchestra—two years earlier, in September of 1984. She had been diagnosed by the orchestra's doctor with mono nine months later, in June 1985. Remarkably, that same month, a second orchestra player was diagnosed with an extremely rare carcinoma of the parotid or salivary gland. The forty-one-year-old man reported no symptoms of illness prior to his diagnosis, but his wife, who also played in the orchestra, had suffered for two years from the same long-term fatiguing illness that had afflicted so many other musicians.

In November, a third member of the orchestra was diagnosed with cancer. The patient was a thirty-eight-year-old woman who had suffered an onset of severe fatigue in August of 1984 and had been diagnosed by the orchestra's doctor with mono in October 1985. The woman, the third player to be diagnosed with cancer in the space of six weeks, had breast cancer.

That same month an orchestra member perusing a recent *Time* magazine cover story on viruses noticed a sidebar account of Seymour Grufferman's investigation of a "contagious cancer" among an American family who had been visited by an elderly South African aunt. The musician was fascinated to learn that the cancer was B-cell non-Hodgkin's lymphoma, since that was the very cancer that had struck a fellow player two months previously. He noted, too, the mention of Epstein-Barr virus as a possible factor in the cancer outbreak. The musician, seeing that Grufferman was at nearby Duke University, decided to call the researcher in the hope that he might be interested in another apparent cluster of cancer concurrent with an outbreak of chronic Epstein-Barr disease.

Grufferman recalled that he was "very, very skeptical" of the reported cluster. But, he confessed, "I love to investigate clusters," and he had a bright third-year medical student at Duke who was eager to take on the orchestra's dilemma as a project. The student, Mary Huang, was by Grufferman's report even more skeptical than he. Grufferman at least believed the chronic disease was a real ailment. Before the project was in full swing, however, he was invited to become the head of the epidemiology department at Pittsburgh University's Cancer Institute. He accepted the job and moved to Pittsburgh, but he was determined to follow the orchestra over time just in case more cancers developed.

Boston, Massachusetts

Michael Caligiuri at Harvard's Dana-Farber Cancer Institute, one of Anthony Komaroff's original "feel the goods" collaborators, completed the first of his natural killer cell studies that fall with dramatic results. Patients from Nevada and New England not only had fewer natural killer cells than the healthy controls, but theirs were less potent as well. Since the cells that natural killer cells target for death are either cancerous or infected with a virus, a reduction in killing power was nearly as worrisome as a shortage of the cells.

"Isn't it interesting," Cheney mused upon hearing the news, "that one of the defects we see in this disease is in the immune system cell that is the first line of defense against cancer and herpesviruses?"

Significantly, AIDS sufferers were known to have a similar natural killer cell defect, although not to the remarkable degree Caligiuri had observed in the Nevada patients. But there were several other serious diseases in which natural killer cell function was awry, and Caligiuri's interest was piqued; he wanted to pursue the matter of the Lake Tahoe disease with an eye toward publication in a scientific journal.

Bethesda, Maryland

A succession of Nevadans, most of them Dan Peterson's patients, were hospitalized at the NIH that fall as a result of conversations between their doctor and government investigator Stephen Straus. Peterson had initiated a series of conversations with the federal researcher about, among other topics, the merit of acyclovir as a treatment for the malady. Straus, who had recently analyzed the data from his own clinical trial of the drug, had little faith in acyclovir, but Peterson was convinced it helped. Hospitalization and intravenous infusion with the drug had resulted in a remission of brain lesions in several of Peterson's worst-afflicted patients. Unfortunately, when the patients were removed from the drug, their neurological symptoms and their brain lesions returned within three months. Yet, in Peterson's view, any relief was helpful to those hardest hit by the disease, particularly when the relief came in the form of reduced brain lesions. "Acyclovir works," Peterson told Straus point-blank. "I can prove it. The brain scans improve."

Straus, Peterson sensed, was tweaked by this observation, but made no further inquiries on the subject; he never asked to see the serial brain scans on patients treated with acyclovir. Nevertheless, Peterson asked, "Will you look at some patients if I send them? To help me out, if nothing else." Straus agreed.

People suffering from all manner of unusual ailments typically were housed in the Warren Magnuson Clinical Center when they turned to the NIH for help. Built upon a rise near the center of the NIH campus, the clinical center—by repute the largest redbrick structure on earth—was a monolithic edifice. Inside, a bewildering maze of research laboratories, boxy offices, and hospital wards, connected by 7½ miles of fluorescent-lit corridors painted in pale shades of enamel, awaited newcomers. To the staff, the clinical center was known simply as Building 10, a designation reflecting its order of construction in the NIH hierarchy of buildings.

The first Nevadan to be studied at the NIH was a middle-aged woman who was in extreme distress about the severity and the tenacity of her illness. She bore many of the classic signs and symptoms of the Tahoe malady, including unidentified bright objects in her brain, cognition problems, immune system abnormalities, devastating physical weakness, and unusual-looking rashes that came and went mysteriously. Nevertheless, the ailing woman returned from

Bethesda after a week's stay with a diagnosis of depression, a characterization that hardly satisfied her.

Peterson, who believed his patient's objective laboratory data offered unequivocal proof of organic disease, grew wary. The second patient he chose to send was more emotionally stable but, like the first, extremely ill. Among other objective signs, she had UBOs and abnormal mental status tests. In addition, she was suffering from an active human B-cell lymphotrophic virus infection, according to blood analyses done in the Gallo laboratory. She, too, came back with a psychiatric diagnosis.

"This was a patient who did very, very well on acyclovir and was a bright patient who I thought would be good to send," Peterson recalled. "Then I started talking to her husband, who began this 'man-to-man'–style conversation with me in which he said his wife had empty-nest syndrome and was always too concerned about her health, that she was sad from her hysterectomy years before and all that." Peterson felt certain the patient's husband, who had accompanied his wife to Bethesda, had shared his views with the National Institute of Allergy and Infectious Disease researchers. "After that," Peterson said, "the damage was totally done. *Totally* done. . . . At NIH she wasn't given a chance to talk about her cognitive function problems or her fatigue. It was just one psychiatrist after another, who kept asking her questions like 'Isn't it hard to be married to an older man?' or 'Don't you miss your children at college?' "

With the cavalier dismissal of his second seriously ill patient, Peterson recalled, "I had learned a lesson. I selected young males to send back."

Richard Pearson (a pseudonym), then a thirty-five-year-old real estate lawyer living in Tahoe City, was among the three Peterson sent next. The lawyer had brain lesions and was grossly abnormal on Sheila Bastien's mental status test. In addition, he suffered from pain in his joints and muscles and overwhelming fatigue. He had been unable to practice law for eight months; his wife had recently left him and was seeking a divorce. The three patients traveled from Nevada to Bethesda together. "We went as a group because no one was really functioning," Pearson recalled. "With three of us, you know, one could read, one could think, and one could carry the bags. I felt like one of Jerry's poster kids."

The three were billeted in Building 10's infectious disease ward on the eleventh floor; nearly all of the other patients on the ward were suffering from AIDS. They were given numerous psychological exams, underwent spinal taps and magnetic resonance imaging brain scans, and had myriad blood samples drawn during the week of their hospitalization. Stephen Straus presented Richard Pearson at grand rounds before approximately fifty NIH scientists. Straus's colleagues seemed far less interested in Pearson's physical symptoms, the lawyer recalled, than in any stressful events that might have occurred prior to the onset of his illness. At week's end, the three were sent home without the results of their tests.

Pearson returned to Nevada with a diagnosis of "neurasthenia, etiology unknown," according to Peterson. In the parlance of contemporary medicine, neurasthenia is little more than a quaint Victorian-era code word for mental illness. "They drew about sixty-eight tubes of blood from each of those patients," Peterson said. "They must have been looking at *something*. But I've never gotten anything back on those people. I don't really know *what* the NIH thought."

When he was asked in person in 1988, by telephone and in writing, Stephen Straus refused to discuss either the nature of the tests performed on Peterson's patients or the results; he refused, too, to release any documents related to these investigations when they were sought under a Freedom of Information Act request, a petition originally made in early 1989 and resubmitted in mid-1991 after the agency failed to comply fully with the original request. In violation of the federal Freedom of Information Act, Straus's superiors at the agency did not force him to comply with either request even when, after an appeal, James Mason, then the assistant secretary for Health and Human Services, instructed them to do so.

It was only by closely following Straus's lectures at universities and hospitals on the chronic disease in the coming years that a member of the press or general public might glimpse a view of Straus's opinion of the handful of Nevada patients whom he had studied that fall, and in his rare references to the Nevadans, his comments were always in the nature of an aside; he failed to provide actual data. In addition, it was apparent that the researcher had used his limited observations of this tiny cohort to form an opinion of the entire Tahoe phenomenon.

Straus, for instance, made the following comments during a grand rounds presentation on the disease in a Silver Spring, Maryland, hospital in 1988: "I admitted a whole series of patients from Lake Tahoe to my service at the NIH ... [Tahoe] wasn't an acute epidemic. Obviously, once it's in the press everybody who's tired comes out of the woodwork. . . . It's clear to me that most of the people there, whatever they had, weren't part of an epidemic. Now, the question is, of those who were there, were they just fatigued and achey and psychoneurotic? Or was this mass hysteria? And we don't know."*

For Straus's purposes, the neurasthenia label did more than just locate sufferers of the Tahoe malady in the never-never land of psychological distress. His diagnosis sent a clear message to other scientists at the NIH and elsewhere: searching for infectious agents in such patients was folly since the condition emanated from the patient's troubled psyche. Straus's nascent theory had crucial implications for the future of government spending, too. As long as a neurasthenia theory was in vogue, research dollars would be reserved for scientists studying "real," transmittable diseases.

Three more ailing Nevadans made the trip to the clinical center later that fall. This group, unlike the first, was invited east by federal researchers Paul Levine and Robert Biggar, epidemiologists from the National Cancer Institute who had met the three in Yerington in October. In return for being "guinea-pigged to death," as the father of Jimmy Dunlap characterized his son's experience, the government paid their transportation costs, an accommodation not extended to the patients from the Alder Street practice.

Sally Bentson of Yerington and her mother, Martha James, were selected because their illness had struck Biggar and Levine as severe and because they were related. Ironically, both women were beginning to feel improved that winter.

* Later in his lecture, speaking about sufferers of the disease in general, the government's expert elicited laughter when he glibly speculated, "Maybe these are the individuals who, you know, they just don't want to drive their BMW unless they feel up to it, and they need our help to get behind the wheel." He also said, after cautioning his audience that he wouldn't "go into this in detail," that "there's a large history of psychiatric problems in these patients."

Bentson, who had been the more debilitated of the two, was actually feeling better than her mother. They arrived in Bethesda early in December and were assigned a room in Building 10's infectious disease ward. During their four-day stay, they underwent numerous tests and an extensive psychiatric evaluation.

The younger woman found the trip to be generally uneventful but for her final day. Both women were unusually weak on tests of muscle strength, but Bentson proved to be weaker than her mother; given her youth, the scientists had expected her to be stronger. Straus asked Bentson if she would agree to undergo a biopsy of the muscle in her upper arm. The night before the procedure, Marinos Dalakas, a muscle expert at the National Institute of Allergy and Infectious Diseases and a Straus collaborator, explained that the incision would need to be made without the benefit of anesthetic; he did not want the muscle fiber to be altered in any way, he said. He promised Bentson the scar would be a short, fine line and barely noticeable. The following morning the biopsy surgery turned traumatic. The pain was extraordinary as the knife sliced through Bentson's skin down to the muscle; Dalakas took one, then two samples of live muscle with a sharply honed tweezer-like device. He then asked Bentson, "Can I get one more piece?" "No!" Bentson pleaded. Dalakas ignored her and excised a third sample from her arm. The doctor stitched the wound, and Bentson and her mother left Building 10 that afternoon, bound for the Nevada desert. The flight to Reno, Bentson recalled several years later, was excruciating due to the untreated pain in her injured arm.

As weeks, then months passed, neither Stephen Straus nor anyone else at the federal clinic informed the women of their test results. In addition, Dalakas's stitches had left a sizable jagged scar rather than the short white line Bentson had been promised. The cut was conspicuous enough that people expressed concern when they saw it. Self-conscious, Bentson kept her arm covered. Her mother, Martha James, was disturbed by the scar as well. "It's a white kind of lumpy thing," James said some years later. "I would have thought they could send her to a doctor who would repair it." Eight months later, on July 17, responding to a letter from Bentson, Straus informed her that there continued to be a number of test results that were outstanding, including the results of her muscle biopsy. Antibodies were detected "in an experimental serological assay" for "the new human B-cell lymphotrophic virus," Straus told her, but he added there was "no evidence [her] illness was due to HBLV."

"It is my belief that your chronic illness was triggered by an acute infection whose nature is uncertain," Straus wrote. "Unfortunately, we lack an adequate understanding of the imbalances that presumably exist in your immune system that make you feel the way you do, nor do we have therapies that I feel are likely to benefit you." In conclusion, Straus wrote: "I apologize for the scar that remains from your muscle biopsy. It should lessen in time. Dr. Dalakas is an international expert in muscle diseases and not a plastic surgeon."

Bentson never learned the results of tests that were pending, including the results of her muscle biopsy.

As he did when asked for his findings or conclusions about the patients referred by Dan Peterson, Stephen Straus refused to reveal his research protocols or findings on the Yerington patients. In addition, the government investigator has never published any findings related to his research in Building 10 on any Nevada epidemic patients, in spite of his no doubt costly investigations, except to report, in the context of a broad overview of the disease in 1988, that he had been unable to find unidentified bright objects by MRI scans in the brains of "most" Nevadans.

By that spring, federal scientists' interest in studying victims of the Nevada epidemic seemed to evaporate altogether; they extended no further invitations. According to cancer epidemiologist Robert Biggar, the Bethesda researchers had concluded by then that the Nevada phenomenon was overblown. Cheney and Peterson's insistence that UBOs were a common finding among victims of the disease seemed to be the rallying point on which the federal scientists focused their disdain. Only one of the Nevada sufferers, the first of the two women sent by Dan Peterson, had demonstrated evidence of UBOs when she underwent a brain scan in the magnetic resonance imaging machine at the Warren Magnuson Clinical Center.* Unfortunately, the MRI apparatus in use at the Bethesda hospital in 1986 was of an earlier generation and significantly less sensitive than the machine at Reno Diagnostics, where approximately 70 percent of the Nevada patients already had been found to have multiple small brain lesions.

"Well, they didn't do them on *exactly* the same machines," Biggar conceded when he was asked about the grade of the clinical center's MRI scanner. "But the fact is that you would think if there's something there, that they could find it objectively at NIH, and they're not finding it. So the bottom line of all of that is that we have pursued these things to the extent that we consider reasonable."

Centers for Disease Control, Atlanta, Georgia

In September, Gary Holmes submitted his paper to the *Journal of the American Medical Association. JAMA,* as the magazine is known, was then number two among medical journals in world circulation; it was published in six languages other than English.

Holmes titled his article "A Cluster of Patients with a Chronic Mononucleosis-Like Syndrome: Is Epstein-Barr Virus the Cause?" On November 18, *JAMA'*s senior editor, Bruce Dan, wrote Holmes an encouraging letter. "We've completed our preliminary review of your paper," Dan said, "and are interested in it." Dan already had sent the paper to at least two reviewers, whose anonymous comments he included. "The editorial group felt that you needed to address their comments before we could make a decision on whether we could accept the paper," Dan explained, and asked Holmes to revise the paper where appropriate, and return it to *JAMA.*

Each of two reviewers, whose critiques were obtained through a Freedom of Information Act request, expressed strong criticism. One of them, puzzled by the absence of a full description of the disease itself anywhere in the paper, wrote in

---

* Straus had concluded she could not be suffering from the Tahoe malady. Another researcher at the federal institution who, with Straus, analyzed the Alder Street patients, recalled that the woman's symptoms had suggested either hysteria or heavy metal poisoning to Straus. "Steve and I were convinced that she did not have the syndrome," this researcher said. "Although," he conceded, "she is considered to be a classic case by Anthony Komaroff. She *did* have an abnormal brain scan," the researcher continued. "And I remember she had had a seizure," he mused. "She was a very interesting case of *something!*"

part: "After reading the paper, one is left wondering if an epidemic *is* taking place in the area. More information should be provided about the case cluster, about the patients and their community. This would include relevant demographics and additional clinical details. The authors have had to grapple with the difficult problem of choosing a case definition, but have done so in such a restricted way as to leave a very small number of patients for comparison. The cases differ from the non-cases by the severity of fatigue. Many other characteristics such as the duration of fatigue could have been chosen."

The second reviewer was harsher, suggesting that the report should not be published: "Given the confusing information that the investigators report, it is not wise to report this information in its present form," the reviewer cautioned, adding, "Much confusion prevails regarding the subject and this would only add to further confusion."

Although not unsympathetic to the problems Holmes had faced in his attempt to define and measure the disease in Tahoe, the second reviewer was deeply unsympathetic to Holmes's methodology. "This manuscript is a result of an extensive study to try to define a syndrome among a very confusing group of patients. Resulting is a confusing report," the reviewer wrote. "The multiple tables comparing the results from the different laboratories are difficult for the reader to follow. It seems that this report might be better published in a clinical pathology or medical virology journal."

The second reviewer was struck, too, by the absence on the paper of the names of the doctors who had reported the cluster to the government, Dan Peterson and Paul Cheney: "This reviewer is perplexed that the two clinicians referring the patients for study were not included in the manuscript."

As the holidays loomed, Holmes wrestled with his Tahoe manuscript, attempting to respond to the criticisms.

The young investigator was struggling on another front as well. By November, he and Carlos Lopez, who ran the herpes research laboratory at the agency and had evinced an interest in the new disease, had developed a cursory "case definition" for it. Hewing to the name "chronic mononucleosis-like syndrome," or CMLS, Lopez, accompanied by the agency's Jon Kaplan, presented the definition in Austin, Texas, on November 6 at a scientific gathering of Epstein-Barr virus experts. At meals and in between sessions, Lopez met the authors of the 1985 papers on the disease, James Jones and Stephen Straus. He also met Harvard's Anthony Komaroff and Nathaniel Brown, an infectious disease specialist with an expertise in Epstein-Barr virus who was then at UCLA. He promised to send each of them a first draft of the agency's case definition for their comments. No draft was promised to Paul Cheney. Cheney was also present and addressed the gathering, describing his findings from the Tahoe epidemic. Years afterward he could still recall that when he began to describe the immunological abnormalities and brain scan results in Tahoe, he looked up to see Kaplan's smirking expression and to hear the low, derisive laughter shared by Kaplan and Lopez, seated together.

Irrespective of his contempt for Cheney, Lopez was suitably impressed by the disease itself. A week later, on November 12, 1986, upon his return to Atlanta, Lopez described the conference in a two-page memo to Albert Balows, a senior virologist who later retired from the agency: "Dr. Komaroff presented an amazing observation: 21 percent of unselected persons visiting a medical clinic in Boston gave a history of the fatigue syndrome. The definition was not strict and might have included other reasons for fatigue, but the percentage was much higher than expected. . . . The meeting turned out to be an excellent opportunity for the major participants in this field to meet and discuss current work. . . . In addition, close ties were established for future studies in this field. We will take a leadership position in the development of a case definition and in the study of the etiology and epidemiology of this syndrome."

Beginning in December, Holmes and Lopez began to hear from a handful of people to whom they had sent a draft of their working case definition. One of them was Elliot Kieff, a respected herpes researcher who was then head of infectious diseases at the Pritzker School of Medicine at the University of Chicago.

"We figured if we could get Kieff as a collaborator on the case definition," Gary Holmes recommended later, "that would lend some weight to the disease. And it was partly for the challenge of it. It wasn't surprising that he wouldn't do it," Holmes continued, "but it was the forcefulness of his beliefs that struck me. He's one of those very highly respected, highly placed individuals in major medical centers who basically say it's a disease of neurotic women. Kieff said, 'I don't want to have anything to do with a case definition—it's all a bunch of garbage.' He's not a clinician now," Holmes added. "He hasn't seen patients in years."

Kieff wasn't as graphic in his written response to Carlos Lopez, but his scorn for the disease and its sufferers was readily apparent. He suggested the agency include a measurable, objective parameter in their absolute criteria, such as a specific lymph node measurement. Absent such parameters, Kieff wrote in his brief letter of December 15, patients would quickly learn how to hoodwink doctors into rendering the diagnosis, thus gaining "membership in this new group."

NIH scientist Stephen Straus, to whom Lopez and Holmes had sent their proposed case definition, weighed in with his views as well in a letter dated December 17. "Allow me to make the following changes in your proposed CMLS case definition," Straus wrote Holmes. "I would not list seizures or paresis [muscular weakness caused by a disease of the nervous system or partial motor paralysis]," Straus wrote, "these being exceedingly unusual in my patients, and to me more suggestive of other organic etiologies."

In his letter to Holmes, however, Straus revealed the circular logic that characterized his own system of defining cases. Straus recommended excluding from the definition any patient who exhibited symptoms or signs (an objective abnormality such as a rash or an aberrant lab result) seen in other serious diseases. A patient with seizures, for instance, would be considered to have a seizure disorder. For Straus, in effect, the new disease was by definition a subjective condition, able to be perceived by the victim and no one else.

Incline Village, Nevada

For the past eighteen months, Paul Cheney and Dan Peterson had been carefully monitoring the symptomatology of the disease in their own practice, entering every complaint they heard described by more than three patients, as well as physical signs, into their computer's database. During the first week in November, Cheney created an exhaustive sign-symptom complex for the disease in north Lake Tahoe. Importantly, he also computed the percentage of total patients suffering from each symptom or sign. In all, the doctors listed forty-three signs and symptoms. There were, in addition, a number of subcategories, bringing the actual number higher. Under "parasympathetic nervous system effects," for instance, there were twenty listings, ranging from tinnitus (ringing in the ears) to aniscoria (asymmetrically dilated pupils) to dysarthria (difficulty pronouncing words intelligibly) to seizures.

Some of the more unusual observations were that 70 percent of all patients experienced a sizable weight change, with weight *gain* more frequent than weight loss; a quarter of all patients had metabolic rate disturbances, most frequently in the form of startlingly low metabolic activity, accompanied by low body temperatures; 10 percent of male patients reported they were impotent; more than half of all patients reported intolerance to alcohol; 25 percent of sufferers, most of whom were adults, were stricken with acne; another 25 percent had discoloration of their tongues; one-third were suffering concurrently from other herpes infections such as shingles and herpes simplex; four out of seven pregnancies among afflicted women ended in miscarriage; all of the babies that made it to term were of a clinically significant low birth weight; and so far 1.5 percent of the epidemic population—three people—had lymphoma.

At a grand rounds presentation on the epidemic disease at the Washoe Medical Center in Reno on January 13, 1987, Cheney held back little from the assembled specialists and general practitioners, beginning with Peterson's original hypothesis that their patients were suffering from the malady described in the early *Annals* articles, which suggested that chronic activation of Epstein-Barr virus was the cause of the disease. The hypothesis had seemed reasonable to both doctors until the epidemic became apparent, Cheney explained. "It seemed like they were coming out of the woodwork," he told the audience of Reno doctors.

He described, too, Gary Holmes and Jon Kaplan's disappointing investigation. "After the frustrations of the CDC's visit," he said, "we decided this might be caused by something new."

The doctor struggled to convey the unusual quality of the fatigue patients described: "They'll say, 'It's like an anvil on my chest,' or 'It's hard to lift my coffee cup.'" And he described the curious sleep disorder people complained of—vivid dreams, nightmares, insomnia. "In some patients it was a kind of sleep deprivation syndrome," Cheney said. "They were like soldiers who hadn't slept in two weeks coming out of a war zone."

Cheney also displayed his voluminous sign-symptom complex to the audience. "It's quite likely there are things on this list that may not have anything to do with this syndrome. It just seemed that if you saw something more than three times, you should note it, and rule it out later," he explained.

He also reported the most recent information on cancers, seizures, and other ominous developments among the epidemic patients: "Frank lymphomas have been seen in three patients," the doctor said. "Five patients have had a complete loss of B-cells. Twenty-five out of thirty-three have a natural killer cell dysfunction. There have been three strokes, five grand mal seizures, and five cases of encephalitis. We have seen lesions in two-thirds of sixty patients who have been tested on magnetic resonance imaging brain scanning. We have done lumbar punctures [spinal taps] on seven patients," he added. "Only two of them had normal opening pressures." (Abnormal opening pressure on a spinal tap was often diagnostic of brain swelling as a result of either infection or head trauma.)

It would be difficult to know just where along the way Cheney lost his audience, but by the time he began describing the suspected Burkitt's lymphoma cases and explaining Sheila Bastien's neuropsychological research, the Reno doctors were glassy-eyed and, as evidenced by their questions afterward, openly hostile.

One of Reno's three infectious disease specialists, Stephen Parker, who was present at the meeting, analyzed the conflict later: "Unfortunately, Cheney just created more confusion, because he was very intimately involved with this disease and knew the ins and outs, and we were still trying to understand the basics. He was, you know, describing the fine intricacies and the physics of how an engine ran, and we were just trying to understand what an engine was. . . .

"The majority of people didn't believe it, or continued to be skeptical. But you know, you didn't want to call him a quack and find out that he was right, and you didn't want to say that he was right, because he might be a quack. We just didn't know if he was blowing smoke or not. Certainly," Parker added after a moment, "Cheney got crucified in the papers up there, and that was, I guess, horrible. I mean, he didn't deserve *that*."

Dan Peterson, seated in the audience—fists clenched in empathetic tension—as his partner struggled to convey the dimensions of the hydra-headed disease, was embittered by the Reno medical establishment's response to Cheney. "There wasn't an ounce of interest," Peterson said later. "It was just a pound of tearing down."

Cheney's unabridged revelations before the Reno doctors angered Anthony Komaroff. As an academic whose career was vitally dependent upon publication in medical journals, Komaroff was sensitive to the need to keep scientific findings secret until they were in press. The Harvard doctor had high ambitions for the Tahoe investigation; he hoped one day to see the research in the *New England Journal of Medicine*. Cheney had allowed the grand rounds presentation to be videotaped as well, which established a verbatim record of the scientific data that had been collected over the previous two years; the video could serve as a road map to other investigators and might even be obtained by lay reporters. Scientific data that appeared in the lay press before being published in a medical journal, Komaroff knew, was considered tainted by medical journal editors. As it happened, however, there was no press coverage of Cheney's remarks, and almost no one in the medical community in Reno found the phenomenon worthy of further investigation.

In the history of the Tahoe epidemic, only one person from the region's medical community stepped forward to actively defend the two internists against their vociferous and increasingly confrontational enemies in Nevada. "I could not be pushed into agreeing it was bunk," recalled Tom McNamara. McNamara was chief of radiology at Lakeside Community Hospital in Incline Village. He also practiced at the Washoe Medical Center in Reno, was a clinical professor at the University of Nevada Medical School, and was the most respected radiologist in the state. "Nor could I be pushed into agreeing that Peterson and Cheney shouldn't be pursuing it," he added.

McNamara had worked with both doctors at the Incline hospital in the years prior to the outbreak. As it happened, McNamara was also the chairman of the hospital's Quality Assurance Committee during the years of the epidemic. In that capacity he served as a lightning rod for the hostility toward the young internists that was rife among the medical brotherhood in the affluent town. By the winter of 1986, a period during which the doctors were hospitalizing severely disabled victims of the epidemic in order to treat them with acyclovir, that hostility had coalesced into a campaign that McNamara was forced to confront.

"There was a movement to prevent them from admitting patients to the hospital with the diagnosis," McNamara recalled. "And then there was a wider movement to prevent them from admitting *any* patients to the hospital and, further, a movement to try to stop them from carrying out their clinical investigations on these people. I was not sympathetic to these requests," McNamara added. "It seemed to me they were based more on fear and lack of information than on scientific fact.

"I was forced, by being the chairman of the Quality Assurance Committee, to investigate this," McNamara continued. "I needed to establish to my own satisfaction that this disease was real. So I spoke to Cheney and Peterson at length. And having myself done clinical research, I was able to assess how they had approached the problem in terms of whether they had valid grounds to be suspicious that this was indeed an entity."

In an effort to make peace, McNamara asked the internists to meet with the hospital committee. In that forum, Cheney and Peterson were able to address a number of concerns, especially ones about the possible spread of the disease to staff and other patients.

"After [the doctors] had had an opportunity to tell what they knew, it was apparent that to exclude those patients from admission was an overreaction," the radiologist said.

Had he not intervened, McNamara admitted, "it could have been steamrolled. And I had to be cautious about how I helped them, so as not to antagonize the other physicians on the staff, in that I'm dependent upon them totally for those patients who come to me directly."

For the moment, the two sides achieved a delicate balance. But by then McNamara himself was hooked on the medical mystery that had ensnared his younger colleagues. For weeks prior to the face-off with the hospital committee, the radiologist had immersed himself in the disease, with Cheney and Peterson as his tour guides. Quite naturally, the magnetic resonance imaging scans of patients' brains held a special fascination for him. "I reviewed virtually all of the MRI reports and many of the MRI scans," McNamara recalled.

Initially, the radiologist considered that the lesions were simply the normal results of aging, since similar lesions are occasionally seen in the elderly. However, when he learned the ages of the patients, he wasn't so sure. One of the things that most impressed him was the fact that in several patients the lesions appeared to change over time. He was especially struck by the fact that in some patients the scan was negative at onset, then turned positive later in the disease, and that patients treated with acyclovir often changed from positive to negative.

"Peterson and Cheney did repeat scans on many patients," McNamara said. "It's the changeability that would make one very suspicious that one is dealing with some infectious process or some reversible demyelinating disease which is, to my mind, otherwise unheard of. And [the lesions] struck me, some of them, as being very unusual in their size and their immediate subcortical location. . . . We were quite suspicious that these lesions seen on the MR were directly related to the disease."

Having found a convert, Cheney was quick to engage the radiologist in a collaboration. He proposed to the specialist that, together, they analyze the magnetic resonance imaging data in order for McNamara to present it at the American Society of Neuroradiology meeting in New York later that winter. The plan was to attempt to correlate all aspects of the syndrome—the magnetic resonance imaging scans, Sheila Bastien's mental status test results, and the clinical portrait—in a way that would be comprehensible to an audience of neuroradiologists. McNamara entered the partnership eagerly and, years afterward, looked back on the project with obvious nostalgia, relishing even his memory of twice navigating the mountain pass from Reno in the middle of driving snowstorms to reach Cheney's rented house on the lakeshore. "We sat up very late a few nights, until two or three A.M., stoking the woodstove from time to time and going over data," he recalled. "We worked at his dining room table, showing slides of the scans on a sheet hung on his dining room wall with the wind and snow blowing outside. It was a wonderful experience."

"Now, Cheney," he continued, "was a person trained in investigation. He has a Ph.D. in atomic physics, is a very bright man, and had a keen interest in pursuing this entity at the expense of diminishing his own practice. They were both pilloried in that community. It's surprising and unfortunate that these things occur. I think if their motivation was to increase revenue, they would have quickly changed their tune, and they did not. Dr. Peterson is a quite skilled clinician and was willing to let their office income and practice really suffer. It wasn't that they were being stubborn. They thought quite sincerely that their observations were honest ones and therefore couldn't—shouldn't—be abandoned. That's where the conflict came. It's caused a lot of hard feelings in the community."

New York City

In early December, McNamara spoke for five minutes before an audience of three hundred specialists at the annual American Society of Neuroradiology meeting in New York City. "We just wanted the neuroradiologists in the country to be aware of this as an entity and to open it up for input from other people who could then say, 'Yes, by golly, I've seen that!' " McNamara recalled. Instead, his data were met with incredulity. The brief discussion afterward, McNamara reported, was mostly limited to whether the Tahoe patients might simply be AIDS sufferers whose disease had been misdiagnosed.

Later, McNamara was evenhanded in his evaluation of the session. "We were suggesting these patients had dementia, had an immune problem, and had abnormal MRI scans. Those things *are* also in AIDS, so I suppose it *was* a valid question," the radiologist said. Another query from the floor suggested the unidentified bright objects were merely normal aging changes sometimes seen in older brains. "I think that was a valid concern," McNamara continued. "However, it was my impression that in many of those patients who had repeated MRs, their initial MR was normal, then they developed these findings on repeat MR. And then in a few patients who wound up having subsequent MR scans after that, the lesions had proved to be reversible."

Speaking of the disease's doubters in general, McNamara added, "I think it's good to be skeptical, but it seems they've gone too far. I think they actually have a bias. They're not neutral in bringing scientific skepticism to bear. I get the impression they've really made a decision, which is that this is not real, and I think they are not open-minded."

Incline Village, Nevada

In December, formerly subtle conflicts between Peterson and Cheney came to a head under the strain of operating a busy practice amid an extraordinary medical crisis. Peterson's style, early on, had been expansive. His initial success in the well-heeled town had led him to enter into a five-year lease in one of the most costly buildings in the region soon after Cheney joined the practice as the junior partner in 1983. "And then we bought all this high-tech equipment," Cheney recalled. "In effect, Dan sort of mortgaged our future, betting that I would become as busy as he was and that, if that happened, we could afford to have all this overhead and still make healthy incomes. What happened was EBV hit. And when it hit, rather than my income going up, it went down. It was never that we didn't have any patients," Cheney continued. "We had more than we could possibly deal with. It's just that EBV patients are not getting treadmills. They're not getting sigmoidoscopies. They're not generally going into the hospital. They're just tying you up for hours on end. And," he added with characteristic candor, "you cannot make it in medicine by listening to people. Or at least, not with the overhead we had."

Peterson bore the brunt of the lab expenses, which in the case of Specialty Labs in Los Angeles, had risen to $200,000 by that winter. The practice's Federal Express bill had ballooned to $9,000, primarily due to the cost of shipping blood overnight to the Gallo lab in Bethesda for human B-cell lymphotrophic virus assays and to collaborators in Boston. And although the once-thriving practice was crashing financially, Peterson's workload had increased. He typically saw thirty patients a day, Cheney ten. At the height of the epidemic, however, Cheney began to cut back his patient load while Peterson, loath to abandon his comparatively healthy patients, was forced to expand his to accommodate the victims of the epidemic. Unlike Peterson, who owned the practice, Cheney's paychecks were proportionate to the degree to which his activities enriched the enterprise. Even so, and in his effort to learn more about the disease, Cheney often spent as much as two hours with each epidemic patient.

Both doctors, in short, were hurting; Cheney, in fact, was increasingly hard-pressed to pay his rent and utility bills. The two began to have a series of conversations about the problem. The more they talked, the more intractable their conflicts became. "My paychecks began to decline below a point where I could meet my monthly payments," Cheney remembered. "There was no clear way out that I could see." Peterson, for his part, could not see a way to raise Cheney's salary. "As time went on, it felt more and more like an endless treadmill," Cheney said. "And I perceived that if we were to stay, we'd have to have very thick skin," the doctor continued in a reference to himself and his wife, Jean. "So I began looking for a way out." Cheney's out came in the form of an offer from the Nalle Clinic in Charlotte, North Carolina, fashioned after the Mayo Clinic and the largest such medical center in the Southeast. He gave notice just before Christmas.

Dan Peterson was struck to his core when his energetic, brilliant collaborator quit at the end of the year. The relationship between the doctors, whose training and intellectual gifts had blended so remarkably to foster an increasingly sophisticated understanding of the disease, never fully recovered. Peterson, Cheney once noted, "doesn't like or dislike; he trusts or distrusts." For the handsome, brooding midwesterner, Cheney's decision to leave the practice wasn't a business decision; it was a betrayal. "I felt abandoned. There's no doubt about that," Peterson said later. "He took off for greener pastures, leaving me with a mess. He gave very short notice, and I wasn't prepared. I think that was probably the low point for me."

Before he left, Cheney's patients and their families held a dinner in his honor at an elegant restaurant set on one of the highest vantages in town, with a panoramic view of Lake Tahoe; it was the same restaurant where Dan Peterson had treated Jon Kaplan and Gary Holmes to lunch thirteen months earlier. Toasts were made to the intense, absentminded clinician whose impending departure seemed, to many, almost beyond imagining. Chris Guthrie and several other heartbroken patients wept. His contributions had been made at the intimate level of a doctor caring for patients in extraordinary distress, and at the public level of an uncommon intellect struggling to forge a paradigm shift in American medicine.

1987
THE FLAT
EARTHERS

Locke's remark that "Truth scarce ever yet carried
it by vote anywhere at its first appearance" is borne
out by the history of all discoveries of the first rank.

—Sir William Osler, *An Alabama Student
and Other Biographical Essays*

10

"You Have Been Blackballed"

National Institutes of Health, Bethesda, Maryland

Real or not, the epidemic disease was a problem that simply wouldn't go away. By 1987, the lavishly funded Bethesda agency was receiving an extraordinarily heavy volume of letters from people claiming to have the disease and from members of Congress making inquiries on behalf of constituents who were ill. By that year, the number of public inquiries about the malady was second only to the public's inquiries about AIDS. The letters often landed at the National Institute of Allergy and Infectious Diseases. Specializing in transmissible diseases, NIAID was the third-best-endowed institute, after the National Cancer Institute and the National Heart, Lung and Blood Institute, on the Bethesda campus, a status it had achieved as a result of the AIDS epidemic. Scientist Anthony Fauci headed the institute. Fauci's staff routinely referred the letters from Congress about chronic Epstein-Barr virus disease to his deputy, James Hill, over whose signatures the letters would be mailed. Of necessity, Hill's staff developed form letters, each tailored to a particular category of inquiry.

Responses to senators and representatives, particularly those who sat on the subcommittees with funding or oversight powers over the National Institutes of Health, usually contained lengthy, mind-numbing descriptions of the agency's intra- and extramural research projects on Epstein-Barr virus. Although by then no one in the scientific community—including the NIH's own Stephen Straus—continued to believe that ubiquitous herpesvirus played a causative role in the disease, the bureaucrats and public relations experts in Bethesda continued to tout the agency's long-standing scientific investment in Epstein-Barr virus as evidence of their commitment to the new problem. On close examination, it was apparent that nearly all of the dollars were being spent on Epstein-Barr virus research projects that had been in place for years. Legislators and their staffs were hardly equipped to decipher the scientific sleight of hand in these letters, particularly since the name "chronic Epstein-Barr virus syndrome" had by then become rooted in the public vernacular. "In conclusion," Hill's upbeat formula letters typically ended, "NIAID is vigorously pursuing the complex questions related to chronic EBV syndrome on many fronts, both basic and applied."

Patients' lengthy accounts of the disintegration of their previously intact lives, frequently bolstered by sheafs of medical records, garnered inversely brief responses: "Researchers at the National Institute of Allergy and Infectious Diseases (NIAID) have been in the forefront of research on the debilitating symptoms attributed to chronic Epstein-Barr virus (CEBV) infection," the government's form letter began. "With continued research, we hope to better define the illness and discover an effective treatment." The patients were then referred to the Portland-based national patients' association "for further information."

Despite James Hill's formula replies describing "vigorous pursuit" of the problem, the only research under way at the National Institute of Allergy and Infectious Diseases was that being orchestrated by Stephen Straus, who had begun in earnest that year to recast his original observations about the disease, moving the debate from the realm of medicine to the realm of psychology. In a highly impolitic slip during an interview in 1991, in fact, Deputy Director Hill clarified the true extent of his agency's commitment to the disease when he said, "If it weren't for Steve Straus and his interest in chronic fatigue syndrome, there's a very real possibility that we would have *no* intramural efforts in chronic fatigue syndrome. Steve is the only person that we have in our institute—within NIAID—who is interested in this particular area." Straus's efforts in Bethesda were costing about $800,000 dollars a year, in contrast to the approximately $45 million or more touted in the agency's letters to Congress that year.

By early 1987, Straus himself felt almost intolerably burdened by the demands of an increasing number of people suffering from the disorder and their doctors. His nurse, Janet Dale, tried to protect her boss from the onslaught. "We've had literally thousands of referral letters from doctors and patients, combined," Dale said that winter. Although Straus had decided to limit his studies to people whose chronic disease had begun with infectious mononucleosis, a decision that put the great majority of sufferers out of the running for evaluation at the NIH, he continued to be inundated.

"At this point," the scientist commented that January, "I have evaluated here at the clinical center probably about a hundred patients with the syndrome, and I probably turn away a dozen or more referrals a day. It's very distressing to patients," he added. "There are those who are relatively poor and can't work and have few support systems who write me or call me up and are quite desperate. And there are people who have extraordinary resources—very successful, accomplished individuals who feel they have a right to be seen by so-called experts—who call me up and are quite desperate. The problem is, I can't do much for any of them."

"I don't know if it's an epidemic," Straus said in response to a question. "What I can tell you is that my phone rings off the hook, that we get a tremendous number of letters that distract me from doing things I'd like to do, that very many critical, imaginative, scholarly physicians and scientists around the country also are seeing patients with this disorder."

Before year's end, Straus attached an answering machine to his office telephone, forwarding all calls from the public to the public affairs office of the National Institute of Allergy and Infectious Diseases.

Straus's shift to psychiatry to explain the malady was telegraphed that year to his NIH colleagues, with the result that attitudes in Bethesda—attitudes that had never been fully formed to begin with—were molded and hardened. Paul Levine, the epidemiologist from the National Cancer Institute who, four months earlier, had gone to Nevada in search of the epidemic, confirmed that by 1987 a potent mind-set about the disease permeated the Bethesda campus. In a moment of candor several years later, Levine admitted, "At that time, everyone here was saying, 'It's psychological.'" Levine disputed his peers on the issue: "I said, 'I don't believe that.'" But he found little support for his ideas.

Since their return from Nevada, Levine's travel companion, Robert Biggar, had dropped the disease without regret and resumed his AIDS research. Levine's fascination, driven primarily by his curiosity about the disease's neurologic component, persisted. In an effort to accommodate the views of his skeptical colleagues, Levine hypothesized that investigators were dealing with at least two kinds of patients, the Tahoe type and the non-Tahoe type. He proposed that the true Tahoe types would have no existing or preexisting psychological problems, but that the non-Tahoe types might indeed be suffering from a psychological disorder. The Tahoe types could be identified by evidence of sudden onset of disease; those who had insidious, gradual onset with more ambiguous symptoms were of the non-Tahoe type.

Levine began a study of Straus's patients to see if they had a different psychological profile, but it was never completed. Other diseases and other projects intervened, he explained; he could afford to spend just 10 percent or less of his time on the Tahoe malady, and, in point of fact, unless there emerged irrefutable proof that the disease was in some way related to the development of cancer in its victims or their contacts, it would be difficult for him to justify continued work in the field.

Nevertheless, Levine's theory, though unpublished, held a certain irony for investigators outside Bethesda in coming years. Over time, Straus's increasingly belligerent statements about the disease struck some independent researchers as being so far afield that they wondered privately if Straus was studying the wrong patients—in other words, the non-Tahoe types—or, more generally, whether the government's expert even knew how to recognize a true case—that is, a Tahoe type.

In mid-1987, CDC principal investigator Gary Holmes received a call from a representative of Pan Am, Mayhugh Horne's employer, seeking the agency's assistance in determining the cause of illness among stewardesses who flew Pan Am's U.S.-Africa route. Holmes confirmed that the symptoms being reported by the stewardesses were consistent with a diagnosis of CEBV, but the agency did nothing to investigate the outbreak.

"Doctors call to report these clusters—we get these calls all the time—but they don't go anywhere because I don't have time to pursue them," Holmes explained early that year.

On an average day, Minann, Inc., Chicagoan Ted Van Zelst's philanthropy, received one or more accounts of cluster outbreaks of the disease, usually involving fewer than fifty people. These reports, Van Zelst noticed, were most common among people who labored in confined workplaces such as sealed office buildings, post offices and schools with heating systems that recycled air, and airplanes. Flight attendants seemed particularly vulnerable. The reports suggested a route of transmission scientists called "aerosol," meaning the inciting pathogen was transported on the very air its victims breathed.

Often, when he read a description of an outbreak that seemed especially persuasive, Van Zelst alerted the CDC. On April 23, for instance, he wrote to Carlos Lopez about an outbreak of CEBV syndrome in Crescent City, California. "It is reported that twenty-six out of thirty workers in a post office apparently have symptoms similar to the CEBV syndrome," Van Zelst told Lopez. Van Zelst also notified the agency of a purported outbreak of the disease among members of the University of Washington's Department of Zoology and Microbiology in Pullman, Washington. The Minann president had also been corresponding with members of a New Jersey–based union for airline flight personnel; some union leaders suspected an outbreak of the disease was under way in the airline industry in the Northeast.

So far as Van Zelst was able to determine, not one of these outbreaks was ever investigated. "They really could have cared less about this disease," he recalled.

If American health agencies were loath to acknowledge the rise of an infectious brain disease, U.S. health insurers, in contrast, gave every indication of having recognized a looming financial disaster. Despite the government's silence on the subject, many major health insurers had modified their applications by 1987 to include questions that would ferret out people suffering from symptoms of the chronic affliction Cheney and Peterson had described to the CDC in 1985. Beginning in 1987, it became impossible to obtain medical or disability coverage from major carriers if the applicant had been diagnosed with chronic mononucleosis, chronic Epstein-Barr virus syndrome, or chronic fatigue syndrome—a policy that continues to the present. Applications frequently were denied even if the applicant claimed to have recovered. Merely having had the Epstein-Barr antibody test, without a diagnosis, created risk.

Patients fortunate enough to be insured at the time of diagnosis became vulnerable to losing their insurance. One sufferer, who had been covered by a private policy for five years before falling ill, was dropped by his insurer, Mutual of New York, within months of his diagnosis that year after missing a premium payment. Were he to apply for coverage with the company a second time, an insurance broker warned him, he would be rejected because of his CEBV diagnosis. After having paid out more than $5,000 in premiums during the years of good health that preceded his illness, he found himself disabled, deprived of health insurance, and uninsurable.

Medical coverage and medical care were denied in more subtle ways as well. Reimbursement for drug therapy was routinely withheld; this was easily accomplished, since no federal body officially recognized the Tahoe malady as a disease. Health maintenance organization members often discovered that they too had been cut off from medical services when their internists referred them to their HMO's psychiatric clinic. "A referral to a mental health department . . . could, of course, signal the doctor's recognition that . . . you need someone on your side who will listen and help," wrote Susan Conant in her 1990 book on coping with the disease.[1] "In practice, it means . . . just what [the patient] understood it to mean: you have been blackballed."

Patients too ill to work frequently had just one option: seeking help from the Social Security Administration in Baltimore. The agency was duty-bound to provide monthly support payments to disabled Americans who had contributed some portion of their wages into the multibillion-dollar fund during their productive years. But the Social Security Administration lacked a classification for the Tahoe malady on its disability forms. And, just as in the private sector, doctors contracted by the agency to examine disability candidates did not accept the disease as bona fide.

Charlotte, North Carolina

By late January, Cheney had begun building a new internal medicine practice within Charlotte's upscale Nalle Clinic. For the moment he was enjoying his hiatus from the emotion-roiling subject of the epidemic disease. During the second week of February, however, Cheney's idyll ended abruptly with the arrival of a packet from Gary Holmes. In a pro forma gesture, the Epidemic Intelligence Service officer sent the doctor a copy of the *JAMA* manuscript with a letter inviting him to be a coauthor. The doctor read it once, then a second time, to be sure he had comprehended it fully. He was appalled: like the *Morbidity and Mortality Weekly Report* on the subject, the article implied that no epidemic had occurred.

On February 23 Cheney sent a letter to the editor of *JAMA* and a copy to Holmes in which he explained why he was declining the "honor" of being a coauthor on the Tahoe report.

The doctor was particularly incensed by Holmes's comment that "of the 134 respondents, 101 described illnesses that resolved in less than one month." Cheney contrasted Holmes's statement with the conclusion of the Harvard study then under way: that the mean duration of illness for 178 Tahoe patients was thirty n.onths; in reality, more than half of those people had been ill *longer* than thirty months. He also cited an October 22, 1985, letter from Holmes to the Nevada state epidemiologist in which Holmes reported that 70 percent of the Incline patients had been ill *longer* than one month.

"Dr. Holmes's report is inconsistent not only with the Harvard study but with *his* own raw data," Cheney wrote (Cheney's italics). In addition, he enumerated a number of other serious problems with the data. The doctor ended his letter with an unequivocal challenge: "I can promise you that if this article is published in the *Journal of the American Medical Association,* I will do everything in my power to bring this fact to light. Dr. Holmes et al. conducted a superficial study, as the Harvard study will show; they used an inadequate assay; their article has, in its current form, no business being printed in a major medical journal."

Incline Village, Nevada

Peterson, too, was offered an opportunity by Holmes to be included as a coauthor and, like his departed colleague, declined. Evidently the defection of the Alder Street clinicians was of no consequence to *JAMA*'s editors. On January 29 senior editor Bruce Dan wrote to Holmes: the journal had accepted for publication the Epidemic Intelligence Service officer's paper about the famous outbreak.

While Cheney was enjoying, however briefly, his freedom from the medical quandary that had consumed him in Incline, Peterson was struggling with his conscience. Alone now, the young doctor mulled dropping his investigation of the disease. Peterson had hoped that with the departure of his outspoken partner, antipathy for him and his patients might abate; instead, the conflict was escalating. Not long after Cheney's departure, the local *North Lake Tahoe Bonanza* published a comprehensive chronology of the Tahoe malady in Incline Village. Businesspeople were stung by the article's timing; it appeared on one of the year's prime ski weekends. The article sent a wave of apprehension through the tourist industry along the lake's north shore. A dismal snow season that winter compounded the Lake Tahoe tourist industry's woes and seemed to shatter hope for a reconciliation between the well and the sick. "The battle lines were drawn," recalled Bill Rulle, a thirty-nine-year-old resident of Incline Village who had been stricken by the disease the winter before. "Everything in Incline is highly leveraged, and if things are going badly, you need an excuse. We were the excuse."

The sentiments of Don Steinmeyer, chairman of the Incline Village–Crystal Bay Visitor and Convention Bureau, were typical of local business owners. Perturbed by the persistent news coverage, he complained, "I'm appalled that a country doctor in a community our size would tackle that kind of a problem. . . . There are other doctors in town who have very successful businesses in this town who think it's a real crock," he added. "And quite frankly most of those doctors are pretty close personal friends of mine and I have a high regard for them."

In spite of such discouragement, Peterson could not back away. "I don't give up on causes," he would say bluntly when asked why he had persevered. "But I decided that I either had to get out of this business or I had to get some allies. Because it was all-consuming. I was burning out. Ten percent of my patients had the syndrome, but they were consuming seventy percent of my time and ninety percent of my energy."

Late in January the doctor received a call from Ray Swarts, the senior of three infectious disease specialists in Reno. Swarts had attended Paul Cheney's grand rounds at Washoe Medical Center and shared the hostile reaction of the city's medical establishment. He told Peterson that he wanted to come to Incline on sort of a fact-finding mission. He brought with him Trudy Larson and Stephen Parker, the other infectious disease specialists from Reno.

Peterson was uneasy. "I remember I felt great trepidation," he recalled, "as I sat there in front of these infectious disease people who had been very critical of [me], very critical of Paul, very critical of the patients. I just started from the beginning, going back to the first patients and describing what we had observed. I mean, I had lots of answers, if people would only listen to some of this stuff."

"I call it a tribunal," Swarts recalled later. "I basically asked Dan every rotten question I could think of for two hours. He didn't flinch. He started dropping some data on me. He told me about the acyclovir protocol. He convinced me."

Swarts's colleague Trudy Larson, who was also the communicable disease consultant to the county health department and, as such, reported to health officer Michael Ford, was impressed as well. "We were looking at records; we were doing chart reviews. We became believers that this was really unusual," Larson said afterward. "There was a lot of physical evidence to back it all up. But the thing that got our attention was the fact that they had these people with abnormalities in their brains, and the head and neck cancers—this really got our attention."

Perhaps it was Peterson's self-effacing style that won over his small audience; perhaps it was his tendency to adhere strictly to the hard data, avoiding speculation about what the data might mean, as Cheney had been inclined to do in a style cultivated and prized among physicists but anathema to medical doctors. Whatever the reasons, the response was less contentious than before. Swarts prevailed upon Peterson to share his findings with the medical professionals in Reno; perhaps he could succeed where Cheney had failed. Peterson recalled later: "I thought, I know I'm right about this. I'm going to present the data. If they spit in my face, *then* I'll drop it."

Swarts set up a meeting at Saint Mary's hospital in Reno. He promised to offer approaches for working up patients suspected of having the disease. "There were about eighty people—seventy doctors and some laboratory people," Swarts remembered. "We had a really hostile atmosphere, which was great, because it held the audience's attention. I told them, 'I don't give a damn if you believe me, but you will never, *ever* be able to say again that you've never heard this.' "

Trudy Larson sensed a sea change among the city's medical practitioners that evening. "That was a kind of turning point in the [medical] community as far as them thinking Peterson and Cheney were a couple of quacks with these chronically depressed women," she remembered. "We were able to answer a lot of questions and turn things around. And for a while I saw a lot of people with this complaint referred from other physicians in the Reno area—about three new patients a week. Most had been ill for two months to a year."

Larson's meetings with her first victims unnerved her. Although Peterson had described to her the intense and peculiar quality of sufferers' distress, particularly their cognition difficulties, Larson was emotionally unprepared for the reality. "The first patient I saw came in with this long list," Larson said. "And she said, 'I'm sorry about this list, but I forget all the time. So I made up this list of what has happened in the last two weeks.' And she *would* forget. She would be talking and she would totally lose her train of thought. She would use words inappropriately. Also, sometimes [the patients] bring their spouse or another family member—whoever lives with them—and it is an objective observer who is under extreme stress because of all these changes, who is saying, 'I can't deal with this anymore!' You can just feel the frustration. It is absolutely palpable in the room."

University of Nevada, Reno

Virologist Berch Henry, a professor of microbiology at the University of Nevada medical school in Reno, had been following the Tahoe epidemic through newspaper accounts. He was frankly puzzled. Henry's expertise was Epstein-Barr virus. He had done his postdoctoral work at Duke with Joseph Pagano, one of the country's top Epstein-Barr virus specialists. Nothing he read about the disease at the lake made sense to him. "EBV just doesn't do the things that this disease—this syndrome—was purported to do," he said.

In early February infectious disease specialist Ray Swarts, who had a joint appointment to the medical school, called Henry and tried to interest him in the problem. The virologist thus became the fourth person from Reno to undertake a fact-finding mission to the lake that winter. "I decided, Well, hell, I want to talk to Peterson and find out what's going on," Henry remembered. "I didn't know whether Dan Peterson was a quack, a knight in shining armor, or something in between, but I spent an hour and a half with him and I could not *believe* the information those two doctors had gathered. Once I walked out of there, I was a believer, no question. I mean, it's just a matter of sitting down and talking with him."

Henry agreed to serve as the microbiologist in the collaborative group being formed by Peterson and Reno's three infectious disease doctors. "I'm sitting here an hour away, and if [Peterson is] having problems with the CDC and Gallo," Henry said, "then it seems ridiculous that the school of medicine is sitting on our thumbs, not doing anything."

That same month the dean of the University of Nevada's medical school in Reno, Robert Daugherty, flew to Washington to discuss the epidemic disease with Nevada senator Harry Reid. The dean, a tall, silver-haired man who had become concerned about the spread of the disease in his state, asked Reid about the possibility of obtaining federal money to fund the school's research into the outbreak, which appeared to Daugherty to be statewide. Daugherty, who knew Congress had asked the CDC to undertake surveillance of the disease, also proposed that Nevada be the site of a major surveillance program. The senator was supportive. He asked the medical school dean to draw up a proposal enumerating the costs.

University of Pittsburgh Cancer Institute, Pittsburgh, Pennsylvania

Seymour Grufferman, recently ensconced as chairman of the epidemiology department of the University of Pittsburgh's prestigious Cancer Institute, had not forgotten the North Carolina Symphony. A questionnaire he devised with his former medical student Mary Huang had generated some interesting results. Paul Cheney had told Grufferman that the mean age of the Tahoe patients was thirty-eight years; the mean age of the afflicted musicians in the orchestra was thirty-eight as well. A majority of the cases were women. There was no evidence that the ailing musicians were suffering from any traditional form of depression. If they were depressed, it was not a classic clinical depression—not one that could be diagnosed by standard tests, at any rate. The once-skeptical Mary Huang was growing more curious about the chronic illness.

Grufferman by now had met an immunologist at the University of Pittsburgh who expressed an interest in collaborating on the orchestra investigation. He was Ronald Herberman, one of the first scientists to identify the natural killer cell in the late 1970s. Herberman confessed to Grufferman he knew little about the chronic disease that had struck the orchestra, but he and a group of Japanese collaborators were studying an illness in Japan that sounded similar. One of the major clinical symptoms of the Japanese disease was severe, protracted fatigue. Herberman and his collaborators had found a dramatic drop in natural killer cell levels in their Japanese patients. The finding was so pronounced, in fact, that they named the disease "low natural killer cell syndrome," or LNKS.* Herberman proposed that Grufferman measure natural killer cell function among orchestra members to determine if there were differences between the unaffected, or well, members of the orchestra and those with the chronic malady.

Grufferman welcomed Herberman's interest. Eventually, in fact, Grufferman and his collaborators in Pittsburgh studied several more parameters of immune system integrity as their interest in the orchestra's dilemma mounted. Their experiments were predicated on the theory that well orchestra members would serve as controls for the unwell members, and the researchers were elated to have such an unusually well matched control population. "We thought we would have the luxury of studying a comparable group of people who work side by side with the cases," Grufferman recalled. "Here you've got comparability—you've got a series of people affected by the syndrome and a very similar group of people not affected."

As sometimes happens with the most reasonable hypotheses, however, the researchers' expectations turned out to be based on faulty assumptions.

Harvard Medical School, Boston, Massachusetts

Although the early Jones and Straus articles on the disease had appeared in the *Annals of Internal Medicine,* Komaroff had bigger ambitions for his investigation of the Incline Village epidemic. On February 3 his manuscript was delivered to the offices of the *New England Journal of Medicine* in Boston, the most prestigious medical journal in the world.

The Tahoe manuscript, as it would be known by its authors for the next several years, was a rich and complicated article. Laboratory and clinical data from several subcategories of patients were reported, including evaluations of cerebrospinal fluid from spinal taps performed on patients who had developed acute neurological changes such as "confusion, marked cognitive deficits, delirium, ataxia, transient paresis, or primary seizure." Komaroff also included the results of magnetic resonance imaging brain scans on nearly thirty patients. The paper included, as well, the results of Sheila Bastien's four-hour battery of neuropsychological tests on twenty-two patients.

In the draft submitted to the Boston journal that winter, Komaroff wrote: "The most disturbing clinical manifestations of this illness have been its neurological features, including the cognitive impairment. While some of the measured deficits may have been influenced by depression, the focality and laterality of dysfunction in most patients [are] more consistent with an 'organic' brain syndrome. . . . Also consistent with an 'organic' hypothesis are the magnetic resonance imaging findings suggesting focal demyelination [lesions] and/or edema [swelling] . . . typically in the subcortical areas [of the brain]. These findings almost surely represent real, acute pathology."

* The year before, Michael Caligiuri, Anthony Komaroff's collaborator at the Dana-Farber Cancer Institute at Harvard, had discovered that a sampling of patients in Tahoe and Boston had strikingly low natural killer cell counts and reduced efficacy among the killer cells that remained, but the finding remained unpublished awaiting Caligiuri's evaluation of more patients.

Lyndonville, New York

More than a year after it struck the village of Lyndonville, the bizarre, debilitating illness had yet to abate. In fact, the roster of patients with the malady in David Bell's practice was expanding rather than attenuating. "By late 1986, it was very obvious to us that this was something that was quite widespread," David Bell recalled. At least fifteen more people had been stricken in the past year, including an eight-year-old-boy and a forty-seven-year-old woman; seven of the new victims were children. It was clear the doctors had a problem in their little town that was not due to yersinia or to any other infectious disease with which they were familiar.

That fall, Karen Bell and three of her colleagues in the infectious disease department at Strong Memorial in Rochester, the primary teaching hospital of the University of Rochester medical school, called the CDC to discuss the Lyndonville malady. According to Karen, the CDC staff said the Lyndonville disease "sounded interesting," but they warned her they would be unable to perform their own investigation unless the New York State Health Department invited them; in New York, as in a number of other states, the health department's policy is to perform its own investigation before seeking help from Atlanta. The health department asked the Bells to perform "a full workup" on several of the children who were ill. EIS officer Gary Holmes, meanwhile, requested that a group of Lyndonville children suffering severe underarm lymph node pain undergo lymph node biopsies. Bell arranged for the excruciatingly painful procedures on the children. The biopsies revealed nothing at all to the Strong pathologist who analyzed them.

Quickly the state health officers became suspicious that the town of Lyndonville was suffering from "hysterical neurosis," according to David Bell.

"It was very clear to us right from the start that the CDC had absolutely no intention of looking into it," David Bell recalled later. "It was clear [that] if anything was to be done, we were going to have to do it. If we could crack this illness and prove exactly what it was and how it was transmitted and how to treat it, *then* the CDC might look at it. But the days of clinical medicine are over. You need to have the organism before you can talk business. Once the CDC gets a bug, fine; they're very happy and they'll look into as much as they're required to. But until then, their job is just to stall."

Charlotte, North Carolina

In February, Marc Iverson was interviewed by the *Raleigh News Observer* for an article about the chronic disease. News coverage of the topic was building as it became fodder for health magazines and its victims were profiled in the Lifestyle sections of newspapers. While reading the *Observer* article, Iverson was surprised to learn that one of the clinicians from Incline Village, Nevada, who had originally described the disease was now practicing in Charlotte. Iverson made an appointment immediately. His meeting with Paul Cheney was a milestone for the former banker. Cheney took Iverson's history, looked at him brightly, and said, "You're classic."

The doctor had a constellation of fourteen laboratory markers for brain and immune system integrity, including MRI brain scans, that he ordered on suspected cases; if more than seven of the tests were in the abnormal range, Cheney felt comfortable giving the diagnosis. Iverson proved to be a very interesting patient to the clinician: he was the first person in whom all fourteen markers were positive.

"After I got a brain scan," Iverson recalled, "Cheney told me there were punctate lesions high in the white matter. When I left, I was depressed. I thought, Holy shit, this is my brain! I went to Toys "R" Us and bought four hundred dollars' worth of toys for my children. It was this unconscious thing—I thought I was dying, and I thought, I'm going to have some fun with my kids. After that, I started having lunch with Paul. I realized what an incredible asset he was for us in Charlotte. But there he was, seeing people with colds and sore throats! It was such a waste. I said, 'What can I do for you?' "

Centers for Disease Control, Atlanta, Georgia

On March 3, Gary Holmes wrote a letter to Paul Cheney in response to the vehement epistle against Holmes's *JAMA* paper that Cheney had sent to the journal's editor.

"Once again, I am disappointed we have not been able to see eye to eye on the Lake Tahoe investigation," Holmes wrote. He defended his paper against Cheney's criticisms, and added that he had "discussed your letter with [*JAMA*'s editor], who feels, as I do, that if you still wish to write a letter to the editor, it would be appropriate to [do so], as do other readers who wish to respond to articles in the journal."

University of Pittsburgh Cancer Institute, Pittsburgh, Pennsylvania

The laboratory results on the North Carolina orchestra members were "very, very puzzling," Seymour Grufferman reported that spring. Still operating on the reasonable assumption that the orchestra was composed of cases and non-cases, Grufferman and his colleagues had begun their comparison. The only aspect of immunological health that was consistently different between the sick and well members of the orchestra had to do with natural killer cells, the immune cells responsible for fighting cancer and viral infections. The sick musicians had markedly fewer natural killer cells than they were supposed to have.

After that initial observation, however, the tidy logic of the study began to disintegrate. After studying his data for several weeks, Grufferman drew his conclusion: "Perhaps we are dealing with a very poorly defined assault on the immune system, a sort of global immune dysfunction, that leads to reactivation of Epstein-Barr in some subjects, leads to high T-cell helper-suppressor ratios in other persons—but there is no consistency," except, of course, for reduced numbers of natural killer cells.

As Grufferman and his associates knew, the only logical explanation for the immune dysfunction among both the sick and the well musicians was that everyone had been exposed to some infectious, immune-altering pathogen; a minority had become ill. This pattern—widespread exposure resulting in overt symptoms of disease among only a portion of those infected—was the standard outcome of nearly all known transmissible agents.

University of Nevada, Reno

As far as Cheney and Peterson were aware, most patients whose blood had been sent east were positive for human B-cell lymphotrophic virus, as were about 30 percent of the healthy controls. The discovery that the new herpesvirus had infected large numbers of healthy people was the first glimmer anyone yet had that it might be a common virus, widely distributed among the population. Should that be true, it would seem unlikely that it was the agent that caused the Lake Tahoe disease, and for the same reason Epstein-Barr virus had been eliminated: ubiquitous viruses are not thought to cause outbreaks. Nevertheless, there was a paucity of alternate candidates. As a result, University of Nevada virologist Berch Henry, a new recruit in Anthony Komaroff's collaborative effort, chose the new virus as his research target. His task: to move beyond finding antibodies to the new herpesvirus and actually isolate the bug in patients with the disease.

By June, Henry and his lab assistant, Ron Ota, were having good luck with their efforts to culture virus from patients of Dan Peterson known to be positive for the human B-cell lymphotrophic virus. As he had been warned to expect, Henry found little but cell debris in his cultures by the end of the second week. "This was just chewing the B-cells all to hell," Henry said. "I'm telling you, there are some pretty bizarre tissue culture effects on these cells. We're talking about something that goes in and totally ravages the cell—totally destroys it. I've never seen anything like it."

Whether or not HBLV was the culprit, Henry and Ota were highly suspicious that the agent of the disease was in the blood samples they were analyzing. By midsummer, the thirty-one-year-old Ota had begun to develop symptoms of the Tahoe malady; by early fall, the former jogger and weight lifter was forced to work half days; some days he couldn't even make the twenty-five-minute drive from his home in Carson City to Henry's lab at the university. Ota had worn gloves only infrequently while handling the green-topped tubes of fresh blood. Late in the spring, he had accidentally broken a tube of fresh blood and spilled it over one hand. Laboratory technologists, like dentists, suffer from chapped, cracked skin because they must wash their hands scores of times in a day; to some viruses, an imperceptible crack in human skin is a Grand Canyon–size portal. When Henry tested Ota's blood for evidence of the virus he was finding in the Tahoe patients, he found that Ota was positive—apparently floridly infected, in fact. Unfortunately, Henry was unable to draw an etiologic relationship between Ota's illness and the infection, since Ota's HBLV status prior to the blood draw was unknown. In addition, there were so many sick Carson City residents—the local support group numbered in the low hundreds—that Henry and Ota could hardly exclude the possibility that Ota had contracted the disease through casual contact with another sufferer in Carson City.

11

Antecedent Epidemics

One pressing question circulating among interested researchers in 1987 was the matter of the disease's age. Was it a new disease, as AIDS was believed to be, or an ancient one that had gone undetected until the Tahoe outbreak drew attention to its existence? Some believed the lines of the argument needn't be cast so starkly: perhaps the disease was old, occurring rarely and in isolated outbreaks, but had only lately reached pandemic status.

By 1987, the government's Stephen Straus had articulated his and, by inference, the government's view: the disease was an age-old problem—neurasthenia—merely highlighted by press accounts, a tenet that would be increasingly useful in preventing panic in the years ahead. It was Paul Cheney's heartfelt belief, in contrast, that the disease which had struck Incline Village—and indeed the nation—was new. "How could we have *possibly* missed this disease for all these years?" he asked that year. "Although a large number of patients are subtle and may not be that sick, there are a significant number of patients who are really quite incredible, and I just can't believe the medical profession could have watched this—*missed* this—for decades, or millennia. It's too striking."

Certainly few clinicians of Cheney's generation were aware of any such virulent, fast-spreading disease existing in earlier decades. But a handful of more senior medical investigators, whose expertise bound them together in what amounted to a kind of secret fraternity, were amply aware of previous outbreaks of illnesses that seemed to presage the Lake Tahoe disease. If one were to undertake a review of the medical literature under such headings as "epidemic neuromyasthenia," "encephalomyelitis," "atypical poliomyelitis," "epidemic vegetative neuritis," or "benign myalgic encephalomyelitis," approximately thirty listings would appear, each of them describing mysterious outbreaks of a disabling disease, most often in institutional settings like hospitals or convents, whose sufferers described symptoms bearing more than passing resemblance to the complaints of patients in northern Nevada decades later. Even more articles would tumble off the shelves of medical libraries if the location of the epidemic was named, since witnesses to these outbreaks frequently named the affliction after its city, its county, or even its institution of origin, as had happened with the Tahoe malady. Hence one found the Icelandic disease, which broke out among 1,000 residents of Akureyri, Iceland's second-largest city, in the fall of 1948; the Royal Free disease, named for a 1955 outbreak in London's Royal Free Hospital, which felled 292 staff members; Punta Gorda fever, a perplexing malady that affected 150 residents in the south Florida town in 1956; and Newcastle's disease, which derived its name from an outbreak among 48 student teachers in Newcastle upon Tyne, England, in 1959.

It is instructive that, in every case, the investigators who studied these outbreaks firsthand became convinced an infectious pathogen had caused the disease although they were unable to name the germ and they lacked the sophisticated diagnostic technology of contemporary medicine. These hands-on investigators of the 1930s, 1940s, and 1950s determined by a process of careful observation that a disease was contagious. In rare cases, those who did the investigating became victims themselves. J. Gordon Parish, for example, a British doctor in Newcastle upon Tyne, became ill during the 1959 epidemic and remains ill to this day.

One of the best-documented investigations of these outbreaks in the United States was undertaken in Punta Gorda, Florida, in the mid-1950s by a team of government scientists headed by Donald Henderson. Today Henderson is senior science adviser to the office of the assistant secretary of health, but in 1956 he was the chief of the Epidemic Intelligence Service at what was then called the Communicable Disease Center of the U.S. Public Health Service (later the Centers for Disease Control). Henderson's Punta Gorda experience led him to coin the name "epidemic neuromyasthenia" for the disease. It was a hybrid of the terms "neurasthenia" and "myasthenia," implying brain and muscle involvement. "Use of the word 'epidemic,' " Henderson explained in a 1959 article on the subject, "emphasizes the need for epidemiologic as well as clinical appraisal of cases."[1] In other words, diagnosing people whose disease appeared outside the context of an obvious epidemic was almost prohibitively difficult.

Henderson had been alerted to the outbreak by the Florida state epidemiologist, who bore the auspicious name James Bond. Bond's letter on the subject landed on Henderson's desk in Atlanta on May 9, 1956. Henderson dispatched a gifted young EIS officer named David Poskanzer to Florida to investigate. Poskanzer remained in Punta Gorda for a week, then returned to Atlanta in time to present his preliminary findings at the agency's annual Epidemic Intelligence Service conference—the same annual conference where, thirty years later, Gary Holmes would discuss the Incline Village epidemic. Henderson described the events that followed to medical reporter Berton Roueche of *The New Yorker,* who later included the story in his 1965 book, *The Orange Man*: "[Poskanzer's] report was a feature of the meeting. One thing that particularly struck him about the disease was its enormous and confusing array of symptoms. They were protean—absolutely protean. He stressed that over and over again. I thought I knew what he meant. That is, the point had been emphasized in all the literature that I'd read. But I was mistaken. The symptomatology of epidemic neuromyasthenia is extremely hard to picture. You really have to see it for yourself. Well, I got to see it a few days later."[2]

Henderson recruited a small team of experts to accompany him to Punta Gorda for what he promised would be "a comprehensive clinical and epidemiological study." The team arrived in Punta Gorda on May 27, staying for four days on their first visit. They returned twice, five months later and then a year later. During their first visit, the federal team undertook a door-to-door survey in an effort to measure the breadth of the disease in the bayside town of 2,000. Aided by neighborhood volunteers, they talked to nearly half the population. Sixty-five cases had already been diagnosed; they turned up an additional sixty-two cases of the disease. As Henderson explained to Roueche, "Medical records are only an indication of the scope of an epidemic. There are always a number of victims who can't or won't see a doctor. This was especially true in Punta Gorda."

Like everyone who ventured to investigate the disease, the CDC investigators were stymied by the multiplicity of symptoms. As Henderson later recalled, "The principal presenting symptoms were recurrent sharp pains in the muscles of the back and neck, severe headache, disturbances of coordination, and some transient motor and sensory dysfunctions. Plus a strong emotional overlay—tension, anxiety, depression." Recent disturbances in memory were included in the criteria. Henderson related one example:

> I was in on several of the interviews, and I can testify that we managed to get the facts—one way or another. I remember one case in point. It was a preacher—white, middle-aged, married. . . . He had been sick, and his symptoms were generally provocative. Except on the emotional side. He insisted that there was nothing wrong with his mind or his memory. As we rose to go, the interviewer asked him if she could have a glass of water. Of course, he said, and left the room. But almost at once he was back. The interviewer had asked him for something—what was it? She told him. Oh, yes. He started out of the room again, and then stopped and called upstairs to his wife. Where did they keep the ice cubes? She told him, and he went on out to the kitchen. But a moment later he called her again. This time he wanted to know just how many cubes should go in the glass. We added him to the case list.

The four investigators struggled, as the next generation of federal scientists would, to arrive at a case definition. In spite of his best intentions, Henderson's defining criteria "fell a bit short of scientific excellence," he admitted in his conversations with Roueche: "Epidemic neuromyasthenia is a most ungrateful disease in that respect. Its manifestations are subjective rather than objective. . . . There was practically nothing that we could see or touch or measure. I mean, there were no lesions to examine, no big livers or tender spleens to feel, no jaundice, no classically paralyzed limbs, no laboratory data to analyze. We used to sit in my room at the motel after dinner and puzzle it over and over. None of us had ever seen anything like it. We just couldn't put it together. It was bizarre. . . . I tell you, we began to feel that we were living in the bughouse."

In time, Henderson and his colleagues began to entertain the notion that the patients, too, might belong in the bughouse. "Depression. Terrifying dreams. Crying without provocation. Nausea and headache and diarrhea. Back and neck pains. Imaginary fever. Problems of memory and mentation. Vertigo. Hyperventilation. Menstrual irregularities. Difficulty in swallowing. Fatigue. Fast heart. Imaginary swellings. Paresthesia [transient numbness and tingling]. And paresis [extreme muscle weakness]. . . . You can see why the possibility of a psychoneurotic explanation came readily to mind," Henderson said.

Ultimately the scientists dismissed the bughouse theory because the facts of the epidemic could not support it. The cases had occurred in scattered, random fashion from February to June rather than simultaneously; additionally, Henderson noted, "nothing had happened in Punta Gorda that could have excited a mass reaction." In fact, he pointed out, "there was hardly a ripple of apprehension among the general population of the town. . . . It was just the reverse of a panic situation." But having dropped the bughouse theory, the researchers were again without a hypothesis to explain the outbreak.

"If it wasn't a question of mass hysteria," Henderson said, "what was the anatomy of the epidemic?"

After eliminating the possibilities of insect-to-man transmission, common exposures to a toxic product, and contamination of water and food supply sources, the team arrived at the only remaining possibility: "It was also, of course, the likeliest explanation," Poskanzer reported to Roueche. "The pattern of epidemic, the apparent absence of any common exposure factors, and the high incidence of illness among medical and hospital personnel were consistent only with an infectious disease transmitted from person to person. Just how the microorganism responsible might travel from one person to another was not at all clear. It is still wide open to conjecture. We were able, however, to postulate the general nature of the microorganism. It was probably a virus."

The fact that the team tested the Punta Gorda patients for several viruses with negative results hardly dissuaded Henderson. He noted that infection might occur very early in the disease; by the time the symptoms arise, the patient could have ceased to "excrete" the virus, a phenomenon common to many viral illnesses. Additionally, Henderson explained, viruses "are hard enough to find . . . in the best of circumstances. . . . They're extremely numerous, too. Umpteen new ones are discovered every year."

Having winnowed the possibilities down to viral infection, however, the team could go no further: "We still know painfully little about epidemic neuromyasthenia," Henderson said. "But Punta Gorda gave us at least some sense of what it is and what it isn't. . . . I wonder if there will ever be a next time."

Henderson and Poskanzer published their Punta Gorda findings in the *New England Journal of Medicine* one year after the Florida outbreak.[3] In the same issue of the journal, an epidemiologist working at the NIH, Alexis Shelokov, published an account of his own investigation of an outbreak of epidemic neuromyasthenia among the nursing staff in a private psychiatric hospital in Rockville, Maryland.[4]

Shelokov's expertise had been sought in 1953 by the administrators of the Chestnut Lodge Hospital, an institution, still in operation in Rockville, that catered to members of Congress and other Washington notables. Because of the virulence of the affliction, which caused a near-paralytic weakness among several of its victims, and its wildfire spread, polio was suspected. This was not the first time the disease had been confused with polio. Iceland's Akureyri outbreak initially had suggested polio to its investigators as well. Shelokov was a polio expert, but it was rapidly apparent to him that the Chestnut Lodge nurses were suffering from something other than polio. "I had never *seen* anything like this, never *heard* anything like this. So I started searching the literature, and in those days it was by hand, in the library. I started to look for any polio epidemic that didn't smell right."

Shelokov's epiphany occurred when he discovered A. G. "Sandy" Gilliam's ninety-page monograph of the Los Angeles County General Hospital outbreak of 1934.[5] That, too, was thought to be polio until Gilliam, a Johns Hopkins–trained epidemiologist who had been sent from the NIH to Los Angeles to investigate, made his canny assessment. Gilliam called the new affliction "atypical polio." More than 198 of the 1,531 doctors and nurses were afflicted. Polio had ravaged the city's children that year, but an outbreak of polio among adults was highly unusual. In addition, the attack rate in the county hospital was, as Donald Henderson would eventually note, "without parallel in the history of poliomyelitis." The Los Angeles epidemic turned out to be the most scrupulously documented outbreak of the disease, thanks to Gilliam's perspicacity and skill.

"[Gilliam] saw there was a clinical pattern that emerged," Shelokov recalled. "He said, 'These people have things which we have *never* seen before with *any* described condition. It's an unprecedented'—and these are the words that he finally used—'it's an unprecedented outbreak, unknown to medical science.' Now he was objective. He had been convinced *against his better judgment*.

"As you read [Gilliam's monograph]," he continued, "the picture emerges. And if the people who think this is just a bunch of hysterics—if they would take the time to read [Gilliam], they would realize that as early as that outbreak, there was a methodological expert who settled the question."

According to Shelokov, Gilliam's paper was "suppressed" for nearly four years by his superiors at the NIH who continued to believe the Los Angles outbreak was an atypical form of polio rather than a new disease. The most formidable resistance came from James Leake, a medical director of the Public Health Service.*

In 1959, Donald Henderson and Alexis Shelokov collaborated on an article about the disease for the *New England Journal of Medicine*. Written by Henderson, the article reviewed the scientific literature describing several similar outbreaks and struggled to impose order on the seemingly innumerable and often

---

* In 1988 the Canadian doctor and researcher Byron Hyde managed to locate a handful of the doctors who had fallen ill during the Los Angeles outbreak fifty-four years earlier. Hyde, who had studied Gilliam's monograph with an intensity equal to Shelokov's, believed the L.A. outbreak was the same disease he had begun to see in his Ottawa internal medicine practice three years earlier. In 1989, writing in a quarterly newsletter he published for Canadian victims of the disease, Hyde noted, "Many of the staff doctors never returned to full employment, although they were all very young at the time. The nurses in particular were all treated as having hysteria and as late as 1955 Dr. Alberto Marinacci writes tongue in cheek that all of the nurses affected in the 1934 epidemic had been hysterectomized as a technique to treat their hysteria, and that the surgery had not helped." (Marinacci studied CFS-like illnesses in the 1950s.) Hyde added that there had been no medical follow-up of any of the cases, which he suspected was the result of a legal settlement between the epidemic victims and the hospital. A condition of the settlement was that the victims refrain from discussing their ordeal publicly. "The one hundred ninety-eight staff members sued the hospital and eventually settled for six millions dollars in 1939, which, divided among the group, would have purchased three houses for each victim in the best section of Los Angeles. Contingent on receiving the payment was non-publicity of the epidemic."

strange symptoms of the disease itself.* Shelokov and Henderson took the position that the epidemics probably represented the same clinical syndrome and may even have shared the same causative virus. They noted the marked susceptibility of nurses and doctors, which they believed was the strongest evidence for person-to-person transmission. They were particularly impressed with the preponderance of the disease among young and middle-aged adults and by its tendency to afflict women by a ratio of at least 1.5 to 1; the severity of the disease had been "considerably greater" among females in most epidemics, they noted. They were also struck by the extraordinary attack rates, usually 6 to 7 percent of the population, which were remarkably consistent among epidemics. These rates, they proposed, intimated that the causative pathogen was one to which the communities affected had no previous immunity.

Significantly, the epidemiologists attempted to describe the confusion and emotional turmoil the disease inspired in its victims, symptoms a later generation of government investigators would dismiss as unrelated to any organic disease and, in fact, proof of the lack thereof: "Depression, tension, and emotional instability have been impressive and among the most incapacitating and persistent symptoms. Repeated episodes of crying without provocation, insomnia, terrifying dreams and difficulty in concentration are probably secondary phenomena. . . . Mild confusion, impaired memory for recent events, alterations in personality structure, euphoric behavior and tendencies to transpose and 'stumble over' words have frequently been observed during the more severe acute phase and during recrudescences [relapses]. . . . Malaise and fatigability are particularly pronounced and persist long into convalescence."

Henderson and Shelokov attempted to address the issue of recovery as well. Because few of the epidemics had been well followed over time, recovery rates remained a nebulous area of study, but it was apparent that for some the disease could last for years, if not the remainder of their lifetime. "The protracted debility engendered by the illness is illustrated by studies from several epidemics," Henderson wrote. . . . "A six-year follow-up study of thirty-nine cases from the Icelandic epidemic . . . revealed that all patients had returned to work, but only 13 percent considered themselves free of symptoms."

As the next generation of researchers would do in the 1980s, Henderson and Shelokov debated the matter of the disease's name. Unlike their successors in the 1980s, whose focus would be on immunology and virology (and, of course, psychiatry), Henderson, Shelokov, and the other epidemiologists who investigated outbreaks were more clinically oriented; they listened to the patients' complaints, which focused their attention on the central nervous system and the muscles.

"To date, there is no agreement on a name, almost every epidemic receiving a different designation. For purposes of referencing and indexing, this creates a chaotic problem. Until an etiologic agent or agents are identified or until the underlying pathophysiologic processes are defined, we recommend use of the name

---

* Theirs was one of two overviews of the subject in a major journal that year. The second: E. D. Acheson, "The Clinical Syndrome Variously Called 'Benign Myalgic Encephalomyelitis,' 'Iceland Disease,' and 'Epidemic Neuromyasthenia,' " *American Journal of Medicine* 26 (1959): 569.

'epidemic neuromyasthenia.' . . . Diagnosis of a single, sporadic case of illness marked by a protean symptomatology without pathognomonic [distinctive] physical or laboratory findings and presenting many of the features of psychoneurotic illness," Henderson wrote with sage understatement, "is fraught with difficulty."

Indeed, in 1970, David Poskanzer, who was then a professor within the neurology department at Harvard Medical School, reiterated Henderson's warning in a letter to the *British Medical Journal*: "It is clear that sporadic cases of this disease cannot be readily identified. It is only in the epidemic form that the distinctive epidemiological features allow characterisation."[6] Poskanzer went on to propose the following remarkable hypothesis, one that no doubt would be scoffed at by today's federal investigators: "Instead of ascribing . . . myalgic encephalomyelitis to mass hysteria or psychoneurosis, may I suggest [that researchers] consider the possibility that all psychoneurosis is residual deficit from epidemic or sporadic cases of . . . myalgic encephalomyelitis?"

Henderson and Shelokov ended their 1959 discussion of the disease with a prediction that more epidemics were likely, an assumption they based on the plethora of epidemics reported in recent years. The article concluded with the following call to arms: "Although from current reports, these illnesses do not appear numerically important on a national scale, the long-term morbidity among those who are ill and the very large percentage involved in a single outbreak indicate a need for intensive, comprehensive investigation and surveillance of outbreaks as they occur."

Donald Henderson never personally investigated, nor did he supervise from his post at the CDC, another investigation of the strange epidemic disease, although at the time, he described to *The New Yorker*'s Berton Roueche his optimism about studying the disease in the future:

> We'll know it the next time we see it. And we'll have some new approaches to employ. . . . We're ready and waiting. But Punta Gorda happened quite a few years ago, and I must say I'm beginning to wonder. I wonder if there will ever be a next time. The last reported outbreaks of epidemic neuromyasthenia occurred in 1958 in Athens, and in a convent up in New York State in 1961. Neither of them was recognized for what it was until it had almost run its course. We haven't heard even a decent rumor of it since then. It seems to have disappeared.*

---

* Henderson's protocol for conducting such an investigation languished for the next three decades somewhere in the CDC's records. Gary Holmes, assigned to what was then known as chronic Epstein-Barr virus syndrome in the late 1980s, searched for Henderson's protocol in 1987 but was unable to find it.

In an October 19, 1992, letter to this author, Henderson expressed dubiousness that the disease that by then seemed so widespread could possibly be the same illness that he, Shelokov, Poskanzer, and others had investigated with such rigor forty years before. Yet, he continued, "What is disturbing to me is to discover how little progress has been made in achieving even a primitive understanding of the pathophysiology, let alone the etiology." He concluded, "I believe our concerns of 1959 are as valid today as they were then and that we were as confidently knowledgeable about the syndrome then as we are today."

If epidemic neuromyasthenia and the Tahoe malady were one and the same, what event or series of events in the 1970s and 1980s—the "new dynamic," as Paul Cheney had described it—had transformed a disease once thought to be, in Donald Henderson's words, "[not] numerically important on a national scale" into what some clinicians were beginning to suspect was the most common chronic disease of young and middle-aged adults?

Portland, Oregon

The Portland patients' organization, staffed by three full-time workers and a number of volunteers, was receiving from fifty to two hundred letters and an average of seventy phone calls each working day from people suffering from the disease. In March the group released a survey of six thousand respondents. Victims seemed to be clustered in occupational groups. Gidget Faubion, the organization's president, reported that a surprising 50 percent were nurses, 90 percent of whom worked in hospitals. Another 10 percent worked in the health care field in other capacities; 20 percent were teachers; 10 percent worked as pilots or flight attendants; and the final 10 percent worked in myriad other fields. Faubion had attempted to share this information with the CDC, without luck. "My calls are not returned," she said that spring.

New York City

In March of 1987, Andrew Kopkind wrote a "Letter from California" for *The Nation*. Kopkind, whose story bore the headline "Down and Out in L.A.," launched his tale of left-leaning politicos in Los Angeles with the following lines: "A mysterious and debilitating virus is ravaging the older ranks of Los Angeles' liberal west side just as the political season opens. The inopportune infection—featured on [20/20] and no doubt the subject of a made-for-TV movie already in development—is not known to be fatal, but it is no laughing matter. Fortunately for the local medical establishment, the malaise, variously called adult mononucleosis, the Hollywood blahs and Epstein-Barr virus syndrome, is undiagnosable, incurable and chronic, thus offering endless possibilities for expensive and unverifiable therapies." Kopkind went on to describe a doctor's furtive delivery of gamma globulin to the hotel suite of one sufferer who was a wealthy contributor to liberal candidates.

In fact, no one in the television industry was planning a disease-of-the-week movie about the chronic affliction spreading through Hollywood. And hardly any of the celebrity sufferers of the disease—by 1987, a list that allegedly included James Garner, Robert Wagner, Gilda Radner, Morgan Fairchild, Alana Stewart, Cher, Carol Burnett, David Puttnam, Kirstie Alley, Cathy Lee Crosby, Randy Newman, Ted Turner, *Los Angeles Times* publisher Otis Chandler, and Nicollette Sheridan—would speak publicly about their misfortune. Only Randy Newman, who commented to one journalist that it was not until he became ill that he noticed his driveway was on an incline, admitted to having the disease that year.

As the affliction spread through the entertainment industry, so did the knowledge of its major symptoms: short-term memory loss, intellectual diminution, and disabling fatigue. One episode of *L.A. Law* opened on a staff meeting during which a senior partner reported he had fired an accountant suffering from "Epstein-Barr" because her math errors were destroying the firm's payroll records. Cher, who was filming the movie *Mermaids* that year, became so ill that production was halted for nearly a year before the star could resume work. With movie insurance policies becoming increasingly restrictive for all major stars, any mention of symptoms that even hinted of the disease could preclude a movie contract.

Just one filmmaker, Blake Edwards, tackled the subject, although in a veiled fashion. Convinced he had beaten the disease that had upended his career and personal life during the previous three and a half years, the filmmaker released *That's Life,* his first movie since the Ted Danson vehicle *A Fine Mess.* Edwards filmed it in his own Malibu house.

"As I began coming out of the disease that first time," Edwards recalled later, "I was so relieved and in such a state of exaltation that I didn't want to do anything typically commercial. I wanted to make a home movie." To the uninitiated, the film could be easily viewed as the story of a middle-aged man coming to terms with mortality. In fact, it was a classic case history of a victim of the chronic illness spreading through Hollywood and elsewhere.

Edwards's wife, Julie Andrews, plays the wife of Edwards's stand-in, actor Jack Lemmon. As the movie begins, Lemmon has been stricken by an unnamed malaise so severe that his career, his marriage, and his relationships with his adult children are disintegrating. "Everything aches!" he complains to his wife upon arriving home one afternoon in a state of near-collapse. Angrily he describes his conversation with an orthopedic doctor earlier in the day: "I said, 'Why the hell do all my muscles ache, all the extremities, all the joints? I've never had pain in my *toes* before!' " The specialist tells Lemmon he may be suffering from stress. "A couple of hundred dollars—and he says I've got stress," Lemmon sputters. "*Everybody's* got stress. Stress is *normal.*"

His wife, the personification of patience, responds in a manner familiar to most sufferers of the disease: "I know you feel lousy, but you've never looked better." She complains privately that her husband has undergone a personality change. "He's not been himself at all lately," she tells the family doctor. Eventually, the husband sees the family physician, who concludes, "There is absolutely nothing wrong with you physically whatsoever." The husband responds, "You're a great doctor, and I love you, but you're missing something. Because every bone in my body, every muscle, every fiber, every nerve—*everything!*—Jesus, I feel terrible all the time! I'm depressed, I have headaches, I can't function. On top of everything else, I think I'm impotent." The doctor counters his outburst: "You need to see a psychiatrist."

Critics panned *That's Life* with a vehemence akin to mainstream medicine's rejection of the disease.

Washington, D.C.

In the absence of evidence that the CDC was establishing a reporting system for the disease, members of Congress began to lean on the agency's administrators. On March 25, for instance, John Porter, the Republican congressman from the tenth district of Illinois and philanthropist Ted Van Zelst's representative, wrote a letter to James Mason, then head of the Atlanta agency. After opening pleasantries, Porter wrote: "Last year, as you know, the Subcommittee report accompanying the annual appropriations measure instructed the Centers for Disease Control to establish a reporting protocol for CEBV. Your budget submission, however, indicates that you only intend to establish a . . . case definition. . . . I want to encourage you in the strongest possible terms to initiate a reporting protocol for the symptoms of the disease. I would very much appreciate knowing the particular reasons why a reporting protocol cannot be established in FY 1987."

And on April 21, Alaska Senator Ted Stevens, at Ted Van Zelst's prodding, wrote to the assistant director of the CDC, George Hardy, asking for an update on the agency's work in the area of the Tahoe malady. Stevens reminded the bureaucrat that "The FY '87 Labor, Health & Human Service, Education and Appropriations Act asked the CDC to establish a protocol for reporting the incidence of CEBV by physicians."

Gary Holmes responded to Stevens on April 30 in a letter sent over James Mason's signature. When the case definition is completed, he assured the senator, "we will develop and submit for approval to the Surveillance Committee, Council of State and Territorial Epidemiologists, a formal case reporting system. We plan to begin with a trial system in four or five states; and if that proves successful, we plan to expand it into a national reporting system. We hope to have a pilot system designed and functioning in several states by fall."

The promise Holmes made to Senator Stevens about developing a case reporting system would never be kept, never even attempted, in fact. As for the pilot program, when Holmes wrote his letter to the senator, his boss, Larry Schonberger, was simultaneously mulling a plan to limit surveillance to two counties.*

Centers for Disease Control, Atlanta, Georgia

On April 27 agency scientists held the First International Symposium on the Immunobiology and Pathogenesis of Persistent Virus Infections. Infectious disease scientists from the NIH attended, as did a number of academic researchers. The symposium's planners clearly viewed the outbreak of neuromyasthenia, or the Tahoe malady, or whatever one might call it, as of such minor importance that it failed to merit its own session. One agency scientist, herpes expert Carlos Lopez, invited several eminent scientists to stay after the official symposium and attend a roundtable discussion of the disease, but many of those invited had airline connections to make and were in taxis bound for the Atlanta airport when the meeting began. Two who attended were J. Gordon Parish, the British researcher who had studied the 1959 epidemic in Newcastle upon Tyne, and the Salk Institute's Alexis Shelokov, who with Donald Henderson had named the disease "epidemic neuromyasthenia," also in 1959.

Shelokov felt the meeting was controlled by novices in the field, people like Holmes and Lopez. "By the time the meeting began," he complained later, "many of the people who would have critically contributed were gone. It was dominated

---

* In a draft memorandum the year before, Schonberger had written to his colleagues, "We propose that CDC surveillance of chronic EBV be done within an experimental context."

by these other people, who played ball with each other. Then, when someone like Gordon Parish—who truly is a world authority, *has* this disease, and really knows what he's talking about—when *he* tried to open his mouth, one of these guys would look at him and say, 'Yeah? Well, that's very interesting. Thank you very much.' I just said, 'Jesus, it's no use wasting my time here,' and that's how Gordon felt. But we stayed politely until the thing was over. Afterward I said, 'Gordon, what do you think?' He said, 'I think they're going off in the wrong direction.' "

Three days later the *Journal of the American Medical Association* published the CDC's Tahoe study, which focused on the 15 patients deemed by Holmes and Kaplan to have suffered from the mystery disease longer than one month.[7] Those 15 had higher levels of antibodies to Epstein-Barr virus than 119 patients with "less severe illnesses," and 30 presumably healthy controls. However, Holmes reported, those 15 patients also had "significantly higher" levels of antibodies to two other herpesviruses, cytomegalovirus and herpes simplex, and to measles. Holmes drew no conclusions about this ominous finding and concluded his article by suggesting that "physicians caring for patients who are thought to have this syndrome should continue to search for more definable and often treatable conditions that may be responsible for their patients' symptoms."

Not long after its publication, Holmes's partner, Jon Kaplan, the second author, conceded that the paper's message was not very strong. "Here we were saying we didn't know what caused [the disease]; nor were we totally sure whether it existed, but there seemed to be some sense that there is a group of patients who are different from another group. That's not a best-seller," Kaplan said, laughing. The limited case-control study that had formed the basis for the paper, the epidemiologist added, had "ended up being about as nebulous as the whole situation out there to begin with."

Dan Peterson and Paul Cheney weren't alone in their dismay over the Holmes and Kaplan *JAMA* report. "It's awful—oh, it's awful," Denver researcher James Jones complained. "The CDC has a reputation for presenting accurate information, but this time it was *way* out of line. . . . It trivialized the whole thing and fueled critics of the disease. Holmes and Kaplan don't know what the hell they're talking about. I mean, the only patients they saw were the ones they interviewed out there, and then they picked the wrong ones. Their choice of controls was terribly shoddy. They proved absolutely nothing. People who are interested students of this disease I don't think are very impressed, but you know, everybody else thinks it's the gospel."

Harvard's Anthony Komaroff was more temperate, but he volunteered he had never quite understood Holmes and Kaplan's analysis of the Tahoe epidemic: "This has always been sort of a mystery to me," the doctor mused. "How is it that—I mean, they talked to the same patients that *we* talked to. They came away with a very different impression as to how many people were—currently viewed themselves as—sick and debilitated." In apparent bafflement, Komaroff added, "I frankly just don't understand *what* goes through their heads."

Komaroff's intellectual distance from the government's epidemiologists had been even more evident when his study of the frequency of the disease in his general medicine clinic at the Brigham and Women's Hospital in Boston appeared in the same issue of *JAMA*.[8] The doctor's earlier hunch that the number of people with the disease in his clinic was rising had turned out to be correct. During a six-month period, 21 percent of five hundred patients interviewed at random as they sat in the Brigham clinic waiting to see a doctor were found to be suffering from symptoms Komaroff believed "were suggestive of CEBV infection—i.e., severe fatigue for at least the past six months with associated symptoms of sore throat, myalgias, or headaches, and without any known chronic disease." Of these patients, 45 percent were periodically bedridden, Komaroff reported, and another quarter to three-quarters had recurrent swollen lymph nodes, joint pain, difficulty concentrating and sleeping, and parasthesias (numbness and tingling in their limbs). The patients had suffered from the illness for a median period of sixteen months, meaning the majority had fallen sick in either 1983 or 1984. Komaroff's team found no incidence of psychiatric or any other chronic diagnoses in the medical histories of the patients.

Many clinicians who had been tracking the upsurge of the mysterious disease in their own clinics were impressed by Komaroff's statistics. Among them was Mark Loveless, an infectious disease specialist at the Oregon Health Sciences University in Portland. Loveless's clinical practice included not only a large contingent of AIDS sufferers but also several chronically ill patients whom Loveless originally diagnosed with AIDS-related complex, or ARC. When Loveless began educating himself about the new disease, he had switched their diagnosis. He noted that when Komaroff's numbers were extrapolated to the larger universe of Americans, the attack rate of the chronic malady was striking. "We are probably dealing with a syndrome that is fairly prevalent," Loveless said.

Incline Village, Nevada

Cheney had made it out of Incline with his career intact—barely. Peterson, left with the "mess," as he described it, was faring less well in spite of newly confirmed believers at the University of Nevada. An Easter weekend report on the Tahoe epidemic, this one on the front page of the *San Francisco Examiner,* fanned local entrepreneurs' slow-burning resentment. The *Examiner* reporter, Lisa Krieger, noted that "[Dan] Peterson himself is infected. So are his wife and most of his nurses and lab technicians." Krieger painted a grim picture of the disease, describing brain lesions and dementia. "A suspiciously high number of patients develop a rare cancer of the immune system called non-Hodgkin's lymphoma," she wrote.

Gary Holmes's *JAMA* paper and ensuing news reports, arriving on the *Examiner* article's heels, let loose a new round of strife in the little town. After considerable complaints from real estate agents about the news coverage, the convention authority decided to hire a Reno ad agency, Dunn, Reber, Glenn, Marz, to deal with a problem they clearly viewed as attributable to Dan Peterson and his former partner rather than to a natural catastrophe. Ultimately, they paid the firm a reported $50,000 to handle the story that refused to die. The firm's copywriters composed a 350-word white paper, which drew heavily from CDC statements about the disease. Like government scientists, the white paper authors blamed the epidemic on the press. "Regarding Lake Tahoe," the document said, "the Centers for Disease Control and a doctor at the National Institute of Health [Stephen

Straus] have suggested some of the EBV cases may have been psychosomatic—that is, people were feeling fatigued, read about EBV in the paper, and then asked for EBV tests. . . . In fact, based on research findings by the Centers for Disease Control, one can conclude there never was a great danger."

Absent from the document's logic, of course, was the fact that most of the Tahoe cases were diagnosed long before any press coverage had occurred. Incline's local office of tourism distributed the white paper freely to skiers and other vacationers; it was routinely mailed to journalists and used by real estate agents and casino managers to soothe their patrons' fears.

On May 6, the *North Lake Tahoe Bonanza* quoted resort owner Don Steinmeyer saying at a meeting of the convention authority that Peterson's investigation of the Tahoe disease was "a sophisticated form of quackery." Steinmeyer's comments devastated Mary Peterson but they shored up her husband's resolve. "I told my wife multiple times that is *not* what was going to get me out of town," Peterson said that year, anger creeping into his voice. "If I decided to leave because I couldn't take it anymore, that was okay. But I wasn't going to be driven out of town by idiots—by people who knew *nothing* about viruses, *nothing* about MRI scans, *nothing* about patients, *nothing* about *anything* and didn't give a damn! They were *not* going to be the ones who got me out of town—and Steinmeyer represents that class."

Komaroff made his second visit to Nevada just as Dan Peterson was accused of quackery on the *Bonanza*'s front page. Komaroff, who was himself featured along with Dan Peterson in a photograph on the newspaper's front page on May 8, told Jean Lamming of the *Bonanza* that he believed Dan Peterson to be "a fine doctor." He added, "There is no doubt from the study our Harvard team has done that there is a real illness." Significantly, in her article headlined "Harvard Wants In-depth Fatigue Study," Lamming documented a rise in hotel room bookings in Incline Village and neighboring Crystal Bay that year.

Komaroff spent an afternoon at Reno Diagnostics with Royce Biddle, looking at the brain scans from the Alder Street practice. By then more than seventy scans had been ordered, some serially; approximately three-quarters of them were marked by multiple punctate lesions, or UBOs, in the white matter tracks of the brain. Komaroff was concerned that Biddle was the only neuroradiologist reading the scans. In order for the findings to be meaningful, Komaroff believed, there needed to be some way to control for bias in the interpretation of the scans. He proposed engaging a Harvard neuroradiologist to read the same scans in a blinded fashion—that is, without prior knowledge of Biddle's calls. Biddle welcomed the opportunity to have his professional judgment certified by a Harvard expert.

News of the disease was entering the public's consciousness that summer through mainstream publications with readerships numbering in the millions. In June, *Vanity Fair* interviewer Stephen Schiff explored Gore Vidal's ennui:

> The bulk of Gore Vidal crumples into a couch in his suite at the Beverly Hills Hotel, and if the couch looks tattered, so does its occupant. . . . Vidal is tired, as friends say he so often is these days. His face, which is the color

of January tomatoes, sags; and the familiar verbal torrents have slowed to a dribble.... He turns to Howard Austen, his companion of thirty-seven years. "I'd like a little bit of whiskey and a lot of soda water," he groans.... "I'm full of gamma globulin at the moment."

Vidal, it seems, has contracted Epstein-Barr, Hollywood's most fashionable and mysterious disease, which counts among its putative victims every third screenwriter, movie director, and studio executive in Los Angeles; its most common symptom is fatigue unto death.

"It's something about the T cells—God knows what they are," Vidal intones. "And it's like jet lag ... you just cannot move. Just total inertia."

"Research is difficult," Vidal commented later on in the article. "I read slowly, I've got no memory, and I can't seem to keep notes properly. Whenever I write a date, I get it wrong."

Slightly less than a year after *Newsweek* published its first article on the disease, *Time* entered the fray. Calling it the "yuppie disease" in a subhead, *Time* illustrated the story in its medicine column with a cartoon of a young man in black tie who has fallen asleep at a formal dinner, his head on the arm of the jewel-laden woman seated next to him; a butler stands at the ready in the background. The magazine reported uncritically the CDC's findings—that only 15 of 134 patients at Lake Tahoe suffered "severe, persistent fatigue." And it quoted the NIH's Stephen Straus, who said, "There certainly are people who are ill and who can be disabled by this, but the percentage is relatively small compared to the claims." The newsmagazine reporters apparently accepted Straus's statement at face value despite the fact that the only published prevalence study so far—Komaroff's recent *JAMA* study—found that one-fifth of five hundred visitors to a general medicine clinic in Boston had symptoms that were highly suggestive of the disease. Moreover, so far, no studies had indicated that the disease was being overdiagnosed, that more people were claiming to have it than actually did have it, or that it was less severe than its victims claimed. The anonymous *Time* writer's glib phrase "yuppie disease" marked a pivotal moment in the history of the epidemic.

In July articles about the disease appeared in two more national magazines, *Hippocrates* and *Rolling Stone*. The first, by journalist William Boly, described the Tahoe epidemic and the intricate scientific issues it raised. Boly's perspicacious conclusion: "Incline Village got the brunt of the publicity; the nation got the disease." Boly, in addition, hinted at federal negligence: during an interview, Gary Holmes had told Boly that he was the only person at the CDC who was working on the Tahoe malady on a regular basis. "On any given day," Holmes added, "it's second or third on my list." *Rolling Stone*'s two-part series, by this author, was a survey of scientific opinion on the disease and a personal account of the illness.

On July 28 the *New York Times* joined the fray. "Fatigue 'Virus' Has Experts More Baffled and Skeptical Than Ever" was the *Times* headline. The subhead: "Some Believe Patients Have Succumbed to Latest Health Hysteria." Elliot Kieff, who was now head of infectious diseases at the Brigham and Women's Hospital in Boston and a professor at Harvard Medical School, told science writer Philip Boffey, "A lot of illness that is now being associated with chronic Epstein-Barr virus infection is probably ordinary neuroses which are manifested nowadays as tiredness. It's a disease mostly of younger adults who are having difficult phases of life," Kieff went on. "These people are very unhappy, and it's often very difficult to sort out how much of their psychological problems come from their illness and how much is the cause of their illness. Most of them do not want to see a psychologist or a psychiatrist. They're looking for a physical cause of their illness, and a relationship with their physician."

If Kieff offered factual support for his comments, it failed to appear in Boffey's story.

The NIH's Stephen Straus, characterized by Boffey as "one of the nation's few experts on the illness," asserted that the disease was "not new": "What these patients complain of has been described for over a century. In each generation, people have a different idea of what it might be and what might cause it." In a reprise of his comments to *Time* magazine, he added, "I don't think there's much evidence that it's expanding."

Gary Holmes of the Centers for Disease Control had a lot to say as well. The Epidemic Intelligence Service officer, sitting in his Atlanta cubbyhole with the "Mono Man" placard on his wall, told Boffey, "A lot more is being made of this by the lay press than it probably deserves." Farther down in the article, Holmes talked about Nevada. "We had an understanding that over one hundred patients were severely affected by this syndrome," he said. "But when we got there, we found that . . . they really did not have any major signs of illness." Nevertheless, Holmes admitted that "something striking" was occurring in some of the Tahoe patients that was "not a figment of these people's imaginations." He also told Boffey, "When you get called by people who say they used to run marathons and participate in iron man triathlons and now can hardly get out of bed or brush their teeth, you realize that something is happening."

Anthony Komaroff was quoted as contradicting Holmes's version of the Incline epidemic, saying that "quite a number" of the Tahoe patients had been fully or partially disabled and that only one-third had reported improvement so far. The Boston doctor said the symptoms of the disease were "hard to attribute to a psychological cause."

On August 10, ABC's *Nightline* weighed in with a report. "The question," intoned ABC's in-house doctor-correspondent, Harvard Medical School alumnus Timothy Johnson, "is whether the cause is biological or emotional." Stanford's Tom Merigan was interviewed for an opening filmed segment. The infectious disease specialist expressed deep skepticism that this newly described phenomenon was actually a single disease; he suggested that those huddled under its catchall label were suffering from any number of known ailments and psychological problems.

"What you've got are individual people with individual problems that have been kind of clustered together and forced into a cause," Merigan told his interviewer, reporter George Strait. The doctor, wearing a crisp-looking white lab coat, was seated next to a row of X rays attached to a backlit screen; his "Baffle 'em with bullshit" plaque was nowhere visible. "People need an explanation for their . . . anxiety," Merigan continued, choosing his words with delicacy while dispensing a meaningful look at Strait. "And they will reach out for it." Strait seemed to accept Merigan's opinion uncritically.

Strait had gone to Incline Village, too, and had interviewed Don Steinmeyer, the resort owner who had accused Dan Peterson of "a sophisticated form of quackery." Steinmeyer, wearing dark aviator glasses and grinning, told Strait, "I'm told it's just as important to have EBV as it is to have a BMW—or an IBM." Steinmeyer later complained that he made the comment only after Strait assured him the camera was turned off.

Anthony Komaroff was interviewed on air by Tim Johnson, as was the Portland patient organization's president, Gidget Faubion. When Johnson asked Komaroff point-blank if there were "brain problems" in the disease, a topic raised by Faubion, Komaroff said only that it was true that some patients experienced dizziness. The neurological aspect of the disease was never discussed again on the show. Komaroff's restraint on the subject was a glaring omission, given his statements to the *New England Journal of Medicine* in February. But the Harvard doctor hardly wanted to divulge information that might upset his relationship with the august publication, which was in the process of reviewing the Tahoe manuscript. The journal's well-known "Ingelfinger's rule," named for one of its strong-minded editors, Franz Ingelfinger, banned publication of findings reported first in the lay press.

Miami, Florida

Mayhugh Horne was still flying 747s from Miami to South America and Europe for Pan Am that summer, but the task of piloting transcontinental flights was now Sisyphean. Exhaustion, headaches, and intellectual sluggishness, his companions to varying degrees since his airbus training in Toulouse two years earlier, were increasingly debilitating. Whenever his symptoms became wholly unmanageable, he canceled; he was beginning to miss almost as many flights as he was able to make.

One evening, Horne's wife looked into his face as he was packing to leave for Miami to fly a 747 to Buenos Aires. "You can't go," she told him.

"I know," he said, after a moment.

Not long afterward, Horne's wife happened to watch a summer rerun of ABC's *20/20* 1986 segment about the epidemic in Incline Village, Nevada. That's *Mayhugh,* she thought. She arranged for a tape of the show to be sent to her, and after viewing the piece, neither she nor her husband had any doubt that the disease at Lake Tahoe was the same affliction Horne had been fighting.

Horne called Anthony Komaroff, who suggested the pilot send his blood to the Henle lab in Philadelphia. The pilot forwarded the results of the Epstein-Barr virus antibody assay to one of the medical professors he had seen at Duke the year before. "I've never believed in self-diagnosis," the professor told Horne when he phoned a week later, "but you did it. It looks to me that you are in this EBV situation." He also recommended that Horne not fly anymore; the doctor even said he would not want to be on a plane that Horne piloted. Horne was devastated.

The pilot was obsessive about following FAA and Pan Am safety regulations. Although he received his diagnosis on the eve of a Labor Day weekend, he called Pan Am to report his condition. "I felt this was a situation like a heart attack—I felt I should turn myself in. I fully expected to lose my job," Horne said. Instead, Horne recalled, "I got laughed at. The Pan Am doctor said, 'Well, if you don't feel good, Mayhugh, don't fly. But when you're okay—fly!' He said, '*Everybody's* got that EBV.' I knew then I was talking to an idiot," Horne continued. "By this time I had talked to so many doctors I could tell when I was talking to another idiot."

Delta Airlines, Atlanta, Georgia

In the space of four weeks in late June and early July, eleven Delta airline pilots made serious in-flight errors. The errors included, in one case, landing at the wrong airport and, in another, a near-miss midair collision with another commercial jetliner. Spokesmen for the airline were unable to explain the pilots' behavior.

Los Angeles, California

That summer two more women cyclists who had been members of the 1984 U.S. Olympic team were sidelined by the disease. Jack Harvey, a doctor and then the medical director of the International Bicycle Classic race and an editor of *Physician and Sportsmedicine* magazine, said that "fear of catching the EB virus is rampant among elite cyclists," who typically traveled together, shared hotel rooms and, most particularly, water bottles.

Herman Falsetti, a cardiologist and consulting doctor for the 1984 U.S. Olympic Bicycling Team, who saw about 70 percent of the licensed cyclists, both male and female, in his practice in Irvine, said he had tested and confirmed "chronic fatigue from Epstein-Barr virus infection" among 3 to 5 percent of these athletes, or almost one in every twenty competitors. That number, he added, included some elite men's team riders and male triathletes.

Lyndonville, New York

Increasingly frustrated by the New York State Health Department's indifference to the epidemic in Lyndonville, Karen Bell, with her husband David's help, devised a questionnaire that was distributed to the 914 children in the Lyndonville Central School District to determine how many were suffering from the mysterious chronic disease.

Slightly more than one-half of the questionnaires—561—were returned. Among the students who responded, 21—or 4 percent—had the distinctive symptoms of the disease. Three-quarters of the victims said they had fallen ill in 1985, the year David Bell observed the outbreak in his own practice. Interestingly, a number of parents and siblings who lived in households where at least one child had the disease were also said to be suffering from some or all of the same symptoms. In several households, every member of the family had the disease.

University of Pittsburgh Cancer Institute, Pittsburgh, Pennsylvania

Seymour Grufferman and his associates continued to be concerned by their findings among members of the North Carolina Symphony. "This pattern of inapparent infections in people who are never symptomatic," he said during an interview, but who have the same "screwy, inconsistent pattern of laboratory abnormalities" as the sick people, needed to be confirmed in another cluster outbreak. The epidemiologist, who found cluster investigations the most fascinating aspect of his work, let it be known he was looking for a second outbreak of the disease.

Through his conversations with leaders of patient organizations, Grufferman quickly learned about a recent outbreak among students and teachers in an elementary school in Chillicothe, Ohio. Because of a shortage of money, Grufferman was able to perform laboratory analysis only on samples taken from teachers. Even without testing the children, however, he found the results troubling in the same way they had been troubling in the orchestra. Immune dysfunction was apparent in teachers who were sick, an outcome Grufferman had expected. But the dysfunction was present in healthy teachers, too. Natural killer cell activity was abnormally depressed in both groups, but virtually rock bottom in "cases" and their close contacts.

"This is not a chance occurrence," he said. "This is analogous to apparent and inapparent infections seen with many other infectious diseases."

Raleigh, North Carolina

In June, a fourth member of the North Carolina Symphony, a forty-six-year-old cellist, was diagnosed with cancer. Although this woman had none of the signs of the debilitating, long-lasting form of "mono" so many of her colleagues had suffered, her antibody levels to Epstein-Barr virus were the highest of any member of the orchestra. In addition, she shared many other immunological abnormalities with her well and sick colleagues in the orchestra, all of whom, it was increasingly apparent, had been exposed to the same immune-harming pathogen. Her cancer was a glioblastoma multiforme—a malignant tumor of the brain.

Grufferman and his collaborators were astounded. The rate of cancer among this small group of relatively young musicians over a two-year period was *eighteen times* higher than would have been expected among people of similar ages and sexes during the same time period.

The cellist died three months after surgery.

Charlotte, North Carolina

In his first ten weeks at the Nalle Clinic, Cheney identified forty patients with the Tahoe malady. By midsummer the number had increased to seventy-nine. With the help of a $16,000 donation from Nevada philanthropist and Tahoe malady victim Paul Thompson, Cheney engaged a research assistant, premed student Susan Dorman, to create a patient database. In addition to information supplied by patients on a long questionnaire that Cheney routinely administered, Dorman methodically entered technological data—like MRI brain scans and a host of Cheney's own clinical observations—into the computer.

A final category of information Dorman added to the data pot was relatively banal, consisting of the results of routine laboratory tests, including blood sugar level tests for diabetes and a test to determine thyroid hormone levels. Cheney also measured the blood sedimentation rate, which indicates the degree of separation between the fluid and blood cells. Oddly, rather than being too high, the sedimentation rate was too low.

Measuring a person's "sed" rate was a relatively primitive assay: the patient's blood sits in a tube for an hour, after which a technician determines the degree of separation between the fluid and blood cells. As one doctor said of the test, "It is like watching cream separate from milk, certainly not sophisticated, but useful nonetheless."[9] Normal sed rates were from 10 millimeters to 30 millimeters an hour; Cheney commonly measured sed rates of 0, 1, or 2 millimeters an hour in his patients. Curious about the finding, he took to reviewing the Nalle's sed rate log, pages on a clipboard maintained by the clinic's lab technicians. A total of eight doctors—internal medicine specialists, pediatricians, and gynecologists—routinely ordered the tests, which, when high, can signal cancer or an inflammatory disease such as arthritis. "Over a period of several months," Cheney recalled later, "I would go in on a daily basis and look at those sed rates." Every abnormally low sed rate the doctor saw, with the exception of those of very young children, in whom low sed rates are not considered pathological, turned out to be a Tahoe malady patient in his care.

For some months, Marc Iverson and Alan Goldberg, an accountant in his mid-sixties who had fallen severely ill after a ski vacation in 1985 in Incline Village, Nevada, had been meeting with other Charlotte patients. These meetings were informal affairs. Usually, they were held in Iverson's living room; some nights, the group numbered just four. In mid-August, the two men organized their support group's first official, public meeting. To their surprise, 150 people crowded the room in the church where the meeting was held. Like Goldberg, the vast majority of them had become ill in the previous two years. A local television crew arrived to film them. In spite of the cameras and lights, emotions spun out of control.

"It was a raucous meeting," Iverson said later. "People just wanted to cry and tell their horror stories."

Adelaide, Australia

That August the provocative findings of a group of Adelaide researchers published in the British journal *Lancet* shed light on the bizarre sed rates in Cheney's patients.[10] The Australians who, like British and Canadian researchers, were calling the disease myalgic encephalomyelitis, or ME, reported that the red cell membrane of such patients frequently exhibited an unusual globular shape and sickled appearance. The changes became apparent during flare-ups of the disease and regressed when the patient was feeling better. Red blood cells carry energy-giving oxygen to muscles.

A prominent tissue pathologist at the Adelaide Institute of Medical and Veterinary Science who analyzed red blood cells from ME patients for the Adelaide group, recalled that when he first observed the samples one Saturday morning, he almost fell off his chair. "I had never seen anything like this," he said. Some 80 to 90 percent of the red cells were "wildly abnormal."*

Harvard Medical School, Boston, Massachusetts

By late August one of Anthony Komaroff's colleagues, Ferenc Jolesz, had studied each of the magnetic resonance imaging brain scans shipped to him from Reno Diagnostics. Jolesz, an assistant professor of radiology at Harvard and director of clinical magnetic resonance imaging of the head at the Brigham and Women's Hospital, had been told absolutely nothing about the disease itself or about the clinical status of individual patients. Komaroff sought to avoid creating bias. Nevertheless, Jolesz achieved a remarkable degree of concurrence with Royce Biddle's findings; the two were in agreement 96 percent of the time.† Biddle turned out to be the more conservative of the pair: where Jolesz had called five scans positive for lesions, Biddle had called them negative.

In all, 88, or 77 percent of the 114 patients had magnetic imaging brain scans that were positive for punctate lesions.

The experiment produced other interesting findings:

- Single lesions occurred in only three of the eighty-eight cases; the other eighty-five patients had multiple lesions.
- The lesions could be seen only when the most sophisticated generation of scanner, the 1.5 tesla, was used. When scans were performed on the .5 tesla—the same tesla grade used by researchers at the National Institute of Allergy and Infectious Diseases to study Dan Peterson's Tahoe patients—the lesions were not detected.
- The appearance and distribution of the lesions were, Jolesz observed, "distinctly different from white matter lesions seen in chronic deep white matter infarcts [strokes] or multiple sclerosis." Eighty-five percent of the lesions were distributed within subcortical white matter; the rest were seen in deep white matter regions.
- Of thirty-five patients who were tested serially, the majority showed no change, about 35 percent developed additional lesions, and 9 percent improved over time.

---

* The following year, Anthony Komaroff and his associate Dedra Buchwald told an audience of doctors and researchers at the University of Washington in Seattle that approximately 40 percent of patients with the disease had abnormally low sed rates. "With the exception of sickle-cell disease," Buchwald said, "we've never seen sedimentation rates that are consistently zero, one, or two, with any other illnesses. We have speculated that these patients may have difficulty in forming red cell membranes, as is the case with sickle-cell disease, because of a distorted red cell pathology." Two years later Canadian clinician Byron Hyde reported in the fall 1989 issue of his newsletter to sufferers, "To my knowledge, there are only five diseases that have a pathological low sedimentation level: myalgic encephalomyelitis [the British, Australian, and Canadian term for the chronic illness], sickle-cell anemia, hereditary sperocytosis, hyper-gammaglobulinemia, hyper-fibrogenemia."

† In an unpublished Harvard study of concurrence among radiologists reading chest X rays, specialists disagreed in their interpretations 25 percent of the time—nearly six times as often as did Biddle and Jolesz.

Shinrakuen Hospital, Niigata, Japan

In June, Ron Herberman, who was helping Seymour Grufferman analyze natural killer cells in members of the North Carolina orchestra and the Chillicothe elementary school teachers, published his paper on the Japanese disease he called, for lack of a better name, "low natural killer cell syndrome." All of the patients described in the article were Japanese and ranged in age from 14 to 77, although the median age was 36.5 years.[11] Their symptoms, lasting six months or more, were "uncomfortable fatigue," depressed natural killer cell activity, unexplained fever, and a "lack of interest in mental as well as physical activities," a symptom translated from Japanese as "uncomfortable general dullness."

Herberman had first heard of the Japanese syndrome in 1985 when a Japanese researcher, Tadao Aoki, called to say he was seeing a number of patients with a bizarre idiopathic illness. "People had gone to doctors for months or even years without a diagnosis," Herberman said some years later. "Often they were considered by their doctors in Japan to have some psychiatric condition. [Aoki] characterized their complaints as a 'generalized dullness.' These people just weren't energetic, or able to do anything very well. As Aoki would describe it, they had difficulty getting out of bed, needed to take several naps during the day. There were other complaints, too—fluctuating fevers, flu symptoms. But Aoki focused on the natural killer cell problem. And when he sent me his data, we decided between us that we should call this low natural killer cell syndrome."

12

Fatigue unto Death

Centers for Disease Control, Atlanta, Georgia

By late summer, Gary Holmes had received a new round of responses to the revised case definition he had drafted at the end of June. He was, he told his respondents, hoping to publish the consensus definition in either the Centers for Disease Control's *Morbidity and Mortality Weekly Report* or a major medical journal.

Harvard's Elliot Kieff continued to be critical of the definition. In his letter of August 24, he reiterated his belief that the Centers for Disease Control's definition lacked hard, measurable criteria. He stated bluntly that he was opposed to publishing the diagnostic criteria unless in the *Morbidity and Mortality Weekly Report,* and only then for the purpose of making the disease a reportable one. He added that he believed the entire dubious exercise was an instance of clinicians "writing the script for patients to play out."

Stephen Straus had responded to Holmes's second draft in mid-July. Straus argued against publishing the CDC's diagnostic criteria *anywhere.* The definition should be "circulated freely among investigators with an interest in this syndrome," Straus wrote. If it was published, the federal researcher warned, practicing clinicians might use it as a tool to diagnose patients. Since the disease was not being taught in medical schools, and since no formal diagnostic criteria existed aside from the CDC's, Straus apparently didn't want anyone to make the diagnosis except him and the people on Gary Holmes's mailing list. Of course, few on that list were actually practicing clinical medicine.

Nathaniel Brown, who was now chief of pediatric infectious diseases at the North Shore University Hospital at Cornell, was against publishing the definition as well. His primary concern appeared to be for health insurance companies who might be required to reimburse patients for medical treatment or provide disability payments if diagnostic criteria should lend the disease legitimacy.

People with the chronic malady were "quite verbal" and typically availed themselves of the medical literature, Brown wrote Holmes on September 2. Doctors who appropriated the government's definition to diagnose such patients in private practice would only compound the problem. After all, the government's diagnostic criteria were to be used only as a research tool to identify homogeneous groups of patients for further study. Should the government's criteria be widely disseminated, Brown warned, "the field could change from an epidemiological investigation into a health insurance boondoggle/nightmare for various interested parties."

Disregarding his critics, Holmes incorporated the suggestions sent to him by his small network of investigators into what was now a true consensus definition of the disease. He sent the draft out for final comments on August 12, for the third time. Seeking to capitalize on Elliot Kieff's prestige in the infectious disease realm, Holmes tried a final time to engage Kieff as a coauthor on the definition. Kieff's last letter on the subject was downright crabby, expressing continued perplexity over the government's dogged and ill-conceived effort to formally define the disease. The great bulk of people suffering from the condition, Kieff insisted in a letter to Holmes on October 26, had no physical disease. "Is the intention to add a new psychiatric classification?" Kieff asked. Any effort to study such a wide and varied mix of patients would be exorbitantly expensive and add nothing of value to medical science, he told Holmes. He ended by advising Holmes that he preferred not to be named among the definition's authors.

In his second letter to Holmes, on October 29, Cornell's Nathaniel Brown wrote that he wanted to be included on the coauthor list in a medical journal. But Brown continued to be preoccupied with the costs that published criteria might pose for health insurance companies. He suggested that Holmes include a disclaimer in the definition alerting doctors that disability claims could not be based on the government's diagnostic criteria. "It might discourage chronic reimbursements for the diagnosis—(i.e., long-term disability)—until more is known," Brown wrote.

A few contributors to the consensus definition were in favor of publication, however, precisely because published criteria would aid doctors in the trenches. Not surprisingly, those in favor were practicing clinicians. Atlanta internist Richard DuBois urged Holmes to submit the definition to the *Annals of Internal Medicine* or the *Journal of the American Medicine Association.* "If publication can be accomplished in one of those two journals, we will certainly reach the population of physicians that we would like to reach," DuBois said. Denver doctor James Jones, too, prodded Holmes toward publication in one of the large journals read by internists. "Actually," Jones wrote, "since the definition is not the result of experimental work, but an attempt to inform physicians of the effort to standardize evaluation of these patients, any vehicle (or vehicles) that is (are) well read by the target audience would be satisfactory." Savita Pahwa, chief of pediatric immunology at Cornell University, was another clinician who had seen a number of patients suffering from the disease. He wrote, "We see a lot of patients who are carrying the diagnosis of chronic EBV syndrome. . . . I feel it is essential that this information be disseminated to all physicians who have to deal with this entity."

Holmes also sent the definition to Alexis Shelokov, who was then at the Salk Institute, and to the British myalgic encephalomyelitis expert J. Gordon Parish, for their signatures as authors of the paper. Neither man signed the definition.

Of course, in addition to setting forth a working case definition, Holmes needed to choose a name for the disease. Virtually all of his respondents wanted to scrap the CDC's proposed name, "chronic mononucleosis-like syndrome," not because it was unwieldy but because it persisted in linking the disease to Epstein-Barr virus. Ultimately the majority ruled in favor of "chronic fatigue syndrome," since it was agreed among the group that fatigue was the cardinal feature of the disease. In truth, while "fatigue unto death," as *Vanity Fair* had characterized sufferer Gore Vidal's misery, was a symptom reported by virtually every patient, the cardinal feature of the disease—the central aspect that defined the illness, that was at the heart of its victims' disability, and that was the most disturbing to sufferers—was brain dysfunction. In 1987, however, few of the clinicians and researchers on Gary Holmes's list, and certainly none of the staff at the CDC, were about to implicate brain involvement in the disease.

In his letter to his collaborators, Gary Holmes had written, "Please include your preferences. . . . Names that we feel to be descriptive but not overly specific include: myalgic encephalomyelitis (the British term), neuromyasthenia, chronic mononucleosis-like syndrome, chronic fatigue syndrome, postviral fatigue syndrome, and chronic viral fatigue syndrome—but feel free to add your own ideas." "Chronic fatigue syndrome" triumphed over minority suggestions of "post-viral fatigue syndrome" and "chronic viral fatigue syndrome." In nearly every case Holmes's collaborators voiced their antipathy toward lending the disease a presumed viral etiology when factors like depression and other psychiatric illness might turn out to be the cause. Clearly it was more politic to err on the side of mental illness rather than infectiousness.

For the next several years the euphemistic, benign-sounding name suggested a trivial, volitional disability, one that could be shrugged off with vitamins, aerobic exercise, stress reduction, a good night's sleep, or sheer willpower. By casting its victims in the role of shirkers who chose to defy the nation's Protestant work ethic, the name, in addition, had the subtle effect of inspiring hostility toward the victim. As one psychologist well versed in standardized systems of evaluating the psychological import of words noted, " 'Chronic fatigue syndrome' has a real negative impact. The word 'chronic' is associated with chronic complainers, chronic whiners. And 'fatigue' is even worse."

More profoundly, the name camouflaged the nature of the illness itself: the fatigue in "chronic fatigue syndrome" was merely a symptom and, compared to the neurologic dysfunction resulting from the structural damage to the brain in the early phases of the disease, a sometimes unimportant one at that. Diseases, after all, are not primarily identified and defined by universal qualities they share with other diseases but rather for the qualities that distinguish them. If diseases were named after symptoms, leukemia too might well be called "chronic fatigue syndrome" and diabetes "chronic thirst syndrome." The government's choice of names was so inept, in fact, that many observers came to view it as a deliberate effort to defuse the potentially panic-inducing issue of the eruption of a life-altering infectious disease. "Chronic fatigue syndrome," after all, hardly sounded "catching."

Miami, Florida

Fully half of Nancy Klimas's immune deficiency clinic patients at the University of Miami were now people suffering from the chronic disease she once had longed to believe didn't exist. "As you get interested and do all these lab studies," Klimas said that fall, "if you're a physician-scientist like me, then word of mouth spreads that there's an EBV researcher in Miami, and all of a sudden you've got a three-month waiting list in your clinic. I don't have *any* available appointments. If I wanted to open up an EBV clinic—if I was that kind of soul who had that kind of energy and time—I could open one up tomorrow and I'd be busy all day, every day."

The immunologist found herself wading deeper into the mystery. She was committed, she said, to getting a federal grant to study the disease. In fact, she hoped she would be able to win several eventually, and she had little reason to believe she would be unable to achieve her goal. "I've got a *dozen* research interests in this particular field now," Klimas said, "from basic science to psychosocial to clinical."

National Institutes of Health, Bethesda, Maryland

Federal grant money awarded by scientific review committees at the NIH are the lifeblood of medical research in the United States. The agency's grants account for nearly half—or around $3 billion—of all medical research under way in universities around the nation. So far, however, only one scientist investigating the new chronic disease was receiving federal support in the form of a grant: *Annals* author James Jones. The National Institute of Allergy and Infectious Diseases, or NIAID, tried to end Jones's funding that year, but when the Portland patients' association alerted its membership to the imminent cessation of Jones's research, two thousand victims of the disease wrote to NIAID's administrators to complain. Purely by coincidence, the agency bureaucrat in charge of such grants assured this writer, Jones's grant was renewed. Giving the lie to the grandiose letters to Congress touting its heavy investment in the new disease, Jones's modest $158,471 grant for fiscal year 1987 was the extent of the NIH's support of independent research.

Responding to congressional pressure that fall, NIAID at last issued an announcement to universities of its intent to fund extramural grants to explore the epidemiology of chronic fatigue syndrome. The announcement, written by the newly appointed administrator of the new grant program, Ann Schleuderberg, explained that applicants should prepare proposals for "population-based epidemiologic studies of chronic fatigue syndrome . . . in order to assess the burden in the general population." Schleuderberg warned that "the complexity of the problem is such that . . . expertise will be needed in epidemiology, medicine, virology, immunology, neurology and psychiatry."

Virologist Berch Henry and his collaborators in Nevada were energized by the announcement, as were Nancy Klimas in Miami, Jay Levy and Carol Jessop in San Francisco, and a number of other scientists and research-oriented clinicians. They interpreted the government's invitation as the launch of a new era, a sign that the federal institution was at last taking leadership in the epidemic and was eager for their contributions. Another researcher with an equally avid interest in obtaining federal support, Seymour Grufferman, was immediately critical of the manner in which the agency was approaching the problem, however. An experienced grantsman who had obtained a number of well-funded grants from Bethesda and who chaired the agency's panel that ruled on some of the biggest AIDS grant proposals, Grufferman quickly located a significant flaw in the plan, and he did not hesitate to pierce the bubble of optimism the announcement had generated.

"The best [that NIH] has come forth with is a so-called ongoing program announcement," Grufferman said that fall, "which is a statement by NIAID that they are *interested* in stimulating grants in this area. But there is no set-aside of dollars." Without a specific set-aside, Grufferman added, the government would be under no obligation to give a green light to research proposals. Schleuderberg's announcement, Grufferman suspected, was cosmetic—yet another effort to appease a troublesome constituency.

Time would reveal the program announcement to be—as Grufferman immediately recognized—a public relations subterfuge, just another item in a phony portfolio that agency administrators submitted to congressional appropriations committees every spring. Contrary to Grufferman's prediction, however, the announcement kindled enormous interest among researchers, even without set-asides. In the next five years, dozens of scientific collaborative groups would apply repeatedly for federal support to study the disease, without success. Only one grant would be funded under the program during that time, for a total outlay of less than $1 million—a figure that can be given perspective by comparison to the annual research outlay of the Department of Health and Human Services, which is more than $11 billion. That grant went to Anthony Komaroff.

Centers for Disease Control, Atlanta, Georgia

When the scientists in the nation's premier retrovirology laboratory announced their discovery of the sixth human herpesvirus, scientists in the Centers for Disease Control's herpes branch were skeptical and not a little jealous. But the Atlanta agency's virologists, as well as herpes experts around the world, had been looking at the sixth human herpesvirus for years without comprehending its novelty, mistaking it for either Epstein-Barr virus or cytomegalovirus, two better-known members of the herpes family. The Gallo team's *Science* article forced the Atlanta scientists to reach deep into their freezers.

The CDC was a storehouse for one of the world's most valuable collections of human blood specimens, some of which had been gathered and stored since the early 1950s. In a room off the "host factors" corridor in the administration building, tall, freestanding metal racks supported thousands of vials filled with blood drawn from at least two generations of agency scientists, their lab technicians, and anyone else who was handy. John Stewart, who headed the viral immunology lab for the herpes branch, turned to this source, as well as to hospitals, general medicine practices, schools, and venereal disease clinics.

In time, Stewart unearthed evidence that the virus had been present in the population for decades. "I was intrigued to find out that I have been positive for H-six for twenty-five years, since I first came to CDC," he noted that fall. Overall, he added, the positivity rate of all populations averaged out to somewhere between 40 and 60 percent. In addition, Stewart and his associates had discovered to their surprise that the infection rate of the virus was extremely high among very young children: as many as half of all children had antibodies to the bug, suggesting the virus could be transmitted casually. But another group with high rates of infection was composed of patrons of sexually transmitted disease clinics, prompting Carlos Lopez to conclude that "this virus appears to be a sexually transmitted virus infection" as well as a casual one.

As the government's assays for the new herpesvirus became more sensitive, the case for its etiological role in the new brain disease was growing flimsier and flimsier. Although it was newly discovered, the virus was not new—an enormous distinction. Old viruses don't cause sudden widespread epidemics, or pandemics, of new diseases; only new viruses do that. Yet an intriguing question remained: why were the numbers of antibodies in people with the new disease so consistently and remarkably high?

An August 15 letter in the *Lancet* from British scientists proposed in print for the first time what a number of other thoughtful researchers were beginning to suspect: "One wonders whether the isolation of this [virus] from immunosuppressed patients could represent reactivation of a latent infection."[1] If the British speculation was correct, then human herpesvirus 6 was merely another red herring—the second, after Epstein-Barr. By September more than a few scientists were privately exhuming the retrovirus theory.

On September 26, Robert Gallo and his scientists conceded in print that their original name for their virus—human B-cell lymphotrophic virus—was inappropriate and suggested it be renamed human herpesvirus 6.[2] CDC staff had never called the new bug by its NIH-given name; herpesviruses are named either for the disease they cause or for the order in which they are found, and the Atlanta scientists had always preferred the more credible nomenclature. In explaining why they were making the change, however, the Gallo team revealed a fascinating discovery: "We have shown that HBLV can infect several . . . human cell lines, including [brain and immune system cells]. . . . This . . . suggests the possible direct role of the virus in various hematological and neurological disorders." The news that HHV 6 could thrive in brain cells as well as immune system cells led some CFS investigators to wonder if the virus could be causing the multiple lesions visible on brain scans of sufferers.

A week later, on October 6, Zaki Salahuddin and Carlos Lopez addressed the twenty-seventh Interscience Conference on Antimicrobial Agents and Chemotherapy on the topic of human herpesvirus 6. The gathering was one of the biggest yearly scientific meetings in the country. Infectious disease specialists and virologists dominated the attendance roster, but the conference attracted a wide range of clinical specialists, pathologists, pharmacologists, and scientists interested in infectious diseases and the drugs that might cure or ameliorate them. Hundreds of lively symposia were held over a period of three days and in such rapid-fire succession that participants often literally sprinted from one to another. Presentations by Salahuddin and Lopez were the centerpiece of a session called "New Viruses and Viral Syndromes." An audience of two thousand infectious disease specialists packed the room.

Although both scientists described the high rates of positivity among children, gays, and heterosexuals suffering from sexually transmitted diseases and immune system cancers, Salahuddin and Lopez assiduously avoided mentioning the fact that they had tested patients with the newly named chronic fatigue syndrome and found them to have the highest seroprevalency rates of all, with antibody levels rivaling those of AIDS and Burkitt's lymphoma victims.

Afterward an audience member strode to the microphone placed in the aisle to ask: "Have you done seroepidemiologic profiling of the outbreaks in Nevada and the other putative chronic viral fatigue–chronic EBV kinds of syndromes, looking at increased prevalence of this virus?" The inquiry offered the federal scientists an opportunity to educate an influential audience about the sweeping positivity rates of the new virus among people with the perplexing disease. One infectious disease doctor who was there remarked later, "You could have heard a pin drop."

Neither scientist dared take the plunge. Gallo's lieutenant, Salahuddin, deferred to Lopez. "Those kinds of studies are in fact ongoing," Lopez said, "but they are very preliminary, and far too preliminary to discuss now."

San Francisco, California

Unlike the federal scientists, who were starting with a virus, Jay Levy, working independently in his tiny laboratory, was starting with a disease. He had chosen a rockier path by far, and the strain was showing. "It's been very frustrating," he said early that October. "*Extremely* frustrating. I'm just happy it's not killing [its victims], because we'd be in terrible shape." Levy, who had never seriously subscribed to the theory that human herpesvirus 6 was responsible for the chronic disease, was studying cell cultures made from patients' serum in search of an entirely new virus. "If [the disease] was caused by a known virus," he said, "it already would have been found by *lots* of people."

The scientist had observed a few instances of cell death, but when he studied the cells under an electron microscope, a half-million-dollar device able to magnify objects 100,000-fold, he was unable to detect further evidence of viral infection. Discouraged, he wondered if he was seeing the right patients at the right time; once the disease had begun its chronic course, the virus might go into hiding. "We don't know the risk group," the scientist said. "We don't know the people who have it. And we are probably getting in there too late—they're already suppressing the virus." A third imponderable: maybe the pathogen wasn't even in the blood tissue. An alternative hiding place, Levy suggested, might be the brain.

Evelyne Lennette, Levy's Berkeley collaborator, was similarly discouraged: "One thing that is unusual about these persistent viruses," Lennette noted that fall, "is that most of the time they do not exist as virus particles. They are much more clever than that. Part of the viral genome—the *only part* that is required to propagate—is integrated into the whole cells. So you can't see them."

The bug had proved so difficult to find that out of sheer discouragement Levy and Lennette had dropped the project for the last several months. Not surprisingly, the scientists' interest was revived by the NIH grant announcement that fall. Early in October, Levy and clinician Carol Jessop met for the first time in nearly a year to talk about new approaches. They were joined by Don Yoshimura, a neurologist from the UCSF medical school who had agreed to be a consulting brain expert.

The three gathered in an empty classroom in the medical school across the hall from Levy's lab. Levy stood on a platform in front of the blackboard, chalk in one hand, a pointer in the other. Jessop sat in a student's chair in the front row, but it was she who launched the discussion with her evolving theory that the disease might be an autoimmune illness like lupus or multiple sclerosis in which the immune system malfunctions and attacks the body's tissues. She proposed to Levy that the autoimmune syndrome might be triggered by some common virus.

"If it's a common virus, then why haven't we seen this disease before?" Levy asked. Jessop quickly assured Levy that nearly all of her patients had become ill since 1983 and that, in her view, the disease was new and caused by a new agent; it was simply that the virus might now be common in the population. "*I* think it's new," Levy concurred. "If it's *not* new," he added, sounding almost petulant, "I don't want to be bothered with it." Ultimately the team decided to study just ten patients intensively, assuming they could be identified in the acute phase of illness. "*That's* different," Levy said. "It hasn't been done yet, and we could get it published."

Ironically, just as Jessop renewed her connection with Levy, she gave up her post as an associate professor of medicine at the university and joined a group practice of general medicine in El Cerrito, a working-class community immediately north of Berkeley. It had been an agonizing decision for the clinician, whose lengthy education had amounted to a concerted effort to prepare herself for a career in academic medicine. Until her research interest became widely known, Jessop had been a respected and popular professor at the medical school. "I was basically a teacher—that was my real forte," Jessop said later. "But I was also expected to do research, and the areas in which I wanted to do research were not considered priority. There wasn't any support all the way around, and I felt I could do more for people when I wasn't hampered by the boundaries of an academic faculty that wasn't open-minded."

Asked some time later how Jessop's interest in the disease had affected her career at the university, Jay Levy responded diplomatically, "I can't comment on that, but I can say with some certainty that if you dedicated your whole career to this disease, you couldn't survive here."

Scottsdale, Arizona

On October 9, Reno doctor Royce Biddle, speaking at the Western Neuroradiological Society's annual meeting, held in Scottsdale, described the experiment he and Harvard's Ferenc Jolesz undertook on the Tahoe brain scans. His audience included nearly all of the academic and many of the private practice neuroradiologists in the western one-third of the United States. Among them were all of the staff neuroradiologists from Stanford, UCLA, and UCSF as well as the president of the American Society of Neuroradiology, Michael Huckman.

Biddle had eight minutes to present his findings, and at the end there was time for only three questions, which Biddle later characterized as "pointed, hardball questions." One of the questioners, a neuroradiology fellow from the University of California at San Francisco named William Dillon, told Biddle that at his institution "we see these [punctate lesions] . . . and I just read them as normal."

"The main point of this presentation," Biddle responded, "is to raise the possibility to radiologists that these findings are *abnormal* and should not be dismissed as normal."

One year after Biddle's presentation, Dillon was still a disbeliever. "We see [UBOs] in patients who are normal sometimes," Dillon explained. "The problem I had with his data, though, is he really didn't have any good control group that he compared patients to. That's my big complaint with his project."

Dillon's objection to the absence of healthy controls would haunt Komaroff, Jolesz, Biddle, and everyone else who tried to study the brain lesions in the disease in the years ahead.

Despite the skepticism of his peers, Biddle continued to believe that year that his findings were abnormal and related to the disease, even though, as he readily admitted, he occasionally found UBOs in patients who did not have symptoms of the disease. "There's no doubt about that," he said. "Except—what does that mean? Is it possible that UBOs might indicate some kind of a subclinical viral infection that might be present in a lot of symptomless patients? I think that's a real possibility.

"And then the other thing that's interesting about this syndrome is that . . . the symptoms include things like headache, disequilibrium, vertigo, seizures—and those kinds of things are exactly why other doctors order MR scans on their patients. So it makes you wonder—could there be some kind of an underlying viral illness that could be in a large proportion of people in this country without having any overt signs of fatigue?

"As far as whether these things are normal or variants of normal or some kind of genetic thing, I don't think so," he added. "However, we have to always keep in mind that every MR scan abnormality has to kind of be weighed in view of the patient's signs and symptoms at the time. Basically we're getting into a real big gray area, and this Tahoe outbreak has just brought it to the forefront."

Berkeley, California

While the controversy over brain lesions persisted, neuropsychologist Sheila Bastien and her associate, Bob Thomas, continued administering their mental status tests to sufferers in Incline Village. By the end of the year the team had tested nearly two hundred people with the disease. Most of them were patients from Dan Peterson's practice, which was becoming inflated with out-of-state sufferers who had read about the doctor, but clinicians from all over were referring patients directly to Bastien's Berkeley office. Internist Paul Simpson in Juneau, Alaska, had sent a score of patients to them during the summer; the team was also testing patients from Albuquerque, Boise, Gainesville, Springfield, Minneapolis, and smaller towns in between. They were excited by their results: the out-of-state victims were demonstrating a pattern of dementia identical to that seen in Nevadans.

"I have never seen this pattern before," Bastien commented that fall. "Never."

From patient to patient, she continued, the only permutation had to do with severity. "On the one extreme, we see people come here who have to be helped in by their spouse or a friend. They literally have difficulty walking. So at least on a motor level, they're that severe. They also test out with very severe memory problems. And then it runs to the other extreme, as with a woman we saw yesterday, who really only manifested about fifty percent of the clinical symptoms and she could articulate very well. She had no problem walking. She didn't even have extreme fatigue. But she had some memory deficit, some concentration problems, and she was getting some muscle weakness."

By October, Bastien had a personal stake in her own research: her college-age son, who helped manage her office and had frequent contact with the Tahoe sufferers, had developed the disease.

Lyndonville, New York

By early fall, David Bell had identified slightly more than one hundred people in his practice who were suffering from the mystery ailment, and he realized his original perception—that the malady was exclusively a disease of children—had been incorrect. In fact, he suspected that adults were more likely than children to be affected.

On the evening of September 8 the Bells called a community meeting in Lyndonville's Yates Town Hall, a two-story redbrick building with white columns flanking the entryway, to describe their findings. A reporter from nearby Medina covered the meeting for the newspaper; that article was picked up by the Rochester and Buffalo papers, as well as by other regional publications. David's homey practice was swiftly inundated with callers from Buffalo, Rochester, and other towns in upper New York State who had read about the "Lyndonville disease." Most of them had been to clinicians who had made the diagnosis of chronic Epstein-Barr virus disease. After meeting and examining several of the out-of-town sufferers, Bell was rapidly persuaded the similarities weren't coincidental.

"Our symptoms in Lyndonville were picture-identical to what these patients were experiencing," Bell recalled. "They had the same clinical illness. It was clear to me then that what we were seeing in Lyndonville, was just another outbreak—one of many around the country."

Portland, Oregon

Neither David Bell nor Paul Cheney had the faintest idea who the other was when they saw each other at the first conference on the disease. The often clamorous, emotional event, convened by the Oregon-based national patient group, was held on November 5 and 6 in a Holiday Inn near the Portland airport. Launched two years earlier from a nucleus of seven women who met periodically in the living room of a wheelchair-bound nurse, Portland's patient association was now twelve thousand strong. Approximately five hundred sufferers attended the conference, many of them support group leaders from around the country, along with the score of researchers and clinicians who addressed the group. A sense of urgency infused the proceedings: how to persuade the medical establishment of the legitimacy of their concerns, particularly in the absence of leadership from the federal government; how to provide solace, however modest, to victims.

Years later, Bell would recall his curious premonition when he saw Cheney, surrounded by a small crowd of patients, standing on the opposite side of the hotel ballroom during the first morning of the conference. Harboring a strange certitude that their futures would be linked, Bell studied the tall towheaded man. In truth, the Lyndonville pediatrician was in a state of high emotion throughout much of the two-day conference. He had been invited to speak less than a week earlier and, only two weeks before that, had come to the conclusion that the disease that had felled so many of his school-age patients was the same disease the press had recklessly dubbed "yuppie flu." Now, in the space of hours, he was being exposed to rapid-fire descriptions of cluster epidemics that seemed to mirror the Lyndonville outbreak and to expansive clinical descriptions of the disease he had studied so exhaustively without realizing it was everywhere outside of Lyndonville, too. Perhaps the most unsettling aspect of the event was Bell's emerging sense that he had been floating upstream on a small raft in his search for a bacterial etiology, while alongside the river a streamlined locomotive had been coursing steadily along the rails in the opposite direction, its occupants discoursing on viruses, especially the newest discovery from the Gallo lab.

Bell found the patients remarkable to observe, too. A majority of them were women; a few were in motorized wheelchairs; a handful, including the association's president, Gidget Faubion, walked with canes as a result of vertigo. Bell noticed that several wore wigs: a great many were overweight. He was most impressed by their ashen pallor and the seemingly numb, unchanging set of their faces. He had noticed the same quality in the faces of his own patients; it was as if they were simply too tired to alter their features. In medical parlance, the term was "myopathic facies." "It's a nonspecific physical finding," Bell would say later. "It's a very tired, bland-looking face. You see it in other diseases—myasthenia gravis is one. These people sort of lose the vitality of expression. They look washed out. A lot of people with this disease have this facial configuration. I think it's characteristic."

In his own formal talk, Bell described the Lyndonville outbreak in some detail, noting the poverty that haunted the town and the outlying farms. "I mention this because chronic fatigue syndrome has been called the 'yuppie disease,' " Bell said. "I do enjoy, however, telling some of my patients, especially the farmers, that they will now be considered yuppies. . . . Originally we thought this was a very isolated outbreak of an obscure illness," he added. "Now we are convinced this is a widespread outbreak of an obscure illness."

At the end of the first day the two men talked for hours in a hotel room reserved as a lounge for the conference speakers. Cheney, too, was exhilarated by the event and curious about Bell, whose Harvard education and medical sophistication seemed to belie his eleven years of general practice in an impoverished town of 1,300 on Lake Ontario's shoreline. Cheney was particularly struck by a graph Bell had prepared that tracked the emergence of the disease in Lyndonville by month and year. When Bell showed him the Lyndonville curve, Cheney stared for a moment, then slapped his forehead and said, "Oh, *Jesus!*" The flow of the Lyndonville graph was identical to the one Cheney had created for Lake Tahoe's north shore. The two missed much of the conference the next day, sitting instead in the Holiday Inn's coffee shop, their chili and hamburgers congealing on their plates.

"It's almost as if nature is saying something and it won't let go," Cheney said that afternoon. "The gibberish which should be coming out of this if it's nothing is not coming. Things are matching up; hypotheses are coming true. And as long as that keeps happening, I cannot accept the proposition that this doesn't exist. . . . I'm really talking about the issue of whether those patients in there have disease," he said, gesturing toward the ballroom where the conference was under way. "*That's* the issue I'm dealing with. And I'm sure that they have disease."

"These people who are attempting to prove this is a psychiatric disease are just dinosaurs," he added. "They're like the people who tried to prove the world was flat. They'll write their peer-reviewed papers, and one hundred years from now their graves will be desecrated."

Seymour Grufferman made his debut in Portland, too, and he used the Portland forum to propose a new medical name for the malady: "chronic fatigue and immune dysfunction syndrome," or CFIDS.

"You are not going to get a fair shake if you call yourself the Chronic Fatigue Syndrome Association, because that carries with it a judgment," he said to the audience. "Your group should be renamed as well as the disease." Grufferman also warned the association about the downside of advertising that the disease was infectious. In so doing he opened a ponderous matter that would remain the single most divisive issue among patient organizations in the years ahead.

"How do you get chronic fatigue syndrome?" Grufferman asked his audience. "Do any of you *know* how you got it?" he persisted as a hush seemed to fall upon the room. "Why are stewardesses and perhaps yuppies at increased risk? Is it because they both breathe recirculated air on airplanes? Yuppies tend to work in those lovely enclosed glass towers. . . . Am I at risk because I am in this room? . . . Think about your own experiences. Did you come in contact with somebody [who had] this [disease]? Why are you people affected and not other people? . . . Second, if it *is* catching, how is it caught? Should you be taking any special measures to prevent this entity from being transmitted? Maybe you ought to wear masks," he added, his tone suddenly flip. "I don't have any answers—nobody does. But I think you have to be very careful about this, because you don't want to become pariahs."

In spite of his obvious commitment, the combative epidemiologist failed to endear himself to anyone, patients or doctors. He threw down the gauntlet, frankly describing the political nature of new diseases and exhorting the patients to become more politically sophisticated. Grufferman told his audience that when he revealed to his academic colleagues that he was planning to address the patient organization, "they thought I was losing my mind. This is not an accepted disease entity in the mainstream of academic medicine or clinical medicine. I tell you this honestly because I think it's important for you to know, because you are potential leaders who play a very important role in focusing the public's attention on this important syndrome and in trying to get some research dollars headed in this direction. *I* believe that the disease is a real disease and of great public health importance, and that's why I'm here today. . . . You may not like what I have to say, but I think you need to hear it."

Grufferman hardly needed to remind his listeners of the contempt in which they were held by the medical profession. But he went further, chastising them for seeking care from purveyors of alternative medical therapies. If patients continued to put themselves in the hands of fringe practitioners, he warned, they would never gain credibility among the mainstream practitioners.

Grufferman was even harsher on the doctors present, publicly chastising Cheney, in particular, for presenting his "unscientific" survey that reflected an exponential rise in cases of the disease starting in the early 1980s. In private, Grufferman's complaint with the doctor was not about the data itself as much as the fact that Cheney had presented it in a public forum where journalists were present and prior to formal peer review and publication. The epidemiologist also predicted that, unlike the work of the small-time doctors gathered in Portland, his own data would survive peer review and be published. "When I got involved in this [disease]," he said, "I was extremely skeptical. But we came up with results that will withstand scrutiny. The peer review process is fair most of the time. The quality will be evident in what you do. I think I have a reputation for very rigorous research. There's no problem getting superb collaborators when you do that. It's a matter of style. We bend over backwards to knock it down ourselves."

Although Grufferman portrayed himself as a sophisticate in the charged arena of the new disease, one who possessed the skill to manipulate the system advantageously, it soon would become apparent that he had underestimated the magnitude of the problem.

Grufferman wasn't the only one in Portland who was concerned about the disease's name. Members of the Portland association and approximately fifty support group leaders from several states had met on the eve of the conference to discuss the matter, unaware that Gary Holmes and Stephen Straus and their collaborators had already chosen "chronic fatigue syndrome." All present agreed that the government's choice trivialized the disease, but reaching a consensus on alternative names proved difficult. Gloom settled as the discussion wore on. Interestingly, although Grufferman would not make his proposal until the next day, the name "chronic fatigue–immune dysfunction syndrome" assumed a place at the top of the list of suggestions; a second favorite was "persistent viral syndrome." The group could not agree on a third option. In a move that few seemed to find ironic, chairwoman Gidget Faubion called the meeting to an end before the problem was solved, citing the participants' exhaustion. "It is clear we are all too tired to continue this discussion tonight," Faubion said.

The group failed to assemble again. When the two-day conference ended, however, thirty support organization leaders from several states met to discuss a topic that, for them, carried higher priority even than the name of their disease. Nearly every leader present reported deaths by suicide among members of his or her organization. For three hours they discussed recommendations for counseling suicidal patients.

Harvard Medical School, Boston, Massachusetts

On November 15, Michael Caligiuri's investigation of natural killer cell function in patients with the chronic disease was published in the *Journal of Immunology*.[3] It was the first time a case-control study that found a particular class of abnormalities distinct to the disease had appeared in the medical literature. It also represented the first time such dramatic natural killer cell defects had been recorded in *any* disease. Caligiuri had run his tests on thirty-two patients from the Incline Village epidemic and about half as many patients from Anthony Komaroff's practice at the Brigham in Boston.

Despite the significance of Caligiuri's discovery, skeptics in academia and elsewhere were unmoved. Tom Merigan, Stanford's chief of infectious diseases, was typical. Two months earlier, Merigan had conveyed to a network television audience that the disease was an expression of the sufferer's anxiety. The doctor was asked his opinion of the *Journal of Immunology* paper soon after it was published. Merigan said he had not read the paper, but he admitted, nonetheless, to being "unimpressed" by its purport after it was described to him. He pointed out that natural killer cell abnormalities are seen in malignancies and suggested that other diseases, such as cancer, could be causing the dramatic abnormalities. When he was told that the patients in the study had had all other diseases ruled out, he said, "I'd like to see [the findings] confirmed in other laboratories." He added that the *Journal of Immunology* was an "esoteric" publication.

▦

Not long after the publication of the natural killer cell study, Komaroff received word from the *New England Journal of Medicine* that the Tahoe paper had been rejected. The journal's editors had held the manuscript for six months, an unusually long interlude, before rendering their decision. The paper had been sent to five reviewers, which, according to Komaroff, was an unprecedented number; usually the figure was three.

Years later Cheney would recall that Komaroff respected the reviewers' comments on that first publishing attempt as legitimate demands for scientific rigor. Privately, Komaroff placed the blame for the flaws on the Nevada clinicians rather than himself. While applauding their "intelligence and dedication and courage," Komaroff noted that Cheney and Peterson, in the thick of an epidemic, had failed to collect data in a systematic manner.

"I'm sorry to sound so lacking in humility," Komaroff said, "but I don't think anyone could have done anything more to beat this into reasonable shape. . . . Given the kind of study it was—the fact that we came onto the scene late in the day and tried to reconstruct a lot of things that had been done, and we could only do that to a limited degree—there are flaws in it. The question that has to be asked is, do those flaws really affect the main message of the paper, or are they blemishes around the margin that don't really matter that much? And my judgment is that they don't matter."

News of Komaroff's rejection by the *New England Journal* hit the Reno team hard. Early in November, Reno infectious disease specialist Ray Swarts proposed to Royce Biddle, Berch Henry, Dan Peterson, and Reno's two other infectious disease specialists that they prepare their own paper on the subject for the British journal *Lancet*. His suggestion was met with enthusiasm. "We've got everything we need to study and understand this right here— banked sera, people who are knowledgeable about the disease," Swarts said. All they lacked, in fact, was Komaroff's clout, and it was painfully apparent to all that the Harvard magic had failed to work its way at the *New England Journal of Medicine*.

Santa Ana, California

Romy Zarit had been a flight attendant for PSA for eight years when she became disabled by the chronic disease in 1985. Zarit, a self-described "aerobics addict," fell ill suddenly; like most people in her situation, she assumed she had caught an unusually virulent flu bug. Within weeks, she was barely able to care for her two toddlers. Zarit's IQ, as measured in high school, was 140. Mental status testing two years after she became ill revealed it to be 105. Her husband, a minister, had taken over the household chores and child rearing, but by the winter of 1987, he was beginning to show signs of the disease, as well.

Zarit, who had been active in the PSA employees union, knew a number of flight attendants from PSA who were similarly afflicted. (She also knew, she confided to this writer, at least two PSA pilots who were suffering from symptoms but were still flying because the airline was denying all disability claims for the disease.) Through her union work, Zarit had met Chris Larson, a TWA flight attendant and union representative. Larson was sick, too, and had been on medical leave since January 1985. Together, Larson and Zarit hoped to survey members of both unions in order to determine how many of their fellow workers had been stricken. Zarit suspected that if the disease was casually transmitted, like colds and flus, its agent of infection could be spread through airplane filter systems. (The Portland patients' organization had determined that one-fifth of its members were employed in the aviation and travel industries.)

By December, with the help of Seymour Grufferman, whom they had met at the Portland conference, Zarit and Larson formulated a questionnaire to be sent to PSA and TWA flight attendant union members. Although PSA was a relatively small company, TWA was not. "Seven thousand people at TWA alone will be reached by this survey," Zarit said. The questionnaire invited airline personnel afflicted with CEBV "to participate in a nationwide survey for medical research in an effort to establish a possible industry-related connection between the illness and specific work environment." Zarit and Larson asked for responses by the following March.

Centers for Disease Control, Atlanta, Georgia

On December 7 the government's principal investigator into the new epidemic disease, Gary Holmes, replied to a letter from Denver patient Craig Barshinger about possible nomenclature for the disease, which the patient organization might then adopt. Holmes's response, in which he alerted Barshinger to the fact that a name had already emerged—chronic fatigue syndrome—revealed the degree to which the government viewed the disease as a social and political problem rather than a medical one. He assured Barshinger that the name was a good one because it avoided "a specific association with any known etiologic agent" and because "it is brief. . . . We believe the addition of terms such as 'postviral' imply more specificity than is currently warranted and that the use of such names as neuromyasthenia and myalgic encephalomyelitis is overly complicated and too confusing for many nonmedical persons." It is difficult to imagine other situations in which scientists' criteria for a disease's name included a stricture that it not be "overly complicated" or "too confusing" to the lay public.

Barshinger's Denver foundation and the Portland patients' association gingerly embraced the government's new name. Neither organization was pleased with the choice, but they acquiesced to the government's will in a submissive gesture of respect and goodwill, a mode of behavior that would characterize most large patient organizations well into the 1990s.

In an age of AIDS activism, the passivity of people suffering from the new disease might have seemed puzzling. Unlike the gay AIDS activists of Act Up, however, victims of the new disease were generally people whose first experience of disenfranchisement had come with the acquisition of a disabling medical disease the government was working to establish as sociopathology. Within this vast and varied constituency the only commonly shared life-defining experience was the disease itself. As University of California epidemiologist Warren Browner noted that fall in response to a query about risk factors for the disease, "The most we can say about people who get chronic fatigue syndrome is that they're people." Lastly, members of this informal confederation lacked the strength to march on Washington or to perform acts of civil disobedience. Neither did they have well advocates who were willing to be stand-ins. Generally speaking, they had no advocates at all.

New York City

In 1987, CBS launched a new magazine show that featured a cadre of fresh-faced correspondents reporting on subjects demographically attuned to the thirty-something prime time TV audience. The show was a marriage of *Entertainment Tonight* and *60 Minutes*. On December 10, *West 57th* tackled the disease about which so much had been written lately in the lay press: the controversial yuppie flu. The segment led the Saturday night show, with reporter Steve Kroft narrating.

As he began his report it was evident Kroft had set out to debunk what he perceived to be a bogus disease. Instead of focusing a journalist's healthy skepticism upon an imperious medical establishment, Kroft turned it on the victims of the disease. In a teaser segment before a commercial, Kroft was seen in a story meeting discussing the disease with his fellow correspondents. The journalist tapped his forehead and, winking at his colleagues, said, "Some doctors think it's all up here." Soon afterward, having launched the piece with the question "Are you tired? I mean, *really* tired?" Kroft and producer Christine Weicher introduced their medical expert, Richard Jacobs, an associate clinical professor of infectious disease at the University of California in San Francisco.

Jacobs began by saying that "this is a trend. It's a real fad, just like other things have been a trend and a fad lately. I think people have jumped on the bandwagon because there's been a lot in the lay press. There's been a lot of sensationalism involved with this—how EB virus ruined my marriage and my life. That kind of sensationalism is what sells newspapers."

Kroft's piece was marked by factual errors, innuendo, and unsupportable generalizations. He attempted to establish Jacobs's credentials in his introduction of the doctor, for instance, by saying the specialist had seen "hundreds of patients who think they have a chronic case of Epstein-Barr. He thinks it's less a malady than it is a movement." In the course of an interview soon after the broadcast, however, Jacobs confessed that he himself had probably seen no more than twenty patients with the disease. In addition, he told Kroft on camera that the symptoms of the disease were "identical to things that you see in clinical depression."

"Could they be suffering from depression?" Kroft prodded.

"Yes, absolutely," Jacobs answered. When queried later, however, Jacobs professed unfamiliarity with the range of symptoms suffered by victims. "I am ignorant of the disease" is how he described his degree of familiarity.

In Portland, Kroft confronted Gidget Faubion, the patient organization's president, with the question "You think you're ahead of the medical profession on this?" When Faubion answered, "Yes. Definitely," Kroft replied, "Maybe you've got it a little backward. The doctors are supposed to diagnose the patients, not patients telling doctors that they've got this wrong with them. Isn't that right?" When one patient told Kroft, "I think the CDC is doing a cover-up job," the newsman seemed barely able to hold back his laughter. "But the CDC is an organization that's supposed to protect the public health!" he rejoined.

Kroft characterized the typical sufferer as "a professional woman in her thirties with a high-pressure job." When he sat in on a support group meeting, however, none of the members looked like fast-track yuppies. Many were gray-haired; several were overweight, their facial expressions classically myopathic. "You all know, I'm sure, that there are a lot of doctors who think that CEBV probably has nothing to do with what's wrong with you," Kroft began. The patients nodded in quiet assent. "I look around the room," he added cagily, "and actually—you look great! I've been with Gidget all day and, I'm telling you, I'm a little tired."

And on it went for twelve minutes before an audience of seven million people, as reporter Kroft relegated one of the country's most controversial medical stories to the realm of an amusing trend piece. He ended his piece with a pregnant comment from infectious disease specialist Jacobs: "People divide their diseases into one of two categories," Jacobs said, "that is, either 'I'm sick' or 'I'm crazy.' And I think most people would rather be sick than be crazy."

Centers for Disease Control, Atlanta, Georgia

The day CBS broadcast its report on the disease, Edward Huth, the editor of the *Annals of Internal Medicine,* sent Gary Holmes a Mailgram informing the Epidemic Intelligence Service officer of the journal's intention to publish the consensus definition of the disease. "Thank you for the privilege of publishing this highly important paper," Huth wrote Holmes.

Wylie, South Carolina

In less than two years Mayhugh Horne had gone from being one of Pan Am's most skilled and experienced pilots to being a broken, confused invalid. Much in the manner of a stroke victim, the fifty-four-year-old cried with abandon at the slightest provocation—and occasionally for no apparent reason at all. He cried while attempting to explain to his two young boys why he had decided to stop flying. He cried sitting by himself next to the pool behind his custom-built "dream house" in South Carolina, where he had hoped to enjoy his retirement. He cried at the increasingly large and tumultuous patient support group meetings in Charlotte. He cried in church on Easter Sunday, and he cried while dining out with his wife. "This was really wild for a grown man," Horne recalled later. "My crying phase lasted a good year."

Horne's wife, Hannelore, was deeply distressed by her husband's decline. "He's been the best of the best. And now his job, his prestige, his friends, his social standing—they were gone. And then to have a disease that has no name, no number—nothing anyone can look up in a book. And you can't explain this disease to anyone—they just don't understand unless they've gone through it themselves."

Pan Am's medical officers refused to accept the pilot's contention that he was suffering from a disease of the brain. "They would say, 'Come on back!' " Horne remembered. "They said I was 'too consumed' with this disease. They said, 'Get your mind off it and you'll be all right.' Several of my pilot friends said, 'Mayhugh, the best thing you can do is get off your ass and come back to work.' "

Additionally, Pan Am officials made it clear they would not pay out on the pilot's disability plan. Within months of his self-grounding, Horne's wife remembered, "We went from a six-figure income to very few figures at all." Without his salary, Horne was facing destitution, yet a resumption of his work would mean imperiling hundreds of lives with every flight.

Horne saw Paul Cheney for the first time that winter. Cheney ordered a magnetic resonance imaging brain scan of Horne's brain. The scan picked up the tiny multiple lesions that Cheney had come to believe were classic for the disease. He then suggested Horne be evaluated by neuropsychologist Sheila Bastien in Berkeley, who saw in Horne the pattern of brain dysfunction she had come to expect in victims of the disease, deficits that were particularly worrisome in a commercial pilot. Horne's ability to send messages between his brain and his hands—his textual kinesthetic ability—was severely impaired, Bastien discovered. She also found profound deficits in short-term memory, abstract thinking, logic, and visual perception. Other aspects of Horne's intelligence, particularly his verbal IQ, were less severely affected. "This localization and lateralization [one-sidedness] cannot be explained by depression or anxiety," Bastien wrote in her final report, which Horne presented to the airline.

Pan Am was unimpressed with either the brain scan or Sheila Bastien's findings. In December the airline asked Horne to go to the Mayo Clinic for an evaluation.

"I showed [the Mayo doctors] my MR scan with the lesions. They said it was 'of no significance,' " Horne recalled. "The neurology exam was a farce. The neurologist said I was trying very hard to 'prove' I had a lack of concentration. The infectious disease specialist admitted to me that the disease existed, but she wouldn't put it in writing. And she said she could not find any basis for it in my immune system. I had all the high-tech blood work from Cheney with me, of course, and they just pooh-poohed that. They seemed to think Paul Cheney was some kind of nut."

Like all patients suffering from the disease who wound up at the famous clinic, Horne was asked to take the Minnesota Multiphasic Personality Inventory test. The Mayo psychiatrist told Horne that his MMPI results evoked the portrait of a typical medical student who is overworked, under stress, and unduly worried about his health. Afterward, reading directly from the Mayo psychiatrist's written assessment, Horne reported that the Mayo had found him to be "egocentric, suggestible, and demanding, mildly depressed and pessimistic." The Mayo psychiatrist diagnosed the pilot with "atypical depression." The Mayo neurologist's report stated that Horne "appears to be a patient of average intelligence with a memory disorder that could be due to depression but is more commonly seen in association with diffuse cerebral impairment." (A finding that Horne was "of average intelligence"—which by definition means having an IQ of 100—was worrisome on its face, since Horne's IQ was 160 prior to his illness.) The neurologist continued, "[Horne's] impairment becomes most obvious when he must recall divergent or unrelated information after a time delay."

Ultimately, the primary doctor in charge of Horne's case at the Mayo Clinic wrote to Pan Am that the pilot was "deconditioned and probably depressed." The doctor suggested to the airline that Horne could return to work as soon as he felt better.

University of California, San Diego

On December 19, a front-page *New York Times* story reported that the U.S. military was removing all personnel who were HIV-positive from "sensitive, stressful" jobs. The decision to do so came upon the publication in the December issue of the *Annals of Internal Medicine* of a study by investigators at the University of California at San Diego, which proved that people infected with HIV are frequently mentally impaired, in many cases even before they begin to show symptoms of AIDS-related complex or full-blown AIDS.[4]

Military doctor Edmund Tramont, an infectious disease specialist and the director of the clinical research program on AIDS at the Walter Reed Army Medical Center, told the *Times,* "We have recommended that people infected with the virus be taken out of positions where they could be harmful to themselves, to other people, or to the mission of their military units. If a person's brain is not functioning correctly, you do not want him flying high-performance aircraft, decoding sensitive messages for the president, or driving tanks in combat."

"The commonest changes detected by MR imaging," the San Diego authors wrote in *Annals,* "were . . . multiple small lesions of high signal intensity . . . in the subcortical white matter. . . . The neuropsychological disturbances," the authors continued, "included subtle decrements in abstract reasoning, reduced speed of information processing, and . . . difficulties in learning and remembering."

Paul Cheney in Charlotte and researchers among the Reno collaborative group were riveted by the study because the San Diego researchers had used a combination of magnetic resonance imaging brain scanning and neuropsychological testing similar to that used by Sheila Bastien to arrive at their conclusions about brain dysfunction in AIDS. As far as Cheney and the Reno researchers knew, this was the first time anyone had published a study that utilized the two technologies in tandem to document central nervous system deficits—and it was precisely the same technology they were using. Even more striking, the findings of both technologies—MRI brain scans and neuropsychological testing—were virtually identical to what the doctors were finding in patients with the disease in Nevada and North Carolina.

〖田〗

Several of the contributors to the San Diego study, interviewed in La Jolla immediately after their paper was published, were fascinated but only mildly surprised to learn that researchers elsewhere were documenting brain lesions and intellectual impairment in chronic fatigue syndrome victims. "The bottom line," said J. Allen McCutchan, an infectious disease specialist at UC San Diego who collaborated on the study, "is that this is a productive approach to trying to correlate functional [brain] problems with structural problems. I think it's something that somebody *should* pursue with respect to whatever agent is in [chronic fatigue syndrome]. I certainly believe that the syndrome exists," he continued, unprompted, "and I believe there is probably an infectious agent behind it. We certainly end up seeing a number of such patients, and they don't seem any crazier or more neurotic or anything else than a lot of other people."

John Hesselink, the University of California neuroradiologist on the study, expressed his view that neuropsychological testing was more sensitive even than MRI scanning in detecting structural damage to the brain, a point of view certainly held by most neuropsychologists, Sheila Bastien among them.

"For a long time," Hesselink said, "we radiologists would look at these white spots, and if the patients didn't have any obvious neurological deficits, we would say, 'Well, it's just nothing. It's a little water there, or a little breakdown of the blood-brain barrier, but it's not a lesion.' But we've never done careful neuropsychological testing of these same patients. We would just look for neurological signs—weakness in an arm or a leg, or sensory disturbances. And I think neuropsychological testing would be more sensitive [than MRI scanning] for detecting organic structural abnormalities in the brain."

Hesselink, in addition, commented that he was increasingly convinced that UBOs were not normal structures in the brain. His belief had come in part from his observations of the tiny lesions in people infected with HIV and in part from another finding made by his radiology group at the university but so far unpublished: that UBOs were commonly present in people with bipolar disorder, otherwise known as manic-depression.

"*I* think they mean something. We just don't yet know what," Hesselink said.

1988

IN THE

BUGHOUSE

[A]ll science is in the facts or phenomena of nature and their relationships, and not in the minds of men, which discovers and interprets them.

—Sir William Osler, *An Alabama Student and Other Biographical Essays*

13

Salami Science

Centers for Disease Control, Atlanta, Georgia

As a result of Chicagoan Ted Van Zelst's lobbying efforts, Congress at last awarded the Atlanta agency a dollar sum to investigate the disease in 1988. By contemporary biomedical research standards, the amount—$407,000—was a paltry one. For patients, it was a watershed. For the first time, Congress had done more than merely suggest to federal scientists that they pursue the disease; lawmakers had apportioned money to ensure that the work was done. Specifically, Congress asked the CDC to institute a disease surveillance system and to assign at least two full-time investigators or "the equivalent" to conduct research— meaning the agency could ask four people to devote 50 percent of their labor to the project, or even eight people to commit a quarter of their time.

Monitoring the spread of infectious diseases and controlling those diseases was, historically, the fundamental role of the Centers for Disease Control in the public health arena. However, the legislature's directive to set up a system whereby doctors could report cases of the newly renamed chronic fatigue syndrome did not sit well with agency staff. Hardly anyone employed in Atlanta that year believed the affliction was a coherent disease entity like, say, syphilis or tuberculosis or AIDS, all of which were reportable diseases. Nor did anyone believe it was flourishing in epidemic form. Agency staff considered the CFS phenomenon to be media-driven mass hysteria; they expected that only a tiny percentage of cases would be found to have documentable organic disease. As Jon Kaplan said, "I don't think you'll find anyone here who really thinks that there is an epidemic of this. That's real popular in the lay media, but not here." Finally, with the exception of virologist John Stewart, who actually had corresponded and conversed in some depth with sufferers, no one in Atlanta understood the disease to be a crippling, life-destroying condition; it was simply "chronic fatigue," and as one agency scientist said with a shrug, "Hell, *I'm* tired!"

Scientists along the viral diseases epidemiology corridors, in particular, regarded the congressional subcommittee's request as a bothersome demand destined to siphon money and manpower from important agency business. Congress had been duped, they believed, by an unusually aggressive group of people obsessed with a phony disease. The patients' very desperation and demands were viewed as symptomatic of the pseudo-affliction itself rather than as a reflection of bona fide need. Jon Kaplan's comments were typical. "One of the ironies in this whole thing is all these people who call us and think they have this," he said. "And they complain of fatigue, and yet sometimes you think they have an incredible amount of energy. They call us, they write us. They write their congressmen. They've got more energy than *I* do! . . . But there's no way that all the people who call us and who think they have this could all have the same thing," Kaplan continued. "It's absolutely impossible."

No one was more troubled by the sudden encroachment of Congress on the agency's management of the disease than Larry Schonberger. His Viral Exanthems and Herpesvirus Branch, after all, was linked to the amorphous affliction by virtue of the Nevada investigation, performed under his authority. Should surveillance ever be launched, the onerous chore would fall to Schonberger and his staff. As a result of patient lobbying, in fact, Schonberger was facing that very actuality as the new year began.

Schonberger's skepticism about the psychiatric integrity of people who claimed to suffer from the idiopathic affliction was increasingly apparent to at least one of his colleagues, agency veteran Walter Gunn, who had observed with quiet dismay the hilarity that the subject inevitably aroused in his boss and among his younger colleagues. The epidemiology chief, Gunn recalled, was visibly distressed at the thought of being forced to perform surveillance on a non-disease. Schonberger, Gunn remembered, struggled to come up with a restrained, piecemeal plan that might satisfy legislators. Ultimately, Schonberger calculated he could hold Congress at bay by setting up a limited surveillance in just two counties; he presumed the harvest from such a small surveillance would be so disappointing as to discourage further efforts. He put Gary Holmes in charge of the project.

San Francisco, California

By 1988, California had at least thirty-four support organizations for victims of the brain disease. Their members were scattered from the populous southern regions, where a group in Riverside numbered more than a thousand, to the northern communities of Carmel, Santa Cruz, Monterey, Fresno, Stockton, Sacramento, Sonoma County, and Paradise. Given that participation in support organizations by victims of diseases historically accounted for only a tiny percentage of the total number of victims, the explosive growth of these sizable groups suggested that the epidemic was particularly severe in California. In fact, half of the 12,000 members of the national organization based in Portland were Californians.

One California sufferer, Jan Montgomery, was increasingly dismayed by what she viewed as the ineffectiveness of her state's local groups and the national organization in Portland. "The Portland organization," Montgomery said that winter, "as good-hearted as it is, is not making it. I just got a thirteen-page newsletter from them. It doesn't even mention the fact that this is an infectious disease. I don't think they're going to be the political arm of the movement."

In the months since the San Francisco Health Commission hearings on the disease, Montgomery had organized a small group of activist patients in San Francisco and the East Bay cities of Berkeley and Albany. "Our intention is to become political," Montgomery said. "We can't waste our energy on support groups. The problem is too overwhelming. We're right where the AIDS epidemic was in the second year. The only thing that really moved it ahead was that there was a possibility that a great number of people were already infected—they realized it was a time bomb. Unfortunately, with this, people are hoping it will go away tomorrow. We've decided to radicalize," she continued. "We've decided to break the silence. We're starting to say, 'AIDS is a major epidemic, and there is another—that's what we have.' "

Montgomery's group petitioned the city's health department to begin tracking the disease in San Francisco, using the AIDS reporting system of the Centers for Disease Control as a model.

Charlotte, North Carolina

In January, Marc Iverson launched publication of the *CFIDS Chronicle,* described on its cover as a journal of "Advocacy, Information, Research, and Encouragement for the CFIDS Community." Iverson took the title from the name Seymour Grufferman had proposed at the Portland conference: chronic fatigue and immune dysfunction syndrome. The first isue of the *CFIDS Chronicle* was a stapled four-page publication mailed to approximately five hundred people, most of them in North Carolina.

By the end of Paul Cheney's first year at the Nalle Clinic, his internal medicine practice included 140 patients suffering from the disease. So far, none of his associates had expressed to him even a modicum of curiosity about either the disease or the famous Nevada epidemic, behavior Cheney found strangely troubling. Instead of discouraging him in his research efforts, however, his colleagues' apparent indifference galvanized him further.

Cheney was struck by the essential sameness of his Charlotte patients and those he had known in Incline Village. "The pattern of this disease is so interesting, and so clear as time goes on, that I'm having an increasingly harder time thinking of this as multiple diseases mixed together," the doctor said that winter. "Clearly, there are some that might be mixed in with it, but it's like predominantly white paint, and perhaps there are a few specks of brown that don't belong, but the thing is white mostly."

Yet, just as in Incline, there continued to be unforeseen, clinically remarkable developments in a few people. In January, for instance, he discovered the first malignant tumor in a Charlotte patient. The tumor, which was successfully removed by surgery, occurred in a twenty-eight-year-old high school teacher who had been ill for one year. Another patient, a twenty-five-year-old kindergarten teacher named Tracy Watson (a pseudonym) who had been bedridden for one year, developed a sudden pronounced weakness in her right arm. Focal weakness was a symptom Cheney had observed among a subset of his Nevada patients, beginning with meter reader Chris Guthrie. But when Watson's symptom began, Cheney was attending the Portland conference. In his absence, the Nalle Clinic routed the patient to a neurologist. Lacking any particular knowledge of chronic fatigue syndrome, the neurologist suspected Watson had suffered a stroke; he ordered a magnetic resonance imaging scan of her brain, unaware that Cheney had ordered the same test a month earlier. The original scan had revealed a single small lesion in the white cortical matter of the teacher's brain. The results of the second scan were more consistent with the majority of patients with the disease: the teacher now had multiple lesions. There was no evidence of stroke. More recently, Watson had developed a mass on her lung.

Cheney was used to patients with the disease reporting bizarre symptoms. Increasingly, he was learning that most of the reports, however fantastic, had some basis in reality. That winter, for example, even a patient who complained that she had lost her fingerprints since becoming ill turned out to be telling the truth. On examination, it was apparent to the doctor that the woman's fingertips had become absolutely smooth except for occasional deep vertical cracks in their surface. To test his own subjective perception of the phenomenon, Cheney sent the woman to the sheriff's department with a request for fingerprints. She returned with a series of ghostly gray smudges on police documents. They were, the police sergeant told Cheney, completely worthless. "What's wrong with the lady, anyway?" the sergeant inquired.

A fingertip exam became a routine element of Cheney's workup. In the next several months he sent a steady stream of patients with the fingertip abnormality to the sheriff's department to corroborate his observations. In addition, the doctor ordered fingertip biopsies to be performed on fifteen badly afflicted patients; he discovered that a majority were suffering from lymphocyte vasculitis, an inflammation of the microscopic blood vessels in the fingertips. Cheney hypothesized the condition was impairing the supply of nutrients to the skin. In time it became apparent that approximately one-quarter of his fatigue patients were missing their fingerprints, a rather fiendish consequence, the doctor mused, of a disease that so powerfully stripped its victims of their identities.

"This whole disease still remains very patient-oriented," Cheney said that winter. "If you're not patient-oriented, you won't get anywhere. You don't learn anything, except from the patients."

University of California, San Francisco

Carol Jessop had been in private practice in El Cerrito for six months. Her caseload of sufferers was close to five hundred. "Everything I know about this disease," Jessop commented that winter, "I have learned from my patients.

"I see very strong patterns now," she continued, "from predisposing problems that might make people more likely to get this, to sequelae of problems that occur down the line. And I hear these patients—people who don't know each other—use almost the same words to describe what it's been like for them. Like 'When I wake up I feel like somebody has been beating me all night with a baseball bat.' Now, I've been in practice for quite a while," Jessop continued, "and that's not a complaint you hear every day, or even every year. But it's very characteristic of what you hear from these patients."

Like Paul Cheney and Dan Peterson, Jessop was discovering that miscarriages were common. Frequently, women referred to her for symptoms of fatigue and spontaneous abortions turned out to have the disease. In addition, every woman under Jessop's care who had been able to carry a baby to term had required a cesarean section. "They did not have the energy—they just didn't have the muscle energy to give birth," Jessop said. "And when they had the C-section, they all received epidural morphine, which is used very consistently in C-section deliveries. And all of them had abnormal reactions to the painkiller. It was as if they had gotten an overdose, even though their dose was typical for their weight. It's like they had an overreactive autonomic nervous system reaction to medications."*

As Peterson and Cheney had observed, Jessop, too, noted that the children born to these women were of clinically significant low birth weight. As Jessop followed her burgeoning patient group, she also noted that within a year's time more than half became allergic to a variety of animals, foods, and chemicals; another 40 percent developed an unusual form of hypothyroidism that failed to respond to synthetic thyroid hormone. Yet another sequela Jessop observed was an intractable depression. "It's a biochemical depression," the doctor said. "It is not present in the beginning of the disease. This depression doesn't go away. In fact, it seems to get worse and worse."

As the gulf between her and her former colleagues at the University of California widened, Jessop remained disturbed by the stance of academics. "It's amazing to me," she said, "that doctors would think people would want to make this up— that people would *want* to feel so bad. I don't understand why people who are so skeptical and negative would go into medicine. A patient comes in and says, 'This is what's going on—help me.' You sit down and you try to figure it out. Sure, we all run into obstacles. We're never quite sure, and sometimes we can't figure it out. But . . . to *invalidate* somebody," she continued, incredulity edging into her voice. "I see so many people who have been absolutely *devastated* by this illness, and I think it's been a very poor showing by physicians."

University of Pittsburgh, Pittsburgh, Pennsylvania

After the new year Seymour Grufferman learned to his dismay that disabled flight attendants Romy Zarit and Chris Larson would be unable to distribute their questionnaires among PSA's and TWA's employees. Under pressure from airline management, the company's unions refused to cooperate with Zarit and Larson. Grufferman was unsurprised. "Someone probably got scared off by the notion of liability," he said. "This has happened before." In the past year, the epidemiologist had been approached by a nurse employed in a Pittsburgh hospital who described a cluster epidemic of the disease within the hospital. Grufferman was eager to pursue her report. The second time he spoke to the nurse, however, she explained she

---

* Jessop's observation would eventually be expanded to include all pharmaceuticals. Doctors who saw large numbers of victims were becoming aware that, for reasons that remain unclear, such patients were exquisitely sensitive to medication of any kind and were at risk of adverse reactions from even the lowest recommended doses; patients with the disease who were facing surgery for any reason faced higher risks than otherwise healthy people from anesthesia and related drugs.

had been placed under a gag order by the hospital's management as part of her disability settlement and was no longer free to discuss the outbreak.

University of Nevada, Reno

The government's announcement of its intent to fund research sharply focused the attention of scientists and clinicians interested in the disease. Alliances were forming, and a multitude of ideas were in play among the coterie of researchers who saw in chronic fatigue syndrome a wealth of scientific pursuits.

During the winter of 1988, Harvard researcher Anthony Komaroff, who had been one of the first scientists to apply for a grant, awaited news of the fate of his proposal. In the interim, he was rewriting the Tahoe manuscript, which had been rejected by the *New England Journal of Medicine,* for submission to the British journal *Lancet,* this time with Robert Gallo as coauthor. (He was unaware that his collaborators in Tahoe—Royce Biddle, Berch Henry, and Dan Peterson—by then had written their own paper, a case study of twenty local victims, for *Lancet.*) Komaroff had also initiated a ten-year prospective study of the Tahoe epidemic victims using money donated to him that winter by a rich patient in Incline Village. Finally, by 1988, the Harvard doctor had no fewer than sixteen individual "feel the goods" investigations under way in Boston and elsewhere. Yet Nevada continued to be Komaroff's anchor; because of time-space clustering, the Tahoe epidemic offered the most compelling evidence so far for the existence of a disease his peers in academic medicine considered chimerical.

Although Komaroff had sought to claim the Tahoe epidemic as his own, a new, independent-minded network of investigators was emerging in Reno that winter. Its members believed they had both the expertise and the moral authority to pursue the disease, not only because of their immediate proximity, but by virtue of the scientific legacy left them by Paul Cheney and Dan Peterson. The *New England Journal*'s rejection of the Tahoe manuscript had revealed Komaroff's vulnerability, and they were frankly indifferent to his participation in their efforts. Most of all, they were eager for federal money that would allow them to make their contribution. By mid-January, this network, based at the University of Nevada, had expanded to include not only Berch Henry, Dan Peterson, neuroradiologist Royce Biddle, and Reno's three infectious disease specialists but also Sandra Daugherty, the chair of the university's epidemiology department and wife of the medical school dean, Robert Daugherty, who was an enthusiastic supporter. Dan Peterson, Berch Henry, and Royce Biddle held positions in the new collaborative effort and in Komaroff's Tahoe projects as well.

Giddy optimism suffused this group after the new year. Infectious disease specialist Ray Swarts had mailed their in-depth evaluation of twenty local cases to *Lancet* immediately after Christmas—all twenty cases had brain lesions, T4–T8 ratios of at least ten to one, low or absent natural killer cells, and exceedingly high levels of antibodies to human herpesvirus 6—and on January 7 virologist Berch Henry had his first conversation with Ann Schleuderberg, the administrator from the microbiology division of the National Institute of Allergy and Infectious Diseases in charge of extramural research funding for chronic fatigue syndrome.*

---

* A T4–T8 ratio of two to one is normal.

Henry described to her his efforts to identify human herpesvirus 6 in Nevada patients. "I've never seen anything like it," he told Schleuderberg. "In two weeks they become the dominant cell type in the culture. They just blow up big as a balloon. I mean—these are *big*. And they lyse [destroy the cell]."

Berch Henry was buoyed by the call. "It's not every day you get a call from an NIH grant officer," he said cheerfully after he hung up.

More than two hundred patients had passed through Berch Henry's lab at the medical school. The once-skeptical investigator had embraced the disease with the conviction of the born-again. For him the prospect of being on the cusp of the discovery of a new infectious disease, perhaps even being a member of the team to crack it, was heady indeed. Henry was eager for government support to pursue his work, and Schleuderberg, who had promised to come west to observe firsthand the microscopic violence under way in Henry's cell cultures, might be the key.

On January 12, Schleuderberg, a small middle-aged woman with large rimless spectacles and cropped red hair, arrived at the Reno airport. She made her way down the noisy concourse, where gurgling melodies from slot machines competed with the theme from *Bonanza* on Muzak, to the baggage carousel. Henry collected her in his sixties-vintage Mercedes and escorted her to his lab. There Schleuderberg studied the bizarre-looking B-cells, which Henry felt reasonably certain were infected with human herpesvirus 6. Afterward she reported that she had been impressed by the dying cell colonies. "It was exciting to see cytopathology [cell death]," she said. "It was a real, tangible thing."

Schleuderberg's Nevada trip generated high spirits among the Reno team, whose members knew NIH grant officers rarely made on-site visits. Although she had made no promises, they believed her interest guaranteed at least a fair hearing for their proposal, which they intended to submit by June. Privately, Schleuderberg was guardedly enthusiastic about the Nevadans, her interest driven almost exclusively by the cell death Henry had been able to demonstrate. Researchers elsewhere might be more sophisticated in the realm of epidemiology, Schleuderberg commented after her visit, but "the people in Reno have the other most important thing: they have their hand on an agent. . . . You don't just get a new virus out of someone's lymphocytes every day of the week."

Seymour Grufferman, the Pittsburgh cancer epidemiologist who was at least as eager for federal support as the Reno investigators, had also been host to Schleuderberg, who had stopped in Pittsburgh on her way to Reno. Grufferman told her he wanted to explore the affliction's relationship to cancer as well as its routes of transmission. Afterward, during her nearly five-hour flight to Reno, the federal scientist had studied the pages of immunological data gleaned from Grufferman's investigation of the North Carolina orchestra.

In spite of such enthusiasms, Schleuderberg revealed herself that winter to be an unshakable proponent of the "wastebasket" theory of the disease. "I will stake my children's lives on the fact that this is not a single disease but many," she said. Her posture created obstacles even to discussing the disease since, in her view, its existence as a discrete entity was unproven. "Forgive me," she would interject when people were described as suffering from CEBV, the name in use that winter, "but don't say that. What [the patients] have is something that's very *compatible*

with what has been called CEBV." In spite of her certainty on many subjects relating to the disease, Schleuderberg confessed she had never even met anyone
who suffered from it.

Schleuderberg was quick to defend her agency against Seymour Grufferman's
criticism that without a specific set-aside of dollars, routine in priority research
projects such as AIDS, it would be difficult to lure scientists to undertake the time-
consuming task of applying for grants. "Some people say you don't get responses
to announcements that have no hard money behind them. I say that you can," she
said. "It's a staging kind of thing," she said of the agency's grant strategy. "Because there is still so much uncertainty, because the science doesn't seem to be
ready, we wanted to see what an announcement could do by itself—let the scientific community come in by themselves without direction from above. It was logical that [my superiors] said, 'Don't do anything further. At the end of a year, let's
see where we are and reevaluate this and see whether we might not want to go further.' If it becomes apparent in workshops convened to discuss the matter, for example, that there are specific areas that need further pursuit," she continued, "I can
go to the Board of Scientific Counselors and we perhaps can be more aggressive
in trying to have money set aside."

In effect, administrators at the NIH had found a way to convey a degree of concern without necessarily having to fund research, since they could always claim
that, although they were ready to provide money, in their judgment, "the science
doesn't seem to be ready." (Indeed, at this writing, a decade after the Nevada epidemic, the NIH has yet to set aside hard money for extramural research on the disease.) The lack of commitment on the agency's part became fully apparent when
Schleuderberg was asked to explain the impetus behind her grant announcement
the previous autumn. A concern that the disease constituted a public health emergency apparently played no part in the agency's move. Instead, Schleuderberg
confided, the request had been motivated by "the activity of the [Portland] CEBV
Association, which has resulted in lots of press and lots of congressional lobbying. That's been very effective. And I don't think that having things hit the *Wall
Street Journal* and the *New York Times* and *Newsweek* and *Nightline,* and whatever else it's hit, has hurt." But, Schleuderberg felt compelled to add, her agency
would not allow patient lobbyists to set research priorities. "Obviously the scientific peer groups that help us make decisions are concerned that we don't go off on
a tack at the behest of the CEBV Association telling Congress what we should
do—to put money toward bad science."

For some years to come, any studies purporting to search for the cause of the
disease would be deemed "bad science" by government administrators. Epidemiologist Warren Browner, Jay Levy's associate at the University of California,
called Schleuderberg shortly after she had written and disseminated her request
for proposals the previous September. Afterward, Browner presaged the conflict
that was shaping up between the agency and at least one virologist, his colleague
Levy: "I think what Jay wants to do and what the NIH wants to do are two very
different things," Browner said after his conversation with Schleuderberg. "Jay
wants to find a virus. He's very straightforward about that. He wants to find out
what's causing the problem." "Good science," as interpreted by the grant gate-

keepers, was most frequently that which purported to investigate the psychiatric profiles of people suffering from the disease.

☒

On January 16, four days after Schleuderberg left Reno, the University of Nevada team gathered in a medical school classroom for an intensive three-and-a-half-hour session during which they discussed strategy for winning federal research dollars. The marathon session was a clear view into the extraordinarily complex issues of scientific credibility posed by the disease. It was one thing, as Reno infectious disease specialist Trudy Larson had done, to meet with patients whose distress was "palpable" and be converted with a suddenness akin to spiritual revelation. It was quite another to prove the existence of the disease to antagonists within the federal government and their local colleagues, especially when its cause and mode of transmission remained mysterious. Larson's colleague Stephen Parker poignantly outlined the problem that afternoon: "We can define the clinical disease," he commented. "Our problem is that people don't believe it. What study are you going to have to do to silence the most skeptical of the skeptical?"

Despite the team's best efforts, which included hundreds of hours of data-gathering and proposal-writing, the University of Nevada's proposal to study the spread of the new disease in Nevada was rejected by the government after its submission in June.

Saint Mary's Medical School, London, England

British researchers were following their own instincts. Unlike Americans, who early on had taken their cues from the disease's seeming relationship to infectious mononucleosis and subscribed to a flu-like syndrome as their clinical model, the British had viewed the disease as a neuromuscular disorder from the start. As a result, they failed to share the American obsession with herpesviruses. Several British scientists were exploring enteroviruses, an entirely different class of pathogens that were harbored in the human gut and were known to cause chronic muscle and heart disorders, polio among them. There were scores of enteroviruses, many waiting to be matched with diseases. Recently the English focus on enteroviruses had paid off, and in the January 23 issue of *Lancet,* a team of English virologists and clinicians described their discovery of active enterovirus in seventeen out of seventy-six sufferers of what researchers chose to call "postviral fatigue syndrome."[1]

Enterovirus investigations aside, the larger English medical establishment more typically viewed the disease with the same lack of curiosity evinced by its American counterpart. One measure of English medicine's indifference was the fact that the enterovirus research performed at Saint Mary's had been paid for by patient organizations. Nevertheless, there were hints that the malady had taken hold on English soil. Like similar associations in the United States, the United Kingdom's Myalgic Encephalomyelitis Association was undergoing explosive growth. It had expanded from 1,900 members in January of 1987 to 10,000 members by early 1988. British medical journals and the English lay press commonly estimated the number of Britons affected at 100,000.

Incline Village, Nevada

No one could have predicted that hostilities would break out between Anthony Komaroff and his Tahoe collaborators when he visited Nevada late in January. Dan Peterson had invited the Harvard doctor to Incline Village on the twenty-sixth for a dinner in Komaroff's honor. The next day, Komaroff would leave for Seattle, where he was to present a grand rounds lecture on the disease before an audience of doctors and scientists at the University of Washington, his medical school alma mater. Komaroff's schedule was tight. He spent an afternoon in the Alder Street clinic going over data, huddling with Dan Peterson, and for the first time meeting Berch Henry. That evening a group of twenty, including a number of wealthy patients who had contributed money to Komaroff's research efforts, met at the Incline Village Hyatt, site of a cluster outbreak among casino and hotel employees two years before.

Over drinks, Komaroff was quizzed by computer prodigy Paul Thompson. "Why is mainstream medicine so resistant to the idea that this disease is real?" Thompson asked, honestly perplexed.

In a rare moment of candor, Komaroff talked about his skeptical peers in academic medicine. "The *real* story," he said, "will be to follow the turnaround of certain big figures on this disease." When the truth surfaced, Komaroff predicted, academic heavyweights like Stanford's Tom Merigan would behave as if they had known it all along. Only their subordinates would remember the original hip-shooting stance taken years before. "They won't say anything, but Merigan will see it in their eyes," Komaroff continued, pointing to his own narrowed eyes.

Though he rarely spoke of it, the personal costs of his involvement in the disease weighed heavily on Komaroff. Near midnight, as the doctor made the icy journey over Mount Rose in his rented sedan to Balley's Hotel in Reno, he talked in subdued tones about the problem: "When the thing that you're pursuing is something that many of your colleagues are skeptical about, that takes a toll because that's a measure of their respect for you and what you do and how you spend your time," he said. "Another part of the toll is trying to reconcile the time and energy needed to do the research with the time and energy called for from patients, other doctors, and the media. Most people who do scientific work have the opportunity to sort of pursue it unmolested until and unless it gets important or visible or whatever, at which time they deal with the problem."

At 6:45 A.M. the next day, Komaroff was seated at a booth in one of the casino's fluorescent-lit coffee shops. Opposite him were Berch Henry and neurologist Royce Biddle; the pair looked sleepy. A fiftyish woman in a ruffled mini-jumper moved among the tables selling keno tickets to gamblers. Komaroff had asked for the meeting, which began amiably enough with a discussion about choosing controls for MRI brain scans.

"I would shy away from choosing people who either worked or played together," Komaroff cautioned. "We need to avoid picking what turns out in retrospect to be a hotbed of subclinical infection."

Later Komaroff directed his comments directly to Biddle, suggesting that, just as it had been helpful to have two independent investigators read the brain scans of diseased patients, at least two independent investigators should read the brain scans from healthy controls as well. "Let's assume we get all those [control] scans and indeed there are very few UBOs," Komaroff said. "Then let's have them read by a second guy, like Ferenc Jolesz. If these were large patchy splotches, like multiple sclerosis, it wouldn't be a problem, but these tend to be small, and the interpretation can be subjective." Biddle agreed.

"We've got to be quick," Komaroff continued. "I've heard through the grapevine that at least two radiology groups are chasing this now—a group at UCSF and a group in San Diego." Biddle expressed surprise that anyone at San Francisco would be interested, given his cool reception by the medical school's contingent at the Western Neuroradiology Society conference in the fall. "Either they're genuinely skeptical, or they're trying to throw you off the scent," Komaroff responded, "so I think we should move fast. The database is all set up in Boston. We'll have computer analysis of the location of lesions in the brain."

The upbeat mood was suddenly destroyed when Henry made an offhand reference to the Reno team's recent submission of their twenty cases to Lancet.

"Wait—am I to understand that you have actually sent a paper to Lancet?" Komaroff demanded. Henry, looking equally surprised, confirmed that the Reno group had done just that. "But Dr. Gallo and I have sent a paper to Lancet," Komaroff said, his expression stony.

During the next several minutes, Komaroff appeared to expand with anger, peppering Henry and Biddle with questions about their paper, chastising every response.

"This is salami science—do you know what that is?" Komaroff continued after a moment. Henry and Biddle glared at him wordlessly from across the table. "It's when you take the same data and slice off a little piece here and a little piece there. This duplication will make the academicians look very foolish to the Lancet editor in England."

Soon afterward, announcing that he needed to catch his plane to Seattle, Komaroff departed abruptly. But he didn't go directly to the airport, which was five minutes away. He went to a pay phone somewhere in Balley's vast flocked-velvet lobby and dialed Dan Peterson, reaching him at home in Incline Village. For the next thirty minutes the Harvard researcher vented his displeasure.

Later that morning, in the familiar territory of his lab, Berch Henry was still angry. "I've absolutely had it with all this subterfuge. This is not the way science is done. This is not the way medical problems are unraveled."

Ray Swarts, perhaps because he had not been stung, like Henry, by Komaroff's condescension and ill temper, was calmer in his view of the matter, but no less cavalier. "Komaroff needs us more than we need him," Swarts said.

Peterson, for his part, insisted he had written to Komaroff weeks before, telling him about the paper. "Of course he knew about it. I got an acknowledgment, in writing," Peterson said. "He did not tell us about his paper, so exactly what he accused us of, he was guilty of. . . . And now I see why he's so upset, because our little paper—talking about the same patients with HHV-six infection from Reno—went into Lancet first and scooped him. Well, I'd be pissed, too, if I were him."

University of Washington, Seattle

Grand rounds presentations are an ancient tradition at medical schools, an opportunity for faculty and students alike to keep abreast of new phenomena in the medical cosmos. Komaroff's reception at the University of Washington's medical school was more a reflection of the skepticism of his academic colleagues than a demonstration of their intellectual curiosity. The title of Komaroff's lecture, which had been posted on signs around the medical school, was "Chronic Mononucleosis: Fact or Fiction?" At the appointed hour, 8:00 A.M., when Komaroff stepped up to the lectern, the medical school auditorium was jammed with more than five hundred professors of medicine, bench researchers, residents, and medical students, many of whom lined the aisles and competed for standing room at the rear.

Komaroff began by admitting that the disease was mired in controversy, but he said, "I do believe that there is a real entity, a real organic disease, that produces fatigue and associated symptoms." The Harvard investigator talked for forty-five minutes. It wasn't until he related the case history of a Tahoe patient that his audience registered any visible reaction. "This is a thirty-two-year-old woman," Komaroff said, pointing to a slide covered with numbers. "Her measured IQ was 134. She was a good student who went to work in 1982 at the U.S. Post Office as an accountant. At that time she took a battery of civil service tests and placed in the top rank nationally in terms of her arithmetic skills. She then went on to handle over $100,000 a week in transactions for four years without any problem. In January of 1986 she developed an acute viral syndrome, followed by months of chronic fatigue, cognitive symptoms, and the other symptoms that we've mentioned. She tried to return to work, but found herself making errors on even simple tasks. . . . When she was retested with the battery of tests four months into the illness," Komaroff continued, "her IQ was 103. Her . . . arithmetic skills were at the fourth-grade level, or the fourteenth percentile."

With the hard numbers before them on the slide, several members of the audience shifted in their seats or exchanged glances with their colleagues.

"These patients are remarkable, the neuropsychologists tell us," Komaroff continued, "because of the *focality* of the deficit—impairment of visual processing with preservation of verbal processing, for instance. And these consulting neuropsychologists feel that these test batteries are consistent with an organic process."

Nevertheless, during the ensuing give-and-take, it became apparent that Komaroff had been unable to persuade even a minority present of the validity of the disease. One skeptic noted that most of the Tahoe cases were diagnosed in a single medical practice, a circumstance that to him suggested a false epidemic. Komaroff explained that the majority of patients he saw in Boston were referred to him from other practices and that 75 percent of the Tahoe patients, too, originally had no relation to the Alder Street practice. "I'll add that several members of the medical staff in Tahoe became ill," Komaroff continued, but as he attempted to finish his sentence, his words were drowned out by laughter, which seemed to explode from the audience as if a great tension had been expelled. Apparently, the first half of Komaroff's comment was interpreted as proof that the Alder Street clinic staff, too, had been caught up in the mass hysteria. Hardly anyone heard the second half of Komaroff's reply: "Two with primary seizures and two with ataxia."

National Institute of Allergy and Infectious Diseases, Bethesda, Maryland

On February 1, seven grant proposals to study the chronic epidemic disease arrived at NIAID for processing. Ann Schleuderberg referred the applications to the institute's large epidemiology study committee for review. No one on the twenty-two-member committee possessed even a passing familiarity with the disease. None of the proposals received scores high enough to be funded, including those proposals from immunologist Nancy Klimas at the University of Miami and Seymour Grufferman at the University of Pittsburgh, each of whom had been awarded numerous federal grants to study either AIDS or cancer in past years.

Grufferman, particularly, had a long string of NIH-supported research projects in his background. He was less than placid when he received his pink sheets, the standard forms on which the agency's reviewers typed their criticisms. In fact, for years afterward, Grufferman's ire could be aroused with a mention of that early review process. "I *never* got scores like that before," he said as recently as 1991. "My pink sheets were *atrocious!*" Grufferman fired a letter to Schleuderberg protesting the selection of the review committee. "I'm probably the only one with the guts to do it," he commented at the time, which was a true statement. He also wrote to Anthony Fauci, Schleuderberg's boss and the chief of the National Institute of Allergy and Infectious Diseases. By law, Grufferman scolded Fauci, federal grant review committees are required to be composed of true peers—scientists and clinicians who have some knowledge of the subject they are reviewing.

Some years later Grufferman characterized the tone of Fauci's response as "nasty." "I chair a grant review committee for the National Institutes of Health," Grufferman said, "so to get one of their own saying these things really bothered them. [Fauci] assured me my review was fair."

Lastly, Grufferman filed a formal appeal with the agency, an action that helped the researcher to vent his anger but which afforded no practical relief.

Nalle Clinic, Charlotte, North Carolina

Paul Cheney saw his most interesting patient, Cliff Harker, every three months. A former technical sergeant from Montgomery, Alabama, Harker had been prematurely retired from the military after a near-twenty-year perfect service record for psychiatric problems after testing positive, then negative, for AIDS. His misfortunes had begun after contracting what seemed to be genital herpes during what Harker characterized as a one-night stand. In addition to suffering myriad symptoms of viral illness, Harker had developed a case of oral thrush and a rare pneumonia peculiar to birds and victims of AIDS. Although he recovered from the thrush and the pneumonia, he continued to be troubled by night sweats, fatigue, lymphadenopathy, and fevers. He also underwent an odd, almost violent deterioration of his personality that included intense anxiety, depression, embarrassing crying spells, and tremendous mood fluctuations. For a while, he had ataxia. He suffered, as well, from peculiar visual aberrations in which he would see black spots or "floaters" in his periphery and, occasionally, flashes of light just slightly above the object of his focus. Strangest of all, he began to detect electrical sensations in his teeth. In time, convinced he was dying anyway, Harker attempted suicide. As a result, in an ordeal that might impress Franz Kafka, Harker was housed in a military psychiatric facility from October 1987 to April 1988: the more emphatically Harker tried to impress air force psychiatrists that he was physically ill, the more protracted his stay. Ultimately, Harker realized he would win his freedom only by denouncing his claim to physical illness, thereby persuading psychiatrists he had forsaken his preposterous fantasies and was now "well." Years later, he would recall gathering in a hospital meeting room with his wife, his sister, and a psychiatrist, the latter of whom sonorously intoned, "I want to assure you that there is nothing wrong with Clifford."

"I'm sitting there in the nuthouse with this psychiatrist telling my wife there's nothing wrong with me," Harker said of the moment, "and I'm seeing sparklers coming out of the tops of their heads!"

Harker remained mute throughout the meeting; the military placed him on "temporary duty retirement status," a nebulous rank he would hold for five years until he was officially discharged as a psychiatric case. Upon winning his freedom, Harker found his way to Charlotte after reading about Cheney's expertise in the new chronic disease.

On Harker's fourth visit to Cheney in early February, the patient had two new complaints: his left forearm was shrinking, he told the doctor, and his right leg had a dent in it.

Set against Cheney's three-and-a-half-year odyssey, Harker's report of a shrinking forearm and a dented leg was just another curiosity in a vast museum of curiosities. Nor were Harker's complaints entirely new to the doctor. Cheney already had observed that in a subset of his patients one forearm shrank on occasion, a sign of apparent muscle atrophy unrelated to the general loss of muscle experienced by sufferers over time. But Harker's forearm was the most disturbing example Cheney yet had seen. In the doctor's words, the forearm "was just wasting away in all these little muscle groups—there were holes in his arm where his muscles had just atrophied." Cheney had witnessed nothing quite like the indentation in Harker's right leg, either. It was in the gastrocnemius muscle, which forms the greater part of the calf; the doctor was able to insert the plump part of his thumb into the cavity. These developments brought Cheney to a diagnostic impasse. For some time, the Tahoe malady label had fit. Now patient and doctor were veering into uncharted territory.

There were others among the brain syndrome patients in his practice at the Nalle who, as Cheney phrased it, seemed to be sinking into "fairly severe clinical holes." But it was Harker who seized Cheney's imagination, who kept him awake nights. Two aspects of the man's case focused his thoughts: Harker's extreme myopathy, or muscle wasting, which after a year's time remained the only significant deviation from the classic brain syndrome profile, and the patient's false-positive AIDS test. The doctor began to wonder if, in fact, Harker had an altogether different affliction.

Cheney knew there was a central nervous system disease marked by muscle-wasting, weakness and, in severe cases, a spastic walk, that Japanese and American scientists had recently linked to the first human retrovirus, human T-cell lymphotrophic virus, type 1. The disease, which was extremely rare in North America but more common in the tropics and in Japan, was known as TSP, for "tropical spastic paraparesis."* Perhaps Harker had been infected with HTLV1 by a sexual partner who was infected with the virus. If that was true, Cheney postulated, Harker's positive AIDS test might have been an instance of HTLV1 responding to the chemical reagents used to test for its sister virus, HIV.

Once the idea occurred to him, Cheney had difficulty banishing it, even though TSP was thought to respect rigid demographic and hemispheric boundaries that, prima facie, appeared to eliminate Cliff Harker. The virus infected primarily black inhabitants of the Caribbean and South America and intravenous drug abusers in blighted northern cities like Newark and New York.†

Robert Gallo, whose team at the National Cancer Institute discovered HTLV1 in the late 1970s, had originally linked it to T-cell leukemia. But Gallo had repeatedly stated that the virus was potentially more important as a cause of central nervous system diseases than cancer. Elaine DeFreitas and Hilary Koprowski's work on HTLV1 and multiple sclerosis was the first study to draw the link Gallo predicted. The link between HTLV1 and TSP was reported a year later, in 1987.

Having formulated such a hypothesis, Cheney put himself in the position of making a difficult phone call. There was just one scientist in the country Cheney trusted to do the HTLV1 assay, and he suspected she would not be eager to hear from him again.

Harvard Medical School, Boston, Massachusetts

Anthony Komaroff's fury over his Nevada collaborators' move to publish independently of him was dispelled considerably in the last week in January when the Reno team heard from *Lancet*: their article, a detailed description of twenty cases, had been rejected. University of Nevada infectious disease specialist Ray Swarts was philosophical. "One thing this paper did is bring this issue into focus in Reno," Swarts said. "I mean, no other institution in the country has this many people thinking about the same thing. We'll have our day in court. The data is going to get out eventually. In the meantime, as I told Dan the other day, now I know what it's like to feel like Dan Peterson!"

Soon afterward, Komaroff heard from the anonymous reviewers at the *Lancet* on the matter of the manuscript he had submitted with Robert Gallo as one of several coauthors. Clearly the Nevada epidemic continued to generate extreme wariness among the biomedical community. Paramount among the reviewers' complaints was the matter of magnetic resonance imaging scans. The manuscript described 175 patients seen by Paul Cheney and Dan Peterson in their Alder Street practice between 1984 and September 1986. All of them had been subjected to numerous immunological and neurological tests, including brain scans. *Lancet*'s re-

---

* In Japan the disease had been called HAM, for HTLV1-associated myelopathy. Although TSP and HAM were once thought to be different diseases, researchers more recently had come to believe they were the same affliction and, in fact, frequently referred to the malady as "TSP-HAM."
† Harker was white.

viewers rejected the brain scan findings, citing a lack of control scans from healthy people and the fact that the same UBOs were occasionally seen in the brain scans of "normals." But there were other complaints, cumulatively reflective of a wholesale incredulity.

"They can't believe one disease does all the things we're saying it does, or that this many people are sick," Cheney said.

In spite of the negative review, Komaroff was determined to press on with the effort at *Lancet*. The editors held out hope for the manuscript if Komaroff and his collaborators could find ways to resolve the reviewers' doubts.

National Institutes of Health, Bethesda, Maryland

By the end of February the number of calls coming in to the NIH each day from people seeking help or information about chronic fatigue syndrome was equal to the number of calls from the public about AIDS. Judy Murphy, the deputy chief of the office of communications at the National Institute of Allergy and Infectious Diseases, reported that she was fielding hundreds of calls on the subject each month; one-quarter of all calls from the public to Murphy's office pertained to CFS, in fact. Each week she and her staff were mailing out several hundred agency-authored backgrounders on the disease in response to written inquiries. Like the form letters sent to members of Congress seeking information about the disease on behalf of their constituents, the agency's letters assured the public that NIH scientists were "at the forefront" of the research in the field.

University of New Mexico, Albuquerque

On February 8, Dan Peterson flew to Albuquerque. Officially his purpose was to share his clinical experience and research in the brain disorder with infectious disease specialists and other doctors at the University of New Mexico. Unofficially, Peterson had a more pressing objective: he was concerned about one of his patients, Albuquerque resident Nancy Kaiser. "I thought she might become my first fatality from this disease," Peterson said.

Before her illness began more than a decade earlier, Nancy Kaiser had been a happy, even pampered upper-middle-class housewife with a passion for golf. Now, much of the time, she was incoherent and disoriented. She suffered from burning pain throughout her body, blackouts, seizures, and deteriorating eyesight. She had been bedridden for nearly ten years. She already had spent more than $400,000 in her search for a name for her disease, and she had been brushed off by the most prestigious medical clinic in the country, the Mayo, as a hysteric with a psychosomatic pain syndrome. She was referred to the Nevada internist by Wistar Institute director Hilary Koprowski, whom she phoned after her husband read a newspaper article about Koprowski's interest in chronic neurological diseases. Peterson was the two hundred eleventh doctor she consulted. "The general consensus among two hundred and ten of those doctors," Kaiser recalled some years later, "was that I was mentally ill."

Kaiser met with Peterson for the first time in August of 1987, after which she began making monthly pilgrimages to Incline Village. Peterson hospitalized Kaiser and prescribed intravenous acyclovir and, later, when that drug failed to force a remission of symptoms, gamma globulin. Initially, Peterson had been impressed by the degree of Kaiser's intellectual impairment and the duration of her illness. But as he followed her over the course of the fall, he was most acutely impressed by the fact of her rapid deterioration. Most days she was too weak to lift her head from her pillow; her speech was slurred. Her immunologic tests were comparable to those of patients in a terminal state of AIDS. Her IQ, formerly 140, had been measured recently by Sheila Bastien at 85.

Since the local epidemic, Peterson had been an avid reader of the AIDS medical literature, scouring journals for studies about the better-studied immune disorder in hope of finding therapies for his own patients. Sensing Peterson's interest in potential drug therapies, cardiologist Jake Lindsay had been sending him information about Ampligen, a drug undergoing clinical trials in AIDS sufferers. Ampligen's creators claimed the drug stimulated natural killer cells, but it reputedly had additional immune-modulating properties as well. In 1987 a paper appeared in *Lancet* touting the results of the first AIDS clinical trial using the drug.[2] Ampligen's promise seemed so great that shortly after the paper's publication, DuPont, the giant pharmaceutical firm, invested $30 million in HEM (Human Ethical Medicine) Pharmaceuticals, the Philadelphia-based manufacturer of the drug. The two firms entered into a partnership to test the drug in expanded trials. By early 1988 the larger trials had begun, but so far no results had been released.

Aside from Ampligen's apparent clinical safety, Peterson noted that the test subjects who fared best were those who had yet to advance to full-blown AIDS— the AIDS-related complex sufferers—whose clinical symptoms were virtually indistinguishable from those of chronic fatigue syndrome sufferers. When Lindsay suggested to Peterson that he might want to experiment with Ampligen in some of his sickest Tahoe patients, Peterson thought of Kaiser. To do so, however, would require the cooperation of the Food and Drug Administration. Under its "compassionate care" rule, the agency allowed doctors to give experimental drugs to critically ill patients who had failed to respond to traditional therapies.

Executives and scientists at HEM Pharmaceuticals in Philadelphia were receptive to Peterson's proposal. The company had suspected for some time that chronic fatigue syndrome sufferers might be a potential market for Ampligen. Nancy Kaiser's case revived that interest. After talking to Nancy Kaiser, HEM's medical adviser, Hahnemann University oncologist David Strayer, called Peterson in Nevada. "What's this patient like?" he asked.

Peterson sent Strayer a lengthy clinical summary of Kaiser's case, from which Strayer began writing an experimental treatment protocol for submission to the Food and Drug Administration. In the interim, Kaiser was trying to enlist the aid of New Mexico senator Pete Domenici and her Albuquerque gynecologist, John C. Slocumb. Another Albuquerque doctor, University of New Mexico infectious disease specialist Frederick Koster, who had been following Kaiser for more than two years, was critical to Kaiser's success in obtaining the drug, since he was considered her primary care doctor. Unfortunately, Koster was among the 200-plus doctors seen by Kaiser during her decade of illness who preferred a psychiatric diagnosis. Peterson's mission in Albuquerque was to convey to Domenici's staff, Slocumb, and Koster the seriousness of Kaiser's condition and the hope offered by Ampligen.

"We've had people with this disease become demented nursing home patients," Peterson said during a meeting with Slocumb and an aide from Domenici's office the morning of February 8. "My argument about Nancy is, she's rapidly approaching that group of patients. So, failing to accept that, which, I promise you, is going to be the natural outcome, then I'm willing to do something more drastic. I am willing to try Ampligen. It's available for AIDS and should be available for this disease under the [FDA's] compassionate care clause if we do it correctly. The problem is, I'm not her treating physician of record, so I'm not in a position to be any more influential in this particular case. Koster is," Peterson continued. "So he has to be the one to apply for this, be willing to do all the paperwork—and the paperwork is just astounding on compassionate care."

In self-defense, Slocumb, Kaiser's gynecologist, had invited Peterson to speak to internal medicine and infectious disease specialists at the medical school. Slocumb was increasingly convinced of the disease's epidemic nature; he had, in his clinical practice, several score of women suffering from the malady. His conviction was generating friction between him and his colleagues akin to that which internist Carol Jessop had encountered at the University of California.* In a gesture of solidarity, Peterson, accompanied by Berch Henry, described the Incline Village epidemic to the Albuquerque academics, drawing a clinical portrait of the disease while his audience ate catered sandwiches. Frederick Koster attended, taking notes on a small pad and squinting at Henry's slides of human herpesvirus 6 causing human white cells to explode. The week before, Koster had given his own grand rounds on the disease before infectious disease specialists at the medical school. Koster was, in addition, in the process of preparing a research proposal for submission to the NIH.

Portland, Oregon

For months the Portland patients' association had been running a deficit. The cost of responding to inquiries routinely outstripped income from the $12 membership dues. One recent newspaper article alone had generated 20,000 requests for more information about the disease. In February the organization reported in its newsletter that it was launching a search for a new executive director, someone more experienced than Gidget Faubion in federal politics and the financial management of large organizations. The thirty-eight-year-old Faubion was unable to travel on behalf of her organization, as well; because of a severe balance disorder, she could neither fly in planes nor drive a car. In general, the association's newsletter reflected the strain imposed by its organization's monumental growth. "Overwhelmed, understaffed and underfinanced" was how Faubion described the

---

* In fact, in 1990, Slocumb left his academic post in New Mexico to become a medical professor at the University of Colorado. In 1993, he was named chief of general gynecology and obstetrics and head of the gynecology residency program there. "I find a more supportive environment here," Slocumb said in 1995, adding, "but it continues to be difficult because the symptoms of CFS are not thought of as a discrete entity and the scientific data is so complex that, ironically, they are ignored." Nevertheless, Slocumb reported he was "trying to teach residents and medical students about this disease. If they don't want to deal with it in their practices, at least they'll have some idea of who to refer these patients to."

situation in her column, adjectives that characterized the seemingly intractable conditions that would burden advocacy groups for some time to come.

Centers for Disease Control, Atlanta, Georgia

Gary Holmes's name was the first among thirteen authors listed on the paper, "Chronic Fatigue Syndrome: A Working Case Definition," when it appeared in the March issue of *Annals of Internal Medicine*.[3] From that point onward, he was inextricably linked with the government's official diagnostic criteria for the disease. In fact, in the future, the government's definition was known simply as "the Holmes criteria." By 1993, Holmes himself acknowledged that the article had become one of the most cited papers published in clinical medicine.*

The definition itself was reminiscent of a Chinese menu, with a multitude of criteria, major and minor, from which to choose. Major criteria included the new onset of fatigue serious enough to cause a 50 percent reduction in daily activities, persisting for at least six months, "that does not resolve with bedrest." The eleven minor criteria included "unexplained generalized muscle weakness," sleep disturbances, sore throat, painful lymph nodes, low-grade fevers, and generalized fatigue lasting for at least twenty-four hours after exercise "that would have been easily tolerated in the patient's premorbid state." To qualify for the diagnosis, patients needed to exhibit at least eight of the eleven minor criteria and all of the major criteria.

Widely reported in the lay press, the government's definition perpetuated the logic of skeptics like Holmes's superiors Jon Kaplan and Larry Schonberger. Kaplan, in fact, took personal responsibility for the inclusion in the definition of a voluminous list of psychiatric and medical disorders that needed to be ruled out, and for a catalog of twenty-two lab tests that were required prior to rendering a diagnosis. "If any of the results from these tests are abnormal," the authors of the new definition wrote, "the physician should search for other conditions that may cause such a result." In other words, if the patient bore any recognizable signs of disease, the patient, by definition, likely did not suffer from chronic fatigue syndrome.

Hennepin County Medical Center, Minneapolis, Minnesota

In 1988, Philip Peterson, who headed the infectious disease department at the county medical center in Minneapolis, launched a one-day-a-week clinic for chronic fatigue syndrome patients. The medical center was the state's largest public hospital and was also a teaching institution affiliated with the University of Minnesota Medical School. Within a few weeks, four hundred patients from Minneapolis and Saint Paul were enrolled. (By comparison, in Minnesota, which had a population of four million, there were an estimated 350 AIDS cases.)

Peterson's blend of judiciousness, clinical skills, and curiosity had allowed him to recognize the emergence of the disease four years earlier among patients seek-

---

* Holmes's source was the Institute for Scientific Information, a Philadelphia company that tracked and analyzed the flow of bibliographic information in scientific articles and published *Science Citation Index*.

ing care at the medical center. He had formed a collaborative network of a dozen immunologists, infectious disease specialists, and neurologists at the university. He also wrote letters to the approximately twenty infectious disease specialists in private practice in Minneapolis alerting them to the symptoms of the disease and asking them to report cases to him. Though dismayed that his peers at the Mayo Clinic, just two hundred miles south in Rochester, were operating under a conviction that the disease was a form of psychoneurosis, Peterson was convinced that, in time, "the Mayo Clinic doctors will have their views altered along with the rest of us. They're entitled to their view," he added, "but they're dead wrong." For the interim, he continued, "I've had to tell my patients not to go to Mayo."

The clinic's clout hardly worried him, nor did the potential damage to his credibility within the city's medical community. "I could care less what my colleagues think," the athletic-looking, prematurely white-haired Peterson said, "because I know it's an enormously interesting illness, and it becomes more intriguing all the time.

"I can't tell you if there has been an epidemic," he added. "What I can tell you is that none of my clinic patients got ill before 1980, and most of them fell ill in 1984 or later."

The governor of Minnesota, Rudy Perpich, was one of Peterson's biggest supporters. Perpich's twenty-eight-year-old son, Rudy Junior, had been stricken by the disease four years earlier while in his second year of law school at Stanford. Disabled, he was pursuing a reclusive existence in the governor's mansion; his rare lonely walks on the mansion grounds were reported in the local papers almost as if they were UFO sightings. As speculation grew in the local media that the ailment was actually mental illness, the young man's affliction, already a family tragedy, was becoming a political liability.

Like many other investigators with an interest in the disease, Philip Peterson was troubled by the absence of federal support for research. Without federal dollars, his own research, certainly, would be limited. On March 4, the doctor made his concerns known to the Subcommittee on Health and the Environment of the House Committee on Energy and Commerce, chaired by Henry Waxman. "I believe a greater commitment to CEBV research by the National Institutes of Health is warranted," the doctor told the congressmen. Like cancer epidemiologist Seymour Grufferman, Peterson also noted that the agency should earmark money for the disease.

He proposed a series of small grants worth $50,000 to $100,000, "beginning with perhaps $500,000 in the first year and increasing as the CEBV research infrastructure develops to several million dollars a year. . . . By the standards of NIH," he said, "these are relatively small grants, but I believe that these funds would allow a great deal to be accomplished. The research standards of NIH would not be compromised. . . . [The grants] would encourage those researchers already involved in these studies as well as provide impetus to starting new research."

Last, in what was perhaps his most important point, Peterson drew the committee's attention to the deleterious peer review process at the agency. Reviews of these small grants, the doctor said, "should involve researchers knowledgeable about CEBV so that an effective peer review can be made, rather than a review by a committee who may not even be aware that the disease exists."

The NIH spurned Peterson's idea for a series of modest, expedited grants to researchers already performing research in the field; agency officials contended that the mechanism in place was adequate. In addition, Peterson's and his University of Minnesota colleagues' multiple applications for federal support to investigate the cause and natural history of the disease would be rejected for several years to come.

14

Viral Vicissitudes

Since his 1985 article in the *Annals of Internal Medicine,* in which he suggested the disease was either a form of chronic Epstein-Barr virus infection, or an immune dysfunction syndrome of unknown origin, Stephen Straus had given a number of lectures on chronic fatigue syndrome at medical schools across the country—from Washington University's medical school in St. Louis to the Cornell Medical Center in New York City and Harvard Medical School in Boston. The engagements bolstered his image as the national expert—he was, after all, the primary investigator into the disease at the nation's premier biomedical research center—and provided him an opportunity to influence a vast number of medical professionals eager for definitive information on the controversial disorder.

The mantle of expertise rested comfortably on Straus's shoulders. He was a Massachusetts Institute of Technology graduate who had earned his M.D. degree at Columbia University in 1972, after which he had pursued a fellowship in infectious diseases at Washington University in St. Louis. He went immediately from his fellowship to Bethesda, where he worked as a research associate in the Biology of Viruses laboratory within the National Institute of Allergy and Infectious Diseases. In 1979, he was named senior investigator of the medical virology section in the institute's Laboratory of Clinical Investigation. The scientist's sartorial trademarks were tassel-topped loafers and a flawlessly tailored tweed sports coat punctuated with a bow tie. He brushed his wavy red hair back from a lightly freckled pale forehead. Even in casual conversations, he spoke in measured, evenly modulated phrases, his diction precise. He was regarded throughout NIAID as a "good scientist," high praise in Bethesda.

But between the winter of 1985 and the spring of 1988, something had happened to Straus to provoke a radical reassessment of his views of the disease. There were rumors about his sea change among the two dozen patients who had participated in Straus's acyclovir trial. Anyone who attended the huge, twenty-seventh annual meeting of the Interscience Conference on Antimicrobial Agents and Chemotherapy in New York City the previous fall would have noted the turnabout, too: Straus unveiled his new position on the disease in a formal address there. In March 1988 the widely circulated *Journal of Infectious Diseases* published Straus's New York lecture, after which the full force of his reversal began to be felt in the biomedical research community.[1] His article discrediting acyclovir as a treatment for the disease was already in the publishing pipeline, as was his spin-off article, a psychiatric evaluation of the twenty-eight patients in the acyclovir trial. He alluded to these studies in his lecture, referring in parenthetical asides to "unpublished observations," but avoided specifics.

In less than three years, Straus had come to the conclusion that the chronic ailment he described in 1985 was in fact a psychiatric disorder. "It is impossible to completely dispel the notion that the chronic fatigue syndrome represents a psychoneurotic condition," he wrote. "On the contrary, there are observations that support the hypothesis." The scientist's support for his claim seemed thin, indeed. He cited decades-old papers that suggested recovery time from flu and mono might be affected by the patient's psychological state and the "unpublished observations" of NIH psychiatrists who had discovered that some among Straus's patient cohort were depressed. He proceeded to enumerate—and then to discard—evidence of organic illness among people suffering from the disease, including the lesions on Tahoe patients' brain scans, natural killer cell deficiencies, T-cell and B-cell abnormalities, and aberrant antibody levels to Epstein-Barr virus. In spite of these signs of disease, Straus insisted, "ultimately, any hypothesis regarding the cause of the chronic fatigue syndrome must incorporate the psychopathology that accompanies and, in some cases, precedes it." No hard scientific data supporting his claim of psychopathology, either preceding or accompanying the disease, were offered.

At least two patients monitoring events at the NIH were immediately aware of the political implications of Straus's turnabout. Marc Iverson, newly appointed president of the CFIDS Association of Charlotte, now approximately a thousand strong, recognized that Straus had imbued the psychoneurotic theory of the disease with the patina of scientific credibility. With his *JID* position paper, the government's expert had removed the lid from the boiling controversy, loosing upon sufferers the rage of an overburdened medical establishment. Complained another, thoroughly enraged sufferer who had been among Straus's acyclovir patients, "[He] couldn't find out what was causing this illness, and instead of admitting that, he called us psychoneurotic."

Centers for Disease Control, Atlanta, Georgia

Straus's *Journal of Infectious Diseases* editorial was carefully perused by epidemiologists along the Viral Exanthems and Herpesvirus Branch corridor, where the letter lampooning victims of chronic fatigue syndrome still hung. Straus's paper seemed to give them permission to articulate their stereotypical, even hostile, view of sufferers with less fear of reprisal.

"I liked the paper," Gary Holmes said. "Straus said it in such a way that he thinks this is what is going on—that it's psychological. . . . And there is, in talking to hundreds of people with this," Holmes continued, "there is a definite personality." When pressed to describe that personality, he proceeded, somewhat warily: "They're very aggressive. They're very defensive. These people are—I've never really tried to put it down in words, but I can picture the typical person. Frequently they make their symptoms sound so much worse than you would imagine from looking at them. These people are not your average American citizens," he added after a pause. "They are out to get things done—and fast. They're very compulsive. They're very aggressive people. And they want this disease cured."

Indeed, records from the agency reveal that by the end of that year staff in Atlanta were highly focused on the possibility that the disease was actually a kind of character defect. One typical memo proposed "[organizing] an effective battery of psychological tests aimed at assessing possible roles of personality type" in the disease.

Holmes's boss, Larry Schonberger, took Straus's paper as an encouraging sign that the resources of his epidemiology division might not have to be squandered on a non-disease after all. "People like Straus who devote a significant portion of resources and their career [to CFS] are coming up with not too much to show for it at the present time," Schonberger said. "They end up with the negative. So you can understand how people might not think that this is the best way to devote their limited resources. . . . It's cut and dried."

Nalle Clinic, Charlotte, North Carolina

Paul Cheney hadn't spoken to Elaine DeFreitas in fourteen months. When he called her early in March, he avoided all references to chronic fatigue syndrome. Instead he described technical sergeant Cliff Harker's shrinking forearm and atrophied calf muscles. He gingerly proposed his theory that Harker was suffering from tropical spastic paraparesis, a disease recently linked with the first human retrovirus, HTLV1, the virus DeFreitas was tracking in multiple sclerosis. DeFreitas stunned the doctor with her avid interest.

The Wistar scientist's change of heart was attributable to the fact that in recent months she and her associates had turned their attention to studies of tropical spastic paraparesis precisely because of its association with HTLV1. It was the view of her boss, Hilary Koprowski, that several neurological diseases, multiple sclerosis and TSP included, would be found to be closely related to retroviral etiologies. In addition, DeFreitas now had more and better technology in place for studying retroviruses in her lab than she'd had a year before. She was intrigued additionally by Cliff Harker's name, which suggested Harker was outside TSP's known risk group.

"Paul mentioned the fellow's name. It was some very English, Anglo-Saxon name," DeFreitas said later. "I was excited, because I knew he was a non-Hispanic Caucasian. I thought this could suggest infectivity other than what was presumed for TSP, since most TSP is acquired either mother-to-child or from blood donations—it has very, very low frequency sexual transmission." DeFreitas told Cheney she wanted to talk to Harker before the sample was sent. In a telephone call, she questioned Harker directly about his sex life. "The point is," DeFreitas commented later, "he wasn't a monk."

Susan Dorman had been Paul Cheney's research assistant for six months when he asked her to pull a sample of Cliff Harker's blood from the Nalle Clinic's freezer and prepare it for shipment to Philadelphia. Dorman took more than a casual interest in her assignment. For some time, at Cheney's invitation, the shy young woman had been sitting in on his consultations with CFS patients, listening to the doctor take medical histories. "I had a sense of these patients by then," Dorman, who was bound for Duke University's medical school in the fall, said later. "At first, I had been uncommitted, or you could say I had a healthy skepticism. I'm not sure what changed my mind, except seeing the same laboratory tests over and over and hearing the same stories from them over and over. This was a disease that was only starting to be understood, and it would have been hard for me to prove to someone else that it was real. . . . In the meantime, people were suffering in so many ways, I couldn't *believe* the disease was being brushed off."

Dorman liked Cliff Harker. She remembered him as an expansive, affable man of six feet who towered over her desk and, drawing upon a black comedic sense, frequently made her laugh. "He was really nice," Dorman emphasized, "but labile. We were never quite sure what he was going to do. He liked Cheney—I think he trusted him. But I remember he was very emotional." Dorman had not viewed the disease as something that could affect her or other people she knew, however, until she began to meet patients closer to her own age. She was particularly struck by a fourteen-year-old Raleigh girl and a sixteen-year-old Charlotte boy. The girl had suffered from the disease for two and a half years; her parents brought her to her medical appointments in a wheelchair; she had missed two years of school.* The boy had been a star athelete on his high school soccer team and an honor roll student until he fell ill at the start of his junior year. Unlike the fourteen-year-old, he was able to walk, but his health had deteriorated so quickly that it was becoming apparent that he, too, likely would not graduate from high school if his illness continued.

"I had more empathy for the teenagers," Dorman admitted. "I knew you were not supposed to feel like that when you're fourteen or sixteen. The kids really got to me."

Dorman listened carefully to Cheney's TSP postulate. Soon afterward, when she went to the clinic's freezer to extricate Harker's serum from Cheney's vast collection of blood samples, she obeyed an impulse: after pulling the vial filled with Harker's blood from the misting interior of the stainless-steel pantry, she searched for and found the serum of the two North Carolina teenagers. Then, after pausing for a moment, Dorman began searching for a blood sample from another patient—Marc Iverson, whose philanthropy was paying part of her salary. Now she had four frozen vials in her hand. She reached in and grabbed a fifth; it turned out to be a sample from the high school teacher who had undergone surgery for the removal of a malignant tumor from behind her eye.

Dorman followed the doctor's instructions for shipping human tissue samples, packing the clear plastic vials in dry ice in a Styrofoam box. She did not tell her boss about her initiative. After taping the bulky container, she immediately carried it to her car and drove to Federal Express. The package arrived in DeFreitas's lab in Philadelphia early the next day. None of the samples bore identifying markers

---

* Before Cheney became the child's physician, her parents had taken her to the prestigious medical center at Duke University in Durham, where specialists had rendered a psychiatric diagnosis. "She was bedridden," Cheney reported, shaking his head, "and they told her parents she was crazy."

of any kind; the Wistar scientist assumed the extra tubes were control samples drawn from healthy people.

Centers for Disease Control, Atlanta, Georgia

In gayer times, Gary Holmes and his fellow epidemiologists had occasionally indulged in rubber-band fights along the viral epidemiology corridor in Building 6. That spring, however, a grimmer Holmes was mired in responsibilities. His office walls remained enlivened with the satirical commentary on the chronic malady of which he had been designated principal investigator. Increasingly, however, instead of supplying divertissement, the issue was turning his days into a private hell. Mostly, he occupied himself by fending off telephone inquiries from journalists, doctors, and sufferers. The reporters' inquiries were the worst because the stories they wrote based on his interviews generated even more calls. In the late afternoons, before departing for home in suburban Atlanta where his wife and two toddlers awaited him, he would leaf through the accumulated yellow message slips from journalists littering his desk, his unlined, youthful face a study in frustration. "Every time I do an interview," he would complain, "I get, like, a *hundred* calls."

As a result of the case definition's publication in the *Annals,* March was turning out to be a particularly bad month. Complaints from patients and their advocates about the government's new name for the disease were so numerous that Holmes was forced to draft a form letter explaining the decision had not been his alone but a consensus name chosen by eighteen researchers. At mid-month, *Redbook*'s April 1988 issue appeared on the newsstands with a lengthy article on the disease informed by several quotes from Holmes. *Redbook* supplied an address at the CDC where readers might write to obtain additional information. Inquiries were so voluminous that staff operations in two divisions at the agency were disrupted within days of the magazine's distribution. Holmes's boss, Larry Schonberger, hired two temporary secretaries to help his branch's full-time clerical staff respond to the deluge. Within five weeks agency staff had mailed five thousand "fact sheets" about the disease to *Redbook* readers. Requests for information continued to arrive for the next eight weeks.

Holmes himself received so many requests for interviews during the next several weeks that he complained of being unable to do any scientific work for days at a time. "I get ten times as many phone calls as anybody else on this corridor," he said. He spoke enviously of Stephen Straus, his counterpart at the National Institutes of Allergy and Infectious Diseases in Bethesda who, Holmes just learned, recently had installed an answering machine on his line.

One year before, Holmes had told *Hippocrates* magazine that on any given day the disease was "second or third on [his] list [of priorities]." That spring, Holmes said, "I probably spend maybe 75 percent of my time on one aspect or another of CFS. But, without me, *nothing* would be being done." Although Congress had enjoined the agency to engage two researchers to work full-time on the disease the previous fall, a job opening for an epidemiologist had gone unfilled for several months. "We had one guy who was vaguely interested," Holmes explained. "But at the last minute he decided to go elsewhere because he didn't want to get stuck in an area that might be a dead end."

That Holmes lacked the temperament required to cope with a public health crisis, counterfeit or not, of such magnitude was glaringly apparent that spring. Nevertheless, the disease, however bogus, was responsible for his job. "It's what's keeping me here," he said. "Nobody else wants to touch it with a ten-foot pole. I get constant jokes about this, you know—'Oh, I'm so tired, maybe I've got chronic fatigue.' *Nobody* wants to fool with this." Although the agency had failed to award him with a permanent post after his two-year Epidemic Intelligence Service stint, it had extended his temporary status two years in a row. Apparently, as long as Holmes was willing to suffer the slings and arrows that the public and his own colleagues were heaving at him, he had a home at the agency in Atlanta.

Aside from his public relations duties, Holmes did have scientific assignments. Schonberger had assigned to the Texan the work of devising a surveillance strategy to count victims and developing a protocol to compare people with the disease to healthy people—a case-control study. Neither project was close to the launch pad that March, however, and as time passed, the likelihood of their implementation seemed to recede as Holmes witnessed the money Congress had appropriated to the agency for these undertakings—$407,000—mysteriously disappear. He discussed this development in a remarkably candid fashion, his tone suggesting honest bewilderment. His revelations began when he was asked why his superiors were advertising for just one epidemiologist when Congress had mandated that the agency hire two full-time epidemiologists to investigate the disease.

"The problem is," Holmes began, "the money [for salaries] comes out of the money for surveillance—out of the $407,000, see—and it's already down. The $407,000 was immediately chopped up, *sizably,* as soon as it hit the door. From all the way at the top on down, people are chopping out little sections for their own use. And it just goes on apparently all the time. I'm sitting here, and I'm just watching it disappear!"

Holmes was asked who was taking the money and for what purposes.

"I don't know what it's going for," he responded. "I just know that it keeps getting zapped. See, it's appropriated for surveillance. But apparently it's just common practice, when some division gets one of these things, that people who have little pet projects who need some money, they chop out sections. I don't really know who has been chopping what. I get the impression that it's fairly high level."

Was the money that was getting zapped being used to investigate diseases other than chronic fatigue syndrome?

"*Completely* different."

Because the appropriation was shrinking, Holmes continued, one plan to undertake surveillance in five or six cities needed to be revised. "As it is now, we're going to be working on three counties for surveillance, is what we're talking about for surveillance."

Incline Village, Nevada

In March, another patient suffering from chronic fatigue syndrome in Dan Peterson's practice developed B-cell lymphoma. Since the Tahoe epidemic began in 1984, Peterson had witnessed the development of four salivary gland tumors and now five B-cell lymphomas among victims of the disease or their close contacts.

"This is way above normal for a community of eight thousand, I can tell you that," a distressed Peterson said that spring. "We have about forty times the amount we should have."

Denver, Colorado

On March 24, an article by Denver researcher James Jones was published in the *New England Journal of Medicine* on the subject of chronic fatigue syndrome and cancer.[2] Three of his patients with severe chronic Epstein-Barr infections had developed T-cell lymphomas. One of the lymphoma victims was an eight-year-old; all of them died. The doctor cautioned against drawing any conclusions about the chronic disease and cancer, but he told a reporter at the time, "I have an obligation to advise the scientific community that the spectrum of EBV disease is broader than previously expected. The syndrome encompasses a lot of different evils." Jones also said that two of his Denver CFS patients had killed themselves that year.

Centers for Disease Control, Atlanta, Georgia

On March 8 microbiologist Berch Henry, who was continuing to explore the degree of human herpesvirus 6 infection in chronic fatigue syndrome sufferers, left Reno for the uncertain territory of the CDC. Having abandoned an effort to obtain viral samples from the Gallo lab, the virologist had turned to Carlos Lopez, the herpes expert who was heading up the CDC's human herpesvirus 6 research. By March, Lopez and his associates had managed to nurture five different strains of the virus. Lopez invited Henry to Atlanta for a three-day stay during which the Atlanta scientists would give Henry samples of their live virus cultures, and would teach him their methods.

Working side by side with the agency's bench researchers, Henry found himself clamming up on the subject of the disease he and his collaborators were studying so intently in Nevada. He was sensitive to his position as "one of those crazies from Nevada," as he phrased it. He kept his mind on the work at hand—the feeding and handling of the new virus—and avoided being baited about the Nevada epidemic, feigning indifference. Upon his departure, the Nevada scientist's relief was conspicuous.

"I came back to Nevada with the realization that they have no knowledge of this," Henry said later. "I mean, I thought maybe they had a bunch of studies back there that show this is a pipe dream. But what they've got is nothing, basically. They're saying it doesn't exist or it's psychological, because they don't know any better. They're ignorant. . . . Bias—that's the one thing you can't experimentally disprove in a lab."

The agency might have been ignoring CFS, but its virologists were pursuing the new human herpesvirus with vigor. Agency scientists were attempting to unlock the pathogen's genetic sequences. During the week Henry was in Atlanta, animal handlers injected it into two marmosets; one of the two monkeys developed mouth lesions and swollen lymph nodes within five days; the other remained symptomless; eventually both monkeys were found to have become positive for the virus. Carlos Lopez, the scientist spearheading all these efforts, was poised to leave the agency, however. "I have the kind of offer one sees about once in a life-time," he said that March. On April 1 he would become head of the viral labora-tory of Indianapolis-based Eli Lily, one of the largest pharmaceutical companies in the world. When he left Atlanta a few weeks later, he took with him any re-maining enthusiasm for pursuing the vital questions posed by the new brain dis-ease. He gave his bulging file on the subject, stuffed with ambitious but perpetually unfunded "CFS initiatives," to Larry Schonberger, who would now be the sole overseer of epidemiology on the disease.

Longworth House Office Building, Washington, D.C.

Republican congressman John Porter of Illinois was startled to learn in April that the Centers for Disease Control had yet to assign two employees full-time to the Tahoe malady and that the $407,000 appropriation, which Porter had been instru-mental in providing, had been whittled down substantially before surveillance had even been launched. The silver-haired legislator was perplexed, too, by the news that several epidemiologists had turned down the assignment. "But why?" he asked, sincerely puzzled. "It's a great opportunity for someone to make a contri-bution!"

Porter had received more than a thousand letters about the disease from people who had targeted him because of his seat on the subcommittee with appropria-tions power over the NIH and CDC. They constituted the largest collection of let-ters the congressman had received on a single subject during his twelve-year tenure in the House. Porter's staff organized the letters by year and stockpiled them in deep filing cabinets; letters from constitutents were flagged. Rob Bradner, the congressman's aide, reported that the letters arrived at the rate of five to ten a week. "A typical letter is handwritten, at least three pages," Bradner said as he pored over one of the file drawers that spring, thumbing letters from Kentucky, Florida, Missouri, Georgia, California, Minnesota, Mississippi, Oregon, and Col-orado, most of them pleas for research. "They really are dramatic," he continued. "Any idiot can look at this and realize that you've got some very clear symptoms here. I sort of encourage these guys to write to other members, too. You know, it doesn't require pressure for us to work on this. It's something we're interested in."

Wistar Institute, Philadelphia, Pennsylvania

Elaine DeFreitas was fascinated by what she was finding in Paul Cheney's blood samples. She had expected that, at most, she might find one sample positive for retrovirus—that of Cliff Harker—especially since she assumed the remaining four samples had been sent as controls. Instead, using a highly specific test called the "western blot," she found that three of the samples had antibodies to HTLV1. In fact, DeFreitas recalled, the antibody presence in these patients was strikingly familiar to her: the lab results resembled those of her multiple sclerosis patients from Key West.

Intrigued, DeFreitas decided to create cell cultures generated from the samples selected by Susan Dorman. Using this technique, known as in situ hybridization, she found some patients who were positive, as well. DeFreitas tried a third exper-iment, this one to test for the viral protein in the cultures. Again, three of the patients were positive for HTLV1. According to three different tests, then, a majority of the North Carolina blood samples were positive for an exceedingly rare retrovirus.

"We were very excited," DeFreitas recalled.

Charlotte, North Carolina

Three weeks had passed without news from Philadelphia, a period during which Cheney and his assistant Susan Dorman were so busy that Dorman's initiative had simply never been mentioned. Their silence on the subject was broken when DeFreitas called Cheney to tell him three of the five samples he had sent her were positive for a retrovirus on three different assays.

Cheney was momentarily puzzled. "Three out of five what?" he asked.

"Well, you sent me five samples," DeFreitas responded.

"I only sent you one," Cheney said.

"No," the scientist replied, "you sent me five."

Cheney learned at last that his young assistant had sent more than just Cliff Harker's blood to the Wistar lab. He literally jumped into the air in an expression of exuberance after DeFreitas's call.

As DeFreitas later explained in a letter to the doctor, Cheney's patients were the first Caucasians Wistar scientists had found to be infected with HTLV1 who suffered from a chronic neurological disease that wasn't multiple sclerosis. She assured Cheney that her lab considered the matter its highest priority, and she asked him to send ten more samples.

Two weeks later DeFreitas called to report that once again a majority of the samples were positive for the retrovirus. Among the American population, the positivity rate for HTLV1 was .031 percent, according to American Red Cross blood bank officials. In some parts of the country—upstate New York, for instance—the positivity rate was reported to be zero. Unlike the new human herpesvirus, then, which had comparatively high rates of seroprevalency—20 to 60 percent—throughout the population, the virus under study in DeFreitas's lab was exceedingly rare.

Cheney's high spirits were mitigated only by concern about issues of confidentiality. If the news leaked to other researchers before DeFreitas and her Wistar associates were close to publishing, Cheney said, DeFreitas would be hurt. He was particularly worried about Anthony Komaroff. "Tony and I have always shared until now," he said. "But Komaroff is the one person who has the resources to scoop this—if he knew—and DeFreitas deserves all the credit."

Centers for Disease Control, Atlanta, Georgia

By April, Larry Schonberger and his subordinates in the herpesvirus epidemiology branch had settled on three cities in which to establish surveillance; the early plan to study as many as five or six counties, incorporating as many metropolitan centers, had been scrapped. Eventually the team chose Wichita, Grand Rapids, and Atlanta from among ten sites around the nation that had been candidates at one time or another. In defiance of the language that Nevada senator Harry Reid had inserted into the 1988 appropriations bill, Nevada was excluded as a site.

CDC staff members were instructed to keep the sites secret from the press and patient organizations out of a dubious concern that sufferers might move to those cities to be part of the study, skewing any measure of the disease's true incidence in the region. From the beginning, however, three considerably more dire issues jeopardized the study's credibility and ensured that the true incidence of the disease would remain a topic of dispute for some time to come. First, although the agency planned to teach Kansas, Michigan, and Georgia practitioners the new working definition of the disease in a quarterly newsletter so that they might better recognize and diagnose it in their clinics, the agency's definition, itself, was seriously flawed. Virtually every sign of organic illness had to be ruled out before a diagnosis of CFS could be rendered. Second, the system relied on doctors to report cases of the disease to the CDC. But as a telephone survey of doctors in Georgia and Nevada conducted for the agency in two previous years had amply demonstrated, only a tiny percentage of doctors tended to diagnose and report most cases. In both states, a handful of doctors had reported 80 to 90 percent of all cases. In its own official assessment of the survey, the epidemiology branch had concluded that "the data suggest that the geographic clustering of cases may be a function of physician characteristics rather than due to geographic variation in the distribution of disease." Furthermore, as the agency's own Gary Holmes pointed out to Portland patients' organization president Gidget Faubion, "Surveillance programs are notoriously weak in the data that are generated because you are depending upon someone to report the cases. In any surveillance system you expect up to fifty percent of the cases are not reported. Some physicians are very understanding about CFS and do a good job of diagnosing it or ruling it out," Holmes added. "Then there are those who don't diagnose it at all even though they probably see patients who have it."

Third, given the extended schedule for implementation and data-gathering set by the CDC, results would not be available for several years.

In Ottawa, clinician Byron Hyde, who now had several hundred victims in his practice, was particularly scathing in his assessment of the American government's plan. "It is my understanding that, since the Centers for Disease Control has no patient base of its own, has a definition of [the disease] that is not consistent with the clinical approach to the disease, does not intend to examine patients, does not intend to test patients, does not even intend to test patients by their own criteria of exclusion, and intends to avoid known hot spots such as Lake Tahoe, this one-million-dollar study supported by a grant from the United States Congress will represent a major waste of the taxpayers' money. Although perhaps I have misunderstood."

Warren Magnuson Clinical Center, Bethesda, Maryland

Writing about the illness that May in the *Journal of Allergy and Clinical Immunology*, Stephen Straus said: "The demography of this syndrome reflects an excessive risk for educated adult white women. This may reflect either a bias toward the cohort of sufferers who can best afford a sophisticated medical evaluation or some unique constitutional frailty of such individuals. Most patients with this syndrome report excellent prior health. Some had engaged in competitive sports or at least aggressively maintained physical conditioning. A less casual appraisal, however, often uncovers histories of unachievable ambition, poor coping skills, and somatic complaints."[3]

Once again Straus offered no supporting data for his comments and, in a remark that seemed jarringly antithetical to the spirit of scientific inquiry, he added, "It is difficult and at times unpleasant to address the demands of such patients or to test hypotheses as to the etiology of their woes."

Patient organizations were examining Straus's words and actions through an increasingly sharply focused lens. Reluctantly their members were conceding that the scientist who controlled research into their disease at the NIH not only lacked objectivity but seemed also to harbor a degree of hostility to his study subjects, a majority of whom were women.

Furthermore, there was little indication that the situation in Bethesda would improve anytime soon. Just weeks before, Straus's boss, NIAID director Anthony Fauci, had testified before Henry Waxman's House Appropriations Subcommittee. "In the absence of a breakthrough [on CFS]," Fauci told legislators, "we do not know how to proceed."

Washington, D.C.

By the summer of 1988, AIDS patients were represented by nine cooperating national advocacy and information agencies in Washington, each with office facilities and support staff, each fully funded. Writing in the *CFIDS Chronicle* that summer, Barry Sleight, a self-styled lobbyist for victims of the new chronic disease, alerted his fellow sufferers, "In contrast, you have me." Sleight asked for donations to support his efforts. Working out of his apartment, with occasional forays to Capitol Hill, the slight, wan young man, a former bureaucrat, spent his days talking to legislators and their aides about the disease. Often he teamed his efforts with those of Chicagoan Ted Van Zelst.

Privately, Sleight was bracing that spring for what he knew was shaping up to be an ugly battle with proponents of the psychoneurotic theory as articulated by Straus in the *Journal of Infectious Diseases* in March. The federal scientist's article was only one of several broadsides Sleight knew would be fired that year. "There is still a lot of bad research in the pipeline," Sleight warned privately.

University of Connecticut Health Center, Farmington

A trio of Connecticut researchers lobbed the first salvos that summer. More than half of the victims of "chronic fatigue" actually suffered from "undiagnosed mental illness," according to Peter Manu, an assistant professor of clinical medicine at the University of Connecticut, and two of his colleagues, Thomas Lane and Dale Matthews. Manu's findings had been accepted for publication in the *Archives of Internal Medicine* in October.[4] The university's press release resulted in a spate of excited coverage. The headline, "Chronic Fatigue Is Often Mental Illness," which appeared on May 10 in the *Washington Post* above a story by Larry Thompson, was typical.

The mental illnesses identified in patients by Manu and his associates were primarily "major depression" and, to a lesser degree, "somatization disorder," which

Manu defined as a "syndrome of multiple, recurrent physical symptoms" for which no cause could be determined. Eight percent had symptoms of "panic disorder," 6 percent suffered from "dysthymia" (despondency), and 2 percent suffered from what Manu labeled "social phobia." "We believe these people may have an inability to express a psychological or emotional problem," Manu was quoted in the release as saying. "Instead of expressing mental suffering, they do it by pointing to their bodies."

Manu, an internal medicine specialist, had opened a "fatigue clinic" at the university two years before. The doctors ordered the standard round of blood tests on the first one hundred patients to enroll, took their medical histories, and subjected them to the Diagnostic Interview Schedule, a 260-item test devised by National Institute of Mental Health psychiatrists for the purpose of identifying psychiatric disorders. According to the university press release, fifty-nine of the patients who were studied "had one or more mental illnesses" on which Manu and his colleagues blamed the patients' fatigue.

Anthony Komaroff considered Manu's conclusions so wrongheaded that he invited Manu to Harvard for a colloquy on the subject. Manu accepted, but during a heated four-hour discussion in Komaroff's office, refused to back away from his conclusions. In response, the Boston doctor wrote a letter to the *Annals of Internal Medicine,* published in March 1989, in which he noted that, although recent studies "have clearly suggested that mood disorders frequently occur in patients with chronic fatigue," the studies failed to address a "critical" question: "Are the patients fatigued because they have a primary mood disorder, or has a mood disorder developed as a secondary component to chronic organic illness?" He further stated, "It would be inappropriate to conclude from the data of Manu and colleagues that 129 of their 135 patients with chronic fatigue had only a primary psychiatric disorder."[5]

University of Washington, Seattle, Washington

Only days after the Manu results made the news, Seattle psychiatrists Wayne Katon and Randy Riggs released the results of their own research to the nation's press after presenting their data at the annual meeting of the American Psychiatric Association in Montreal. *Newsday*'s story, which was widely syndicated, was typical. "Dr. Wayne Katon and his colleagues found that the majority of people suffering from the latest fad disease—Epstein-Barr or chronic fatigue syndrome—characterized by sheer exhaustion and a laundry list of medical symptoms. . . . may actually be depressed. . . . Patients in the study," reporter Jamie Talan wrote, "complained of eleven different symptoms, despite the fact that detailed and repeated physicals showed hardly any problems. . . . The real differences between patients and the control group emerged from the psychiatric tests . . . 42 percent of the patients were currently experiencing a major depression. No one in the control group was similarly affected." Talan noted that Katon's findings reprised research at the NIH which found CFS sufferers to have "histories of depression, anxiety disorders and phobias."

Katon, who had written frequently about psychosomatic illness, used the same tool for assessing the psychiatric integrity of the twenty patients in his study as did

Peter Manu in Connecticut: the Diagnostic Interview Schedule, or DIS.* This test was the bible of psychiatrists, but it had never been intended for use in assessing the psychiatric status of people suffering from organic, "medical" diseases.

The team had looked for physical differences between patients and healthy controls drawn from university volunteers—medical students, secretaries—and reportedly found none. At least one member of the research team involved, psychiatrist Riggs, had noted profound differences in the day-to-day existences of the two groups, however: "Many of [the patients] couldn't function. They were unemployed or barely able to keep a job," he commented during an interview. "They were having troubles—a *lot* of troubles."

Wistar Institute, Philadelphia, Pennsylvania

Elaine DeFreitas began that summer to discuss her discovery with her boss, seventy-four-year-old Hilary Koprowski, an internationally known scientist who had been on the cusp of most of the great biomedical advances of the last half century. A former president of the New York Academy of Sciences and a onetime Nobel Prize nominee for having created the first successfully tested oral polio vaccine, Koprowski has been jocularly accused of bearing sole responsibility for the European brain drain of the 1950s and 1960s, a period when some of Europe's best scientists came to America. Many of them followed Koprowski to Wistar.

DeFreitas's preliminary evidence of retrovirus infection in CFS sufferers failed to surprise the Wistar chief. Koprowski had long suspected that retroviruses would be found to cause a spectrum of common chronic neurological diseases, including multiple sclerosis, tropical spastic paraparesis, Parkinsonism, and even Alzheimer's. He knew that retroviruses were able to hide in the brain and remain there for years, safely insulated from immune system surveillance, which made them strong candidates for these increasingly common disorders. It was Koprowski's view, in fact, that a biomedical research campaign equivalent to the war on cancer of the 1970s would be imperative to surmount what he believed was an epidemic of related neurological diseases. The malady the government had named "chronic fatigue syndrome" was obviously an infectious central nervous system disease, Koprowski reasoned; it was yet another candidate for retroviral investigation.

DeFreitas knew she was facing a difficult funding problem, however. She had two substantial grants from the NIH, one to study cutaneous T-cell lymphoma, an extremely rare disease, the other to study retroviral infection in multiple sclerosis. She examined the language in her MS grant contract, which authorized her to study the role of retroviruses in "chronic neurological disease." The scientist believed her research on the new disease could be funded legitimately by the government grant, "especially since," she said later, "Cheney was so taken with, and would describe so well, the various neurological deficits some of these people have. I was hearing that from him as an ongoing issue. . . . I decided we could do the chronic fatigue syndrome study under that grant until we had at least enough

---

* Between 1984 and 1995, for instance, Katon authored at least ten articles on psychosomatic illnesses.

preliminary data—actually, *more* than preliminary data; in this disease, you need *hard* data—to get a grant of my own."

Still, DeFreitas was uneasy about committing herself to research in the controversial new field. "It was a risk. I'll be honest with you," she said later.

Miami Beach, Florida

Theories that human herpesvirus 6 caused the new chronic malady were being placed into question by advances in scientists' ability to detect antibodies to the pathogen. By the spring of 1988, researchers at both the CDC and the NIH were persuaded that antibodies were present, to varying degrees, in a majority of healthy controls. On May 10 in Miami Beach, Robert Gallo addressed the annual meeting of the American Society for Microbiology. It was apparent that Gallo's interest in CFS had waned considerably since the early days of his team's Tahoe investigation. The chief of the tumor cell biology lab focused the lion's share of his comments on the virus's behavior in AIDS, suggesting it was a "cofactor" in that disease.

Four days later, *Lancet* published a short article by researchers in Osaka, Japan, that was the first to establish a primary disease association with human herpesvirus 6.[6] The authors contended that the herpesvirus identified by Zaki Salahuddin three years earlier was the cause of roseola, a common baby disease usually lasting three days and characterized by a fever and rash and, on rare occasions, seizures. The scientists had been able to isolate the virus from four babies suffering from the disease, but not from two other children suffering similar symptoms. The Japanese finding met with wide acceptance in the scientific community, but few were satisfied that the virus's mystery had been wholly solved, including the authors of the *Lancet* article. The following year, the same Japanese team described finding HHV6 in the cervical lymph nodes of patients suffering from a degenerative lymph node disease.[7] They went on to ask "whether in patients with [roseola] and in those with HHV6-positive cells the finding reflects primary HHV6 infection or persistent [reactivated] infection."*

In spite of the apparent prevalence of the virus in the population, however, many CFS investigators continued to find evidence for an "association" between it and the disease, even if causation seemed increasingly unlikely. In collaboration with Gallo, Anthony Komaroff reported that, based on an ongoing study of fifty-one New Englanders with the disease, a case could be made for HHV6's role in the disorder. The data, Komaroff wrote in a paper submitted to the Society of General Internal Medicine in late April, "are consistent with secondary reactivation of a latent [HHV6] infection; alternatively, HHV6 may play a role in the pathogenesis of the syndrome, in some patients."[8]

San Francisco, California

On May 23 a group of patients and their supporters in local government met with David Werdegar, the director of the city's public health department, to press their

---

* By 1995 the disease or diseases primarily caused by HHV6 remained in doubt, although the virus continued to be implicated in AIDS, B-cell lymphoma, CFS, and other serious maladies.

agenda. More than anything, the patients wanted the officials to begin to assess the breadth of the epidemic in San Francisco. The advocacy group asked internist Carol Jessop to address the assembled health department officials before they made their pitch. The doctor described the dramatic increase in the number of sufferers in her practice during the previous four years, beginning with twelve patients in 1984 and leading to a crush of 550 sufferers by the summer of 1988. "I have in my ten years in practice seen a lot of things, and I think, besides the AIDS epidemic, this is the most absolutely devastating illness I've ever seen," Jessop told the city's health officers. "People have not expired from this disease but have been known to commit suicide. The morbidity is untold. Jobs lost, relationships lost, suicides, and the cost to the health care system. Most of my patients are on disability. . . . It should be called 'chronic devastation syndrome.' "

Jessop told the health department chief Werdegar that her model for the disease was autoimmunity. Just as other autoimmune diseases like multiple sclerosis, lupus, rheumatoid athritis, and Crohn's disease have their own classic presentation, she said, the new disease sweeping San Francisco would one day be understood to have its own classic presentation, one that would be recognized with similar immediacy by doctors. Unlike other autoimmune diseases, however, CFS was vastly more common. "The thing that is so devastating," Jessop explained, "is that the attack rate is so high. I see two new patients every week, and get calls on a daily basis from everywhere in the United States. I don't have two patients a week with multiple sclerosis; I may have seen five present de novo to me in my entire ten years of practice. I could say the same for lupus, ulcerative colitis, and Crohn's disease—they just don't walk in your door every day." Jessop urged Werdegar to measure the attack rate in the city, as well as the degree of spread to household contacts of victims; she and her collaborator, microbiologist Jay Levy, Jessop said, had laboratory evidence that a virus was likely causing the disease.

Werdegar, in turn, made two commitments to the patients and their advocates that day: his department would randomly survey local doctors about the incidence of the disease in their practices and would convene a medical conference for the edification of the city's medical establishment. Actual surveillance, in which the city would ask doctors to report cases to the health department, was garnering an extremely low approval rating among local health officials, however, and Werdegar avoided discussion of it.

In private conversations, city health officials explained their aversion to undertaking surveillance—or any other public health measures. "I'm personally very interested in this disease, I must admit," city epidemiologist Gisela Schecter commented. "But it's not clear what educational effort would be worthwhile in terms of preventing future cases. With AIDS, it became clear pretty quickly: don't use drugs and don't have unprotected gay sex. With this, what are you going to say, 'Don't shake hands?' Come on—be realistic. I think that's why we're sort of sitting on it."

Fran Taylor, an infectious disease specialist who headed the health department's Bureau of Communicable Disease Control and was Schecter's boss, was unequivocal about her bureau's antipathy to setting up a surveillance system to measure the spread of the disease in San Francisco: "I see the whole thing as too nebulous to deal with," she said. Taylor reported she had been telephoned on occasion by victims of the disease who seemed to her to be exaggerating their complaints. She described them as "clinging . . . which leads one back to the thing that maybe this includes a personality disorder. . . . My gut feeling is that it is a fad diagnosis," she continued, "and the possibility exists that this group of individuals is a social phenomenon as much as a medical phenomenon."

Taylor was surprisingly frank, too, about her own medical bias, which she explained stemmed from her infectious disease training: "I have this job because I don't like to deal with patients," she said. "I can't stand patients who don't get well. I don't want to be their support group. I like to deal with disease *problems.* And you've got a real problem here because if you're going to investigate this as an infectious disease, you've got to have infectious disease specialists involved who don't—who don't particularly want to deal with the patients you're talking about. Now, if and when there is a *defined* disease problem," Taylor added, "then, fine, I'll jump on the bandwagon immediately."

Incline Village, Nevada

The impact of the federal government's stance on the disease was beginning to affect patients in ways that were both broad and highly specific. In Tahoe, for example, where Dan Peterson had identified five lymphomas among his CFS sufferers by that spring, insurers were refusing to pay for the test Peterson frequently ordered to presage the development of lymphoma. Called the kappa/lambda clonal excess assay, the test was typically used by medical oncologists to diagnose and monitor the progression of B-cell lymphomas. Given the apparent high rate of lymphoma among CFS patients in Nevada, Peterson believed the test's expense was justifiable in his sickest patients. He had already discovered lymphoma in one CFS patient using this test. When Peterson wrote to Blue Cross/Blue Shield of Idaho to explain why he considered the test useful in some patients, the insurer sought Gary Holmes's counsel on the matter. Holmes apparently assured the company that there was no place in standard clinical medicine for kappa/lambda clonal excess assays. Citing Holmes's authority, Blue Cross/Blue Shield informed Peterson that it had no compelling reason to reimburse his patients for the test.

On May 30, in an effort to correct the problem, Peterson wrote Holmes, explaining his use of the kappa/lambda assay in certain critically ill patients. "I would like to update you on the current conditions at Lake Tahoe," he began. "We now have five patients who have developed B-cell lymphoma from the original study group. . . . In one case, patient B.C. was followed periodically with kappa/lambda clonal excess, which became positive for marked monoclonal excess. Due to this change and the known prevalence of this finding in B-cell lymphomas, the patient had exploratory surgery with splenectomy and liver biopsy which did document well-differentiated B-cell lymphoma. It is upon this basis that I do find the kappa/lambda clonal excess very useful."

Peterson took the opportunity to tell Holmes about other worrisome developments in Tahoe, and asked Holmes for his suggestions:

Additionally . . . a significant portion of our original group has now developed progressive [MRI brain scan] changes which are being read as:

"large lesions consistent with demyelinating process such as multiple sclerosis." I have attached a copy of the reports in such a progressive patient. These scans have been independently reviewed by other reviewers.

Your opinions in these findings and the way in which we should proceed in the research would be much appreciated. I also have a large stockpile of sera that have been collected over the past three years and I do, of course, have sera from ten babies who have been born to affected mothers. I look forward to hearing your thoughts regarding these matters.

Gary Holmes responded to Peterson on July 7. His letter, in part, follows:

Thanks for your recent letter about CFS. The case histories of the patients who you presented in the letter are quite interesting. However, I believe most of the researchers in the field agree that CFS is a diagnosis of exclusion, and that the identification of other diseases, such as the lymphomas that occurred in your patients, or of MRI abnormalities that are suggestive of multiple sclerosis, moves such patients out of the CFS category. CFS is little more than a collection of symptoms at the present time, and it remains highly likely that many patients' symptoms are actually caused by occult lymphomas, multiple sclerosis, or any of multiple other chronic diseases that may not be diagnosed in the initial evaluation. Continued grouping of patients who have such definitive diagnoses as lymphoma or multiple sclerosis under the title of CFS may artificially imply that such patients have a single cause for their varied illnesses. . . .

Regarding your own research, I can provide no specific recommendations. Probably the best advice I can give is to link up with researchers at the University of Nevada, Reno or at other nearby university medical centers, although I believe you have already done so. . . . With regard to the possible cluster of lymphomas that you mentioned, I would suggest you contact . . . the Cancer Branch, Division of Chronic Disease Control, Center for Environmental Health and Injury Control, CDC. . . . This group has expertise in investigating cancer clusters.

Peterson, not surprisingly, found Holmes's response chilling. If Holmes's agency persisted in this view, the doctor added, its surveillance system would generate meaningless data. "If [Holmes's] criteria is, 'no other disease, no immunological abnormality, no organic brain syndrome,' he's going to find nothing—except crazy people. He's going to prove his own point," Peterson said. "So he doesn't have to spend four hundred thousand dollars proving that. I'll accept that hypothesis before he spends the money!"

Interestingly, the incidence of lymphoma in the nation had tripled since 1950, its rate of increase trailing only lung cancer in women and skin cancer. Therefore, the agency's decision to exclude from its case definition any patient with a malignancy meant that if there was a connection between CFS and lymphoma, it would be missed, since anyone with cancer would be eliminated from the surveillance plan.

But even if the agency did include CFS patients who developed cancer in the surveillance study, a major piece of the puzzle would still be missing. Two of the four cases of cancer that Seymour Grufferman was studying among members of the North Carolina orchestra were people who had never had CFS. One was the spouse of a CFS sufferer in the orchestra; another was an orchestra member who had never had symptoms of CFS. In order to determine whether a rise in cancer was concomitant with outbreaks of CFS, therefore, it was necessary to study not only people with CFS but also the people *around* them.

Mayo Clinic, Rochester, Minnesota

In June, the *Mayo Clinic Health Letter* included its second report in four years on the malady afflicting so many of the people who sought help in Rochester each year. The article carried the headline: "Chronic Mononucleosis: No Disease Underlies this Common Complaint." "Is there a new disease caused by E-B virus?" the authors of the article asked. "We think not . . . If E-B virus is not at fault, how can we explain the widespread reports of these symptoms?" The Mayo authors never answered the question; instead, they cautioned their nearly half a million readers: "Remember, it's just that—a syndrome, or collection of symptoms. In most cases, there is no serious underlying disease causing chronic fatigue syndrome."

Nalle Clinic, Charlotte, North Carolina

By early June, DeFreitas had tested even more of Cheney's patients for HTLV1. The rate of positivity was extremely high for such a rare virus, usually at least 50 percent, and sometimes higher. As DeFreitas pursued her experiments, however, the retrovirus's identity was becoming ambiguous. The epidemiology of the disease simply didn't support a case for HTLV1. It was too rare in the population—.031 percent according to the Red Cross—and almost never found in white Americans unless they used intravenous drugs. In addition, no human retroviruses were thought to be casually transmitted. DeFreitas was beginning to wonder if she had stumbled onto an entirely new retrovirus, the first that could be transmitted casually, like a cold virus.

The scientist's early evidence for the presence of HTLV1 might well have been the result of a related retrovirus's cross-reaction with her chemical probe. Such cross-reactions were common in retroviral research; families of viruses bore certain likenesses to one another and shared common properties, and the probes humans devised to identify them were imperfect.

DeFreitas's investigations were complicated by something else: although positivity rates were high in cell cultures at the end of the first week, positivity rates among the same cultures plummeted by the second, third, and fourth weeks. "It's there, it's there, it's there—it's gone" was how DeFreitas described the phenomenon. The scientist began to look for the virus at regular intervals over time.

"We found that, to be on the safe side, we could only grow the cells for six days," she said, before the cultures turned negative for the virus. "Seven days was the cutoff. Either the cell that supports the virus dies in the culture, which is what I favor as an explanation, or the virus has particular nutritional needs that we're not supplying in our culture system—zinc, cobalt, something very bizarre that we've never needed to add before."

Cheney, too, favored the first explanation, blaming the cell death on the famously lytic, or cell-destroying, herpesvirus prevalent in chronic fatigue syndrome sufferers: HHV6. In a reference to the NIH's Tom Folks, who had searched without success for a retrovirus in patients in 1986 using the same techniques, Cheney noted, "Human herpesvirus six may be the reason no one has found this retrovirus before. What seems to be happening is that HHV-six is co-infecting T-cells—it blows up the T-cells, the cells that would host the retrovirus—so nothing's there. So this is one of those really cruel things where we've been blinded by our technology. It may be that HHV-six plays an extremely important role in modulating the infection, allowing it to further embed itself in the immune and nervous system.

"But—why is this happening?" Cheney asked after a pause. "There is something *unbelievable* going on. The most amazing thing is that I had a hint of this long ago. Elaine [DeFreitas] found it in 1985, but we didn't know what it meant," he continued in a reference to the handful of blood samples from Tahoe that De-Freitas had evaluated late that year, before Cheney's departure from Nevada. De-Freitas had discovered suggestions, though not proof, of retroviral infection in these samples. If the new findings panned out, he continued, "this could be extremely embarrassing to a lot of people." Cheney was thinking about the government scientists who had preferred to promulgate theories about mass hysteria and neuroses instead of vigorously investigating the epidemic.

On May 1, Zaki Salahuddin and his colleagues in the Gallo lab, the discoverers of the new herpesvirus, presented to the American Society for Clinical Investigation a paper that lent credence to Cheney's theory about the role of human herpesvirus 6 in the disease. Their report stated that the virus seemed mostly to infect T-cells in an early stage of development. They suggested for the first time that the virus should be viewed as a potential cause of immune system disorders, "including T-cell disorders." Significantly, the Gallo group had found AIDS patients' T-cells to be co-infected with the new herpesvirus and HIV. Because HIV itself killed only a small number of T4 cells, the herpesvirus might be responsible for the eventual annihilation of T4 cells in AIDS, the team said.

London, England

On Sunday, July 17, the *Times* of London reported that myalgic encephalomyelitis, a.k.a. yuppie flu, was "all in the mind." "The fastest growing 'disease' in the West may not be a disease after all," wrote medical correspondent Neville Hodgkinson in a banner-headlined article. "Once thought to be a shirker's disease, with outbreaks owing much to mass hysteria, ME (myalgic encephalomyelitis) became respectable last year when scientists announced that evidence of a lingering viral infection (enterovirus) was present in many sufferers. . . . It is now said to afflict 100,000 in Britain alone, with similar outbreaks sweeping Australia, the United States, and several European countries."

Irrespective of the enterovirus finding, Hodgkinson continued, doctors in the cardiology unit at London's Charing Cross Hospital had determined that the "viral theory is a red herring." Sufferers were people with "four-star abilities with five-star ambitions" who were "battle fatigued" from trying so hard. The Charing Cross team called the disease a syndrome of hyperventilation "in which the struggling individual unconsciously keeps the body in a hyper-aroused state by breathing slightly faster than normal."

Hodgkinson's story was typical of coverage, occurring on both sides of the Atlantic, that routinely spun readers 180 degrees away from earlier theories without explanation or evaluation. Just eighteen months earlier, Hodgkinson himself had written a *Sunday Times* article that proclaimed in its headline, "Virus Research Doctors Finally Prove Shirkers Are Really Sick." The reporting of journalists in England and the United States was driven mostly by the issuance of press releases written by the public relations staffs of institutions whose scientists or doctors had undertaken the research. As a result, the malady's identity bobbed haplessly like a rudderless boat, vulnerable to every wind and current, "real" one day, imaginary the next.

New York City

Stephen Straus had been effective in disseminating his newfound view of the disease throughout the medical press that year. On July 28, *New York Times* nutrition writer Jane Brody gave Straus a platform in the lay press in her widely syndicated health column. This "problem has been around for at least 30 years," Brody wrote, "and probably for more than 120. . . . In the 1860s, (Stephen Straus) believes, it was known as neurasthenia (a neurosis characterized by weakness and fatigue). In the twentieth century, it has been identified as anemia, chronic brucellosis, hypoglycemia, systemic candidiasis and, most recently, chronic Epstein-Barr virus syndrome. . . . 'It seems quite likely that there is not one cause for chronic fatigue syndrome, but rather a number of different factors that can trigger a similar set of symptoms,' Straus said."

Straus went on to explain that he and his colleagues at the NIH had "demonstrated that many patients were psychologically 'different' long before they developed the syndrome." Brody added that Straus "described some patients as having been anxious and depressed with various neurotic symptoms for years before becoming ill."

Predictably, Straus's comments, published in scores of metropolitan newspapers, served to inflame patients whose personal experience belied the theory he was championing. Sam Josephs (a pseudonym), a former dentist who had been wholly disabled by the disease and who was one of five directors of the Massachusetts CFS Association, wrote a letter of complaint to Anthony Fauci, the director of the National Institute of Allergy and Infectious Diseases and Straus's boss. "[T]his is the most unprofessional statement that can be made by a doctor about an illness without being able to quote any study or specific survey," Josephs wrote in a reference to Straus's contention that patients were "psychologically different" before they ever fell ill. Josephs accused Straus of "grossly misinforming the public, the taxpayers who foot the NIH bill. . . . This is plain malpractice by Dr. Straus. This is a disservice to the American people."

Josephs went on to cite anecdotal reports from support-group leaders around the country of high suicide rates among sufferers, a phenomenon he suggested was incited by the medical establishment's failure to properly diagnose the disease and by its eagerness to consign victims to the netherworld of mental disorders. "[Sufferers] have what we call in the medical profession iatrogenic depression, or depression caused by the physician," the dentist said. "Has Dr. Straus helped to alleviate the depression, this iatrogenic depression that is appearing in CFS patients across America, or has he fostered it? It is obvious he has fostered it. He has committed gross negligence."

Josephs ended his letter by asking Fauci to "take corrective action to discipline Dr. Straus and remove him from NIH at the earliest possible date."

Fauci's response to Josephs illuminated a cardinal moment in the history of the disease. Straus's views, once his own, had risen to the highest levels of the agency, from middle-level medical researcher to agency head. Far from apologizing for Straus's comments to the press or for his agency's research tack, Fauci went on to cite Connecticut doctor Peter Manu's study in support of Straus. The Connecticut researcher, Fauci assured Josephs, "found that half of the patients in his chronic fatigue study were suffering from undiagnosed mental illness." Fauci even thought to enclose with his letter the University of Connecticut Health Center's press release heralding Manu's findings. "If we can be of further service to you, please feel free to contact us. Best regards," Fauci concluded.

Josephs was hardly appeased. He wrote to Washington lobbyist Barry Sleight describing Fauci's letter and expressing his dismay that Fauci was unaware or unconcerned that Connecticut's Peter Manu had failed to select his patients according to any known diagnostic criteria for CFS.

"Dr. Fauci has *no* understanding of the illness," Josephs complained to Sleight in his letter. "This is a major, catastrophic problem for us with CFIDS. When the director of NIAID does not understand an illness and starts misquoting medical articles, we have a situation that must be corrected. We need millions from NIH to combat this disease, but we cannot get far if the disease is not understood by those at NIH who are responsible for doling out the money."

American Medical Association, Chicago, Illinois

As lonely CFS lobbyist Barry Sleight had predicted, 1988 was turning out to be a very bad year for victims of the new disease. Yet another study linking "chronic fatigue" with depression and hypochondria appeared that summer, this time in the August issue of the *Journal of the American Medical Association.*[9] Although the researchers at the Brooke Army Center in Fort Sam Houston, Texas, never claimed to be studying people suffering from the specific entity "chronic fatigue syndrome," recently defined by the CDC, *JAMA*'s press release did not make the crucial distinction, nor did the lay press, which covered the finding as if it were a breakthrough in the search for the cause.

The researchers focused the brunt of their clinical investigation on their subjects' emotional lives, administering numerous psychological tests. "Depression or somatic anxiety or both were suggested by screening. . . in eighty-two fatigued patients, compared with three [of twenty-six] controls," the authors reported. The researchers recommended "psychoactive drugs" and exercise for such patients.

The Charlotte-based newsletter tackled the subject in its fall issue. "There is a raging debate within the medical community as to what chronic fatigue syndrome is and its place in the medical universe," Paul Cheney wrote. "[W]e who believe this is a real disease are almost in a death grip with those forces who would stifle debate, trivialize this problem, and banish patients who suffer from it from beyond the edges of traditional medicine. These individuals and institutions seem to be universally those which have no clear understanding of this syndrome, do not listen to these patients in any numbers, and whether they know it or not, are increasingly at risk of finding themselves on the outside looking in."

Even after venting his dismay in the *CFIDS Chronicle,* however, Cheney found it hard to drop the Texas study. Eventually he compared the Texas patients with his own database derived from 250 patients and discovered that the two groups exhibited distinct differences. Half of the Texans were hypertensive; just 2 percent of Cheney's fatigue patients had high blood pressure. The Texans were also heavier smokers and drinkers; they had more cardiac problems, more diabetes, and less education; and they were, on average, twenty years older. They also had normal sed rates. The point, as far as Cheney was concerned, was made: chronic fatigue was not chronic fatigue syndrome.

New York City

Only one journalist in the country examined the Brooke Army Medical Center study with suspicion: Neenyah Ostrom, a reporter for the *New York Native,* a lively Manhattan-based gay newsweekly whose editor and publisher, Charles Ortleb, was deeply distrustful of the government's handling of the AIDS epidemic.* Ortleb, in fact, increasingly suspected the AIDS outbreak was merely a modest subset of the more pervasive, immune-damaging epidemic disease claiming heterosexuals—chronic fatigue syndrome. In effect, in a logistical leap that was not entirely devoid of merit, Ortleb believed AIDS and CFS were virtually the same disease, with one obvious difference: the outcome. He was further convinced that HHV6 was the primary cause, not the cofactor, as Gallo would argue persuasively in years to come, and insisted that the widespread presence of the newly discovered herpesvirus in the population supported, rather than upended, theories about its role as the outbreak's cause.

Ostrom, whose unusual beat was AIDS and chronic fatigue syndrome, titled her report on the subject, "Chronic Fatigue Syndrome: It's a Dirty Little War." She

---

* The Kansas native, who was thirty-eight in 1988, had been steering his irreverent weekly from its cultural focus toward matters of health and science since the early 1980s, alienating a sizable portion of his readership along the way. Ortleb was nothing if not iconoclastic; even before acquired immune deficiency syndrome had a name, his relentless coverage of the new epidemic was marked by fierce attacks on the government's research agenda. Robert Gallo's announcement in April 1984 that the third human retrovirus was the cause of the malady decimating the gay community failed to impress the publisher. In one memorable issue, Ortleb featured the nation's most famous biomedical research scientist on the *Native*'s cover with a bowl of fruit on his head and hoop earrings à la Carmen Miranda. In spite of, or because of, such antics, the *Native* could often be spied on scientists' desks at the NIH and CDC.

wrote, "The singularly most important aspect of this article is the confusion it creates. . . . At best, it is intellectually sloppy. At worst, it represents a deliberate attempt to convince the medical community that CFS is actually misdiagnosed depression and somatic anxiety."

Incline Village, Nevada

In August, Nancy Kaiser moved from Albuquerque to Incline Village to become "Patient 00" in the first clinical trial of Ampligen in the Tahoe malady. Kaiser had sought to begin the treatment in Albuquerque, but Frederick Koster, her primary care clinician at the University of New Mexico, declined to help. Dan Peterson and his staff in Incline Village took on the task, but Peterson insisted Kaiser move to Nevada for the duration.

Medical oncologist David Strayer, who was overseeing the AIDs clinical trials of Ampligen for its manufacturer, HEM Pharmaceuticals, worked with Peterson to create a formal treatment protocol. "Because the drug is experimental and the disease is so poorly understood," he said later, "we knew the study would have to involve a patient who was at the far end of the spectrum—someone totally disabled who had failed other therapies. The patient had to have brain lesions. [The patient] had to fit the CDC criteria, too, but the biggest criterion was brain lesions."

Kaiser qualified. "She couldn't walk twenty-five feet without having to stop and rest," Strayer said. "She couldn't read. She was having seizures. Her IQ had dropped. We were worried she was going to die."

Strayer flew to Reno soon after Kaiser's arrival, bringing the drug with him from Philadelphia. Ampligen was an extremely fragile substance that needed to be packaged in glass and remain frozen until its use. Even the temperature at which Ampligen thawed was crucial. Taking no chances, Strayer had sent ahead a defrosting machine that was specially calibrated to melt the drug without damaging its molecular structure.

In a quiet, little-used storeroom in Peterson's Alder Street offices, the fifty-three-year-old Kaiser received her first dose on August 9, with Strayer and Peterson at her side. "In retrospect," Peterson said some years later, "the drama was excessive. It took an hour. We monitored her vital signs—her temperature, her pulse. Mostly, I remember being relieved that she could tolerate the drug. Nothing good happened, but nothing bad happened, either."

Strayer remained in Incline Village for several days, carefully monitoring Kaiser's next three infusions, each of them two days apart.

15

Return from the Living Dead

Charlotte, North Carolina

Paul Cheney and Elaine DeFreitas pursued their collaboration into the summer, with Cheney and his assistant, Susan Dorman, cataloging and shipping vials of blood to Philadelphia on a weekly basis. "They went in batches," Dorman recalled. "We would send as many as [DeFreitas] could handle," sometimes twenty-five at a time. Using a centrifuge, Dorman spun the patients' whole blood until it turned clear amber, becoming pure serum. Then she poured the substance into small tubes, corked them with green rubber stoppers, packed them in dry ice and Styrofoam, and dialed Federal Express for immediate pickup. Nevertheless, by July, Cheney was discouraged. Serum samples from 250 patients had been shipped to Philadelphia, but the doctor sensed that "things were not really being pressed." Cheney had hoped to help DeFreitas prepare a paper on the finding by summer's end. Now he worried that DeFreitas was losing interest; she had not even returned his phone calls for some weeks.

In August, Cheney sent Susan Dorman to Philadelphia to spend two days in De-Freitas's lab. "The purported purpose was for us to dump our patient information into their computer," Dorman recalled later, "but in effect, we wanted her to know we were real, that we existed. And I think, ultimately, [the visit] put to rest Cheney's fears that she thought he might be crazy."

U.S. Congress, Washington, D.C.

On August 9 a House-Senate conference committee more than quadrupled the previous year's appropriation for the chronic malady, mandating that $1,182,000 be spent in the next fiscal year by the Centers for Disease Control. The bill specified that the agency expand surveillance and assign eight additional full-time investigators to perform research. As usual, legislators also asked for increased research at the National Institutes of Allergy and Infectious Diseases, but they failed to specify a dollar sum. Finally, the bill asked the Social Security Administration to standardize its guidelines, in consultation with the NIH and CDC, for awarding disability payments to people with the disease. Just how many CFS patients were applying for disability awards from the Social Security Administration was unknown because the agency lacked an official listing for the disease, a situation that remained uncorrected until 1994.*

Chicago's Ted Van Zelst and other patient advocates were jubilant. Eight federal scientists would turn their full-time efforts toward the devastating disease. That not even one person was working on chronic fatigue syndrome full-time, in violation of the previous year's legislation, was of concern to Van Zelst and others, but they expected that to change with the new appropriation. As for the rapid dissipation of the 1988 appropriation, lobbyists and patients were unaware it had occurred.

Charlotte, North Carolina

In August the *CFIDS Chronicle* published an appeal by Denver patient Craig Barshinger to patients and their families for contributions to support the research of Denver researcher James Jones. The desperate Barshinger offered a pathetic promise to *Chronicle* readers: "The government will believe CFS is real if you make a sacrifice."

Dunedin, New Zealand

Increasingly, an emerging pandemic was reflected in medical journal articles from around the world. The enduring mystery—the cause of the disease—was paramount in these reports. At least one group of investigators in Dunedin, New Zealand, was increasingly suspicious that retroviruses were involved. On August 10 the *New Zealand Journal of Medicine* published an article by general practitioner J. C. Murdoch describing immune dysfunction in Dunedin patients with myalgic encephalomyelitis syndrome.[1] Murdoch described a range of immune aberrations, including the same T-cell aberrations already noted by Paul Cheney, Dan Peterson, Seymour Grufferman of the University of Pittsburgh, Nancy Klimas of the University of Miami, and others. Murdoch called T-cell depreciation "the outstanding immune deficit in the disease," a finding, Murdoch added, that "suggests that [ME] may be the result of acquired immune deficiency." AIDS, of course, was one form of acquired immune deficiency. "It is altogether possible that further retroviruses exist causing a spectrum of ill-health in the community," Murdoch wrote. He added that "further investigation of [myalgic encephalomyelitis] . . . might be able to reveal such a factor." Murdoch was unaware that just such an investigation was under way in the United States.

Centers for Disease Control, Atlanta, Georgia

Late that summer, acceding to stepped-up pressure from Nevada's senators, the CDC reversed itself on the matter of expanding surveillance to Nevada. Reno, Carson City, and Incline Village would now be included. Walter Gunn and Gary

---

* In December 1985, administrators in the disability office of the SSA had asked their field officers to make photocopies of claims for the disease and send them to the Baltimore headquarters. According to CFS lobbyist Barry Sleight, who was monitoring the process, "They yelled 'Stop!' when they got to one hundred thirteen. Apparently they had been under the impression it was a rare disease." Out of the 113 claims reviewed by the SSA administrators, only 26 claimants had been awarded disability.

Holmes were to serve as co–principal investigators for the study. Gunn was named project officer in charge of surveillance.

If Americans suffering from the Tahoe malady needed an angel of mercy four years into the epidemic, he came that fall in the form of a prematurely white-haired, avuncular fifty-three-year-old who resembled nothing so much as an Amway salesman. Gunn was a towering former navy officer who had earned a doctorate in psychology before joining the agency in 1972. Innocent of the transforming nature of the work he was about to undertake, he was looking forward to a vigorous early retirement in two years.

In the years ahead, Gunn would suggest that it was the "data" that changed his mind about the malady, a conversion that would mark him as a rogue among his colleagues. But he admitted later that "What colored my view was genuine hands-on experience with patients. You didn't get the picture of malingering or laziness or even depression with these patients. You got the impression of someone who was sick.

"The first patient I met was a young man of thirty," Gunn continued. "He was a corporate vice president in Atlanta. He skied in Aspen and hiked the Appalachian Trail. He was a normal, successful thirty-year-old. But one day, he got the 'flu.' And you know the rest. I just didn't see him as crazy. He didn't say anything bizarre. He didn't have any strange reasons for having the disease. Maybe it takes a psychologist to realize these patients don't have a psychiatric disease."

National Institute of Allergy and Infectious Diseases, Bethesda, Maryland

In the fall of 1988, eight research groups submitted grant proposals to Ann Schleuderberg. Seven of the eight, among them Seymour Grufferman's and Nancy Klimas's, were resubmissions. All seven investigators had carefully reworked his or her proposal to accommodate the criticisms of the agency's epidemiology study group whose members had dismissed their first attempts.

On the second round, every grant was turned down except Anthony Komaroff and Dedra Buchwald's proposal to study the incidence of the disease in a large health maintenance organization in Seattle. The NIH agreed to pay out approximately $800,000 over the next five years to support Komaroff and his colleagues.

Seymour Grufferman was enraged by the fashion in which Schleuderberg had managed the second round of submissions. What dismayed him, in particular, was that the new ad hoc panel assembled to study the second round of grant applications included psychiatrists but lacked an epidemiologist. Grufferman's proposal, like a number of the others, had at the agency's request been oriented along epidemiological lines. "These people simply didn't understand the language!" Grufferman said.

Wistar Institute, Philadelphia, Pennsylvania

As fall began, Elaine DeFreitas was working on several new experiments to tease out the mysterious retrovirus from the North Carolina sera. So far she had tested about 250 samples from Paul Cheney's North Carolina patient cohort. The percentages of patients who were positive for her new retrovirus, based on the presence of antibody, remained stable—50 to 75 percent. DeFreitas and Cheney were confident they had made an important finding, but DeFreitas wanted to move the investigation to a higher level. Until then her tests had been focused on retrovirus antibodies. That fall, as Cheney explained, "we needed to move off of antibody and into looking for the virus itself."

One of DeFreitas's Wistar colleagues had recently discovered that HTLV1 inhabits macrophage cells, a third class—along with B-cells and T-cells—of immune system cell. Manufactured in bone marrow, macrophages have been compared to Pac-Man because they seek out and destroy invading antigens, enveloping and literally consuming them. DeFreitas had been looking for the bug in T-cells. A colleague suggested that she separate macrophage cells from the other cells in her cultures and create separate macrophage-only cultures. DeFreitas tried the new tack and met with immediate success.

DeFreitas was particularly dazzled by the amount of virus the experiment detected. In some of the samples the virus was infecting as much as 3 percent of all the cells, an enormous number, considering that in the Swedish MS patients, by contrast, the virus infected from one cell in ten thousand to one cell in a million. If searching for a novel retrovirus in MS patients had been like looking for a needle in a haystack, as DeFreitas would eventually comment, this was like looking for a Volkswagen in a haystack.

"What that meant," Cheney said, "was that these people were royally infected with that virus. Which means that their symptoms were very likely due to that virus. Elaine and I were excited," he continued, "because this was the first time we had any evidence that the western blots [which detected antibodies] were indeed indicating what we *thought* they were indicating. We were looking at virus."

On September 14, Cheney flew to Philadelphia to meet the scientist he had known only as a voice on the phone since 1985. He arrived at Spruce and Thirty-sixth Streets early in the morning, passed through graceful, tall, wrought-iron gates, and found himself inside the courtyard of the Wistar's three-story brick-and-sandstone Victorian mansion, erected ninety-eight years before.* He made his way through the marble foyer, where glass cases recessed into the walls held silver urns containing the remains of former directors, and proceeded to the third floor, where, at the end of a long corridor, he found Associate Professor Elaine DeFreitas in her lab. Cheney spent the day with the immunologist.

"The laboratory was somewhat in disarray," Cheney recalled. "Elaine is a frenetic woman, and she had too much to do. She had like fifty irons in the fire, and this was just one of them. An important one. But whereas most of her other projects had a postdoctoral fellow on them, this one did not. It had only Elaine, and

---

* Built in 1892, the Wistar was the result of the largesse of a Philadelphia lawyer whose uncle happened to be Caspar Wistar, the first medical school professor of anatomy in the United States; the nephew sought to erect a suitable museum in which to house Dr. Wistar's extraordinary collection of anatomical specimens. In 1957 one of Hilary Koprowski's first directives as chief of the venerable institute was to demand that a massive whale skeleton be removed (to the Field Museum of Natural History of Chicago) and that additional laboratories be constructed in the space left behind.

Elaine wasn't in the position to give it the kind of focus that a postdoc could give it."

The Twentieth Century Club, Pittsburgh, Pennsylvania

A plush private women's club was the site of a two-day government "workshop," formally titled "Considerations in the Design of Studies of Chronic Fatigue Syndrome," in mid-September. The NIH and the University of Pittsburgh were the official hosts, a development that arose from the nascent, and ultimately short-lived, friendship between the grant program administrator for the new disease, Ann Schleuderberg, and Pittsburgh's ambitious cancer epidemiologist, Seymour Grufferman. Schleuderberg explained that the purpose of the meeting was to enable the scientists seeking federal grants—only one of whom, Anthony Komaroff, had so far been successful—to design better research proposals by exposure to scientific bigwigs. Grant applicants, Schleuderberg said, needed a firmer grounding in the tenets of epidemiology and multidisciplinary research. "The idea," she added, "is to have a body of experts—people who are thoughtful, senior scientists—[who] will not have a vested interest in it, so that we have a point and counterpoint opportunity."

As a result, some of the nation's best-known Epstein-Barr virus scientists attended, as did a number of epidemiologists, psychiatrists, and biostatisticans. Lamentably, a majority of the experts who had been invited to speak over the course of two days by Schleuderberg and Stephen Straus, the latter a co-chair of the meeting along with Grufferman, were unfamiliar with CFS. University of Alabama epidemiologist Philip Cole's comment was typical: "I learned about this entity at the time I was invited to speak here."

Attendees gathered on September 15 in the baroque ballroom where upper-class residents of Pittsburgh had held tea dances in the 1930s. The peculiar venue was only one of several curious aspects of this meeting. Schleuderberg and her associates had avoided announcing the meeting in the forums typically used by the NIH to advertise such events to scientists inside and outside the agency, such as the publications "What's Happening at NIH?" and the NIH Calendar of Events. Instead, the workshop was by invitation only, and the guest list, to many observers, seemed prejudicial. One Los Angeles clinician, Jay Goldstein, who had nearly a thousand patients with the disease in his practice, lobbied aggressively for an invitation, even traveling to Bethesda at his own expense for a meeting with Schleuderberg, but was denied admission. "He simply does not have the credentials of someone who's trying to do peer review research," Schleuderberg explained, although specific credentials for grant applicants exist nowhere in NIH guidelines and Goldstein was board certified in psychiatry and general medicine and had every intention of applying for a grant to study the disease. Lobbyist Barry Sleight was invited by Grufferman as a gesture to the patient community. In a private memo some years later on the subject, Sleight confessed, "I was permitted to attend only on the condition that I not say anything." The workshop constituted, de facto, a secret meeting, since all press was barred from attending, although at least half of the money for the event—a sum Sleight estimated might be as much as a quarter of a million dollars—came from public funds. Had the meeting been held at the NIH, the government would have been legally bound to admit journalists to the proceedings. Significantly, the Bethesda scientists, not the Pittsburgh scientists, orchestrated the press blackout.

Stephen Straus launched the conclave with a slide of a Victorian-era woodcut of a young woman reclining on a fainting couch with her hand pressed to her fore- head. Straus, in fact, used the slide as his standard opening in all of his medical school lectures on the disease. "I would like to point out that this is not a new syn- drome," he said, and quoted from an English medical tract, circa 1750, which de- scribed the "Febricula," or "Little Fever, commonly called The Nervous or Hysteric Fever, the Fever of the Spirits, Vapours, Hypo or Spleen."

Hard science intruded on the proceedings when Seymour Grufferman gave a full report of his cluster investigations. University of Nevada epidemiologist Sandra Daugherty, in an overview of the Tahoe epidemic, presented a vivid de- scription of the range and severity of immune and central nervous system abnor- malities documented over the previous three years.

Paul Cheney sat quietly throughout the meeting, his head down as he took co- pious notes. At the workshop's end, Yale Epstein-Barr virus expert George Miller turned in his direction and said, "We haven't heard from Paul Cheney yet."

Cheney stood and began to speak, his tone polite, tentative. "One thing that struck me is that I sometimes think there is something old, something that might best be described as a postviral fatigue syndrome, that is probably as old as man and viruses. . . . And then I think I am seeing something that is new, that I don't think may have even existed before. And I really haven't heard anyone express this concern that we are seeing something new."

Straus was quick to respond. "I don't believe there is anything new here," he said. "I think that everything we see has been seen before, both the endemic and the epidemic patterns. . . . One should not assume that it is a new problem or an explosive problem. It is just that we have the opportunity to interact with more people in our society today than we did fifty years ago. We hear from them, and they hear from us, whereas our predecessors in these disciplines were far more isolated in the past."

Straus ended the workshop immediately afterward with the following com- ments: "We have been deliberating here for a day and a half in a very rarefied at- mosphere. Not forgetting the fact that there are some very debilitated, very upset, very depressed, in some cases, very angry, people in the community who desper- ately hang upon the results of these deliberations, we chose, despite community anger, to keep this a very closed meeting so we can speak freely. But ultimately we have to go back into that community. And we have to realize that in doing so, we face a conflict. And the conflict is between providing care and understanding and compassion for people who have this problem, and for getting solid scientific answers. . . . I don't think that these things are entirely exclusive, but depending upon how one chooses to live with that conflict, one can be more or less success- ful with one side or the other."

Straus's suggestion that choosing science over sympathy put investigators at odds with patients was in character with his own adversarial view of sufferers and his skepticism about the reality of their complaints. If their letters to the agency were any indication, patients were seeking concerted, legitimate research into the cause of their disease, not compassion, from the NIH.*

▧

Cheney, who reported he had found many of the presentations interesting and even helpful, was struck by the forcefulness of Straus's faith in the centuries-old "Febricula" or "Little Fever" diagnosis.

"I actually obtained a copy of [the 1750 medical tract that Straus had cited] and read it," Cheney said later. "Some things certainly ring a little bit of chronic fatigue syndrome," he said, but significant discrepancies made him wonder whether he and Straus were really studying the same disease.

"The febricula, or little fever, is perfectly well described by Hippocrates and is everywhere to be met with," the eighteenth-century treatise began. "It is attended with a great variety of strange and threatening symptoms, than any other fever whatever, even to impersonating almost every other disease. Persons of tender and delicate constitution and those in the decline of life are principally exposed to its attacks."

Cheney knew, however, that athleticism and youth seemed to be predisposing factors for chronic fatigue syndrome. After listing the symptoms of the "nervous or hysteric fever," which included "frequent yawnings with little flying pains" and "unaccountable anxiety," the treatise concluded with the following sentence: "These symptoms more or less usually accompany the febricula, and will last thirty or forty days, unless stupors, syncopes [fainting], and death come on sooner and end the scene." Straus's own patients, Cheney knew from reading the researcher's papers, had been ill for an average of nearly eight years, and none had died.

▧

Upon his return to Charlotte, Cheney determined his next effort had to be an attempt to secure money for DeFreitas's investigation. The Wistar scientist had told Cheney during his visit to her lab that without more money she would be forced to drop her investigation, which required a skilled, full-time postdoctoral candidate to perform essential experiments. Cheney called Incline Village's Paul Thompson, the independently wealthy patient with whom the doctor had maintained close ties. Cheney explained the significance of DeFreitas's findings to him and asked if he could finance a postdoc's salary for one year at Wistar. Thompson immediately donated $30,000 to the Wistar cause. DeFreitas hired a virologist named Brendan Hilliard, a twenty-nine-year-old Irishman. Hilliard's task was to

---

* The NIH's scientific summaries from the Pittsburgh conference went unpublished until February 1991. In the intervening years, only one CFS research proposal was funded; for the second time, the grant went to Anthony Komaroff. Seymour Grufferman, who was among those turned down, commented later that, not only did such workshops function as a substitute for funding research, they could be used to manipulate the dissemination of controversial findings presented at the workshop by independent researchers. "You can whitewash conferences," Grufferman explained. "They're 'show trials.' [NIH administrators] control the invitees, select the speakers and write the summaries themselves. They get 'spin' control."

isolate the virus, characterize it, and determine whether it was indeed HTLV1 or something entirely different.

Los Angeles, California

Singer and songwriter Randy Newman was one of the few celebrity sufferers aside from Blake Edwards to discuss his affliction in a public forum. He agreed to an interview with *Rolling Stone* that fall. After having been ill for three years, Newman, who was then forty-four, reported he was feeling better. In the years leading up to his illness, Newman had created best-selling albums like *Sail Away,* scored sound tracks for the films *Ragtime* and *The Natural,* and written hit songs like "Short People" and "I Love L.A." After contracting the disease in 1986, however, Newman was reduced to living as a near-invalid for eighteen months in his Venice, California, home. He told interviewer Michael Goldberg that when he attempted to perform in concert during that period, the experience was "nightmarish." He made mistakes in songs he had been playing without error for years. Newman had discarded as "worthless" the compositions he wrote while he was ill. It was apparent, too, that despite his wealth and celebrity, Newman had fared no better with mainstream medicine than did the poorer victims of the disease. "I ended up going to people with towels on their head, homeopathic guys, acupressure sort of things. Holistic-worldview counterculture leaders. 'Cause I didn't know what the hell to do," Newman said.

Washington, D.C.

On September 27, one week after he attended the Pittsburgh workshop, Barry Sleight wrote to the Centers for Disease Control's Larry Schonberger, addressing the epidemiology chief in stern language. Sleight was growing suspicious. He reminded Schonberger that "Public Law regarding appropriations for Fiscal Year '89 related to chronic fatigue syndrome is unequivocal that $1,182,000 and eight [full-time equivalents] are for activities . . . related to chronic fatigue syndrome." He added that, in his judgment, Congress "would not tolerate" use of either money or staff time "for purposes other than those very clearly related to chronic fatigue syndrome," nor would Congress tolerate a sluggish pace in filling the new jobs. "At this writing," Sleight concluded, "I know of no public policy or public health justification for having any of the appropriated funds and FTEs used outside the programs, grants, or contracts of the Division of Viral Diseases, Center for Infectious Diseases, and expect them to remain with the CID-DVD."

Sleight cautioned Schonberger, too, about failing to investigate reported outbreaks of the disease. "This [task] falls clearly within the published mission of the Center for Infectious Diseases, and is of great interest at the Congress," he wrote.

Sleight's mistrust had been aroused during a conversation with Walter Gunn, the project director for the surveillance study. "[Gunn] warned me that some of the money might get siphoned off into the 'chronic diseases activity' section," Sleight said later. "That's the section where they study how to get people to quit smoking and wear seat belts. These guys, they just require constant attention," Sleight ruminated. "You have to watch them like hawks. It's a real obstreperous agency."

Cambridge, Massachusetts

On October 6 and 7, Walter Gunn, Gary Holmes, and Larry Schonberger met with eight medical specialists who had been impaneled to help the agency assess the legitimacy of cases referred by doctors into the surveillance system. The group gathered at the Cambridge offices of Abt Associates, the research firm that had won the CDC's contract for performing surveillance.

The original study working group included Susan Abbey, a research fellow in psychiatry at Toronto General Hospital who, at the recent Pittsburgh workshop, had championed the disease as a psychiatric condition; Nelson Gantz, a University of Massachusetts infectious disease specialist who had contributed to the government's case definition; the government's Stephen Straus; Jordan Graffman, a neurology researcher from the NIH whose understanding of the disease had been shaped entirely by Straus; and Anthony Komaroff of Harvard. Gantz and Komaroff were the only members of the group who had any regular clinical contact with patients, and Gantz's contact had been minimal. A history of interaction with people suffering from the disease was considered a disadvantage by agency staff, who felt that such contact might bias investigators toward a conclusion that the disease was real. In fact, according to Gunn, Komaroff's inclusion on the panel was hotly contested by Gary Holmes, who believed Komaroff was, Gunn said, "too close to patients."

"It was almost like having the devil incarnate on the board," Gunn recalled.

Nalle Clinic, Charlotte, North Carolina

From the beginning of Elaine DeFreitas's investigation, it was apparent that some of the patients in Paul Cheney's practice were more virulently infected with the mysterious pathogen than others. One of the worst infected was a wheelchair-bound fourteen-year-old from Raleigh who was among the five original patients whose blood Susan Dorman had sent to Philadelphia the previous March. Cheney was fascinated that a white middle-class child could become infected with a retrovirus—if that was what it was—a germ that, according to scientific orthodoxy, was so fragile it could be passed from person to person only through blood transfusions, syringes, sexual contact, or mother's milk. The doctor had ruled out all risk factors in the child's case. If DeFreitas's findings were real, they posed the grim possibility that the bug was being transmitted casually through saliva, like mono, or even through the air, like tuberculosis.

Cheney began to ponder the possibility of sending more children's samples to DeFreitas. What, after all, would be more suggestive of casual transmission than the discovery of such a virus in children, especially very young children without histories of sexual contacts or drug abuse? During phone conversations and by correspondence with pediatrician David Bell, Cheney was learning more about the children's epidemic in upper New York State. Increasingly, the Charlotte doctor wondered whether blood samples from children who had become ill during a discrete outbreak would demonstrate the same hints of retrovirus that DeFreitas was scrutinizing. Eventually, Cheney confided in Bell, describing his secret collaboration with the Wistar scientist. He asked if Bell would join the effort by contributing blood samples from some of his young patients. Bell agreed without reservation, sending samples from two brothers, the sickest boys in the Duncanson family, to DeFreitas. She looked for evidence of the retrovirus using the western blot test, which measured for the signals of antibodies. The results were dramatic. "One of [the brothers] turned out to have the strongest signal of all the patients," Cheney said later.

DeFreitas and Cheney had yet to discuss the implications of retroviral infection in a population of children who were without traditional risk factors for such agents; the subject was a medical and sociological morass, which Cheney correctly suspected the scientist preferred to avoid for the moment. "Virologists are more interested in getting the bug under glass, and they're less focused on the clinical aspects or the epidemiology aspects or the broader aspects of what the hell's going on and how this all fits together. It's just 'Give me the virus. Whoever's got it is who I want,' " the doctor commented. "So David began sending blood from this entire child epidemic in Lyndonville. Dozens and dozens of samples."

Lyndonville, New York

David Bell was at a low point in his inquiries into the cause of the disease when Paul Cheney called to tell him about the events at Wistar. "I just felt I didn't have the energy to maintain these investigations anymore," Bell recalled. "I knew one hundred things this disease *wasn't* caused by. I remember sitting there in my office feeling that I had no more avenues to explore. Within twenty-four hours of that, Paul called." Cheney's news about Elaine DeFreitas's discovery "immediately made sense," Bell continued. "Of course, Paul told me that if I ever told anyone, I would be shot. And I took that very seriously."

Bell's fealty to the DeFreitas-Cheney collaboration rapidly generated strife between himself and a small coterie of epidemiologists and other specialists at the Roswell Cancer Institute, the cancer research arm of the New York State Health Department, and the Dent Neurological Institute, a research center for multiple sclerosis in Buffalo. In recent months, Bell had found some solace within this group, all of whom expressed genuine interest in investigating the disease flourishing among children in Lyndonville and nearby villages. The researchers met on the first Tuesday of every month to discuss their findings and to plan a grant proposal they hoped would be funded by the NIH; their research focus was on the neurologic component of the disease.

With David and Karen Bell's help, the team was following the Lyndonville epidemic closely. They had determined that 3.6 percent of all children in the town were suffering from the disease. Lending support to Bell's sense that the disease was infectious within families, the team had discovered that having at least one family member ill with the malady greatly increased the risk of acquiring it.

David Bell was referring his most intellectually impaired patients to Carolyn Warner, a regular at the Tuesday meetings and a Dent-affiliated neurologist and specialist in neuromuscular disorders such as myasthenia gravis and multiple sclerosis. Starting in 1987, Warner began to see patients who had been given diagnoses of either atypical multiple sclerosis or atypical myasthenia gravis. "These were very sick people," Warner recalled later, "but their neurological exams were only mildly abnormal, although they had really disabling histories." Warner was fascinated by the resemblance between the new disease and multiple sclerosis, particularly by the manifestation of UBOs in the brain. There were so many similarities, in fact, that the neurologist suspected misdiagnoses of both diseases were probably rampant.

Warner's colleague, cancer epidemiologist Diane Cookfair, concurred: "Half of these people could go to any neurologist in town and get a diagnosis of multiple sclerosis." In an effort to quantitate the degree of disability in the disease, Warner and Cookfair had administered a standardized measure of morbidity called the Sickness Impact Profile Scale (SIPS) to nearly one hundred CFS sufferers. Cookfair was testing Lyndonville patients; Warner was testing patients in Buffalo. "People are scoring off the wall on the SIPS," Cookfair reported. "Chronic fatigue syndrome patients test as high or higher than people with cancer and heart attack."

Given their increasingly sophisticated understanding of the disease, it was probably inevitable that Bell's collaborators would fix their sights on retroviruses, pathogens suspected of causing a range of central nervous system diseases. Said Cookfair that fall: "I've been reading up on the neurological sequelae in AIDS. Chronic fatigue syndrome *could* have a retrovirus cause." In addition, because western New York state had an unusually high incidence of multiple sclerosis, the Buffalo team was receptive to the increasingly serious proposition that MS was an infectious malady. They were following closely the Wistar Institute's work with the retrovirus HTLV1 and MS. Not surprisingly, they began that fall to discuss the real possibility of searching for a retrovirus in David Bell's Lyndonville patients.

Diane Cookfair suggested sending blood samples from that outbreak to Bernard Poiesz at the State University of New York in Syracuse. Poiesz was a refugee from the Gallo lab who was considered one of the best retrovirologists in the country. In 1978 Poiesz had been the first to isolate HTLV1 from an adult T-cell lymphoma case. He agreed to run the assays on patient samples.

"A week later we had our study group meeting," Bell explained. "The whole group was there—about ten people. Our virologist said, 'Okay, let's get some samples.' And I said, 'Wait a minute. I can't send any samples from my patients.' "

All eyes fell upon Bell, who had been providing the team with both the patients and the blood samples for their studies. "I cannot send any samples," Bell reiterated as his collaborators grew silent. "I am already doing these studies with other investigators."

"Who are your collaborators?" Cookfair asked, her tone stern.

"I was asked not to disclose their names," Bell responded.

"That they couldn't *believe,"* the doctor recalled later. "At that point, Cookfair started going through the people she knew, trying to figure it out. Then we got into this whole harangue about loyalty within the group. I said, 'No, I'm being loyal to the people I was involved with before I met you.' We had some very unpleasant conversations. They called me a betrayer and a traitor, and all that. . . . Eventually it was decided they were going to go through Poiesz. If there was a retrovirus, then they would get it through Poiesz."

One issue remained: whose patients would the team use for Poiesz's samples if they couldn't use Bell's? "It was finally resolved that because Carolyn

Warner was seeing a lot of my patients in the course of doing the neurology study, she could send blood to Poiesz from those patients," Bell said. "They would not be Lyndonville patients; they were mostly Buffalo patients who had come to me to be evaluated, whom I then had referred to her. And by then she was beginning to pick [the disease] up in her own neurology practice anyway, so she was starting to have quite a few of her own patients."

Despite the strife it caused within his Buffalo group, Bell was quickly caught in the grip of the Wistar research. "I was very excited," he recalled. "Right from the beginning with those western blots, there was something going on."

Nonetheless, it was apparent the work would not be simple. After Bell sent the initial blood from the Duncanson boys to Wistar, Cheney asked him to send more samples from thirty of his sickest patients. If these sufferers had a retrovirus in their blood, Cheney and DeFreitas reasoned, they would likely have more of it than less sick patients. Bell complied by sending the stored serum from adults he had seen in the last six months.

Cheney called Bell with the results.

"I remember I began to be very disappointed, because [the results] didn't look all that impressive," Bell said. "So-and-so is positive, so-and-so is negative. As he was reading off the names, the negatives and positives were not matching up to the severity of the patients' illness. There was obviously something there, but it wasn't a straightforward relationship. It was not going to be an easy thing."

By the fall of 1988, one of Bell's most seriously ill patients, twelve-year-old Skye Dailor of Rochester, had been out of school for more than a year. The year before, she had been examined by infectious disease specialists at a University of Rochester clinic for adolescents. Unable to determine the cause of the child's complaints, the specialists ultimately diagnosed the seventh grader with "school phobia." It had seemed a bizarre conclusion to Dailor's parents, who had explained to the specialists that their daughter was an A-plus student and had rarely missed school until the onset of her illness the year before. Skye's parents brought her to Bell's Lyndonville clinic soon afterward, and within minutes of meeting her, Bell was certain she was suffering from the illness that had claimed so many children in Lyndonville.

"She was a very beautiful little girl, very bright," Bell recalled much later. "When I first saw her, she was absolutely typical for the disease, although she was depressed and bewildered. She had lost all her friends, had failed a grade in school. It was *that* kind of depression. She definitely had the disease in its severe form," he added. "Basically I wrote some letters and suggested she get home tutoring, at which point the University of Rochester backed off, because whatever they were doing—psychotherapy—wasn't working. They were happy to dump her. She was off school the whole next year—1988."

Bell began seeing the child at regular intervals, carefully following the progression of her disease. By fall, Dailor's T4–T8 ratio had reached the astronomical level of eleven; two was normal. She had almost no natural killer cells. "She had a lot of markers [laboratory abnormalities]," Bell recalled. "I would talk to the others at the University of Rochester who knew about her case. They had absolutely no interest. I am technically on the staff of the University of Rochester," he continued, "and I wanted to look credible. It was frustrating."

That fall, Bell continued, "Skye developed these striae—long purple marks— on her forearms. Striae are markers for rheumatological disease; they're very abnormal. At times she was in a wheelchair. But she was still considered a nutcase at the University of Rochester."

Bell sent Skye Dailor's blood to Wistar. Skye was, as Cheney would eventually say, "royally infected" with the retrovirus DeFreitas was working to characterize.

Rome, Italy

Paul Cheney and Dan Peterson had not seen each other since Cheney's sudden and emotional departure from Incline Village. Peterson missed his colleague. Cheney's energy, his facile intellect, his profound commitment to unraveling the medical dilemma that had altered their lives, were qualities Peterson knew he was unlikely to find again in a partner. On October 3, the two met up at a convocation of European, American, English, and Japanese virologists at the University of Rome. Most of the participants in the Third International Symposium of Epstein-Barr Virus and Associated Malignant Diseases shared a fluency in the language of microbiology. Paul Levine of the National Cancer Institute and Germany's Gerhard Krueger succeeded in securing a ninety-minute slot on the four-day program to consider the "chronic postviral fatigue syndrome." In anticipation of hearing world experts in the molecular biology of Epstein-Barr virus participating in a roundtable discussion on the new disease, most of the major players in the emerging CFS field—Anthony Komaroff being a notable exception—had come to Rome.

When the appointed hour arrived, however, the auditorium, which had seen scientists packed cheek by jowl for lectures on matters of Epstein-Barr virology, was suddenly almost empty. Mark Kaplan, a Long Island infectious disease specialist who often collaborated with the Gallo group, set the tone with his opening remarks. Flanked on the stage by imposing busts of Dante and Leonardo da Vinci, Kaplan suggested that CFS and depression were clinically indistinguishable and called the disease's spread a "pseudo-epidemic."

Within the confines of the Rome conference, it was possible to sample the range of scientific interest and activity swirling around the epidemic illness in Western Europe. Pathologist Gerhard Krueger of Cologne University was the most enthusiastic, and concerned. Krueger had launched a prospective study of the disease in Cologne two years before, enrolling a total population of 1,600 healthy medical students and military personnel. "Among the population in Germany," he explained, "there is tremendous interest in this disease. Among physicians, not so much." Unlike scientists from the National Cancer Institute, Krueger felt free to speculate openly on the link between cancer and CFS. "We have tools today to detect diseases much more early," he said. "Ten years ago, we could only diagnose malignant lymphomas. Today we can define the condition that leads to the lymphoma. CFS is interesting because it may be such a condition that leads to lymphoma, but it is too early to tell." Asked what German researchers called the disease, Krueger smiled. "We call it the Lake Tahoe disease," he said pleasantly.

The liveliest debates at the Rome Conference were carried on in sidewalk cafés. Several conflagrations were ignited by a scientist who had remained in the United States due to illness. Pittsburgh cancer epidemiologist Seymour Grufferman sent a "poster" to Rome, a four-page summary of his findings among members of the North Carolina Symphony. The poster, which advertised an incidence of cancer among the musicians that was eighteen times what might have been expected, was tacked to a bulletin board outside the auditorium and served as a litmus test. Predictably, its most vehement detractors were those who failed to view CFS as a serious disease.

Cheney and Peterson achieved a precarious truce in Rome. At twilight on the first day, they walked up the Valle Policlinico, a broad avenue lined with trees whose branches formed a bower over noisy traffic. They took long, quick strides, rarely looking at one another, but their conversation—their first in two years—was unbroken for the nearly three-mile walk to Peterson's hotel. There, along with Reno microbiologist Berch Henry, they sat in the hotel's subterranean bar, the only patrons, and talked some more. Two hours later, the three men rendezvoused at dinner. Cheney's head was filled with the developments at Wistar, but he withheld the findings from Peterson in Rome, as he would for the next two years. New York pediatrician David Bell, who had been invited to speak about the disease in children at the Roman conference, withheld the news from Peterson as well.

All three doctors, each of whom had been witness to the disease in its purest epidemic form, left Italy abashed. Some of the world's finest scientists had gathered there, yet the fate of the disease that was so patently real to the three clinicians had receded deeper into the gloom. Against expectations, the world scientific community's disharmony and skepticism on the matter had emerged in bold relief.

"The only people who really believe in this disease are the few clinicians who have seen enough patients to have seen the pattern, and isolated clinicians who either have the disease themselves or who have someone close to them who has it," Cheney said. "Once you believe this disease is real, your whole attitude changes. If you get a negative result or an ambiguous finding, you say, 'Well, it's a negative result and an ambiguous finding,' and you keep going, because you know the disease is real. And then you have these other people who are sitting over there and could really be helpful—the bench researchers and the scientists who could supply the objective parameters by which this disease will ultimately be defined—and they don't really believe in this disease," the doctor continued. "So when *they* find a negative result, they say, 'Well, see? It doesn't exist.' We need to have more of those people on our side. I don't know the most efficient way to get them here. Sort of by osmosis and exposure and cross-fertilization, meetings like this, experiences on their own. One day it clicks—their own personal experiences, family members, themselves.

"And one day these people will take us out of this morass. They will lead us out of Osler's web, which is kind of a diffuse feeling that this disease is real, even though we can't find the objective measures. Which is what Sir William Osler was famous for being able to do—defining an illness well enough clinically so that you could study it long enough to eventually ferret out those objective features. The bench researchers are going to take us out of Osler's web. Because I can't do it. I don't know how to do subtle things with MRI scans. I don't know how to do western blots. *They* have to do it."

Albuquerque, New Mexico

Nancy Kaiser moved back to Albuquerque in November after three months on Ampligen. She was remarkably better, though not recovered, and needed to continue infusions with the drug three times each week. For a short period after each two-hour infusion, the drug made her feel worse, but evidence of improvement was accumulating as the weeks and months passed—and not only by the patient's self-assessment. Peterson ordered tests each week that revealed an immune system on the mend; Kaiser's T-cell ratios were approaching normalcy, and her natural killer cell function was up. Berch Henry, who was monitoring Kaiser's antibodies to human herpesvirus 6, determined that antibody levels were dropping, suggesting that infection was subsiding. Kaiser's obvious cognitive improvement was documented on Sheila Bastien's mental status tests: her IQ had risen from 88 to 118.

To those who had known Kaiser before she began receiving Ampligen, her transformation was astounding. "I wish I had made videos of her when she arrived," Peterson said. "She couldn't walk. She could barely speak." Albuquerque gynecologist John Slocumb agreed to continue to give Kaiser the intravenous drug infusions in his office. When Slocumb saw her after her three-month absence, he was deeply affected. "I was in tears. To see her that way after following her for five or six years was quite a surprise," he recalled.

Kaiser said she did not mind being tethered to the drug. "It is far better than being tethered to the disease," she observed.

HEM Pharmaceuticals scientists and executives, as well as the company's private backers, were following Kaiser's return from the living dead with considerable interest. That fall Peterson entered into discussions with a team of HEM corporate officers and the firm's medical adviser, Hahnemann University's David Strayer, about the possibility of performing a pilot study of the drug on nine more patients in his care.

Newport, Rhode Island

Sixty-nine-year-old Claiborne Pell, a distinguished fifth-term U.S. senator and blue blood from Newport, Rhode Island, had not fallen prey to the disease, as some patients began to suspect that year. His attention had been focused on the subject by members of his constituency, Rhode Islanders suffering from the disease. Although the actual number of sufferers in Rhode Island was unknown, one support group in the state had evolved from just five members in November of 1987 to more than five hundred dues-paying members a year later, suggesting an impressive prevalence of the disease in the nation's smallest state.

Brown University's medical school, in addition, had instituted a CFS research clinic at its teaching institution, Miriam Hospital, in 1988. Internist Charles Carpenter, chief of staff of Miriam Hospital and a professor of medicine at Brown, and several of his colleagues had concluded that a discrete, if unknown, pathogen was abroad. Carpenter's certitude was such that when other researchers proposed hypotheses about multiple causes and multiple syndromes, he was quick to disagree. "We're seeing something that wasn't there in the fifties and sixties," Carpenter argued that year. "Most of us feel this is new. If this had been going on in the fifties and sixties, even if we had discarded it as psychiatric, it would have been written about, and it's not in the literature. And that suggests there is a dominant agent that's driving the majority of the cases."

In his role as the second-ranking member of the Senate subcommittee with appropriation and oversight power over the NIH and the CDC, Pell had mobilized support for a medical conference on the disease in Newport where Rhode Island clinicians could learn more about the disease.

The event occurred on October 21–22 in the flashy Newport Marriott on the waterfront. Predictably, the weekend's most revealing commentary erupted over candlelit dining tables and in private rooms, particularly the sparsely furnished, sun-dappled rooms of a Newport mansion that had been rented by CFIDS Association president Marc Iverson. For months, Iverson and other patient organizers had sought to provide an intimate environment where research clinicians like Paul Cheney, James Jones, David Bell, and others might speak informally with government scientists and policymakers. They hoped to inspire a clearer understanding of the disease on the part of the federal researchers by exposing them to the clinical expertise of Cheney and others like him. To that end, Bell, Cheney, Los Angeles clinician Jay Goldstein, Charles Carpenter of Brown University, and others met with the National Cancer Institute's Paul Levine and NIAID's Ann Schleuderberg on the Friday afternoon before the conference began and on Sunday afternoon after it ended. Stephen Straus was invited, but did not attend either the conference or the private sessions.

The private meetings were dominated by efforts by Cheney, Bell, and others to lead the government representatives to an understanding of the disease as a discrete entity with an infectious cause. "I'd like to make an analogy," Cheney gently interjected at one point in the discussions. "Historically, in AIDS, we had a sign-symptom complex where in order to make the diagnosis we looked for evidence of Epstein-Barr, cytomegalovirus, toxoplasmosis, and so on. But this heterogeneity was then thrown out the window when HIV was discovered." Although Cheney did not feel free in these sessions to discuss his collaboration with Elaine DeFreitas, he felt certain it was only a matter of time before the Wistar Institute announced its discovery of the virus behind the disease.

Brown's Charles Carpenter, too, expressed his conviction that the disease was new and likely to be the result of what he called "one dominant agent" spreading through the population. David Bell concurred, pointing out that, as a result of his position as a pediatric specialist in the disease, he had now had an opportunity to see children from all over the country. "They are virtually indistinguishable from the children in Lyndonville," Bell said. "This is such a *dramatic* disease in children," he continued, "that if it existed in the days of rheumatic fever, it would have been described in the literature."

"If it *is* increasing," government scientist Paul Levine commented, on the defensive, "the CDC surveillance will show it."

Claiborne Pell assumed the role of keynote speaker at the conference, but his oratory made it clear that the influential senator was ill informed about the politics of chronic fatigue syndrome. According to Pell, the NIH was preparing to spend $15 million dollars on the disease in 1989. In fact, the figure was one-tenth that: $1.5 million. The CDC, Pell continued, would spend more than $1.1 million and assign between four and eight full-time staff members or their equivalent to the disease in the coming year. Gary Holmes, however, when interviewed privately in Newport, reported once again that his agency's 1989 appropriation was "up for grabs," meaning it was vulnerable, like the previous year's appropriations, to poaching by other divisions within the agency. And if the agency hired eight new staff members, Holmes continued, there would be almost no money left over for research.

When Pell's administrative aid was asked about the dollar sums in her boss's address, her response suggested that Pell's staff found it as hard to pry accurate figures out of health agencies as did patient advocacy groups.

"We made the dollar figures as vague as we could because the appropriations were so vague," Lauren Gross said. "We got the figures from the budget offices at the National Institutes of Health and the Centers for Disease Control. Pell sort of rounded out the numbers, because they're estimates, and ultimately [the agencies] will make the decisions. . . . There's really no way of being absolutely positive what the numbers are," Gross continued. "Even when we talked to two different people in the NIH budget offices, we got two different figures."

National Institute of Allergy and Infectious Diseases, Bethesda, Maryland

On December 2, Stephen Straus was quoted extensively in a long article about chronic fatigue syndrome in *Medical World News,* a biweekly publication mailed to the offices of 130,000 practicing clinicians. "People with the somatic complaints of fatigue that we see in CFS may have coexisting or underlying psychiatric problems," the scientist told the reporter. Straus provided no evidence for his assertions.

Harvard Medical School, Boston, Massachusetts

On December 2, Anthony Komaroff sent a memorandum to the Tahoe Research Group, which included Dan Peterson, microbiologist Berch Henry, neuroradiologist Royce Biddle, infectious disease specialist Ray Swarts, internist Dedra Buchwald, and Paul Cheney. Komaroff's letter was a kind of cheerleading effort, as well as a summary of the status of their difficult and underfinanced research. Komaroff was still laboring to satisfy the *Lancet* editors, who continued to seek better proof for a number of assertions in the Tahoe manuscript.

"The paper unfortunately contains a number of 'holes' which we cannot fill in retrospect, data that should ideally have been collected at the time the patients were seen between 1984 and 1986," Komaroff wrote. "This problem is not really delaying our publication, but it constitutes a weakness of the manuscript that cannot be remedied. Reviewers who have a bias against the paper from the outset can find things to fault."

Komaroff told his collaborators that the British journal had agreed to submit the paper to a second round of peer reviewers if he could provide a full complement of magnetic resonance imaging brain scans on healthy people for use as controls. In an effort to save the manuscript, Dedra Buchwald, Komaroff's Seattle-based collaborator, had located what she believed was an unassailable control group for the brain scans: fifty presumably healthy General Electric engineers from the Midwest. GE was the manufacturer of the magnetic resonance imaging scanner; fifty of the company's engineers had volunteered to undergo brain scans in order to test the machine's calibration. They would use an ultrasensitive-grade scanner like one in use at Reno Diagnostics—a 1.5 tesla.

Lancet wanted incontrovertible proof, too, that the virus infecting the Tahoe patients, which Komaroff and Berch Henry were claiming was HHV6, really was HHV6. So far Henry had demonstrated that the cytopathic effect, or cell-killing pattern, of the virus matched perfectly that described by Zaki Salahuddin, Robert Gallo, and others in their *Science* article about the discovery of the virus. Henry had demonstrated also that when the patient's infected cells were exposed to antisera known to contain a high level of antibodies to the virus, the cells responded, further proof that the virus was HHV6. But, the *Lancet* editors had asked, might there be any other viral antibodies in the same antisera?

"Could it be that the cells are really infected by some virus other than HHV6—call it virus X—and that the antisera which we know contains antibodies to HHV6 also contains antibodies to virus X?" Komaroff wrote. "Hence, what appears to be a result indicating that cells are infected with HHV6 really could be telling us the cells are infected with virus X."

The Tahoe paper had been fraught with difficulties, and the tasks ahead would be time-consuming, particularly for Henry, in whose laboratory more delicate bench work on the herpesvirus would need to be undertaken. So far, however, none of the collaborators had voiced a desire to leave the project, in part because of Komaroff's steady encouragement.

"We should all remember that this is a huge effort, with very little outside research support," Komaroff wrote. "As someone who has done a lot of research for over twenty years, I am amazed at how far we've come. One manuscript—the natural killer cell paper—already has been published, and in the best journal. A second manuscript—the overview paper—has been taken very seriously by two of the best journals—the *New England Journal of Medicine* and *Lancet*—even with its faults and limitations.

"Could we have published more about Tahoe sooner? Probably so. You can usually find some journal to take a paper. But our work is too important to be buried in an obscure journal that no one reads, [especially] if that *prevents* us from publishing the same data, when they are improved, in a top journal [Komaroff's italics]. "This is how I see things, and I welcome everyone's thought."

Komaroff, in spite of his experience, underestimated the depth of the hostility in the medical establishment to the subject of his investigative effort. His struggle to see the Tahoe data published would last another four years.

Public Health Department, San Francisco, California

By December the city's department of health survey of local physicians, launched several months earlier in an effort to pacify an increasingly vociferous patient organization, was complete: 200 Bay Area doctors—internal medicine specialists, gynecologists and family practice doctors—had been queried; 143 responded. Carol Jessop, who had seen nearly 1,000 patients with the disease in her East Bay clinic, and a handful of San Francisco doctors, each of whom was seeing close to 100 patients, were excluded from the survey to prevent a skewing of the statistics. Of the 143 respondents, 50 (41 percent) had cared for at least one patient with the disease in the previous year. Each of these 50 doctors, in fact, had seen an average of 5.8 patients. More than half of those who saw such patients believed there had been an increase in the number of victims in five years.

The health department also surveyed 100 patients and learned that 92 had been employed before their illness; now 65 were employed. Only one patient had recovered. The median age of the patients was thirty-eight.

Boston, Massachusetts

The *New England Journal of Medicine*, having rejected the Tahoe manuscript the year before, published Stephen Straus's long-awaited acyclovir study on December 29.[2] Most in the medical community already knew Straus's conclusions, but the study's publication was their first opportunity to evaluate his methods.

The following April, Straus described his trial at a medical grand rounds at Holy Cross Hospital in Silver Spring, Maryland. He had selected twenty-seven patients with the disease, he told his audience of nearly two hundred, and treated them once with the antiviral drug and once with a placebo. He used the drug "aggressively," he said. "I frankly didn't want to spend three years of my life asking the question and then have someone say, 'You didn't use enough.' So we treated patients for a week in the hospital with 500 milligrams . . . three times a day, intravenously. That is a lot of intravenous acyclovir. And we gave them a month at home with 800 milligrams [orally] four times a day."

In fact, three of Straus's twenty-seven patients had to drop out of the trial due to renal failure when blood levels of acyclovir rose too high. It wasn't the size of the dose, however, that caused the problem, according to Paul Cheney, who with Dan Peterson had treated over sixty patients with the drug at Tahoe; Straus failed to provide enough fluids to his patients while they were on the drug. "Their infusion techniques were wrong," Cheney observed. "We gave acyclovir in higher doses in Tahoe. And we never saw renal failure. Straus didn't give enough water. The mistake was to depend on the patients to drink the fluids, and I can imagine the blood level went really high."

Straus's paper reported only that "vigorous oral hydration was encouraged."

Of the twenty-four patients who remained in the study, twenty-one felt better at some point during the course of the study, Straus told his audience in Silver Spring. "And what's important to point out is that of the twenty-one who felt better," Straus said, "eleven of them felt better while they were on acyclovir and ten of them felt better when they were on the placebo." The comment elicited an outburst of laughter from his audience.

Writing in the *New England Journal,* Straus concluded: "We did find an association between the result of psychological tests and patients' sense of well-being. Significant improvement in levels of anger, depression and other mood states correlated with overall clinical improvement. . . . Our findings are . . . in accord with recent findings that a history of affective [psychiatric] disorders is frequent among patients with the chronic fatigue syndrome."

As usual, Straus offered no supporting data for the last comment.*

In contrast to Straus, Cheney and Peterson had discovered that acyclovir produced a remission in approximately 85 percent of the patients who were infused with it. Unfortunately, the relapse rate when patients went off the drug was 80 percent. They had also discovered that those who responded best were people who had been ill for an average of eleven months; those who had been ill longer than two years received no benefit at all from the drug. "The people that we hit with acyclovir who were within a year of onset—their response to that drug was just astounding," Cheney recalled. The results suggested that the malady began as a fast-burning viral infection that, if caught early enough, could be treated with potent infusions of the antiviral drug, but which changed in time to an auto-immune illness in which viruses played a minor role, if any role at all. After struggling to fight an infection for months or years, in other words, the immune system was now in overdrive and was itself causing many of the symptoms of the disease.

The average duration of the disease among patients enrolled in Straus's acyclovir study was 6.8 years.

In Nevada, Dan Peterson had continued to treat with acyclovir patients who had brain lesions on MRI scans and who displayed obvious neurological deficits. In Peterson's opinion, even though the drug was not a cure, it was better than nothing at all for the most severely ill, many of whom were invalids; not surprisingly, his patients agreed. An official from Burroughs Wellcome Company, the manufacturer of acyclovir, had met with Peterson earlier in the year to discuss a drug trial, but the company seemed tepid in its commitment; word of Straus's failure to achieve results were percolating through the far-flung networks of interested researchers and patients. Once Straus's paper appeared, and in such an august journal, any hope for a new clinical trial withered; in addition, insurance companies, never eager to reimburse the costs of experimental therapies, now refused outright to pay for acyclovir therapy.

Cheney, not surprisingly, considered Straus's article to be destructive in the extreme, setting back the use of acyclovir in the disease for at least a decade. "Traditionally," Cheney said, "there is a bias against publishing negative results

---

* Cancer epidemiologist Diane Cookfair was among a number of CFS researchers who were particularly incensed by Straus's final statements. "Straus took what should have been a straight drug trial and used it to say this disease is psychosomatic," Cookfair complained. "And to talk about mood disorders in this disease without reviewing the chronic disease literature for an assessment of mood disorders in other chronic diseases is unfair. Chronic illness is a very stressful life event. There are mood disorders in every chronic disease."

because it closes the door. Negative studies close off a pathway. And when they appear in the *New England Journal of Medicine,* that pathway could be closed for not just a decade but perhaps a generation."

The *New England Journal* used Straus's acyclovir study as an opportunity to sound off on the disease in its lead editorial that week. "The Chronic Fatigue Syndrome—One Entity or Many?" written by Harvard infectious disease specialist Morton Swartz, concluded that the disorder was likely to have "multiple somatic and psychosomatic causes."

Charlotte, North Carolina

By year's end, the *CFIDS Chronicle* had grown from a four-page newsletter distributed to a few hundred people to an eight-page journal distributed to six thousand. Its subscription list had grown without any systematic publicity. The CFIDS Association had paying members who lived as far away as Peru and the Soviet Union, and received hundreds of letters each week.

1989
THE TEFLON
SCIENTIST

Medicine arose out of the primal sympathy of man
with man; out of the desire to help those in sorrow,
need, and sickness.

—Sir William Osler, *The Evolution of Modern Medicine*

16

Black Jell-O

Berkeley, California

By early 1989, neuropsychologist Sheila Bastien had tested patients from cities as geographically diverse as Boise, Miami, Albuquerque, and Juneau. The pattern of intellectual impairment, as manifested in her battery of tests, was so real to her, so distinctive, that she maintained she could diagnose a person with some confidence merely by studying his or her test scores. Like Alzheimer's, brain tumors, learning disabilities, and toxic chemical exposures, the epidemic disease had its own footprint.

"I realized there was a new pattern very soon," the psychologist said that year, adding, "but it is only after testing several hundred patients that I have a feeling of confidence about that pattern. And, on average, I find two striking things." Verbal memory, the capacity to remember speech, Bastien said, was "always more impaired than visual memory," the capacity to recall images. "I had never seen the verbal-visual memory problem before," Bastien noted.

Disparities in areas of intelligence are diagnostic of structural damage to the brain, since they betoken pockets of damage. In contrast, when memory problems exist in cases of depression, verbal and visual memory deficits are equal.

A second striking impairment emerged on a test requiring blindfolded subjects to identify the shapes of wooden blocks. Were they star-shaped or square? Crescent-shaped or triangular? Normal five-year-olds performed the test without difficulty. Victims of the new disease, many of them adults with advanced degrees, were markedly impaired at this task, particularly in their nondominant hand, most frequently the left. "It's the left hand that taps into the sensory strip in the right parietal lobe, which is the nonverbal, nonlanguage function of the brain," Bastien noted. Again, the unilateral nature of the impairment strongly suggested structural damage.

Bastien had observed one other curious abnormality, and in her interpretation of it, she drew from psychology as well as neuropsychology. "There is a small proportion of patients," Bastien said, "whose figure drawings deteriorate as their disease gets worse and they become more demented. I believe two things happen. One is organic, in that they have spatial perceptual problems, so they can't put the parts together anymore. The other thing, I believe, is emotional," Bastien continued. "There's a subpopulation of patients who draw figures without feet on them." Here Bastien quickly sketched a primitive figure whose legs ended at the bottom of the page just below the knee, as if the limbs had been amputated at mid-calf. "You could argue that they just didn't fit it on the page because of poor planning— the brain isn't working. Or you could say it's a psychological manifestation of helplessness because they have lost their position in life: they've lost their footing."

The first CFS patient the psychologist had observed drawing a human figure without its feet, Bastien added, was the forty-seven-year-old Nevada postal worker who, in the second year of her illness, had been found sitting alone on a curbside, unable to find her house.

Bastien's findings were being reprised at Harvard by Professor Stephen Kosslyn, who was described by his colleague Anthony Komaroff as one of the "world's foremost cognitive psychologists" and who had evaluated a number of Boston sufferers at Komaroff's invitation. Perpetually occupied by the struggle to strengthen the disease's credibility, Komaroff had concluded, "We need to expand these studies . . . to further demonstrate abnormalities which we believe are characteristic of CFS and are not seen in patients with primary psychiatric disorders."

After interviewing nearly forty patients in Nevada and California, government cancer epidemiologist Paul Levine had found the disease's neurologic component to be its most outstanding aspect. "You can just *feel* when you're talking to someone with the cognitive disorder," Levine said later. "It's like a break in an electric current." In an effort to describe their experience, he recalled afterward, patients commonly expressed a sense of having been ambushed or overpowered. "I feel as though I am demonically possessed," said one, words that expressed her sudden loss of control and alienation from her once-competent self, as well as her sense of violation. Said another, "I exist in black Jell-O." She was unable to rely on her senses, which had gone "black," and she was captive in a new dimension, an opaque sludge that impeded her movement in a world through which she once had traveled freely.

The disease's intellectual debilitation, particularly the memory impairment, cut to the core of the patient's identity. By interfering with the victim's capacity for remembering, the disease corrupted personal histories and betrayed the sufferer's sense of the passage of time. Sometimes events were logged into the memory apparatus; sometimes they weren't. Childhood memories and events of the week before acquired equal standing; days were reduced to meaningless white squares on the calendar page, month accumulated upon month, year upon year, with little about them in the victim's memory bank to distinguish one from another. Unlike diseases that were localized—affecting a limb or another organ, for instance—the disease, like most brain afflictions, was a remarkable assault on the foundations of selfhood.

If, as Bastien's tests indicated, the greatest damage had been sustained in the right hemisphere, then the cognitive dilemmas of which CFS victims complained lay within the confines of the most enigmatic, least investigated brain disorders. In 1985, neurologist Oliver Sacks published a collection of case histories in which he sought to describe the impact of profound right brain syndromes upon the lives and personalities of the afflicted. Even the title of Sacks's unlikely best-seller, *The*

Man Who Mistook His Wife for a Hat, conveyed the cryptic quality of such disorders. Their deeply complex nature, according to Sacks, had ensured their omission from the realm of neurologic investigation. Sacks writes:

> One important reason for the neglect of the right, or "minor," hemisphere, as it always has been called, is that while it is easy to demonstrate the effects of variously located lesions on the left side, the corresponding syndromes of the right hemisphere are much less distinct. It was presumed, usually contemptuously, to be more "primitive" than the left, the latter being seen as the unique flower of human evolution. . . . On the other hand, it is the right hemisphere which controls the crucial powers of recognizing reality which every living creature must have in order to survive. The left hemisphere, like a computer tacked onto the basic creatural brain, is designed for programs and schematics: and classical neurology was more concerned with schematics than with reality, so that when, at last, some of the right hemisphere syndromes emerged, they were considered bizarre. . . . And yet . . . they are of the most fundamental importance. So much so that they may demand a new sort of neurology, a "personalistic," or . . . a "romantic," science; for the physical foundations of the persona, the self, are here revealed for our study.[1]

Several of the people whose case histories Sacks describes in his book were so denuded by their neurological disorders that they were institutionalized, their doctors awaiting, perhaps, a "personalistic" or "romantic" neurology to explicate their dilemmas. Many of Sacks's subjects, too, were unaware of their deficits. Victims of the new epidemic disease, in contrast, remained both at large and horribly conscious of their loss. Their freedom was meaningless, in fact, since they were no longer at home in the world. Their "crucial powers of recognizing reality" impaired, their mental competence shattered, they had been pared down to elemental remnants of their former selves.

"This disease erases lives," Marc Iverson often said.

Centers for Disease Control, Atlanta, Georgia

Through no fault of his own, Walter Gunn had inherited an extremely bulky, complicated surveillance project known in-house as Protocol 904, an elaborate blueprint for probing mental illness among CFS patients referred to the agency.

As Larry Schonberger and Gary Holmes had designed it, this surveillance plan involved extensive use of psychiatric tests, the preponderance of which would be administered to patients by nurses hired by Abt Associates. Leading the cumbersome battery was the psychiatric trade's bible, the Diagnostic Interview Schedule.* Patients, additionally, would be entrusted with self-administered psychological

---

* Such was Holmes and Schonberger's zeal that at one stage in the development of Protocol 904 a strategy existed to administer Rorschach tests. The decades-old Rorschach—its inventor, Hermann Rorschach, died in 1922—was a series of ten inkblots once believed to reveal the underlying personality structure of the test subject. Holmes and Schonberger dropped the idea only when they learned that Rorschach data was so unreliable that medical journals had long ago ceased to accept it.

evaluations such as the Critical Events Calendar, on which they were to list every stressful event that had occurred in the year leading up to their illness, and Beck's Depression Inventory, a multiple-choice test devoted to measuring depression.

After this initial investigatory round, which Schonberger and Holmes reasoned would establish baseline psychological status, the surveillance nurses would submit each patient's chart to an agency-tapped Physicians Review Committee, which would meet quarterly in Cambridge. Patients who made the grade would be required to answer quarterly psychiatric questionnaires, and undergo yearly psychiatric interviews with surveillance nurses for four additional years, thus enabling the government to continue its inquiry into their psychological functioning.

Protocol 904 revealed an investigative posture that took no notice of organic disease, an omission that had its own logic within the milieu of the viral epidemiology branch. The agency's own "Holmes criteria," after all, ruled out a diagnosis of CFS if there was evidence suggestive of any other medical disease. Nevertheless, the plan's indifference to assessing patients' bodies, as opposed to their psyches, troubled at least one outside researcher who was privy to the agency's workings: Anthony Komaroff.

"The surveillance study started out as basically a chart review, a psychiatric evaluation and *five hours* of psychiatric testing!" the doctor said later.

In order to proceed, Schonberger needed to submit Protocol 904 to the agency's Institutional Review Board, an internal body charged with approving agency studies involving human subjects. Walter Gunn, who was now the senior investigator on the surveillance project, was the obvious staff person in Schonberger's shop to supply a defense of Protocol 904 to the board. That winter, Gunn gamely set about immersing himself in the disease and the peculiarities of his colleagues' surveillance plan.*

Los Angeles, California

One of many ironies in the discovery process under way was the fact that proponents of the psychoneurotic theory, as wrong as they were, were also partly right. Patients did suffer from extraordinary, sometimes suicidal, depressions. Many previously well-employed, socially competent people also underwent dramatic personality changes, occasionally losing their ability to cope rationally with their feelings of rage and despair. Their relationships eroded, not just because their friends and family failed to comprehend the catastrophic nature of their disease, but also because sufferers often became too angry, suspicious, or desperate to sus-

---

* The Institutional Review Board's written assessment of Protocol 904, issued in 1988 and acquired through a Freedom of Information Act request, indicated that board members were clearly perplexed by Schonberger's byzantine plan, particularly its extravagant array of psychiatric probes. Their first and primary concern had a plaintive quality: "To reach the explicitly stated objective—i.e., estimate incidence—it would seem that a much simpler system could be devised." After all, the agency had its own case definition, they noted. Why not simply ask referring clinicians to "check off which of the signs and symptoms pertained for each potential case? Alternatively," they proposed, "a simple questionnaire or interview dealing only with the signs and symptom list could be given to . . . patients." The board members expressed puzzlement, too, over the questionnaire's detailed queries about sufferers' sex lives. But there was a wealth of bizarre-sounding inquiries posed to patients, covering everything from their bed-wetting histories to their relationships with their siblings.

tain such relationships. Stated bluntly, victims of the disease, particularly long-term sufferers, were altered in ways that transcended the merely physical, and when they were given tests to measure their psychiatric integrity, patients often fared poorly in comparisons with members of the general population who were physically healthy.

Yet, in shearing off the disease's psychological component, the psychoneurotic theorists left the bedrock reality of the disease—its impact on the physical structure and functioning of the brain—hulking and unexamined below the surface. To a degree perhaps unparalleled in the history of infectious disease, in fact, the affliction highlighted medicine's inadequate understanding of the relationship between brain injury, intellect, and mood.

Jay Goldstein, a psychiatrist on the faculty of the University of California at Irvine and a general practitioner with close to a thousand CFS sufferers in his clinic, was the first to instigate an inquiry into these matters. Eventually, he believed, everything from patients' severe exhaustion and depressions to their disordered metabolisms and immune systems would be linked to structural damage to the brain, most probably to the limbic system, a complex brain network that controlled the establishment of memory as well as primitive instincts and mood, including the expression of fear, rage, and pleasure. The psychiatrist was aware of the MRI brain scan findings made by Cheney, Peterson, and Komaroff, but he was frustrated by the lack of specificity of the test. Even if one could prove the patient's brain was pocked with tiny lesions, how did those findings correlate with the patient's intellectual and emotional well-being? Goldstein wondered if a more sensitive technique was available for studying the brain.

That winter he learned that a former colleague, Los Angeles neurologist Marshall Handleman, had emerged as a West Coast expert in a new brain imaging technique known as the BEAM scan. (BEAM is an acronym of "brain electrical activity mapping.") Developed by a Harvard engineer, the technology was a marriage of the computer and the electroencephalogram, or EEG, which measured electrical activity in the brain. The $350,000 equipment added visual and audio stimulation to the EEG test; barely noticeable to the patient, these stimuli were called "evoked potentials." Patients were subjected to the stimuli while a computer simultaneously generated a color-coded topographical model of the brain. A second monitor compared the patient with a set of controls matched by age and sex. Thus the BEAM was able to identify not only whether a brain response was abnormal but also the precise degree to which it deviated from the normal.

Goldstein, eager to see how chronic fatigue syndrome sufferers performed on the BEAM, told Handleman he had collected a group of patients who suffered from memory and mood disorders and asked the neurologist to perform BEAM scans on a few of them. Handleman tested his first CFS sufferer on November 18, 1987.

"Jay told me very little about the condition, but he sent several patients over," Handleman recalled later. "They were college grads, more women than men. They were all very bright, but when they began telling me about their intellectual processing problems, I thought, Gee, this sounds hysterical. Then I tested this engineering professor at UCLA. He got 1600 on his boards. He got a Ph.D. in math at twenty-one. And now he's just barely hanging on to his job." Another CFS sufferer Handleman tested happened to be an oncologist who had asked Handleman for a neurology consult on a cancer patient just four months before. In addition to his prominent and disabling CFS symptoms, the oncologist was experiencing profound depression and panic attacks. "I'm prejudiced," Handleman said. "To be honest, I need to know someone was smart. And now I had two people who met my qualification of being super bright, and something had definitely happened to these people. They were not the same. I thought, Jesus, there must be something here."

By midwinter, Marshall Handleman had performed BEAM scans on fifty of Goldstein's Los Angeles patients.

"Forty-nine out of fifty of these people have abnormal brain mapping," Goldstein reported. "And not just a little abnormal but *real* abnormal—as if they've been hit in the head with a hammer."

In January, Paul Cheney flew to Handleman's West Coast clinic to see firsthand the BEAM technology Goldstein had been describing to him so tantalizingly in phone conversations for the previous several weeks. As the computer identified regions of brain dysfunction in each patient, Handleman drew on his training in both psychiatry and neurology to describe to Cheney not only the intellectual deficits affecting each patient but the emotional and behavioral problems likely to have resulted from their brain injuries as well. What struck Cheney most powerfully that afternoon in January, however, was the objective nature of the fully computerized BEAM system. He left Los Angeles in a state of excitement about the new technology. Tired of the persistent mind-body talk emanating from the NIH's publications and conferences about the new disease, Cheney commented at the time, "The *real* mind-body connection is in that room."

The doctor was further impressed by the superiority of BEAM technology to MRI technology for evaluating brain injury in the disease. "The MRI scan is an idiot savant," Cheney said. "It sees what it sees very well, but does not reflect symptomatology." BEAM scans, on the other hand, drew distinct, unequivocal connections between brain injury and intellectual processing deficits.

Ironically, it appeared, one sophisticated diagnostic technology for the disease was being quietly supplanted by a newer one before the mainstream medical community had even been made aware of the first.

Upon his return to Charlotte, Cheney asked Pan Am pilot Mayhugh Horne to undergo a BEAM scan. Horne had exhibited a dramatic combination of emotional and intellectual symptoms during the course of his disabling illness, and Cheney thought the pilot might make an interesting test case. In addition, Horne was sorely in need of evidence to persuade his employer, Pan Am, that his problems were something more than the figment of a vivid imagination. The airline's steadfast view that Horne's complaints of intellectual deterioration were delusional meant that Pan Am was withholding disability support, leaving the once richly remunerated Horne without an income to support his wife and two young sons. As a result of the company's hard-nosed stand, in fact, Horne was about to lose his house. "I had never anticipated that I would have financial worries," Horne said that year. "It's all the things that come on top of this disease that bury you."

Horne had not flown in almost a year when he agreed to make the trip to Handleman's Los Angeles clinic. While he was hardly eager to hear more bad news, concrete medical evidence to validate his claims might stave off destitution. The pilot felt an instant camaraderie with Handleman, who had been an air force flight surgeon in Vietnam. "Handleman *knows* what pilots have to do," Horne said afterward.

During the three-hour test, a number of deficits in Horne's brain emerged in bold relief, including right frontal lobe lesions that Handleman believed explained the fifty-four-year-old pilot's daily crying jags during the early years of his disease. In one area of Horne's left temporal lobe that correlates with selective attention there was no electrical activity at all. "This would support the patient's claim that he has trouble sustaining concentration," Handleman later wrote in his report. He also wrote that although it had been four years since the initial injury to Horne's brain, the pilot should nonetheless select some kind of job that did not involve "multi-complex tasking" and in which "individual lives would not be at risk." To Horne, the neurologist simply said: "Let's face it—do something else."

When Horne told Handleman that Pan Am was trying to return him to the cockpits of 747s, the neurologist called the airline. "I talked to the Pam Am doctor," Handleman recalled. "I knew Horne's BEAM was off. I told the doctor that I was a Bronze Star winner in the air force, but I still wouldn't want to be on the plane that Horne is flying. I said, 'If he crashes and this report comes up, Pan Am will be up the creek.'" Struggling to convey his concern, Handleman explained the ways in which Horne's brain was not working. "I said, 'It's like Horne is trying to draw up a memory of doing geometry problems that he did thirty years ago. He just can't draw up the file.'"

According to Handleman, the Pan Am doctor asked, "How do you know he's not a malingerer?"

"I said, 'Highly motivated men have a lot of pride in their accomplishments. They're obsessive-compulsive. They're perfectionists. They believe in honor; they don't want their honor destroyed. Pilots are usually honorable men, and air force pilots are the elite of the air force. For them to admit they have a problem is highly unusual.' And then I began to tell him about this guy's BEAM scan."

Even after Handleman submitted his lengthy written report on Horne's extensive brain problems, however, Pan Am continued to suggest to the ailing pilot that he was free to return to work. Additionally, the company held firm in its position that Horne was not entitled to disability support.

By the winter of 1989, Handleman was hooked on the new syndrome of brain dysfunction. He had performed nearly one hundred BEAM scans on Californians with the affliction and found every one of them to be abnormal, sometimes grossly so. "Patients have a variety of cognitive problems," Handleman said that year. "They may have acquired dyslexia with left parietal lobe involvement. They have paraphasias, using the wrong word—like 'table' for 'train.' They can have dyscalculia [math problems], dysgraphia [writing problems], and disorientation. They have decreased acquisition of new language from left temporal and left occipital lobe involvement, and visual-spatial perceptual problems from right parietal lobe involvement. They have attentional deficits—they can't concentrate for a period of time that allows them to program information into their memory. They're not doing well on their jobs because they have injury to their memory mechanism. That's basically the cognitive problems." The neurologist paused for breath. "Now let me tell you about mood disturbances. They are often *very* depressed. Depression tends to come from the bifrontal lobes and right temporal. They have panic attacks, which come from the right temporal lobe. They may have behavioral problems, particularly with right frontal lobe dysfunction. Some of them have decreased ability to anticipate the immediate and long-term effects of their behavior. . . . This disease is getting higher on my scale," Handleman added. "I rate it right up there with AIDS and head trauma."

It was Mayhugh Horne's conflict with his employer, Pan Am, however, that contributed most powerfully to the neurologist's emerging outrage about the apparent disregard with which mainstream medicine, and corporate medicine, had responded to the disease. Horne, after all, had been a top-ranked pilot in both the air force and the U.S. commercial fleet; he was, in fact, like the brave, highly skilled pilots with whom Handleman had flown during the Vietnam War. For Handleman, the awesome reality of the affliction and its resolute epidemic spread was hitting uncomfortably close to home.

"I want them to change the name—stop with this 'chronic fatigue' crap," Handleman said that winter. "It does a *great* disservice to these people. Doctors associate this term with malingering, and doctors work hard; they don't like malingerers. What I'm saying," the neurologist added after a moment, "is that this is just an old-fashioned subacute viral encephalitis. Let's call it what it is, and let's *deal* with it!"

Rocky Mountain Multiple Sclerosis Center, Denver, Colorado

The absence of a scientific basis for the extreme skepticism surrounding CFS research findings was highlighted by the easy acceptance of similar if not identical findings in well-established diseases. No one disputed the intellectual dysfunction that beset some AIDS patients, for instance, although the same technologies—MRI brain scans, mental status testing—had been used to document the problem in both AIDS and CFS. But AIDS was a "real" disease, hence the test results were also "real."

In February, a medical journal article about intellectual and mood disorders in victims of multiple sclerosis—disorders that were powerfully reminiscent of the difficulties faced by CFS sufferers—again starkly illustrated the bias mainstream medicine brought to bear on the newer disease. The observations and conclusions of the study exemplified a rational, levelheaded interpretation of data sorely missing in the CFS field.[2] Researchers Gary Franklin, a neurologist, and his colleagues at the University of Colorado, documented deficits in MS sufferers in the realms of problem-solving proficiency, "visuospatial" ability, attention span, concentration, and memory—the same deficits being documented in CFS. In addition to cognitive dysfunction, the Colorado researchers identified episodes of depression and manic-depression among a majority of their MS cases. Instead of blaming their patients' cognitive difficulties on their shattered emotional states or blaming their physical problems on their psychiatric difficulties, as federal scientists tended to do with CFS sufferers, the investigators hypothesized that intellectual deterioration was "an organic component" of MS, as were depression and manic-depressive cycles.

Wistar Institute, Philadelphia, Pennsylvania

In January, Elaine DeFreitas and Hilary Koprowski strengthened the link between multiple sclerosis and the retrovirus HTLV1. Their first paper on the subject, published three years earlier, had established evidence of antibodies to the retrovirus in patients. Since then a more sophisticated technique for identifying viruses rather than antibodies—polymerase chain reaction (PCR)—had come into play in the top retrovirology labs in the country. Using the new technique, virus hunters could find the agent itself, and in incredibly small amounts. Scientists designed biochemical probes to match the DNA of the virus, then used these probes to identify as little as one virus in 100,000 or more cells. Employing PCR in blood samples from six Swedish patients, DeFreitas and her colleagues had detected genetic components of the virus in every patient. Their study was published in *Science* that month.[3]

Los Angeles, California

On the strength of the initial BEAM results, Jay Goldstein that winter expanded his effort to illuminate the brain injury in CFS, reaching out to two more brain imaging experts in the region. One of them was Ismael Mena, director of the division of nuclear medicine at Harbor-UCLA Medical Center and a professor of radiological sciences at the University of California. Mena was one of the nation's experts in the NeuroSPECT scanner, a new imaging technology to study blood flow in the brain. In normal, healthy people, blood perfused the brain evenly. For two years Mena and his colleagues at UCLA had been evaluating patients with frank neurological ailments such as dementia, Alzheimer's disease, stroke, seizure disorders, brain trauma, and HIV infection—as well as patients with psychiatric disorders like depression, obsessive-compulsive disorder, and psychosis—to learn whether and in what ways blood perfusion was altered. "Every time function is diminished, blood flow is diminished as well," Mena said. "Cerebral blood flow and cerebral function are directly related."

Goldstein referred a group of his CFS sufferers for the test. Mena found that close to 70 percent of them were "*quite* abnormal." In a majority, cerebral blood flow to the temporal lobes was unusually low—most commonly the right temporal lobe. But Mena found other regions of hypoperfusion in several patients.

Goldstein managed to enlist a third expert that winter; he was Steven Lottenberg, an assistant clinical professor and clinical director of the brain imaging center at the University of California at Irvine, where Goldstein was a member of the psychiatric faculty. Lottenberg's expertise was positron emission tomography, or PET, a two-year-old imaging technique that measured brain glucose metabolism and was proving markedly more sensitive than MRI scanning in revealing damaged regions inside the brain. (BEAM scanning expert Marshall Handleman called PET scanning the Cadillac of brain imaging; BEAM scanning, Handleman suggested, was the Chevrolet.)

Lottenberg began his collaboration by performing PET scans on just six CFS sufferers. All six had abnormally low glucose metabolism in portions of their brains, but three of them had frank abnormality in the right middle frontal region. "The frontal lobe is a good one to look at," Lottenberg said, "in terms of any cognitive problems that might exist in these patients."

Lottenberg conceded that the numbers in his random trial of just six patients were too small to enable him to make definitive assumptions. "It's not data you can make conclusions from," he said, "but certainly it's very interesting data." Like Mena, Lottenberg was eager to pursue the research. Together with Goldstein, he began laying plans that winter for including healthy controls in a study of a much larger group of patients.

All three of Goldstein's collaborators—Handleman, Mena, and Lottenberg— although still in the nascent realm of their research, raised the discovery process to a new level. Their technologies differed substantially from MRI imaging and from neuropsychological testing: MRI offered exquisite anatomical views of the brain, providing evidence of *structural* abnormalities, and neuropsychology measured *intellectual* skills; the new imaging techniques provided *physiologic* data— information about the way the brain was working. Additionally, the new techniques were far more sensitive; they furnished evidence of functional problems in the absence of obvious lesions. PET scanning expert Lottenberg liked to cite an example of a stroke patient whose MRI brain scan was normal but whose PET scan revealed "a huge lesion," indicating an area where metabolism simply was not occurring. After testing several of Goldstein's patients, Lottenberg stressed that another distinct advantage of PET scanning over MRI in the new disease was PET's ability to provide "a real, objective evaluation of these patients rather than just a visual evaluation, which is a bit more subjective."

Indeed, removing the subjective element from brain evaluation in the controversial disease would preclude the kind of controversy that had swiftly enveloped the MRI results. In evaluating a BEAM scan, for instance, no one could argue that a black hole in a patient's brain that was bright red in the brains of fifty healthy age- and sex-matched controls was a normal result, or even a variance of normal. And because Goldstein's collaborators had already employed these technologies to explore a range of central nervous system and psychiatric disorders when Goldstein approached them, they had accumulated a large database with which to compare CFS victims.

By February, all three imaging experts were committed to a continued collaboration with Goldstein.

National Institute of Allergy and Infectious Diseases, Bethesda, Maryland

During the week of February 9, an NIH panel met to consider the latest round of CFS grant proposals. It was the sixth time such a meeting had been convened. The committee, a different group from the ad hoc committee of the previous year, reviewed two new proposals and three revisions. None of the grants was approved for funding.

By that winter, cancer epidemiologist Seymour Grufferman's skepticism about the Bethesda agency's declared commitment to funding extramural research on the new disease seemed to have merit. In the nearly two years since the agency's request for grant proposals, scientists around the country had submitted approximately thirty proposals, including resubmissions. All of them except Anthony Komaroff's had been denied funding.* Paul Cheney's assessment of the process was characteristically blunt: "I don't think God could get an NIH grant at this point."

Ann Schleuderberg, the NIH administrator in charge of the chronic fatigue syndrome grant program, seemed impervious to the grumblings in the CFS research community. "Early on, particularly in something as difficult to study as this, it will be hard to get super-duper scores," she said. "But when scores are arrived at that are indicative of really super scores, I expect that funding will become available."

Among independent researchers, the composition of the government's grant review committees was perhaps the greatest bone of contention. At NIH, administrators like Schleuderberg delegated scientists working outside the agency to serve on panels that convened two or three times each year. These committees were usually standing panels, but on occasion they were ad hoc juries. In either case, by law, the panels were to be composed of scientists who might fairly be considered the peers of those scientists whose grant proposals were under consideration and who knew something about the subject of the proposal. This was the time-honored process by which a sizable portion of the biomedical research in the nation was funded. In the case of CFS, however, the process, at least as it was handled by Schleuderberg, was muddied considerably.

The matter of peer review, particularly, was problematic given the tiny fraternity of CFS experts; there weren't very many peers around. Many of the researchers who were convinced the disease was real were submitting grants, a course of action that tended to preclude their participation on a review panel. Theoretically, there existed a corrective mechanism: if a scientist's grant was under consideration and he or she was also a member of the review panel, the scientists simply left the room during the discussion of the proposal. Schleuderberg and her NIH colleagues, however, had already demonstrated a bias against certain researchers who had made strongly worded expressions of belief in the reality of the disease; the participation of these investigators in a review panel seemed to be precluded. Outside the CFS fraternity, of course, there remained a sizable body of scientists who doubted that the disease existed and who—was it mere coincidence?—knew next to nothing about it. Schleuderberg and her colleagues drew liberally from this group in the early years of the smoke-and-mirrors grant program.

Complaints arose about Schleuderberg herself. Many grant-seekers, in fact, suspected Schleuderberg and her superiors of manipulating the supposedly independent peer review process to suit the NIH's bias. An unruffled Schleuderberg

---

* Anthony Komaroff's $800,000 award the previous fall to study the prevalence of CFS among members of a health maintenance organization in Seattle would be paid out once each year over a three- to five-year course. "Komaroff's prevalency study will teach us absolutely nothing about this disease that we don't already know," Cheney observed a few months after he received word of Komaroff's winning entry. "It will show that chronic fatigue syndrome is a common problem. And the results won't be available for three years." In fact, it was five years before the statistics were released.

cheerfully deflected the criticism, portraying herself as a disinterested party, a mere facilitator. Repeatedly, she insisted that she bore no responsibility for the decisions made by the doctors and scientists who convened to evaluate proposals. Although she frequently sat in on meetings of these panels—in an "advisory" capacity, she always hastened to explain—she herself played no role in scoring the proposals. Further, she said, although her role as grant administrator enabled her to make recommendations about who might sit on the study section, she was not officially able to select the panel members.*

Stephen Straus, on the other hand, could very well be asked to sit in on the review, Schleuderberg suggested, and like her, he could propose review panel members. "You might have an intramural expert like Steve Straus—just as an example of an appropriate person to be brought in," she said during a conversation that winter. "It has to be someone doing intramural research in their own little ivory tower." Schleuderberg, however, steadfastly refused to confirm or deny whether Straus actually had been called in at any point so far, either to select panel members or to help them rule on the scientific merit of grant proposals. She deemed that to be private NIH business and not for public dissemination.

▓

Schleuderberg's characterization of Stephen Straus as someone who labored in an ivory tower may have been apt for the purposes of defining the difference between an NIH bureaucrat, like her, and an NIH scientist. But in fact, Straus and his institution, the National Institute of Allergy and Infectious Diseases, were working to engineer a niche for the researcher that was far from hermetic. On February 15 the NIAID public affairs office issued a press release describing a new study by the agency's expert in the February issue of the *Journal of Clinical Psychiatry,* a publication read by some but not all psychiatrists and unknown to the lay public.[4] The article presented the results of psychiatric interviews conducted on the two dozen participants in his acyclovir trial during their hospitalization three years before, and drew some conclusions.

To circumvent the possibility that Straus's observations would go unnoticed by the popular press and the general public, the agency sent the three-page press release by fax or Federal Express to approximately five hundred reporters and news organizations around the country, including the television networks and the science and government writers for every major newspaper and wire service. The press release announced, in boldface capital letters, **"LIFETIME HISTORY OF PSYCHIATRIC ILLNESS IN PEOPLE WITH CHRONIC FATIGUE SYNDROME."**

Recipients of the announcement reacted enthusiastically. Virtually every metropolitan newspaper in the nation reported on the article in the obscure journal, cribbing their headlines from the press release. "Chronic Fatigue Linked to Psychiatric Troubles," topped the *Washington Post*'s story, for instance. In the weeks that followed, the story percolated through the nation's media, from newspapers

---

* That job fell to yet another NIH administrator in the division of research grants. In 1988, Horace Stiles, a DRG administrator, was responsible for assembling at least one of the ad hoc panels that reviewed CFS grants.

to network television to magazines. Almost without exception, most journalists reporting the study failed to interview anyone but Straus. His conclusions about the disease, based on two dozen sufferers, were repeated uncritically; his data remained unexamined.

Straus had ordered that patients in the acyclovir study be given the Diagnostic Interview Schedule during their hospitalization at the Bethesda Clinical Center. The DIS was supposed to measure and quantify depression and other aspects of psychiatric health; it had not been designed to evaluate the psychiatric status of people with medical illnesses. Straus, in addition, used no controls; a suitable control group would have been people suffering from another disabling chronic illness. According to Straus, twenty-one of the twenty-eight patients interviewed "had been or were currently affected by a psychiatric illness."

"This rate of psychiatric illness," according to the press release, "greatly exceeds that reported for the general population."

Fifteen of the patients were said to be depressed; fifteen had other psychiatric problems that were identified as phobias or anxiety.*

For most Americans the news was merely an interesting item in the morning paper, something noted, then stored away until the next wave of coverage of the disease. For sufferers, the government's new tack seemed tantamount to a declaration of war. Common sense suggested that anyone who was chronically ill was bound to be depressed. With his new paper, Straus had moved the goalpost: he was now proposing that there was something psychologically "different" about people with CFS long before they ever fell ill. It hardly mattered that some victims were so sick they could no longer hold a job or function within a family; nor did it matter that some of them were wheelchair-bound or bedridden, unable even to care for themselves. The government's premier health agency was spreading the news: the catastrophic disease from which they suffered appeared to have its roots in mental illness.

Patients felt the impact of Straus's report and the potent NIH-fostered press blitz in the most intimate regions of their lives: it undermined their relationships with their spouses, children, and friends. More devastatingly, it added an immeasurable burden to their struggle for survival in a society that failed to appreciate their dilemma. Confusion and ambivalence about the disease, which already had created ruinous obstacles for sufferers in the realm of jobs and medical care, were intensified. For Straus and his supporters in Bethesda, the paper was an abstract undertaking to advance Straus's career and standing within his institution. For victims of the disease, the paper became a weapon that would be wielded against them at every turn, especially in courts of law and in the de facto courts of American medicine.

In Charlotte, one of Paul Cheney's patients, a former lawyer who had been completely disabled by the disease, felt the brunt of Straus's science immediately.

---

* In fact, eight of the "phobias" that Straus found to predate onset of CFS were common problems few laypeople would characterize as psychiatric disease. One of the acyclovir patients so branded, for instance, confessed that she suffered from a fear of heights. Simple phobias—fear of heights, claustrophobia, fear of snakes, and so on—were so prevalent in the general population that, according to one psychiatrist who evaluated the study, "it is very misleading to call it a predisposing psychiatric problem."

In divorce proceedings instigated by her husband, the young woman sought alimony because she was no longer capable of supporting herself; her husband was contesting her request. "This patient's husband is now trying to prove that she is crazy," Cheney reported that winter. Eventually Cheney found himself engaged in a three-hour deposition with the husband's lawyer. Throughout the grueling session, the attorney quoted again and again from Straus's study and from the scientist's previous articles that insinuated the same general concept: CFS was a psychiatric affliction of women. Cheney struggled to explain the subtleties of the disease and the blowtorch approach to the problem taken by Straus, to little avail. The young woman lost her case and was left to the vagaries of the Social Security system.

Equally serious, Straus's work further alienated mainstream practitioners from the disease and its victims. On the other hand, it was a reassuring balm for the public; citizens now had it on highest authority that the disease was neither contagious nor deserving of significant taxpayer-supported research. In one bold stroke, using American taxpayers' dollars, Straus had managed to brand as mentally ill hundreds of thousands of people in the United States alone.

Asked why her agency felt obliged to trumpet the findings—which, after all, were published in an obscure medical journal and based on a sampling of only twenty-eight patients—as if they were a major scientific breakthrough, the press officer at NIH fell silent.

"Well," she said after a lengthy pause, "for chronic fatigue syndrome, there aren't that many studies that come out of the National Institutes of Health. But it's our second most popular inquiry from the public. It's just behind AIDS. We know there's a lot of interest in it."

17

The Lie

Straus's paper hit the burgeoning Charlotte organization like an electric bolt. CFIDS Association president Marc Iverson, an eleven-year sufferer, was angry. In an editorial in the association's newsletter, Iverson wrote, "[Straus's] studies have grave flaws in experimental design. . . . His conclusions do not follow from his data, his subjects do not all meet Centers for Disease Control criteria. . . . Funds, which are scarce for CFIDS research, should be allocated to those projects most likely to uncover the organic causative agent and the best treatments for this disease."

The *CFIDS Chronicle,* now mailed to more than 15,000 subscribers, also included articles by Paul Cheney and Los Angeles clinician Jay Goldstein, both of whom attacked Straus's methodology.

Goldstein noted: "It is extremely important that the interviewer not be biased. There should be multiple interviewers who are blinded to the disease status of the patients, who should have been divided into three groups: normals, those with an unrelated illness, and those with CFIDS."

He also raised the question of selection bias. "Why did Straus choose so few patients, and what characteristics of these special twenty-eight made him pick them?" Goldstein asked. "The choice should have been random, but one can only conjecture how it was actually made. We are not told in this article." He was also perplexed by a diagnosis of alcoholism in three of Straus's CFS sufferers, since one nearly universal aspect of the disease was alcohol intolerance.

Goldstein was stuck, too, by Straus's extrapolations from his two dozen subjects to the sizable realm of people suffering from the disease. Considering his tiny patient cohort, Straus's assertions began to seem grandiose indeed. As an example, Goldstein cited Straus's "ludicrous pronouncement" that "somatization disorder [hypochondria] and/or antisocial personality disorder are also overrepresented in our female study group participants (10 percent and 10 percent respectively) compared with rates for women in the general population of up to only 1.2 percent in three U.S. sites.

"This axiomatic-sounding statement is based on just two patients being diagnosed," Goldstein complained. "To generalize to the universe of CFIDS patients on this meager sample is sheer folly. . . . To be quite frank, I could not believe a research paper could be this bad and be published."

Paul Cheney was hardly less incensed by Straus's latest effort. "Having been exposed to Dr. Straus's 'mind-body' views of CFIDS at a National Institutes of Health–sponsored workshop in Pittsburgh in September 1988," the Charlotte clinician wrote, "I am not surprised by the appearance of this paper in the medical literature. However, I am surprised by the lack of rigor in a scientific journal concerning an issue which, while a valid subject of investigation, can easily be (and has been) a source of misinformation and misinterpretation, which hurts persons with the disorder and may reduce chances for funding this emerging clinical entity. And I am appalled by the lack of sensitivity and integrity apparent in the National Institute of Allergy and Infectious Diseases press release. . . .

"It is worth noting," he added, "that in a study of AIDS patients the lifetime incidence of depression before (AIDS) symptoms is as high as 70 percent, and at diagnosis (of AIDS), it is greater than 80 percent. . . . Despite these very high percentages, NIH researchers are, with good reason, investing virtually all of their energies in studying the 'organic' components of AIDS. One must wonder why the same is apparently not true for CFIDS."

Privately Cheney complained about what he called Straus's manipulation of data. "The concept that psychological disturbances are major drivers of disease is a valid one, but it applies to *all* illness," the doctor said. "To use that valid data to drive *misinformation* about chronic fatigue syndrome is what I object to. There is a conscious attempt to misrepresent those findings—to *prove* it is a psychiatric disease. Straus's article is an absolute *lie*. He said twenty-one people had a 'life history' of psychological disorder. Ten preceded the disease, eleven came after. But eight of the ten who came before were simple phobias! There is a very conscious attempt to misrepresent the data."

Straus's critics were hardly limited to the patient movement and its clinician-experts, however. The following April, the *Journal of Clinical Psychiatry,* which had published the Straus paper, published letters from other doctors who took issue both with Straus's assumptions and with his paltry patient sample. One of them, George Reiss, a Phoenix clinician, wrote: "I am concerned that these investigators simply do not have enough individuals to reach any conclusion other than for this small group. . . . At present, all that can be said from this study is that in *this* small group of patients with chronic fatigue syndrome, psychiatric diagnoses predated their illness 48 percent of the time. No definite conclusions can be drawn about other patients with chronic fatigue syndrome."

Another doctor, Cecil Bradley of Union City, California, flatly proposed that Straus's conclusions "are not warranted." Bradley noted that many diseases are sometimes preceded by depressive symptoms. With diabetes, for example, especially the insulin-dependent variety, which is "generally considered to be an autoimmune illness occurring in genetically predisposed persons following some insult, perhaps infectious," there is a "33 percent lifetime prevalence of major depression.

"Prior psychiatric illness," Bradley continued, "is not considered likely to predispose people to diabetes. In another autoimmune disease, Hashimoto's thyroiditis, psychiatric symptoms may be the earliest presenting symptoms of the disease. Depression has long been noted to be a common presenting symptom of carcinoma of the stomach." He added that "note should also be made of the study's small sample."

Straus's presumed involvement with the grant-funding mechanism at the NIH protected him from full-out frontal attacks by the majority of researchers committed to unraveling the disease. Anyone trying to win federal research dollars would have been exceedingly ill-advised to publicly condemn either his research agenda or his methodologies. Only those without a prayer of becoming recipients—doctors like Cheney and Goldstein who were tainted by their high-profile association with clinical practices serving large numbers of sufferers—could afford to take such risks. In fact, it was increasingly apparent that, in order to obtain government money to study the disease, investigators would have to pay lip service, at the very least, to Straus's theories and opinions in their grant proposals. As a result, by 1989, Stephen Straus had become the Teflon scientist of the troubled CFS arena.

In the years ahead, patients and their advocates in medicine would engage in a kind of armchair psychoanalysis of Straus and his motives. The activity had its own poetic justice, since Straus, too, was engaging in his articles and lectures in an identical form of idle speculation about victims of the disease. Needless to say, Straus's platform as a federal scientist and presumed expert was wider and vastly more influential than any forum patients could devise. Preeminent among the speculative theories concerning his intellectual evolution toward his "psychoneurotic" perspective was that Straus had become increasingly frustrated, even humiliated, by his inability to explain the etiology of the disease he had described with such authority in the *Annals* in 1985. This seemed especially feasible since it now was apparent that Epstein-Barr virus had been a red herring. Straus, after all, had proposed that the virus might be at the root of the symptoms of the disease. He had also suggested that if the disease was not caused by Epstein-Barr virus, then perhaps it was caused by an unknown pathogen that disrupted the immune system. Either way, the scientist was talking about a transmissible organic agent. In the intervening four years, however, Straus had been unable to prove the existence of such an agent. Most scientists would be able to live with the uncertainty, Straus-watchers argued. James Jones, for instance, had postulated virtually the same theories in the same issue of the *Annals,* but the Denver researcher had hardly launched himself on a psychiatric investigation of his patients in the absence of an etiologic agent. Jones, in fact, was increasingly vocal by the end of the decade about the need for clinicians to reject a diagnosis of depression in patients with CFS symptoms.

Unlike Jones, Straus's critics argued, the thin-skinned Straus could not bear what must have seemed to him to be a public tarnishing when his Epstein-Barr theory failed to fly. According to Susan Simon, a psychotherapist who had been an acyclovir trial participant, Straus suffered a "serious depression" when he broke the code on the acyclovir study and discovered that the anti-herpesvirus drug had failed to ameliorate what he had posited as a potential herpesvirus disease. The patient's source for this rumor was nurse Janet Dale, Straus's assistant. The rumor may have been unfounded, but it reflected an intensifying view of Straus as someone who found scientific ambiguity intolerable and who had a deep emotional investment in his own scientific authority.*

Some suspected that there were darker reasons for Straus's shift, having to do with the government's need to soft-pedal the disease.† Certainly it was vastly easier and required fewer resources to certify depression in these patients than to identify the presence of a rare virus, as Paul Cheney, Anthony Komaroff, Elaine DeFreitas, Berch Henry, and others were trying to do. And, without question, steely nerves were required of anyone who cared to discuss the disease as a bona fide affliction within the increasingly angry, derisive environment of academic medicine. Anyone for whom professional standing was paramount would find it far more rewarding to follow the path being forged by Straus. In fact, Straus's decision to plumb his patients' subconscious seemed to precipitate a similar conversion among other federal researchers whose amateur psychiatry skills apparently were just waiting to be dusted off.

Charlotte, North Carolina

The very day Straus's paper appeared in the psychiatry journal, the *Annals of Internal Medicine* published a letter from David Bell and Paul Cheney.[1] The clinicians reported exceedingly high levels of an immune system protein called interleukin-2 in the blood serum of 104 CFS patients, 51 of them children from Lyndonville, 53 of them adults in Cheney's practice in Charlotte. The finding was remarkable, but it received no publicity of any kind.

During the late 1970s and mid-1980s synthetic interleukin-2—alternatively known as T-cell growth factor because it promoted the proliferation of T-cells—had been touted as a magic-bullet cancer therapy. By the late 1980s, however, the drug was used only in the most desperate cases because of its extraordinary toxicity. For many cancer sufferers, the cure turned out to be worse than the disease. In addition to "severe cognitive changes [with] evidence of cognitive deterioration" and mood changes, researchers had noted decreased energy, fatigue, anorexia, disorientation, chills, heart arrhythmias, and even coma. "Many [patients] likened their symptoms to an influenza-like syndrome," one group of researchers wrote.

Spurred by two 1987 reports describing the toxic side effects of synthetic Il-2 in cancer patients, symptoms that were remarkably similar to the symptoms of

---

* Byron Hyde, the Ottawa clinician who specialized in CFS, recalled some years later that he was seated next to Straus at a 1987 meeting on chronic viral disease at the Centers for Disease Control when Gary Holmes passed out copies of his just-published Tahoe study. While it did little to advance understanding of the mechanisms of the disease, the article certainly cast serious doubt on Epstein-Barr's role in causation. Hyde recalled vividly Straus's reaction to the paper. According to Hyde, Straus began talking to himself out loud as the scientific purport of the paper sank in: "He held a monologue that lasted at least two minutes," Hyde recalled. "I thought he was having a nervous breakdown. He kept saying, 'They've ruined me. What will my colleagues think? These goddamn patients!' He seemed to be taking it personally, and talked as if the patients had banded together to destroy him."
† Commented one sufferer who was among Straus's tiny patient cohort in Bethesda: "This is exactly what happened to AIDS patients. It becomes necessary to psychologize this disease to make us an 'other.' This is not a medical event; this is a political event."

CFS,[2] Cheney had been measuring interleukin-2 levels in his adult patients in Charlotte. He wondered if CFS patients were suffering, in some part, from the effects of an exorbitant rush of the substance in response to whatever pathogen was causing their disease. A search of the literature revealed just four other disorders with such a marker: chronic progressive multiple sclerosis, tropical spastic paraparesis, T-cell lymphoma, and AIDS. Cheney was particularly impressed by the fact that, like tropical spastic paraparesis, the latter two were definite retrovirus-caused maladies, and the first—MS—was a suspected retrovirus disease.

Strikingly, the levels of interleukin-2 in most of Cheney's patients were higher than in people suffering from any of the four diseases described in the literature—and as much as fifty times higher than in healthy controls.

When in June 1988 the *New England Journal of Medicine* published a letter about high interleukin-2 levels in multiple sclerosis patients,[3] Cheney began to wonder if his interleukin-2 findings should be published as well. The MS researchers, after all, had used the same test kit to assay for interleukin-2 that Cheney's lab used, suggesting that the values between the two patient groups would have a high degree of standardization. Cheney was impressed, too, that the interleukin-2 levels in his adult CFS patients were higher than the levels in even the most severe MS cases.

"The average value for rapidly progressing MS is forty-two units of interleukin-2 per milliliter of serum," Cheney commented. "In *our* patients, the average value is sixty, but our highest value is *sixteen hundred* units per milliliter."

Cheney decided to conscript David Bell into his interleukin-2 research. The Charlotte doctor was curious to know whether children with the disease displayed the same abnormality; he also wanted to test patients from a second, geographically distinct location. Bell was immediately amenable to Cheney's overture. The doctors decided to select three categories of children: those who were severely ill with CFS, children who were mildly ill, and healthy children. The well children had normal levels of interleukin-2; children with mild disease had levels ten times higher; children with severe disease had levels higher than any measure Cheney could find in the literature for AIDS, lymphoma, tropical spastic paraparesis, or multiple sclerosis.

The story behind the publication of Cheney and Bell's four-paragraph letter on interleukin-2 levels in chronic fatigue syndrome, which they had sent first to the *New England Journal of Medicine,* was painful as well as emblematic of the medical politics that had thoroughly enveloped the disease by 1988.

Seeking to make his letter rejection-proof, Cheney had carefully modeled it after the MS letter. Cheney's letter, in fact, was even more persuasive than the multiple sclerosis letter in that he provided data on patients from two geographically distinct regions and in two age categories—adult and child—as well as from healthy controls.

"Six weeks went by, and we didn't hear anything," Cheney recalled later. "So we called the *New England Journal* editors up. And they told us they had sent it out for peer review. I understood that to be a good sign," the doctor continued, "because it suggested they liked it enough to have it reviewed. But it was also unusual, because they don't usually peer-review letters. The next thing I heard was when I went to the Rome meeting in October: I heard Stephen Straus was criticizing my letter.

"At first I thought, What the hell does *Straus* know about our IL-two letter? Then I realized the *New England Journal* must have sent it to him. Or it's possible that they sent it to someone else and *that* person called Straus. Straus heard about it through the peer review process, of that I'm sure. And I imagine the *New England Journal did* call Straus because they were considering his acyclovir study at the time my letter was received. So they were considering Straus's acyclovir study and my IL-two letter at the same time," Cheney said, shaking his head.

"When we got back from Italy," the doctor continued, "we called the *New England Journal* again and were told, 'It's back from the reviewer, it's sitting on the editor's desk, we'll let you know by the end of next week.' The end of the next week came, and we heard nothing. So we called back and were told, 'The letter is on its way.' The letter arrived at last, and they had rejected it. It's basically unfair to hang up a major article like [Komaroff's] Tahoe manuscript for thirteen months, and it's unfair to hang up a letter like that for four months. And then you find out at some meeting that someone's criticizing it, and it hasn't even been published!"

Upon receiving the *New England Journal*'s rejection notice, Cheney immediately sent the interleukin-2 letter to the *Annals of Internal Medicine.* "We got an acceptance notice in three weeks," Cheney recalled. "It was published four weeks later."

San Francisco, California

On January 11 the San Francisco Health Commission, which oversaw the city's health department, met and proposed seven priority concerns for the new year. Prevention and treatment of chronic fatigue syndrome were among them.

The week before, Jan Montgomery's task force had met with a health department epidemiologist, aides to city supervisors Harry Britt and Nancy Walker, and several patients. The group began laying the groundwork for a medical conference on the disease to be held in San Francisco in the spring. A representative from the health department suggested that Stephen Straus be invited to speak. "The entire community of people with the illness went crazy," Montgomery reported. "We said, 'It's like having a conference on the Holocaust and inviting someone who believes the Holocaust didn't happen.' " The health department backed down.

In an effort to raise money for the conference, Montgomery wrote to the CDC, which had funds in its budget to support medical conferences on emerging diseases. In a letter dated February 10, the agency's grants management officer, Henry Cassell III, informed Montgomery that her application for a public health conference support grant of $15,000 had been recommended for approval. The bad news: "it was not selected for funding this year."

Montgomery was fascinated by an anonymous agency assessment of her proposal, which she received along with Cassell's letter. In it, CFS was described as a "fairly new disease ... an important issue," and one which "appears to be an emerging epidemic."

Clinical Immunology Society, Arlington, Virginia

The passion that marked discussion of the disease was intense, and more than one clinician drew the analogy of a holy war to describe the division over the disease that had split the medical community. The rough-and-tumble spirit of the dispute was exemplified by an exchange between doctors at a meeting of the Clinical Immunology Society, held that year in Arlington, Virginia. Before giving an overview of the disease at an afternoon workshop, Andrew Saxon, head of clinical allergy and immunology at UCLA, where medical staff were still discouraged from rendering a CFS diagnosis, donned sunglasses, a Hawaiian shirt, and a trench coat. "I might not get out of town alive after I give this talk," he began. "They apparently couldn't get anyone east of the Mississippi to do this, so they had to reach way out to the West Coast to bring in a hit man, and that's me."

In fact, a number of clinical immunologists who had an abiding research interest in the disease were in the audience. Any one of them would have been more qualified to address the subject, and a few of them had sent original research papers on the disease to the organizers in advance of the meeting and been rejected as speakers. Nancy Klimas, the University of Miami AIDS expert, was there, as was Australian John Dwyer, who had served as chief of the clinical immunology section at Yale's medical school before being named the head of the school of medicine at the University of New South Wales in Sydney, Australia, where he had been studying the disease for five years. In a book published the previous year, Dwyer had concluded that "there is no longer any doubt that the syndrome we are discussing is primarily organic, not psychological," and he condemned the "intellectual arrogance" of his peers who continued to deny the existence of the disease.[4] Klimas, who was sitting behind Dwyer during Saxon's talk, recalled some years later that Dwyer's neck veins bulged and his skin reddened as Saxon pressed on, promising to examine the disease "in at least a humorous if not accurate way."

"I have a *major* problem with the idea that this is one illness," Saxon announced. "The second problem I have is with the word 'infection,' which is probably not true. . . . But you *can* catch it from reading the newspaper! The world is in the midst of two great pandemics. One is AIDS. . . . The second great pandemic is CFS. It hasn't struck certain parts of equatorial Africa because they don't read our news in English as much, but most English-speaking countries have been swept away by this pandemic." The disease, he added, was "becoming a form of mass hysteria. . . . What's happened is we've really generated a social issue today."

Saxon also criticized the CDC's case definition because, he said, "it's given the imprimatur that we know what we're dealing with, so patients can be told, 'You have chronic fatigue syndrome.' The doctor's off the hook, the patient has a socially acceptable disease, and everybody's happy."

Addressing the pattern of complaints voiced by sufferers, Saxon observed, "[Patients] don't have a lot of feverishness, a lot of sore throats—" quickly adding, "Well, they didn't used to but they do today—they've *learned* to" in their efforts to escape a diagnosis of depression. The doctor also bet his colleagues a case of beer that no more than 2 or 3 percent of patients would turn out to have symptoms caused by a virus, including Epstein-Barr, cytomegalovirus, or "HTLV1 and HTLV2, the known human leukemia viruses." Instead, Saxon counseled, the correct diagnosis was likely to be psychiatric—a diagnosis he urged his peers to render sheerly by default. "I think you can be right with ninety-five percent of the patients who walk into your office," he said, "and, hell, as a physician being ninety-five percent right is damn good!"

Saxon's address was met with applause, but when the floor was opened to discussion, John Dwyer leaped to his feet in fury.

"Andy," Dwyer began, "when there are so many things that you know so much about, isn't it *amazing* that they asked you to give a talk about something of which you know nothing?" Dwyer continued, "You're so extraordinarily knowledgeable. I've heard you give some wonderful talks. But the only thing I agreed with you about in that talk was what you said about how amusing you were.

"This is a *serious* topic. There is *clearly* a pandemic of this sweeping around the world. I'm seeing people who literally cannot walk from one end of this hall to the other end of this hall without having to rest for four to eight hours. We see patients with quite gross impairments in concentration, people who had wonderful jobs that required great intellectual capacity, who are reduced to being unable to work—"

Saxon, becoming uneasy, interrupted Dwyer: "John, what is the question?"

"I'm making a statement," Dwyer responded angrily, "and then I'm going to give you a question. Now, you take these patients with these gross symptoms, and you send them to a psychiatrist and you tell the psychiatrist, 'I don't want you to send anybody back to me who you think has a primary psychiatric condition.' Then, when you get them back from the psychiatrist, you study their immune system and you find reproducible, demonstrable abnormality in their immune system—and by far the most reliable test we've found is anergy [an inability to marshal an immune system defense against certain antigens, toxic substances such as bacteria]. Then if you take that subgroup, you have a group of people with a homogeneous condition! Now, in a double-blind placebo-controlled trial, we've found these people do respond to—"

"John, stop!" Saxon interrupted again. "You're trying to make this into a controversy. *I* don't know if they're a homogeneous group or not, but you've obviously got a very small group of patients who may have some other disease, or *a* disease."

"We *don't* have a small group of patients," Dwyer shouted. "We've got *hundreds* of patients! Surely that's the whole point! And my question to you is, don't you think we should get an interested scientific group like this to work on a better case definition? Because I think there are hundreds of *thousands* of patients, and if we had a better case definition we could do some good science on this disease."

Before Dwyer could finish his response, the session's moderator abruptly ended the debate by urging the assembled scientists to address questions on other subjects to members of the speakers' panel besides Saxon.

Although the moderator's intervention denied her a chance to express her thoughts, Miami researcher Nancy Klimas was barely less affronted by Saxon's attack on the disease than was Dwyer. "*I* was in the audience," she recalled bitterly some years later. "*Dwyer* was in the audience. There were some very good immunologists in the audience, and none of us were accepted for presentations. But they had accepted a person who has never done a study of this illness to blast it out of the water."

A compulsion to "blast" the disease "out of the water" as if it were some elaborate scientific hoax prevailed among organizers of the annual meetings of other large medical societies as well. Michael Ascher, the chief virologist for the California State Health Department, for instance, expressed the wish that "we could just figure out some way to get the Infectious Disease Society of America [of which he was a member] to talk about this disease at their meetings in some way other than humiliating the most recent version of it—because you sort of come away skeptical."

Prince Henry Hospital, Little Bay, New South Wales, Australia

John Dwyer was among a coterie of medical specialists in New South Wales who had been actively studying the disease since the early 1980s. He and his colleagues in the Departments of Immunology and Infectious Diseases at Sydney's Prince Henry Hospital had noticed the affliction in their clinic in 1982. Denis Wakefield, an immunopathologist in the group, recalled, "We began seeing patients with severe unexplained fatigue after viral infections. It was about the same time that we began to see a lot of AIDS patients. We were struck by the similarity of AIDS to this disease. It was very like the slim disease, as AIDS was then being called, except that these patients didn't waste."

Since 1982, Wakefield's team had identified more than seven hundred Australians with the disease. Although they had yet to evaluate any clusters of the disease in Australia, it was apparent to them that the malady was on the increase. By 1989, Wakefield and his colleagues were seeing at least twenty new patients every month with the disease, most of them from Sydney and neighboring regions in New South Wales, but from every point on the Australian continent, as well. A preponderance of their patients were female; the mean age of the sufferers was thirty-five. Their waiting list at Prince Henry Hospital was a torturous six months. They undertook an epidemiological survey of the disease in the New South Wales region in 1989. Their findings would not be published until the following year, but their preliminary assessment to their data suggested that CFS was commonplace in southeastern Australia—at least as common as multiple sclerosis.

"The doctors in Australia think we're out on a limb," Wakefield said. "There's a lot of skepticism and it's not seen as a common disease." Nevertheless, he continued, there were enough clinicians in Melbourne, Brisbane, Perth, and elsewhere in Australia who found the disease credible that they were helping the team in its research. "We're the group in the country with the biggest interest in the disease, but there are groups of doctors in each of the major cities who are at least interested enough to see the patients and help us with our clinical trials."

One study under way was a trial of large doses of intravenously administered gamma globulin. The substance was manufactured from the pooled blood serum of healthy people and was rich in virus-fighting antibodies. So far, the group was having some success with it. The team had already published a study in the *Medical Journal of Australia* that documented a loss of immunological integrity in one hundred CFS sufferers.[5] Like their U.S. counterparts—Anthony Komaroff, Nancy Klimas, Paul Cheney, and others—Dwyer and Wakefield had found the same immunological problems in Australians, including disordered ratios of T-cell subsets and reduced levels of immunoglobulins, the proteins that make up disease-fighting antibodies. The group's most striking finding was made employing the French Multitest. Developed to track the progress of AIDS and ARC, the Multitest measured the vitality of the body's immune system response when minute quantities of seven different antigens were injected just below the skin surface of the forearm. Among the Australians studied, 33 percent were hypoergic, meaning they had a reduced response; 55 percent were anergic, meaning their immune systems failed to respond at all.

"The findings of reduced responses in 88 percent of patients provides the strongest evidence reported of disordered T-cell function in patients with chronic fatigue syndrome," the scientists had written in their article. By comparison, they added, "One percent of healthy Australian adults demonstrate [this problem] using [the Multitest]."

Charlotte, North Carolina

Paul Cheney was unaware of the Australians' experiments with the Multitest when he decided to employ it in his own practice in 1989. As always when he began using a new technology, he logged the results into his computer. Eventually he tested 149 patients and 22 healthy controls matched with patients for age and sex. Of his patients, 21 failed to register any reaction at all, suggesting anergy. In combination with a positive HIV test, anergy on the Multitest was considered diagnostic for AIDS. Another third of Cheney's patients were hypoergic. Cheney's remaining patients had reactions that were within the normal range on the Multitest.

"It's just so obvious that this disease is an immunodeficiency syndrome of some kind," the doctor commented that winter.

Centers for Disease Control, Atlanta, Georgia

Performing investigations of cluster outbreaks was the best, if not the only, way to gain insight into the cause and mode of transmission of an idiopathic disease. D. A. Henderson, who in 1956 investigated the Punta Gorda outbreak for the CDC, had emphasized repeatedly that his colleagues needed to remain alert for new outbreaks of what Henderson called epidemic neuromyasthenia. The mystery of this devastating illness, Henderson insisted, could be unraveled only by launching an inquiry as early in the outbreak as possible, obtaining blood samples and medical histories in the earliest weeks or even days. With the exception of Walter Gunn, however, epidemiologists employed at the CDC staunchly resisted undertaking any such investigation into the disease they had named chronic fatigue syndrome, either in the second half of the 1980s or well into the 1990s. Certainly there was no shortage of opportunities. By accounts from inside and outside the agency, cluster outbreaks of CFS were being reported with routine regularity to federal epidemiologists. Walter Gunn's conservative estimate put the number of reports his branch was receiving from doctors or other medically sophisticated sources at "at *least*" ten a year.

According to documents supplied through the Freedom of Information Act—documents apparently chosen at random by the agency's FOIA officers—reported outbreaks included a cluster of forty to sixty cases in Doylestown, Pennsylvania (1986); a cluster of five pediatric nurses—one of whom developed nasopharyngeal cancer, a cancer associated with reactivation of Epstein-Barr virus—at Overlook Hospital in Summit, New Jersey (1986); a cluster of more than one hundred cases among staff at an acute care hospital in Quebec, Canada (1986); a cluster of an unknown number of cases in Van Horn, Texas (1987); a cluster of twenty-six out of thirty employees at a post office in Crescent City, California (1987); and a cluster of more than forty policemen as well as some of their spouses and children in Spokane, Washington (1988). One such report was relayed to Atlanta by a small health department in upstate New York, according to Walter Gunn. Fifteen employees worked at the health department; ten of them had developed a disease that met the government's own criteria for a CFS diagnosis.

Gunn noted that the primary opposition to on-site investigations came from his boss, Larry Schonberger. "The resistance I get here," Gunn said in 1989, "is that we don't have a marker. Schonberger doesn't want to respond to outbreaks because we don't have the marker."

Gunn found Schonberger's objection disingenuous. After all, he reasoned, the CDC's own surveillance system had been designed on the principle that agency staff had tools to sort out cases from non-cases, with or without a virus. Gunn proposed to Schonberger that the agency use the same techniques to identify cases in cluster investigations. "I keep saying, 'Why can't we go into the outbreak, using the surveillance team?' " Gunn said. "It's *feasible*," he added, his frustration evident. "I don't understand why they won't do it!"

A few in the community of CFS researchers gamely tried to defend the agency's failure to investigate: "The CDC is a beleaguered federal agency and it gets calls every day from people all over the country who think they've spotted an epidemic of something," Komaroff said that year. "It's like firemen in the firehouse who get nine false calls out of every ten. It becomes tiring."

Yet, by Gunn's account, cluster reports were coming from all directions by 1989. Furthermore, Congress had charged the agency to investigate these reports and had supplied taxpayer dollars expressly for that purpose. On paper, agency administrators paid lip service to the goal: early in 1989, for instance, an agency document listing the agency's "future plans" in the CFS arena included the phrase "[to] investigate suspected clusters of CFS that may be reported to CDC in order to better delineate this illness, clinically, virologically, and epidemiologically." As with so many congressional directives relating to the disease, however, the agency continued to subvert the legislature's intent that year.

Pittsburgh Cancer Institute, Pittsburgh, Pennsylvania

Seymour Grufferman's poster report describing a cancer cluster in the North Carolina Symphony had generated vituperative responses from many scientists who studied the four-page document when it was thumbtacked to a bulletin board at the University of Rome during a medical conference the previous fall. Clearly, the once sane and respectable Dr. Grufferman had gone off the deep end. "Crazy" or "irresponsible" was how some characterized Grufferman's conclusion that the orchestra's CFS outbreak was accompanied by an incidence of cancer eighteen times the predicted rate and by widespread immune dysfunction even among healthy musicians and their close contacts.

With the superb vision of hindsight, Grufferman now regretted his failure to analyze two orchestras at the same time, using a second orchestra as his control group. His own early skepticism about the disease, he reflected, had precluded such a course. "I suspect many cluster investigations evolve the same way that mine did in North Carolina," Grufferman said that year. "You start out not taking it seriously, so you do a cursory investigation. Then you get more intrigued, and you begin to add modules onto it. Ultimately you don't get the same quality of refining as if it had been taken seriously in the first place. And although you now have a full-scale investigation, you've kind of backed into it."

Grufferman, quite reasonably, had assumed that the well orchestra members and their well spouses would be appropriate controls for the CFS victims among the orchestra. Although Grufferman's choices were, epidemiologically speaking, entirely appropriate, few could have foreseen the outcome: 20 percent of the healthy musicians and one-quarter of the spousal controls had suffered immunological damage, in some cases damage that was no less striking than that seen in the orchestra's CFS victims. After making these discoveries, however, Grufferman knew he needed an orchestra free of fatigue cases. In February he began to arrange for a full-scale immunological investigation of the Pittsburgh Symphony Orchestra, none of whose musicians, so far as he knew, suffered from CFS. His prediction: the Pittsburgh musicians would have healthy immune systems.

In spite of his now-keen interest, Grufferman remained hampered by a lack of money. Although a year had passed since he had been turned down for federal grant support to pursue the connection between cancer and CFS, he continued to deplore the NIH's stance. His frustration was exacerbated by his belief that his own investigative approach was unique, likely to yield significant clues to the transmission patterns of the disease as well as its cancer-inducing potential.

Grufferman was the only epidemiologist in the country who was attempting to learn more about the disease by studying cluster outbreaks. In addition to his cluster studies, he was working to set up a research clinic for the disease at the University of Pittsburgh. He also planned to incorporate the disease into the medical school's curriculum. So far as he knew, the disease wasn't being taught in any medical school.

In his own lectures on the topic to audiences of doctors, he pounded home two elemental facts: first, that the disease was a serious pathological disorder rather than a volitional one; second, that exercise, particularly vigorous exercise, was detrimental, sometimes seriously so. Clinicians who based their care of CFS patients on those two principles, Grufferman believed, would at least honor the ancient Hippocratic oath, which began, "First, do no harm."

Incline Village, Nevada

Early that spring, Dan Peterson obtained a brain sample from a living CFS patient who had been sent to Stanford for a "skinny needle" brain biopsy. The patient had severe cognitive deficits, cerebellar ataxia, transient blindness, and a range of other neurologic symptoms. Peterson sent the precious sample, along with a clinical summary, to Stephen Straus's lab at the National Institute of Allergy and Infectious Diseases for evaluation. Straus returned the sample to Peterson. In his letter on the matter, dated June 14, 1989, Straus explained he had neither the time nor the resources to analyze the brain tissue.

Nevada State Senate, Carson City, Nevada

Nevada suffered from its reputation as a center of gambling and legalized prostitution, and its medical community long had resented the perception that the state's health establishment was an equivalent backwater. Many clinicians and health officials in Nevada were beginning to sense that by taking a lead in aggressively investigating the epidemic disease, they could position their state, as one official said, "at the cutting edge."

On February 17, in testimony before the Nevada state senate, Joe Jarvis, the state's health officer, proposed that instead of funding a surveillance study that relied on doctors to report the disease, "a study of a different nature" be attempted. He explained that "population-based" studies, like Donald A. Henderson's 1956 investigation of Punta Gorda in which researchers actively surveyed an entire community for cases, were superior to the doctor-based system the federal government intended to use. "Fewer people are left out; there's less reporting bias," he said, adding, "More information can be gained about such things as transmission, about certain clinical features of the disease, and more hypotheses can be generated about the cause of the illness.

"I am here to support the notion that the state of Nevada should be interested in chronic fatigue syndrome as a problem," Jarvis continued. "For the first several months that I served as health officer, I had daily phone calls from all over the country requesting information about this problem—in some cases even asking whether it was safe to visit Nevada."

Robert Daugherty, the University of Nevada medical school dean, testified in support of Jarvis's proposal. Incline Village, Daugherty said, would be the targeted site. Trained interviewers would be engaged, and their search for cases would involve every household in the town.

"We have identified over three hundred people in Incline Village with this disease," Daugherty said, "and we think there may have been more. . . . This outbreak is a unique event in the history of illness in this country. If valid, scientifically sound information is not gathered soon, then the information will be lost, and the opportunity to develop treatment programs in this state as well as for the population in the country will be lost."

Larry Mathias, the executive director of the Nevada State Medical Association, also testified in support of the proposal. "This disease is a matter of growing concern in the physician community," Mathias said. "There is very little reliable information through the usual medical journals and literature at this point. . . . What we're really talking about is putting Nevada at the cutting edge of finding out just what the source and course of this particular syndrome is."

Coco Crum, a petite, thirty-five-year-old woman, was the only non-medical professional to testify. "My husband has chronic fatigue syndrome," she began, her voice quavering. "Three years ago he collapsed. He had a seizure and began suffering neurological symptoms as well as extreme fatigue." Crum, whose husband had been a computer programmer and an electronics technician, recounted his horrific odyssey through the health care system in Nevada in his effort to obtain a diagnosis: "We saw an internist. He took EEGs, EKGs, and PET scans, and could find nothing wrong with my husband. He told us to return if he had any other symptoms. Jerry continued to have seizures. And so we went to the internist again, who referred us to a neurologist, who referred us to a cardiologist, who referred us to a different neurologist, who referred us to a psychologist."

Crum told the legislators that her husband "began to have, by then, severe neurological problems. We have lived in Carson City for twelve years. He can't find his way to K mart. He cannot find his way to the hospital to get a blood test.

"It took us a year to find a physician who had some knowledge of chronic fatigue syndrome," she said. "But, we did not learn this through the medical community. We learned this through NBC Nightly News. . . . Unfortunately for my husband, his problems became worse. He's had neuropsychological testing, and the left side of his brain functions at an IQ of 130. His right side functions at an IQ of 85. The right side of your brain governs mathematical abilities, reasoning, memory, logical sequencing—which are all the skills my husband needs to perform his work."

Five months later, on June 11, the Nevada state senate approved the proposal, giving the University of Nevada $100,000 to undertake the first community-wide study of chronic fatigue syndrome prevalence in the United States, to be performed in Incline Village.

Centers for Disease Control, Atlanta, Georgia

On April 3, Walter Gunn and Dave Connell, the director of Abt Associates in Cambridge, responded to the Internal Review Board's inquiries about Protocol 904, the epidemiology branch's ambitious, multi-layered surveillance plan. The board had been puzzled by the team's predilection for administering hours of complicated psychiatric tests in an effort to make their own determination as to whether patients had the disease. Why not depend upon referring doctors to adhere to the agency's own diagnostic criteria? The board was particularly worried that such abundant testing would be burdensome to patients. In an effort to justify the plan's extensive data collection, Gunn and Connell set about explaining why doctors could not be trusted as sole reporting agents in a disease so controversial and complicated.

Gunn and Connell, in addition, were forced to make a number of estimates and assumptions about the degree to which doctors would be willing to participate, as well as the degree to which the surveillance would reflect the true incidence of the disease. Abt Associates planned to invite approximately 900 doctors to report cases, a figure derived from local telephone books and medical society directories; most of these doctors would be internal medicine and infectious disease specialists, rheumatologists, and family practitioners. Gunn predicted that 40 percent, or 360, of these doctors, would sign on. As it turned out, his prediction was correct.

Gunn's estimate of the number of CFS sufferers was derived from lobbyist Barry Sleight's list of nineteen support groups in the regions under study, which Sleight had supplied to Larry Schonberger at the branch chief's request months before. Gunn estimated that for every member of a CFS support group there were probably another two people suffering from the disease, an assumption that seemed injudicious; it was hard to imagine any other disease whose sufferers had such a high rate of participation—one of every three patients—in support groups. Gunn and Connell suggested that the agency's system would pick up 80 percent of all cases, a figure that contradicted Gary Holmes's own admission to Gidget Faubion that surveillance was likely to miss at least 50 percent of the patients because it relied on doctors to report cases.

Privately, Larry Schonberger and others of Gunn's colleagues were predicting that no more than 5 percent of the patients referred would be found to be suffering from a disease matching the agency's case definition. If Schonberger was correct, the number of acceptable cases became very small indeed. After eliminating 95 out of every 100 candidates, the agency could expect to unearth only 40 cases a year in the four cities under surveillance, even using Gunn's optimistic estimates of doctor and patient participation.

18

Disappearing Fingerprints

Longworth House Office Building, Washington, D.C.

Since his paper on the psychiatric status of sufferers, Stephen Straus had been under siege, the subject of a reportedly massive letter-writing offensive by patients. (In an interview, Jim Hill, deputy director of NIAID, Straus's institute, suggested that the patients who had sent the "cascades of letters" attacking Straus might be more prone to have "some psychological component" to their disease than patients who supported Straus.) A form letter drafted on Straus's behalf by agency staff made it clear that the NIH had no intention of firing its expert or reassigning him to another area of research, as the letter writers requested. "The agency is fortunate to have a dedicated and talented researcher such as Dr. Straus working in its laboratories," the government reply said, in part. "Dr. Straus has been and will no doubt continue to be at the forefront of research on chronic fatigue syndrome, and we hope that greater understanding of the nature of this illness will result."

Straus himself was less than content with this defense, however. He prevailed on his boss, NIAID chief Anthony Fauci, for additional support.

Accompanied by the distressed Straus, Fauci made the trip from Bethesda to the Longworth Building on Capitol Hill and thence to the offices of John Porter. The Illinois congressman was on the House subcommittee with appropriations power over the NIH and had held a long-standing advocacy position on the CFS issue. He was, in Fauci's view, a key political figure. One of Porter's staff members, who had been close to the appropriations process for several years and was present at this unusual meeting, described it afterward on the condition that he not be named. He said that Fauci and Straus complained to Porter that patients were applying undue pressure on Congress that, in turn, was being felt in Bethesda. Congress, Fauci reportedly reminded Porter, had no business telling scientists at the NIH how to perform their jobs. Straus wanted to be left alone to pursue his research as he saw fit, free from congressional scrutiny and demands.

"Now, John Porter sees Dr. Fauci as a national hero," the staff member explained. "If Fauci comes into John Porter's office and says this is a *scientific* issue and we are pursuing this as a scientific issue, that's the end of it. Who is John Porter to say he's wrong? Porter's not a scientist."

Porter's assistant, however, adopted a slightly more provocative pose with

Fauci and Straus during the meeting. He raised the possibility that Straus was indeed mistaking an organic medical disease for a psychiatric one. He further suggested that people whose private and professional lives were being devastated by Straus's posture had reason to be frustrated.

NIAID director Fauci, in response, expressed puzzlement over CFS victims' vehement reaction to being told their difficulties were psychiatric in origin. "Fauci said, 'Look, if I tell someone they have an ulcer, they don't get upset, but ulcers are related to the brain.'*

"The NIH is frustrating," he added. "You can't stop these guys if they start going down the wrong path. They just go on and on and on. They go down the wrong path a lot, they waste money, but I don't know what you [can] do about it. You can't micromanage the NIH. Patient groups can scream all they want, but Steve Straus is never going to leave NIH. He's got Fauci's backing and, as a pragmatic matter, that's all there is to it."

When asked about Straus's influence, direct or indirect, over the composition of the panels that reviewed research proposals from scientists outside the agency, the staffer responded, "The researchers I talk to think that he screwed them by changing the study groups. . . . I have no way of knowing how venal Straus is. He professes, 'This is not an ego thing.' But even if he is the most venal guy in the world, there isn't any way Congress is going to intervene and dump him."

Patients weren't the only constituency turning to Congress for a fair hearing. Cancer epidemiologist Diane Cookfair, a member of the Buffalo research network who, with her colleagues, had made application to Straus's institute to study the neurological abnormalities in the disease, called Porter's office the same week the NIH scientists had visited. Cookfair, neurologist Carolyn Warner, and their collaborators had achieved a high score on their second grant submission. "If mine doesn't get funded," Cookfair said, "nothing will. It got the highest score after Komaroff's. There's still a chance they might fund [our study] if they feel the heat."

Buffalo, New York

That spring, despite their disappointment over David Bell's apparent betrayal, the Buffalo group remained optimistic about their work. The team was now more focused, having moved away from virological investigations into neurological ones.† These studies had borne fruit, primarily due to the persistence of multiple sclerosis specialist Carolyn Warner. In March, the elfin, dark-haired woman presented the findings at a national neurologic conference in Chicago.[1] In her paper, Warner simply listed the neurologic abnormalities discovered in some but not all of fourteen patients who had been studied intensively. Those abnormalities included indications from spinal fluid samples that something, perhaps a virus, had broken the blood-brain barrier; abnormal brain waves on electroencephalograms,

---

* Actually a common bacterium called *H. pylori* had been identified seven years before as the leading cause of ulcers.

† Retrovirologist Bernard Poiesz of SUNY had been unable to document squarely the presence of retrovirus in eight patient samples he had been sent; only one of the eight was positive for HTLV1 by the western-blot antibody test. Diane Cookfair suspected the wrong probes had been used, but Poiesz indicated to the Buffalo team that he was too busy to pursue the research further.

multiple lesions on MRI brain scans, and evidence of muscle fiber atrophy from muscle biopsies taken from either deltoid or thigh muscles.*

In the brief question-and-answer period, Warner was asked if she might be studying MS patients by mistake. Like all neurologists, Warner was used to diagnostic ambiguity, but the question posed by her peers in Chicago was a particularly difficult one. Neither MS nor CFS had a definitive diagnostic test; each was considered a diagnosis of exclusion. Additionally, there was an array of similarities between the two. Differences did exist, however.

"Chronic fatigue syndrome patients have prominent headaches, joint pain, and muscle pain," Warner said during an interview that year. "These are *not* MS symptoms." Neither were the CFS complaints of sore throat, swollen lymph nodes, and fevers that were frequently prominent in the early months and years of the disease. "But we do see more overt neurological abnormalities in MS," she added.

Although Warner was convinced that CFS was a distinct disease, she speculated, as other CFS researchers had, that "maybe they are sister-type disorders. Maybe if you get chronic fatigue syndrome you're at increased risk for MS."

Multiple sclerosis, Warner continued, "was always a diagnosis of exclusion. But now you've got another vague 'by exclusion' neurologic disease with many similarities. With chronic fatigue syndrome on the horizon, you were probably far safer five years ago making an MS diagnosis than you are now. I don't think *anything* is definitive in the interface between CFS and MS yet."

Charlotte, North Carolina

By springtime, the triad of Cheney, Bell, and DeFreitas was well cemented. DeFreitas had processed nearly three hundred patient samples sent to her by the clinicians. Occasionally Cheney worried that Bell, in his eagerness to track the disease to its source, might use the information he had gained from the Wistar collaboration to help a second retrovirologist, like SUNY's Poiesz, get a leg up. But they were fleeting fears, born of isolation. Mostly, Cheney believed the benefits of collaboration with the Lyndonville pediatrician outweighed any risks.

Ironically, Bell was worried about competition from Poiesz, too, although he avoided verbalizing his fears to Cheney or DeFreitas. Buffalo cancer epidemiologist Diane Cookfair's aggressive efforts with Poiesz had caused him sleepless nights. Bell had no idea whether Poiesz had made progress, and he didn't feel he had the right to ask.

The spread of the disease, and the class of virus DeFreitas was finding broad hints of in patients, made little sense. The premier orthodoxy of retrovirology—upon which the entire public health response to the AIDS epidemic was based—was that retroviruses are not transmitted casually, at least among humans, although a

* In her abstract, Warner noted the following abnormalities: "elevated cerebrospinal fluid (CSF) protein (5 of 13), elevated CSF IgG synthesis (3 of 6), elevated CSF cell count (2 of 13), prolonged visual evoked response latency (2 of 11), abnormal EEG (1 of 13), and MRI lesions 1 of 13)." She summarized: "The abnormalities we found provided evidence for central nervous system and neuromuscular involvement, which may provide clues to the pathogenesis of this syndrome."

number of researchers had proved that retroviruses were casually transmitted among animals.* The transmission patterns of CFS, in contrast, seemed to be far broader and more insidious, encompassing not only blood transfusions and sex but also casual interaction—sharing office space, living together, sitting in the same classroom, playing on the same playground, perhaps sharing a row of seats on an airplane.

DeFreitas, according to Cheney, was having "a lot of trouble with the epidemiology." In fact, given the implications of her work, the immunologist preferred not to think about epidemiology for the time being.

"I don't think Wistar is wedded to any ideology about this syndrome," Cheney added. "First of all, this was always very much a clinical syndrome, and the people who have agonized over it have been clinicians. I think the bench researchers have been largely ignorant of the controversies. They don't have any vested interests. As clinicians, we're more vulnerable to the politics. We sort of have to believe that what our patients are telling us is, in fact, reflective of some underlying process rather than a monster from the id. Bench researchers just aren't into that. They are willing to accept anything that they can see on the western blot. It's the 'altar of technology' phenomenon; it's this 'I'll believe in the devil if it's on the western blot' attitude."

Cheney, no doubt savoring thoughts of the moment when he would cease to be vulnerable, was awaiting a green light from his Wistar collaborator to allow him to break the retrovirus discovery at the San Francisco conference, scheduled for April.

"I really hope Elaine will let us talk," the doctor said. "Of course, it's got to be underplayed, because the power of it is so great. It will be like throwing a bomb into the auditorium."

Cheney's own career at the Nalle Clinic was intact, but he was beginning to feel his colleagues' collective cold shoulder. In fact, he and his intense research assistant, Susan Dorman, were increasingly inhabiting a world unto themselves within the clinic. The two were appropriating an ever-expanding portion of the clinic's industrial-size −70°F. freezer in which to store serially drawn blood samples from most of the doctor's six hundred patients. Dorman's cramped office space—a closet, really—was filled with a computer, a fax machine, two telephones, and voluminous files. This busy hub was populated at any given time by the doctor, his research assistant, his two nurses, and the occasional reporter—sometimes all at the same time—as they pored over computer printouts and medical journals. Not surprisingly, the rest of the clinic's nursing staff abhorred this breach of clinic decorum; Dorman reported that spring that the only members of the clinic staff who were still speaking to her were Cheney's own nurses.

Cheney remained impervious to the bad vibrations emanating from the rest of the nursing staff, but he was aware that several colleagues were professing antipathy to his activities to the clinic's chief executive officer. "I've got support among the top people here, but if enough clinic members become antagonists . . ."

---

* In medicine and science, unlike religion, however, one orthodoxy inevitably gives way to another. As an example, until Robert Gallo identified HTLV1 in adults with T-cell lymphoma in 1980, the premier orthodoxy of retrovirology was that only animals developed disease from retrovirus infection.

The doctor once had dared to hope that, in time, he might establish a clinic within the Nalle where he could care for CFS patients exclusively. By spring, however, he was beginning to suspect his future at the Nalle would hardly be rosy.

Incline Village, Nevada

Nancy Kaiser had been on Ampligen for eight months. Her IQ had continued to recover; it was currently 136, having been 88 when therapy began and 118 after three months of infusions. Kaiser's seizures had ended completely, and her eyesight—she had been plagued by transient blindness—had returned to normal. A multitude of other clinical and laboratory signs revealed improvement, too. On the strength of Kaiser's remarkable progress, HEM Pharmaceuticals had given Peterson permission to give the drug to ten more people.

David Strayer, the Hahnemann University oncologist who would serve as HEM's adviser on the study, was excited. "This is much more prevalent than HIV disease," Strayer said that year.

The protocol for inclusion in the first Ampligen pilot study was rigorous. Patients had to have positive MRI brain scans, drastic diminution of performance IQ and other cognitive deficits as measured by Sheila Bastien's tests, seropositivity for human herpesvirus 6 as measured by Berch Henry's probe, and a wide array of immunological aberrations and physical signs. In all, nearly sixty criteria needed to be met. Peterson had four patients enrolled by early March: former Truckee algebra teacher Andy Antonucci; Amy Long, a housewife; Tom Miller (a pseudonym), a former stockbroker; and Marylou Guiss, a former psychotherapist. Miller and Long lived in Reno; Guiss moved to Incline Village from Santa Barbara. By mid-April, Peterson had selected six additional patients for the trial. They were former engineer Gerald Crum of Carson City; former real estate saleswoman Gloria Baker of Riverside, California, who had been disabled for nearly a decade; former hospital administrator John Trussler of Turlock, California; housewife Ellen Mears of Riverside, California; housewife Billee Reed of Idaho; and Nancy Taylor, the wife of Tulsa, Oklahoma, cable TV entrepreneur Ed Taylor. With the exception of four patients who lived in the area and New Mexican Nancy Kaiser, who was already in residence, all of the patients moved to Incline Village to participate in the sixteen-week pilot trial. All were severely disabled by their disease.

The study began that summer with HEM's blessing. Just weeks into their treatment, however, Peterson found that his patients were complaining more bitterly than ever about their symptoms. Oddly, the drug was making them feel worse, even though their immunological deficits were beginning to improve. After two months of increasing complaints from his weary test cases, the doctor began to hope that Ampligen was like cancer chemotherapy, the purpose for which Ampligen originally was designed: it made patients feel even worse for a while, but cured or at least controlled their disease.

San Francisco, California

Patient activist Jan Montgomery and her supporters moved their agenda along substantially on April 15, when the city's public health department held a one-day chronic fatigue syndrome physicians conference at the San Francisco Hyatt. Five hundred doctors and researchers attended.

Nancy Walker, a city supervisor, launched the Saturday morning meeting with a passionate speech. "The initial public response to this disease," she said, "has placed an almost intolerable burden on patients to stand up in the face of this ridicule and educate the very people whose job it is to help them." She went on to harshly criticize the federal and local health establishments whose members, she said, had responded to the epidemic with "stonewalling and denial."

The event was notable for the public emergence of Jay Levy as a major player in the research arena. Until then the scientist had remained silent about his involvement. His presence would have been enough to lend the problem credibility, but Levy, who was famous in the San Francisco medical and scientific community, stepped up to the lectern and described his research in some detail. He reiterated his belief that CFS was probably caused by a new infectious agent. In some cases, he said, the disease might lead to other progressive autoimmune diseases such as multiple sclerosis. He told his audience that he was searching for a new virus in blood samples from patients with the disease and had found cytopathic effect—cell death from an unidentified pathogen—in eight patients so far.

Paul Cheney described the immunologic and clinical findings he had made during the previous eighteen months in his Charlotte patients, who now numbered nearly seven hundred, only a fraction of whom hailed from North Carolina. Despite his high hopes that he would be able to break the retrovirus discovery in San Francisco, Elaine DeFreitas had insisted she was too far from publication in a scientific journal to take her work public. Instead, Cheney talked at length about one of his findings that had fascinated him for months: the loss of fingerprints in about one-third of his patients. The doctor was teased by friends afterward for his preoccupation with disappearing fingerprints; he responded with a Cheshire cat smile.

The conference generated news stories in the *Los Angeles Times,* the *San Diego Union, USA Today,* the *San Francisco Chronicle,* and the *Boston Globe.* A 2,500-word *Los Angeles Times* story, which was syndicated, included the address of the Charlotte-based CFIDS Association. In the space of two weeks, the Charlotte staff received more than two thousand inquiries.

Jay Levy had not entirely given up his microbe hunt, but he was discouraged. Like DeFreitas, Levy had looked for the retroviruses HTLV1 and HTLV2, but admitted his efforts had been halfhearted because he doubted a retrovirus was causing the disease. "This is an agent that is spread easily," he said.

Levy's torpor on the subject of the disease dissipated shortly after the San Francisco conference, however, when the parent of an afflicted child donated money to his research effort. "We got started again," Levy recalled some time later. Once more, the virologist turned to East Bay clinician Carol Jessop for patients. "I said to Carol, 'Let's try to develop a diagnostic test.' In AIDS, the CD-fours [helper T cells] are down. Does CFS have some immunological markers?" To help him answer that question, Levy called upon immunologist Alan Landay, a flow cytometry expert from the University of Chicago who was spending a year on sabbatical in Levy's lab to study retroviruses. Landay's specialty amounted to literally sorting and counting categories of immune system cells, a skill he had thus far devoted entirely to the study of AIDS.

Levy advised clinician Jessop to disregard all viral signs, such as elevated antibodies to Epstein-Barr virus, and look primarily for what Levy called "the mental problem"—cognitive dysfunction—and fatigue in selecting her patients. Following Levy's directive, Jessop began sending blood samples from such patients to Landay. Soon after their collaboration began, Levy, Landay, and Jessop were rewarded.

"It was a hell of a lot of work," Levy reported later. "But . . . three different markers popped out. These markers indicated to us that a large number of chronic fatigue syndrome patients are chronically activated in their immune system in a way that's very similar to what occurs with a viral disease."

Harvard Medical School, Boston, Massachusetts

In May, Anthony Komaroff lost patience with the CDC's seeming obsession with psychiatric evaluation of patients in its surveillance protocol and sent a strongly worded letter to the agency arguing for the agency to search, even if minimally, for evidence of an organic problem. Panel members ignored Komaroff's suggestion that they look for viruses in patients, but together they arrived at seven basic tests they wanted performed on each patient referred to the agency. These tests— which included blood sedimentation rate, liver function, endocrine function, a renal screen, complete blood count, urinalysis, and a test for autoimmune disease—could be completed for a mere $48.00.

"By the end of the summer, the plan had changed," Komaroff said later. "The psychiatric battery is no less intense. It's just been balanced. And after you do everything man has ever thought of to find psychiatric disease," he added, "you can't find it in these patients."

Yet, in a curious twist, Komaroff's campaign backfired once surveillance got under way in the fall and played a contributory role in what many would come to view as the agency's failure to measure the true prevalence of the disease. The six medical doctors and two psychiatrists on the Physicians Review Committee, whose mission was to meet periodically to adjudicate cases, grew increasingly restrictive in their judgments. According to Walter Gunn, they began to cite any abnormal result on any of the basic tests as grounds for automatic expulsion from the study, a practice that would yield numbers that even Gunn, originally a proponent of the surveillance plan, described as "too conservative." "If there was *any* possibility of an organic sign, the patient was immediately ruled out," Gunn said some years later. "And it was done without ever following up with the doctor who had referred the patient to us. For instance, if he or she had a high glucose level, the Physicians Review Committee would say, 'Well, that patient could have diabetes instead of CFS.' But no one would check to see if the patient's physician had ever *tested* for diabetes and ruled it out. *All* the results had to be normal, and if they weren't, then without *any* further evidence, the patient was gone—history," Gunn said.

"Now, of the patients we found who made the grade," Gunn recalled, "I am certain there is not another medical illness they could *possibly* be suffering from except chronic fatigue syndrome. And that would be fine," he added, "if we were doing an etiological study—if we were going to search for the agent in these patients—because if you're looking for an agent, you want to be absolutely sure everyone you study has exactly the same disease. But that wasn't the purpose of our study. The purpose of our study was to estimate the prevalence of the disease, and [his practice] made our estimates too conservative."

Just how conservative was painfully evident to Gunn by the fourth year of surveillance. The senior researcher frequently attended support group meetings in Atlanta, often to apprise local sufferers of goings-on at the CDC. "There are inevitably two hundred people at these meetings," Gunn reported. And yet in four years only 289 patients had been referred by local clinicians from the five Atlanta counties enrolled in the surveillance network. Of those 289 people, only 34 passed the review committee's screen to be counted as authentic CFS victims. "I always ask how many people in the support group audience are in our surveillance program," Gunn said. "Usually two or three people raise their hands."

Hollywood, California

On April 4 the supermarket tabloid the *Globe* reported that Cher was "battling a baffling illness that's put her career on hold." According to the publication, which regularly publishes stories of dubious veracity, Cher had been suffering for a year and was often too weak to lift her head off her pillow. So severe was her illness that she had been forced to postpone the filming of her next movie, *Mermaids.* "Her life has been a nightmare," one of the *Globe*'s unnamed sources reported. In addition to "numbing fatigue," the source continued, Cher suffered from "aches and pains" and "sore throats so severe she's had to stop singing." Doctors had been unable to diagnose the problem, so the actress was consulting a "spiritual healer."

With the exception of Blake Edwards and Randy Newman, hardly any celebrities suffering from the disease had spoken publicly about their ordeal. Cher's "outing" by the *Globe* in April inaugurated a steady stream of tabloid coverage of her CFS experience, however, which for the next several years left her the most closely examined Hollywood star with the complaint.

On July 4 the *National Enquirer* took up the story: "A terrifying mystery illness has gripped Cher for the last year. Doctors have no idea why she's suffered a string of health problems that have forced her to postpone one show biz commitment after another. What started as an apparent bad case of flu a year ago took hold of the Oscar-winning star and has refused to let her go. Overwhelmed by repeated attacks of weakness and aching, she's been bedridden for weeks on end, put off two movies, delayed filming a music video and canceled an Atlantic City engagement."

Civilian CFS victims watched the drama unfold in the tabloids with a mixture of empathy and fascination. There was talk among patient support group leaders of approaching the actress with an invitation to serve as a national spokesperson for the disease and to testify about her experience before Congress.* And in an open letter to Stephen Straus, published in the *CFIDS Chronicle* that fall, Amy Kritz, a thirty-three-year-old from Brooklyn who had been disabled by the disease for two years, wrote, "I'd like to be in the room when you tell Cher (if she's unfortunate enough to have CFS, which I sincerely hope she does not) that her illness is due to 'unachievable ambitions and poor coping skills.' "[2]

The scope of the disease in Los Angeles remained unknown in 1989. There were hints of its enormity, however. CFS clinics were flourishing. The Southern California CFIDS Support Network boasted more than fifty patient organizations under its umbrella. The film and television industries, more closely scrutinized than any other California industry, likely were reflecting the rise in cases throughout the region.

On May 18, a letter was mailed to the 9,600 members of the Writers Guild of America-West from the trustees of the guild's Health Fund. "Many questions have come to the Health Fund recently about conditions known as chronic fatigue syndrome and/or Epstein-Barr virus," the letter to union members began. "The policy of the Fund towards these diseases or conditions is the same as for any other illness or injury: Benefits are provided only for necessary care and treatment, that is, treatment which is currently accepted medical practice as recognized by an established medical society in the United States. Unfortunately, for those patients diagnosed as having CFS, at present there is no treatment which is currently accepted medical practice. All current treatment for this condition, such as the use of acyclovir and gamma globulin, is still considered experimental." The authors of the letter assured guild members they were "sympathetic" to all those who suffered from the disease, but they continued, "[We] have relied upon the the latest information received from experts in the medical community, including the Centers for Disease Control . . . in formulating [our] guidelines."

The *New York Post*'s widely read Page Six gossip column took up the matter soon afterward: "Lately," the Page Six reporter wrote, "the Writers Guild Health Fund has been deluged with claims from listless, blues-ridden script scribblers who claim they suffer from chronic fatigue syndrome, sometimes known as Epstein-Barr virus. Chastening Tinseltown hypochondriacs, the [Health Fund] memo advised that, 'up to 90 percent of all adults would test positive for the Epstein-Barr virus, yet are perfectly healthy.' "

United States Senate, Washington, D.C.

On May 8, Paul Cheney flew to Washington, D.C., where he presented testimony to the Senate Labor, Health and Human Services Appropriations Subcommittee.

---

* One sufferer, Tucson resident Nomi Antelman, was angry at Cher for her failure to speak out. "In this country," Antelman complained, "your illness is only as important as the celebrity who represents it. Cher could help millions simply by being honest and talking about what this disease has done to her life, but she's promoting cosmetics and health clubs instead—she *can't* be associated with this disease. . . . People with CFS are actually *more* closeted than people with HIV."

"The most remarkable thing about chronic fatigue syndrome," the doctor told the Senate panel, "is that the impetus for its recognition as a defined clinical entity has come primarily from patients. If there ever was a grassroots disease, this is it. What clues there are to this disorder lie presently in listening carefully to these patients. . . . Most of those from the corridors of academia and government research offices have not listened carefully to more than a handful, let alone the thousand or so it would take to get a feel for this both monstrous and subtle disease. . . . The generals charged with developing strategy do not know the enemy. They have not seen its face.

"The CFIDS problem will not go away," Cheney concluded. "It is real. It seems to be on the increase, and if so its relationship to the AIDS epidemic will need to be investigated with great urgency. A problem such as this, which has consistently grown in the face of enormous skepticism within our medical establishment, is most deserving of your attention and serious consideration."

Washington, D.C.

On May 22, Stephen Straus delivered a lecture on the disease to seventy-five congressional staff members in the Rayburn House Office Building. Straus's appearance was billed as an NIH "Medicine for the Layman" lecture and was sponsored by Representative John Porter of Illinois, to whom Straus had taken his public relations woes two months before. According to lobbyist Barry Sleight, who reported on the event in the *CFIDS Chronicle,* Straus indicated during the course of his hour-long lecture that chronic fatigue syndrome was not one disease but "a mixture of things." It affected, Straus said, "those who can afford to take time off" and those "who can admit to this."

"Straus was trying to reduce congressional focus on this issue," Barry Sleight said some years later. "The underlying theme was that the National Institute of Allergy and Infectious Diseases had everything under control and no congressional attention to chronic fatigue syndrome was needed."

Soon after his report on Straus's lecture appeared on the Charlotte-based newsletter, Sleight received a letter from Straus's colleague Ann Schleuderberg, the CFS grant program administrator:

> I was very disappointed. . . . [The report] gives a very false impression and damages the image to the layman of a dedicated, accomplished scientist. This is very sad, because the CFS community desperately needs medical scientists like Steve to pursue their cause. He is far more valuable than a thousand doctors—regardless of their motives—who say what the constituency wants to hear but do not have the skills, motivation and support to find the truth. Your statement, together with those presented in the *CFIDS Journal,* hurt him deeply and ultimately may drive him from this area of research. This would be tragic.

In a manner that, under the circumstances, seemed grossly patronizing, Schleuderberg added: "I recognize your work must be very frustrating and difficult, especially with the personal battles you face. I hope these frustrations won't lead you to alienate those who are in a position to help the most."

Unlike Schleuderberg, neither Sleight nor the constituency served by the *CFIDS Chronicle* found the prospect of Straus's departure from the field remotely tragic. In fact, a rumor, based more solidly in wishful fantasy than in reality, that Straus was leaving the NIH percolated through the patient community in the spring of 1989.

Schleuderberg and Straus were not the only NIH staff members who had begun to find the contents of the *CFIDS Chronicle* disagreeable. After the appearance of the spring-summer issue attacking Straus's article about the psychiatric status of twenty-eight CFS sufferers, publisher Marc Iverson had begun hearing from National Cancer Institute researchers Dharam Ablashi and Paul Levine, who telephoned to suggest that Iverson allow them or someone else at the NIH an opportunity to "peer-review" his entire journal prior to publication in the future. Summoning his finest southern manners, Iverson politely declined the offer. Privately, he joked that he would let government scientists peer-review the *Chronicle* when they let him peer-review their scientific papers.

Harvard Medical School, Boston, Massachusetts

The strife launched by Stephen Straus's research agenda persisted into the summer among patients and their advocates, erupting at the end of June within a nascent organization of doctors and scientists and influential patient advocates who had been conscripted, at the request of patient organizations, to advise patient philanthropies on meritorious research projects. The members of this National CFS Advisory Council included the National Cancer Institute's Paul Levine and Dharam Ablashi; clinicians Anthony Komaroff, James Jones, and Paul Cheney; Minnesota governor Rudy Perpich; and Tulsa TV entrepreneur Edward Taylor.

On June 17, Anthony Komaroff wrote a letter to council members in defense of Stephen Straus, seeking the body's approval for a statement of support. Although the Harvard doctor confessed he was less than pleased with the scientific methods and conclusions of Straus's recent psychiatry study, he was dismayed by the vehemence with which Straus was being criticized.

"The issue is simple," Komaroff explained in a private conversation some months later. "The study published by Straus is a bad study. But that's not the issue. Should people take away the job and livelihood of a scientist who is trying to do good? It's *thought* control," Komaroff continued. "It's an abridgment of the Bill of Rights. It's what you see in a Communist society where many scientists are hounded. That's very different from scientists being critical of one another. I've been critical of Straus before." Komaroff must have been dismayed when he received a peppery response to his letter from Edward Taylor of Tulsa, probably the most generous private contributor to research in the country and a fellow council member.* Taylor's wife, Nancy, had been disabled by CFS for seven years. "I believe your defense of Dr. Straus is both unwise and wrong," Taylor wrote the Harvard investigator:

---

* Years before, Taylor had designed and bankrolled the launch of the Atlanta-based "superstation," and with it the fortunes of Ted Turner. As a result, Taylor was independently wealthy.

One only has to talk to patients to realize the harm Dr. Straus has done by legitimizing the comment "It is all in your head." Patients' friends, families, employers and doctors have turned against them, and now these false friends can point to Dr. Straus as an expert. . . . If you wish to help Dr. Straus, go to him as a colleague and suggest he send an apology letter to CFIDS. . . . He should include a statement of where he does stand. Hopefully, he would support Dr. Cheney's research on a new virus and Dr. Peterson on his Ampligen tests. The public support of Barry Sleight's testimony, asking Congress for $25,000,000 in next year's budget would also be helpful. . . .

Make this your personal plea and leave the Council out of it. . . . If the Council votes for your letter of support for Straus, please consider this letter my resignation and withdrawal of financial support. I will withdraw my personal and financial support. . . .

Nancy and I stand firmly with the patients.

Komaroff's statement of support for Stephen Straus failed to be approved by the council.

Philadelphia, Pennsylvania

During the first week in June, *P.M. Magazine,* a nationally syndicated evening news and feature show, aired a seven-minute segment on chronic fatigue syndrome. Produced by Charlotte affiliate station WBTV, the show, according to the series producer, generated more interest among viewers than any other piece produced in the ten-year history of *P.M. Magazine.* In Philadelphia, the segment aired on the local *Evening Magazine,* generating a record seven hundred calls to station KYW, according to a story in the *Philadelphia Inquirer.*

Lyndonville, New York

Since the Lyndonville epidemic of 1985–1986, David Bell had learned a great deal about the manifestation of the disease in children. "It is a *devastating* illness in children," Bell observed in 1989. "Even worse than in adults."

In private conversations, Bell struggled to explain the tragic proportions of the disease in children. He referred to a study he and his wife had undertaken of thirty-two children and their families. All but one of the children experienced a decrease in their grade average after they fell ill, sometimes as much as three points; a third had missed six months or more of school. "The family disruption is very pronounced," Bell said. "The kids can't participate in family activities. They get labeled malingerers or 'school phobics.' "

One of his saddest cases, Bell said, was an older child who had failed to recover after she was struck in January of 1984, at age thirteen, with a severe flu. "She was a bright child from a healthy, intact family," Bell recalled. "She had boasted the highest grade average in her school and won most of the awards available to students. But she went the usual course, and after she had been out of school one month, the school began to apply pressure on her parents. Eventually she saw ten doctors, most of whom called it 'viral infection' or 'mono.' At that stage, she had fevers, lymph nodes. No one considered psychosomatic illness as a possible explanation. But after three months the school brought charges against the family for keeping their child home. It was a very lengthy and serious investigation. Eventually the school asked a shrink to evaluate her. The shrink made a statement that she was emotionally very healthy. After five thousand dollars in legal costs to the parents, charges were dropped. But the school couldn't authorize home tutoring because she had no diagnosis.

"Over the next two months," Bell continued, "the child had seizures and became increasingly unable to function. She had major difficulty with speech. Overall, she saw twenty-eight doctors who gave her fifty thousand dollars' worth of medical tests, with completely normal results, before her parents read about chronic fatigue syndrome. She hasn't been to school in three years."

By the spring of 1989, so many youngsters in the Lyndonville school district were suffering from CFS that David Bell prepared a form letter children could present to their teachers that explained the learning problems caused by the disease.

Nalle Clinic, Charlotte, North Carolina

By the summer of 1989, Paul Cheney had determined that between 20 percent and 50 percent of his CFS patients were losing their fingerprints. Fully four-fifths of the fingertip biopsies the doctor ordered in such cases revealed an identical vasculitis problem. As the doctor ruminated over this phenomenon, he began to wonder if the disappearing fingerprints might provide a scientific method of proving the disease was a new epidemic. One of Cheney's adolescent patients, an eighteen-year-old who had been suffering from CFS since she was fifteen, had communicated the disease to her mother, who worked as a nurse. The mother, in the course of applying for a job at the Veterans Administration Hospital in Salisbury, North Carolina, was fingerprinted. A hitch arose when the hospital's personnel department asked her to return for a second fingerprint session; the nurse's first set of prints had been sent to the FBI and had bounced. Her fingerprints bounced on the second attempt, too, and an FBI officer was flown down to Salisbury to interview the woman to learn if she had tried to eradicate her fingerprints.

"There are one thousand people employed at this hospital," Cheney said. "Someone should find out how often fingerprints have bounced. If we do see a trend, that might tell us something about the rise of this disease."

Wistar Institute, Philadelphia, Pennsylvania

Hilary Koprowski and Elaine DeFreitas had been perplexed by aspects of the multiple sclerosis outbreak in the Florida Keys from their earliest investigations of it. In the summer of 1989 they began seriously to reassess their Key West findings based on DeFreitas's experiments with blood samples from CFS patients in Paul Cheney's and David Bell's practices.

There had always been something odd about the Key West lab results, particularly when compared with results in the Swedish MS patients. Clinically, too, the Key West MS patients had been a puzzling group to the many neurologists who studied them.

As DeFreitas studied the apparent retrovirus infection in Bell's and Cheney's patients, she realized that, under the microscope, it seemed to mirror the infection in Key West patients. "The antibody patterns looked like CFIDS," DeFreitas remembered later. "It would be very interesting to go back and see if those people have bona fide multiple sclerosis now," DeFreitas said. "I'll bet they don't. . . . The Key West epidemic was never evaluated by anyone with the credibility of a Paul Cheney or a David Bell."

19

The Ampligen Effect

Centers for Disease Control, Atlanta, Georgia

Although trained in internal medicine and infectious disease, Gary Holmes had sought work at the CDC in large part because he had a marked distaste for clinical practice. "Primary care is not my bag," Holmes once remarked. When he took his job in Atlanta, Holmes's career plan had been to parlay his federal credential into a professorial post in epidemiology at a university, thereby escaping altogether the vicissitudes of workaday clinician's life. By mid-1989 his pleasant scenario was fast receding into the realm of youthful fantasy. At year's end he would return to Texas to take a post in infectious diseases at the Scott and White Clinic and Hospital in Temple. There he would be given a beeper and he would be "taking call."

If Holmes's tenure at the agency had been calamitous for CFS sufferers, the disease had been Holmes's personal nuclear winter. The former Epidemic Intelligence Service officer had been badly encumbered as a result of his involvement with the Nevada epidemic and subsequent developments. By early 1988, Holmes himself admitted he was being proffered annual extensions of his temporary position for no reason other than his willingness to field thousands of calls and letters every year and be the agency's point man with the press. Apparently, even such yeoman duty wasn't enough to counterbalance what some on Clifton Road considered Holmes's mediocrity, however.

"CDC has its own environment, and Gary was not succeeding in it," Walter Gunn commented later. "He was not getting promotions or awards. He was just staying where he was. Nobody told him to leave, but he could see the handwriting on the wall."

News of Holmes's departure was received with mixed feelings by patients and clinicians who were monitoring the agency's progress from afar. His tenure at CDC had failed to result in a collective realization that a new, highly infectious and disabling disease was abroad in the land, but Holmes had been, for better or worse, the only person on the case in Atlanta since 1985. Soon the only voice on the telephone who could honestly report that he was studying the problem would be gone.

New York City

On July 16 the *New York Times Magazine* published an article by Bruce Dobkin, a University of California professor of clinical neurology in Los Angeles, titled "Ill, or Just the Blahs?" In the fanciful spirit of a British cardiology team whose members had declared the disease to be a syndrome of hyperventilation a year before, Dobkin suggested to the Sunday magazine's four million readers that the malady was a phenomenon of deconditioning and dehydration that developed when people stricken by a flu or cold indulged in too much bed rest. In support of his theory, Dobkin drew from his own collegiate experience as a victim of the Hong Kong flu in 1968. Recalling his exhaustion, headache, and light-headedness upon being released from his college infirmary, Dobkin wrote, "Years later, as a doctor, I realized that I had become dehydrated and so deconditioned that even minor exertion wiped me out." In his conclusion, Dobkin promoted the Mayo Clinic's dangerous therapy: exercise. "It's worth leaping past notions about the cause, and playing the card of physical reconditioning," he suggested. "The answer for many may lie in a closely supervised program of gradually progressive exercise, with good emotional support and maybe a temporary regimen of antidepressant medication. . . . Perhaps the deconditioned victim will finish the race only if heart, will and legs get back in shape."

No scientists associated with the federal health agencies wrote to rebut Dobkin's analysis, but Harvard's Anthony Komaroff protested, as did a Long Island internal medicine specialist named Paul Lavenger. Lavenger, who had been disabled by the disease and forced to retire from practice one year after his wife had fallen ill, complained: "Dr. Dobkin's comparing his own faltering steps after a self-limiting viral illness, Hong Kong flu, with the protracted debilitation of chronic fatigue syndrome is as unfair as suggesting polio victims get out of their wheelchairs and take a hike."

Said Komaroff: "When a doctor cannot figure out what is producing a patient's symptoms, often he may react by thinking the illness must not exist or that it must be 'psychological.' As doctors, we must avoid that trap."

London, England

War was breaking out among victims of the disease and their advocates in England that fall. Under the headline "Yuppie Flu Sparks Hate Campaign," reporter Jeremy Laurance wrote in the *Sunday Correspondent,*

> Fierce feuding has broken out among people with myalgic encephalomyelitis—the chronic fatigue syndrome sometimes known as yuppie flu—in a row about the true nature of their condition that reflects the widespread public horror of psychiatric illness. A specialist in ME has been sacked, a researcher has received hate mail and abusive phone calls, a campaign is under way to unseat the chairman of the ME Association and an ME pressure group has sought publicity to discredit the chairwoman of a rival group. In the eyes of ME sufferers, believed to number more than 100,000 in Britain, the targets of these assaults have committed a common sin by highlighting the psychological component of the illness.

The English reporter took the side of the medical professionals, whom he portrayed as unfairly under siege. He described the case of a British psychiatrist, Simon Wessely, who promoted the disease as a "disorder of the nervous system with a range of causes" but who had written articles with titles such as "ME Is All in the Mind." Wesseley's efforts had earned him little but abuse from patients, the reporter noted, although he quoted a British sufferer who protested that ME patients "don't have the energy for a hate campaign."

A third faction was the Campaign against Health Fraud, an organization of about two hundred doctors, which supported the psychoneurotic theory of the disease. Its chair, journalist Caroline Richmond, was the author of articles such as "Exercise Is the Key to Fighting ME" and "It's All in the Mind—or in the Media," in which she lobbed wittily denigrating salvos at sufferers, frequently suggesting they were hypochondriacs.

A fourth faction, the ME Action Campaign, was also described in the newspaper article. One thousand British sufferers with CFS belonged to this "pressure" group, including Melvyn Bragg, a well-known British novelist, and David Puttnam, the filmmaker who had produced the Academy Award–winning *Chariots of Fire*. Its members had been known to write letters to journalists complaining about their "inaccurate and sometimes downright nasty articles that had done untold damages to ME sufferers," according to reporter Laurance.

"Boy," quipped Dennis Jackson, a Delaware journalism professor and contributor to the *CFIDS Chronicle,* when he was apprised of the English conflagration that fall. "I'm happy I'm here in America where we *never* fight over stuff like that!"

Lyndonville, New York

Jean Pollard and her husband, Paul, had lived for most of their twenty-year marriage in the rambling house filled with a profusion of comfortable antiques and a kitchen you could roller-skate in. All of their children—Alison; the twins, Meg and Libby; and their youngest daughter, Hannah—had been raised there. Until the fall of 1985 the Pollards and their children had been happy, their life together idyllic. By 1989, however, the tragedy that had befallen the three youngest Pollard girls in 1985 had spread to the eldest. Alison was in her junior year of high school when she was stricken. Not long afterward, Jean and her husband fell ill as well. Now, four years after the Lyndonville epidemic began, every member of the Pollard family was sick. Hospitalizations, innumerable trips to the infectious disease clinic of the University of Rochester teaching hospital, Strong Memorial, and the loss of months at a time from school had defined the childhoods of the Pollard children. Their parents, who had the disease in a more moderate form, were coping, but their powerlessness to end their daughters' suffering was a frustration almost beyond bearing.

Jean Pollard had insights into the disease few others in Lyndonville could match. She was David Bell's office manager and had assisted Bell and his wife, Karen, in their epidemiological studies of the town's children. With the college career of her eldest child, Alison, in jeopardy, Jean Pollard was becoming desperate. On August 24, the mother of four sat down and wrote a letter to Barbara Bush, the wife of the president:

I am writing to you because I know that you have made a commitment to children. I have four beautiful daughters who have chronic fatigue syndrome. Perhaps you have heard of this illness. There has been a great deal of controversy at the government level over this issue. . . .

My daughters became ill in the same week after having the flu, or what appeared to be the flu in October 1985, about the same time as the outbreak in Incline Village, Nevada . . . they never recovered. . . . My children . . . became sick along with five other children from another family who were friends of ours. Doesn't this sound odd? As we began to research this, we found many people in our small community who have the identical syndrome. It was very fortunate for my husband and [me] that I work for a doctor. The girls have missed many months of school at a time and have been tutored at home. They have been hospitalized twice. . . .

In the beginning, the fatigue, headaches, severe eye symptoms and aching, along with sore throats, backaches and lymphatic pain . . . were the most debilitating. Now, as time marches on, the neurologic symptoms have developed into a strong and more frightening syndrome. They have severe memory and concentration loss. They sit in class, listen to a lecture, and come away not even being able to remember an hour later what was discussed. They are not able to read as they once did, and their handwriting is nearly illegible. They have developed severe dizzy spells, some periods of blacking out (possibly petit mal seizures), severe joint pains, and migraine headaches.

Can you understand how very frightened we are?

Our doctor, David Bell, is a pediatrician. His wife, Karen Bell, is an infectious disease specialist. . . . They have been cruelly ridiculed by their peers and coworkers for their belief in this illness. . . . When our children first became ill four years ago, David and Karen Bell made plea after plea to the CDC in Atlanta for help. [The agency was] mildly interested and suggested certain tests be done (e.g., lymph biopsies). They continued to tell Karen Bell that they would come here to Lyndonville if this or that was done. The biopsies were agreed to by my husband and [me] *only* so that the CDC would come and investigate this syndrome. They never came! In fact, they would not return Karen's phone calls or take them. We have done everything that they asked of us.

My plea comes to you not only as a mother but also as a concerned citizen of the United States. This illness is devastating, and no one will listen, it seems. Few, if any, patients ever recover from this. We need some help! We need somebody to step in at a national level and say there has been enough discussion, and to do something. I am so frustrated. That is why I have turned to you, Mrs. Bush. I . . . believe that you care about children and issues that affect them.

Jean Pollard's letter never made it into Barbara Bush's hands. The White House turned the letter over to a public relations staff member at Stephen Straus's agency, the National Institute of Allergy and Infectious Diseases in Bethesda. A response was prepared by the staff member and sent to Pollard over the signature of Jim Hill, deputy director of the institute. The letter, dated September 11, read: "The NIAID supports research aimed at identifying the cause of this syndrome and is vigorously pursuing the complex questions related to CFS on many fronts, both basic and applied. . . . The NIAID is supporting a variety of studies that will contribute to the understanding of this disease."

Pollard had enclosed with her letter several epidemiologic and clinical studies undertaken by David and Karen Bell upon their epidemic population in Lyndonville and surrounding communities. "The reprints of Dr. David P. Bell are useful," the agency responded, "and are being forwarded to NIAID researchers concerned with CFS." In a 1990 interview, Jim Hill acknowledged that the only scientist at the agency interested in CFS was Stephen Straus, the same researcher who had disparaged David Bell and Paul Cheney's research on interleukin-2 levels in the disease.

Centers for Disease Control, Atlanta, Georgia

In September, nearly three years after Congress had asked the CDC to undertake the probe, the agency's surveillance program officially began. Three hundred eighty doctors in four sentinel cities had agreed to refer patients with unexplained severe fatigue lasting six months or longer to the agency, starting that month. For senior researcher Walter Gunn, the surveillance launch was an important line of demarcation.

As a result of his interaction with the hundreds of patients who called or wrote the agency every month, as well as his attendance at support group meetings in Atlanta, Gunn was beginning to sense the imposing outlines of the epidemic. Again and again he asked himself the fundamental question: how could so many people—all of whom told a story that was, with only minor variations, the same— be making this up? The longer he pondered the matter, the more unavoidable his conclusion: they were telling the truth. For the first time during his reasonably happy tenure at the federal agency, the senior researcher found himself quietly at odds with his colleagues. By fall, in fact, Gunn was increasingly uneasy with the surveillance plan he had once helped to defend.

For one thing, the plan as constituted clearly subverted the will of the Congress, which had asked the agency to determine the *national* prevalence of the disease. As things stood, four years hence the agency would be able to provide an extraordinarily conservative estimate of the prevalence of CFS in only a few counties, most of them in areas like Wichita and Grand Rapids, which were hardly considered hot spots, unlike the entire state of California and the Northeast Corridor. "Larry Schonberger wasn't convinced the disease could be diagnosed by *anybody*," Gunn recalled, "so he wanted a doctor-based system, and he wanted just three sites. But in doctor-based systems some people don't get counted for the simple reason that they didn't go to the participating doctors. And then you've got to deal with doctor bias."

The other problem, of course, was that the case adjudication system was far too conservative and would yield, Gunn now suspected, a vast underestimate of the true number of cases in the four regions under study.

Wistar Institute, Philadelphia, Pennsylvania

In the summer of 1989, Elaine DeFreitas asked Paul Cheney and David Bell to begin sending controls from their patient populations. DeFreitas had processed hundreds of blood samples from Cheney's adult patients in the South and East and from Bell's younger sufferers in rural upstate New York as a kind of broad initial foray into the problem. Now she wanted to see what she might find in healthy patients from the same clinical practices. The doctors complied, labeling their controls by a secret code known only to each other and mixing the samples in with the patient samples before sending them.

In September, DeFreitas asked Cheney and Bell to come to Wistar for a conference. She now felt closer to being able to publish her findings. "The feeling we all had was that this paper was just about ready to get written," Bell recalled later. "We felt we were really close—there were a few little odds and ends that needed to be patched up."

DeFreitas's diction and manner were colored by her Brooklyn upbringing. Her *g*'s were hard and her words were punctuated with expressive gestures of her long-fingered hands, which more often than not held a smoldering cigarette from which she would draw deeply, as if taking nourishment. She was of Portuguese descent. The gaze of her enormous, deep-set brown eyes seemed intense enough to burn holes in the object of their focus. Surrounding this striking countenance, a leonine froth of curly black hair, moussed to a patent-leather gloss, shimmered as if weightless.

DeFreitas's exotic, sensual look was completely at odds with her scientific modus operandi. An immunologist by training, she was, by reputation, a perfectionist. In her laboratory in the Wistar building next to the University of Pennsylvania campus, the scientist was positively compulsive in her methods. Seated on her high steel swivel stool, her hands sheathed in a powder-soft second skin of latex, she would stare through the lens of her microscope, her eyes narrowed in concentration. Sometimes she snapped a photograph of what she saw. She hung her evidence—magnified 100,000-fold and printed on glossy paper—on the wall and referred to it throughout the day. Her skepticism, willful as a living thing, was subdued only temporarily. She lay awake at night wondering if her findings might be due to contamination or some other fluke—even, she sometimes wondered guiltily, laboratory sabotage. She drove her postdocs to distraction. Only when she had confirmed her findings in a multitude of ways and on numerous occasions would she concede, "Yes, given the data, it *appears* to be so."

Five years earlier, when she was thirty-six, Wistar chief Hilary Koprowski had recruited her to work in the field of T-cell immunology. DeFreitas, who had earned her Ph.D. in microbiology at Penn State, was working as a postdoctorate fellow in the lab of Jacques Schiller at the National Jewish Center for Immunology and Respiratory Medicine in Denver when Koprowski wandered into Shiller's lab unannounced, looking for her boss. Unable to produce Schiller, who was in Switzerland, DeFreitas answered Koprowski's questions. Koprowski hired her on the spot. "After you see as many people as I do in a lifetime," he recalled later, "it's not so very difficult. I saw in her an extremely clever, inventive, and driving person. She sinks her teeth into a problem. And she's enormously careful."

DeFreitas brought her compulsive methods and excruciating doubts to her collaboration with Paul Cheney and David Bell. One of the sticking points she brooded over that summer was controls. Some of the controls Bell and Cheney were sending her were positive. Given the extremely rare rate of infection with HTLVs in the general population, once one eliminated all possible known risks like blood transfusions or drug use, the only other explanation for the finding was that the controls had picked up the agent from the patients. This was entirely possible since the controls had been deliberately selected from people who knew the victim—colleagues, family members, and school playmates. These healthy exposure controls were, then, analogous to HIV-positive people who had not developed symptoms of AIDS. An unanswered question, of course, was would these HTLV-positives go on to develop the disabling disease that had afflicted their playmates or co-workers?

"In the middle of all this," DeFreitas remembered, "I sort of swallowed hard and said, 'Let's do some controls of our own.' " DeFreitas's husband was a Philadelphian internal medicine specialist. "I gave him the CDC criteria for this disease," DeFreitas said later. "I told him I wanted adult normal controls. And so he asked his patients—he read down the list of symptoms—and he found ten people who said, 'No, I have never had those symptoms.' And he bled those people and sent me the blood. Then I went to a gynecologist-obstetrician friend of mine, and he gave me ten cord bloods, which is the baby's blood that comes out of the umbilical cord. . . . And we ran ten of these normal, healthy Philadelphia controls. And every single one of them was negative.

"I was very reassured by that," DeFreitas said, "because it meant that the controls that Cheney and Bell were sending me obviously had exposure to this thing, even though they didn't get sick."

Los Angeles, California

The disease that had cut a swath through Los Angeles three years earlier at last bubbled up into prime-time network television on September 30. The format was a highly rated situation comedy in its season premiere: *The Golden Girls.* The Bea Arthur character on the show caught chronic fatigue syndrome.

Susan Harris, the creator of the series and its top producer, had spent the summer laboring over a two-part script and attended the live tapings of both shows in Los Angeles. Harris managed to convey the trauma of the disease without sacrificing comedy. No doubt satisfying every sufferer's best fantasies, the barbs came at the expense of a parade of medical specialists who failed to recognize the disease as an organic illness. Before she finally found a doctor who could identify her problem, Arthur's character was told to change the color of her hair, to take a cruise, and to see a hypnotist. The only false note: Arthur had recovered by the third show of the season.

University of Pittsburgh Cancer Institute, Pittsburgh, Pennsylvania

Members of the Pittsburgh Symphony orchestra agreed to be cancer epidemiologist Seymour Grufferman's guinea pigs. His hopes for the project were exceedingly high. He had found, after all, an impeccable control group for the North Carolina Symphony. The demographics of the orchestras were nearly identical in terms of age distribution, income, race, and sex. "This was going to be our brilliant idea," Grufferman said some years later. "We thought it would be a nice, tight match on a lot of lifestyle factors, so they would be comparable."

Grufferman decided to begin with just ten Pittsburgh subjects, analyze the results, the proceed from there. By October, however, the study was yielding surprising results. Several of the Pittsburgh musicians sampled had unusually low natural killer cell activity, signaling immune dysfunction. Two days after the blood draw, Grufferman learned, one of the musicians developed viral pneumonia, which explained his sudden drop in natural killer cell activity, but there was no obvious explanation for the other results.

While Grufferman was mulling over these matters, he received an extraordinary phone call from one of the Pittsburgh orchestra members. "This musician called us up," Grufferman remembered some time later, "and he said, 'You didn't draw *my* blood, and I came from the North Carolina Symphony and *I* have chronic fatigue syndrome." It turned out he had got this bid to make a career jump and join the big-time Pittsburgh Symphony, and he came with his chronic fatigue syndrome from North Carolina to the Pittsburgh orchestra where there were no apparent cases of the syndrome."

In one moment Grufferman's beautiful plan had come to a crashing end. In all likelihood, the Pittsburgh Orchestra members had been contaminated by the North Carolina musician. Certainly the low natural killer cell results in the first ten musicians, selected at random, suggested as much.

"I was amazed," the scientist said later. "Amazed at what a small world it is, number one. And, number two, amazed at just how difficult it is to do this research. It is *so* tough to study this disease! Here we had this great idea and we just fell flat on our faces."

Grufferman's next step was apparent: "We dropped the Pittsburgh group because we thought it was perhaps contaminated. What we *really* wanted was some healthy reference group that was comparable."

So far, Grufferman and his colleagues had found low natural killer cell function and other immunological aberrations in three discrete groups: the North Carolina Symphony, the faculty at a Chillicothe, Ohio, elementary school, and the Pittsburgh Symphony. The North Carolina orchestra and the Ohio school had been hit by CFS outbreaks; the Pittsburgh group merely had been joined by a sufferer from the North Carolina outbreak. Although they were alike in many ways, the Ohio and North Carolina clusters were different in one important way: there was no cancer in Chillicothe.

"Now, how do you interpret this?" Grufferman said. "The answer is, I don't *know* if there is an increased risk of cancer in this disease, but I think we have an urgent need to confirm or refute that finding."

Unfortunately, Grufferman had run out of money and energy for his cluster research. "I really felt kind of paralyzed by the awful reception this [research] got in peer review," the scientist recalled some years later. "I mean, it's kind of crushing. I found this a really painful occurrence," he added, "and it really kind of stopped me from moving forward. It was *so* discouraging to try twice to get grant funding and not be able to get it when I thought I was sitting on top of a potential gold mine of information. So the project just sort of festered and sat on the back burner." He was emotionally drained, too, by the resistance of his peers in medicine to the disease itself. "I've never seen such a violent reaction," he said, adding after a moment, "People desperately want this disease to just go away! Why is there this institutional—it's almost *hostility*—to this disease?"

One success kept Grufferman's hope alive: it was a day-long elective seminar he gave to first-year medical students, which 60 percent of the incoming class opted to take. Grufferman began by describing the body of scientific literature on the subject of chronic fatigue syndrome as well as the affliction's clinical signs and symptoms. Next, the class listened as a CFS sufferer discoursed on her peculiar fate. "She is a very articulate, very unhappy patient who tells us about her experiences going from doctor to doctor and getting no satisfaction, and this sort of downward spiral of her life—losing her social supports, losing her income—and how she came to our clinic expecting us to have magic bullet, and all we did was tell her to stay away from unproven therapies, and how dissatisfied she was with us," Grufferman said. Next, the same patient's doctor described the case from his perspective. "He talks about how difficult it was for *him* to be in this position of having no way of diagnosing it, having nothing to offer and wondering, How do I keep my patient away from quacks?" When the testimony ended, Grufferman asked his students to form small groups with individual psychologists to discuss not the patient's emotions, but their own.

"These students were asked to talk about how, as a doctor, you deal—in terms of *feelings*—with a disease like this," Grufferman said. "How do you comfort people? And the students love it. It is the first introduction to the human side of medicine that they get."

Incline Village, Nevada

By mid-September, Dan Peterson's pilot study of Ampligen was officially over. All the patients had undergone an elaborate series of tests including treadmills, mental status exams, MRI brain scans, and careful assessment for human herpesvirus 6 as well as a wide range of blood tests. Eight patients experienced dramatic improvement by several measures. Their performance IQ levels rose. Consumption of oxygen, tested by walking on a treadmill, increased "markedly," Peterson reported, in 60 percent of the patients, some of whom had greater than 100 percent improvement without engaging in any exercise program. Interestingly, Ampligen also reversed high levels of human herpesvirus 6 proliferation in assays by tissue culture.

Two patients—former stockbroker Tom Miller and former hospital administrator John Trussler—failed to respond to the drug, however. Additional testing revealed that those patients who responded well to Ampligen had a deficit in the body's natural antiviral defense system. David Strayer had found the same deficit in AIDS sufferers who responded to Ampligen. Peterson and Strayer suspected this defect might eventually become the diagnostic hallmark that had been sorely lacking in CFS.

Peterson was excited by the results of the first real clinical trial of Ampligen, but his enthusiasm was tempered by the fact that none of the patients had completely recovered, and a majority of them had suffered an increase in headaches and muscle pain during the trial. He reported, too, that one patient was hospitalized for chest pains after having sex. "But I don't think it was due to the medication," Peterson said, straight-faced, adding that it was the first time the patient, a man, had engaged in sex in the four years of his illness.

Milwaukee, Wisconsin

Eight executives from HEM Pharmaceuticals in Philadelphia, including the chief executive officer and owner, Paul Charlap, converged on the Pfister Hotel near the Milwaukee waterfront late on the evening of October 20. They came to hear Dan Peterson present the results of his Ampligen pilot study at a day-long medical conference organized by a consortium of midwestern CFS patient associations, scheduled to begin the following day. Since his meeting with the HEM board in New York the previous spring, Peterson had been invited back to the company's offices in Philadelphia no fewer than three times. He was developing a sense of the firm and its principals.

"Some rich people have a lot of cars. HEM is Charlap's Porsche," Peterson said that night over dinner in the hotel's pricey dining room as he watched the vivacious chief executive table-hopping among his dark-suited employees.

The kinetic Charlap was sixty-four. He was bald, five feet four inches tall, and jocular and expansive in mood. Paul Cheney compared him to Captain Bligh as he paced outside the conference hall the following afternoon holding animated conversations on a cellular telephone. Charlap's business career had spanned such diverse enterprises as ownership of the Philadelphia-based HEM and the founding of the Savin Corporation, the office machine manufacturer. A University of Pennsylvania graduate, he had attended medical school at Temple University for two years. Charlap's brother, Mark, a Broadway composer affectionately nicknamed "Moose," had written some of the music for *Peter Pan.* By some accounts, Paul Charlap was the inspiration for the song "I Won't Grow Up."

William Carter, Ampligen's co-inventor, had invited Charlap, a friend, to head the company the previous May. By that autumn, Charlap was effusive about Ampligen's potential in treating CFS, AIDS, and other diseases such as cancer and hepatitis B. His commitment to Ampligen had been triggered, he explained in Milwaukee, by his concern about AIDS and his faith in the experimental drug as a potent therapy for that disease. "Ampligen is a very strong immune stimulator. It's a strong virus-killer. In *our* minds, CFS is a virally caused disease. You have to look at Ampligen as a broad-spectrum antiviral drug just like you look at penicillin as a broad-based antibacterial drug. We're going to expand our work in this disease."

Stephen Straus did not attend the Milwaukee conference. In fact, by 1989, no fewer than six such scientific conferences had been held in major cities around the country, and Straus had been absent from all of them. Given the barriers to publishing on the subject, these gatherings were important opportunities for CFS researchers to share their findings. One possible explanation for Straus's reliable absence was provided by the deputy director of NIAID, Jim Hill, during an interview in early 1991: "I'm not surprised that Steve doesn't necessarily want to go to a meeting where the whole purpose of the meeting is going to be to attack Steve Straus."

While Straus's name was rarely if ever mentioned at these conferences by patients or by scientists, Milwaukee turned out to be an exception. Significantly, the criticism of Straus came from perhaps the only independent investigator with the kind of institutional prestige to take the federal scientist on: Anthony Komaroff of Harvard. Komaroff departed from his prepared remarks, a summary of the clinical abnormalities he and others had discovered among CFS sufferers, when he said, "Most of us would agree that many people with chronic fatigue syndrome are depressed, but Straus has gone on to imply that patients and their families have more depression in their histories than the general population." According to Straus, Komaroff continued, "Seven-point-one percent of the [CFS] patients had histories of major depression." But, he added, among the population at large, a history of major depression is present at a rate of 6.9 percent. "There's really no difference," Komaroff said, adding, "Among patients with AIDS, nineteen-point-six percent have histories of major depression. So, nearly twenty percent of AIDS patients have had a major depressive episode—nearly three times the national average. Is there anyone who would argue that AIDS is a depressive illness?"

Houston, Texas

In December, *Aviation, Space and Environmental Medicine,* a magazine for flight surgeons, published an electrifying autobiographical account of a pilot who developed the disease.[1] The revelatory tale was one of the first published accounts ever by a victim who was also a doctor. As a consequence, William T. Harvey's powers of description encompassed an ability to provide a professional as well as a personal self-assessment. He was also the first pilot to write about the devastating impact of the disease upon his piloting skills. Harvey, based in San Antonio, developed the disease in the autumn of 1987, but it was not until late in 1989 that he obtained a diagnosis. In the interim he came close to crashing his plane twice. In one case, after being cleared to land at Moffett Field in Sunnyvale California, he was told to land on the left runway; Harvey thought he was complying with the flight controller's directive when he headed his plane for the right runway. "I had correctly complied," he wrote, "but remained totally confused between left and right. In fact, I had been having difficulty the whole flight remembering my flight plan and recalling common radio phrases familiar to me for twenty-six years!" Harvey landed safely after the flight controller, who began shouting at him, corrected his flight plan. He had been feeling unwell for several months, but this was the first time he had experienced cognitive difficulties in flight. He blamed the incident on the early hour.

"On my very next flight," he continued, "I again became confused in the pattern. This time I also had trouble with concentration, word recall, and word substitution. Fortunately, I survived that flight as well, but this time the controller's frustration got through to me. I understood that something was seriously wrong, and that I must not fly again until I knew what was happening to me."

Harvey had fallen victim to what he assumed was a severe flu in November of 1987. For the next several months he experienced a pattern of remission and exacerbation, although he noted that he never felt "well" again. "In December," he wrote, "my mood began to vacillate wildly, with periods of extreme depression and withdrawal." In January, he began to experience headaches so frequent and severe that he consumed a 1,000-pill bottle of aspirin in two months. "I experienced several episodes of full-blown migraines with scintillating scotomata [areas of absent vision in the visual field, surrounded by normal sight] and gross outbreaks of cold sores at least twice," Harvey recounted. His other symptoms: "mild photophobia, 'head-in-a-barrel' cognitive fuzziness, mild muscle aches, slightly sore throat . . . the 'feeling,' not verifiable, of fever . . . [and] persistent sensory symptoms: a low-grade tinnitus, difficulty with night vision, and decreased acuity in low light. . . . Finally I admitted that the time had come to face my terror, regardless of the consequences."

Harvey's story proceeds to his eventual diagnoses, his experiences echoing those of thousands of patients before him. He saw a multitude of expensive specialists, including cardiologists, neurologists, ear, nose and throat specialists, endocrinologists and rheumatologists, all of whom told him he was healthy but suffering from stress.

After a year, he diagnosed himself when a colleague gave him a transcript of a 1988 lecture on the disease by James Jones. He learned, too, that several other people who worked in the building in which he worked had "the same persistent symptoms that had onset vaguely about the same time mine had."

Harvey lamented the Centers for Disease Control's position that "there are no strong indications that it is easily transmitted to other persons. . . . Meanwhile," he added, "the numbers of us getting the illness seems to be increasing."

The doctor listed the symptoms "common to a majority of CFS patients" that he believed were important to "aircrew functionality."

"One, cognitive: includes attention-span contraction, decreased concentration, sequential memory disturbance, math calculation difficulty, word-recall disturbance, increased response-time, and word substitution. All appear consistent with a chronic, generalized encephalitis. (I can vouch for most of these; I experienced them during much of 1988.)

"Two, neurologic: severe frequent headaches, some classic migraine; dysequilibrium, visual acuity disturbance . . .

"Three, emotional: emotional lability, depression, anxiety, or all three. I experienced all these as well; the first seemed out of control at times and related to the overall severity of the infectious symptoms of fever, sore throat, and lymphodynia (painful lymph nodes). The second and third alternated as I learned I might never recover from this illness, and as I encountered a mostly uninformed and disbelieving medical community."

Harvey ended with an appeal to his audience of fellow flight surgeons: "I hope you recognize the effect this illness may have or already may be having on air crew performance and safety . . . recognize its potential aeromedical consequences, and will follow with interest as the mystery unfolds."

Harvard Medical School, Boston, Massachusetts

That winter the NIH awarded a second research grant to Anthony Komaroff. The Harvard investigator's new proposal was dedicated to probing the neurological manifestations of the disease, with special emphasis on the relationship between chronic fatigue syndrome and multiple sclerosis. With its decision to fund a second research project on the disease, the federal government could and would make political hay, pointing to their support of Komaroff's investigations as evidence of their commitment to the discovery process. But the questions Komaroff's inquiries promised to answer over the course of years ultimately were less urgent than those posed by the many grant proposals the National Institute of Allergy and Infectious Diseases had turned down.

The doctor's second grant—again, under $1 million—was a "prove it to us" setup much like his first (which promised to reveal the number of CFS sufferers in a large HMO in Seattle). The Boston researcher was being paid this time to prove to the disbelieving scientists and bureaucrats in Bethesda that the Tahoe malady was real, that it did what a multitude of skilled clinical observers and bench scientists outside the agency already had documented it did, which was foment measurable—that is, objective—damage to the brain and intellect of its victim.

"In our patient group," Komaroff had written in his proposal, "15 percent have suffered from intermittent periods of disorientation (typically involving time and place) and confusion, as described by relatives and referring physicians . . . acute profound ataxia (failure of muscular coordination) typically lasting 3–14 days, transient focal paresis (weakness or partial paralysis on one side). He wrote that 7 percent had suffered primary seizures and 4 percent had transient blindness "typically lasting six hours to three days. . . . The CFS patients in this study," Komaroff added, "will be especially impaired: recurrently or persistently bedridden or homebound and unable to work."

Discussing his grant privately, Komaroff said, "I've always believed this disease was connected in some way with lupus and multiple sclerosis."

He added that he would be using the federal money to look for retroviruses as well. "The talk of retroviruses had been going on now for over two years," he said. "I'm very dubious that any one agent will be responsible, but I've also said that it's very possible that retroviruses could be responsible for this. We have evidence for retrovirus in some of our patients, but *which* retrovirus? And is it new? Or, like herpesviruses, has it been there a long time? Establishing cause and effect is easy when the virus is brand new to the human race," he added, but pointed out that that was unlikely to be the case in CFS, simply because the odds against it were so high. "The only example of that in our lifetimes," the doctor said, "is HIV."

Buffalo, New York

Cancer epidemiologist Diane Cookfair's grant was never funded, despite continued high scores on each of its two revisions and her congressional lobbying effort the previous spring. Eventually the Buffalo team lost its spirit for the seemingly impossible quest for federal support of their research. Simply rewriting the grant each time required the full-time effort of at least one of their members for six to ten weeks. Gathering data to defend their hypotheses, in addition, was not only time-consuming but expensive, and money was in short supply. By the end of the year the Buffalo group had disbanded.

Within two years, Carolyn Warner, one of the very few neurologists in the country to take a serious research interest in the disease, was forced to drop her CFS investigation entirely when she was offered a post as the director of a Buffalo institute dedicated to performing research and providing clinical treatment for myasthenia gravis.

Centers for Disease Control, Atlanta, Georgia

Four years after their first visit to Key West, epidemiologists Chad Helmick and Matthew Zack's December paper in the *American Journal of Epidemiology* confirmed the substance of what several eminent neurologists and the victims themselves had proposed to the Florida health department and the CDC nearly a decade earlier: "Key West appears to be a high-risk area for multiple sclerosis."[2] In fact, the MS rate in Key West was fourteen times what would have been expected for the region. In addition to the primary risk factor, which was living in Key West, Helmick and Zack determined there were other risks. Two they considered statistically significant were being a nurse and, curiously, owning a Siamese cat.

Elaine DeFreitas, who read the paper with a kind of detached, almost amused curiosity, ruminated on the bizarre state of affairs that would lead federal investigators to document an epidemic of what likely was the wrong disease.

1990
THE
GREEN DOT

The quarrels of doctors make a pretty chapter in the history of medicine. Each generation seems to have had its own.

—Sir William Osler, *Counsels and Ideals*

20

The Sneering Committee

National Institute of Allergy and Infectious Diseases, Bethesda, Maryland

The government's rejection of all but two research proposals after four years of effort by outside scientists was bound to have a chilling effect. By 1990 the Nevada team, having tried three times to win a grant, had given up on the agency even though they had compiled a wealth of important findings. Most significantly, microbiologist Berch Henry, who had isolated from approximately two hundred Nevada patients a highly virulent virus that he was ultimately able to definitively identify as human herpesvirus 6, had begun to do forensic work for the Washoe County Sheriff's office. And infectious disease specialist Ray Swarts, formerly among the most enthusiastic proponents of the Tahoe investigation, was busy writing the state of Nevada's AIDS protocol. By early 1990, only Dan Peterson and University of Nevada epidemiologist Sandra Daugherty, who had won money from the state legislature to pursue her epidemiology research in Incline Village, were exploring the disease with real fervor.

Nancy Klimas, the University of Miami AIDS expert, was probably the most battle-scarred veteran of the grant war, having tried and failed seven times so far to win federal support for her research since the NIH's first invitation to submit proposals in 1987. Klimas had little difficulty winning federal dollars to pay for other projects, particularly her AIDS research. (By 1988 approximately 50 percent of the budget of the National Institute of Allergy and Infectious Diseases was devoted to AIDS research; by that same year the CDC had begun a new accounting system whereby all moneys disbursed were classified as A, for AIDS, or NA, for non-AIDS.) In fact, Klimas managed to support a staff of sixteen in her lab at the university almost entirely on NIH grants. But winning funds for her work in the disreputable CFS field was something else again. She had taken advantage of every opportunity to submit a proposal to study the disease, had met every grant application deadline set by NIAID, and had been shot down every time.

"I've tried from *every* angle," Klimas said that year. "The National Institutes of Health is funding sick dog research at a much higher level than they're funding

362

chronic fatigue syndrome research, and I think maybe they ought to refocus their priorities."

Like most CFS investigators, Klimas had taken seriously the agency's claim that the purpose of the 1988 Pittsburgh workshop was to help researchers design better grant proposals. With hindsight, Klimas saw that event as little more than a sophisticated shell game. The conference had imbued the agency with an appearance of concern while simultaneously deflecting attention from its failure to investigate the epidemic or to provide support to those who were struggling to do so.

"You would expect that out of the next round, *someone* would be funded," Klimas continued. "And did anybody get funded? No, although we all made the adjustments that seemed to have been requested of us by this consensus group. On the *next* round Tony Komaroff got funded, but he was the only one out of God knows—there had to be *dozens* of applications that time. And then more nothing, more nothing, and more nothing."

To support her CFS research, Klimas was cribbing from other sources of funding. "We've gotten some seed money for different things, but I, like every other investigator doing basic research in this area, have depended heavily on the healthy support of our labs from other areas. It is very interesting, fascinating, and completely unfunded work."

In spite of the government's refusal to fund studies seeking to identify the agent of the disease, research was proceeding in some pockets of the private sector with the support of patients. *Golden Girls* creator Susan Harris had become a generous contributor to the North Carolina–based CFIDS Association, her dollars always earmarked for research purposes only. Max Palevsky, Malibu colony resident and occasional movie producer, was sending a reported $50,000 a year to Anthony Komaroff. In early 1990, Paul Thompson of Incline Village provided Elaine DeFreitas with a year's salary to support Brendan Hilliard, the Irish postdoc who was doing the bench work on CFS blood samples in the Wistar lab, and made it possible for her to hire a second full-time lab researcher. Thompson was also supporting Paul Cheney's research at the Nalle Clinic by paying the doctor's salary one day a week to free Cheney from the obligation of seeing patients and allow him to devote at least one of his working days to uninterrupted clinical research. Ed Taylor, the Tulsa TV entrepreneur, continued to be influential among researchers as a result of his support, as did Chicago's Minann foundation, headed by Ted Van Zelst. The wealthy parents of several victims, people like Nucor chief Kenneth Iverson, Marc Iverson's father, were contributors too. By 1990 the CFIDS Association of Charlotte had raised close to half a million dollars to support independent investigator's research. The association's journal, the 100-plus-page *CFIDS Chronicle,* provided a home for independent research findings.

Examining the moral underpinnings of a federal health system that forced victims of an epidemic disease and their families to bear the financial burden of scientific inquiry was an exasperating exercise for these philanthropists, and they voiced their frustrations frequently. Yet it was patently obvious that there would be no research into the cause of their disease unless they paid for it.

Hennepin County Medical Center, Minneapolis, Minnesota

Hennepin County infectious disease chief Philip Peterson, in his testimony before Congress the year before, had asked the government to establish a priority system for funding CFS research grants. In the absence of federal funding, the doctor had continued to pursue his own investigation of the chronic disease in his county hospital research clinic, which opened in July of 1988. With this ready supply of subjects, Peterson engaged his colleagues in the local research community in several small research projects.

"How you approach this disease depends on your subspecialty," Peterson said that winter. "It is, potentially, an immunologic disease. We saw chronic fatigue syndrome as a paradigm illness in which the relationship between the brain and the immune system has gone haywire."

One aspect of the disease Peterson and his colleagues sought to assess was its degree of morbidity: just how bad a disease was it? A majority of Peterson's clinic patients had been highly active, even athletic women in their thirties when they fell ill. "Once they developed chronic fatigue syndrome, roughly half of our patients could walk no more than three blocks. . . . Running was out for all the patients, but for most, even minor exercise, like walking uphill, was difficult. . . . It does appear to be a chronic illness that does not resolve, as least as we've seen it."

Working with a University of Minnesota medical professor, Peterson and his collaborators employed the Medical Outcome Study, which had first been described in the *Journal of the American Medical Association* in 1989, to measure physical suffering. A score of one hundred was "best health" on the study's scale. Peterson's team compared their CFS patients' scores with those of healthy people and people suffering from either myocardial infarction (heart attack) or rheumatoid arthritis. Healthy people scored an average of 75. Victims of rheumatoid arthritis scored in the high 40s range; patients with myocardial infarction scored slightly lower. Patients in Peterson's clinic scored, on average, 16. As far as Peterson and his colleagues knew, such low scores had never before been measured on the scale. When he presented his findings at a medical conference that year, Peterson noted that the disease caused greater "functional severity" than heart disease, virtually all forms of cancer, and all other chronic illnesses. "We really haven't seen anything like it with respect to other medical illness," Peterson said, adding that he had needed to engage an artist to redesign the morbidity graph for the slide he presented at the conference, since no other category of patients had ever scored so low.

Peterson's findings reprised the observations of Portland infectious disease specialist Mark Loveless, an associate professor at the Oregon Health Sciences University, whose primary clinical specialty was AIDS. Loveless frequently administered another test of morbidity, the Karnofsky scale, to both his AIDS patients and his CFS patients. The Karnofsky test, which dated back to the 1940s, was a time-honored measure of a patient's ability to perform common daily activities like bathing and preparing meals. Even in their last week of life, Loveless had noted, many AIDS victims scored higher on the Karnofsky test than did Loveless's CFS patients.

"This is the most frustrating medical condition I have ever taken care of," Loveless said. "It is harder than HIV care, and *that* just grinds down the best of us."*

Miami immunologist Nancy Klimas, who ran a CFS clinic at the University of Miami and an AIDS clinic at the Miami veterans hospital, agreed. Her young children could tell whether she had spent her day with CFS sufferers simply by reading her face when she walked through the door at night. "They'll say, 'It was a chronic fatigue day, Mommy,' or 'It was an AIDS day, Mommy.' They know the difference."

University of California, Irvine

One of the most puzzling aspects of chronic fatigue syndrome, to casual observers, was the contrast between how sufferers claimed to feel and how they looked. Little about CFS sufferers' conditions was more invisible or more difficult to explain than their altered mental states. In a riveting description of his chronic fatigue syndrome odyssey, published in the *Boston Phoenix,* a novelist with the unlikely named Floyd Skloot gave voice to the paradox of appearing normal while feeling "unplugged" and "like a polluted stream."[1] Skloot had come down with the disease—like most victims, literally overnight—in December of 1988. Tellingly, although Skloot, a former marathon runner, addressed the disease's physical pain and disabling weakness, he devoted greater effort to its impact upon his intellect, chronicling in particular the embarrassing wash of intellectual gaffs that marked his daily existence:

> If I see you scratch your head while I'm talking to you, chances are I'll forget what I'm trying to say. When I prepare hot cereal in the morning, I'm as likely to pour my rolled oats onto the lid as into the pot. . . . And the things I say! I ask my wife for a stick of decaffeinated gum, ask my doctor whether the blood tests show "amnesia" instead of anemia, complain to a friend that my hair is leaking rather than thinning. The Xerox machine apparently stands for all machines in my rearranged brain: I ask my wife to reheat my coffee in the Xerox, ask my son to Xerox the lawn, explain to my daughter that the doctor will Xerox her injured arm. My spelling and my math have become utterly original. This is not the way I was before.

Skloot also threatened his readers: "If I hear you call it the 'yuppie flu,' I'll hit you with a Xerox machine."

By 1990, a new player had entered the field with new tools for evaluating the problems Skloot described so helplessly. Curt Sandman, a slim, light-haired man in his early fifties, was the vice chairman of the Department of Psychiatry and Hu-

---

* On May 12, 1995, testifying at a congressional briefing sponsored by Illinois congressman John Porter and Nevada senator Harry Reid (at the behest of the CFIDS Association), AIDS specialist Loveless would tell legislators that a CFS patient "feels every day significantly the same as an AIDS patient feels two months before death." Loveless supported his statement with data from research conducted at his own institution and morbidity data provided by other CFS experts who had compared the two diseases.

man Behavior at the University of California at Irvine. He was a clinical psychologist who, in addition to his work at the university, was chief of research for the State Developmental Research Institute, a small group of select scientists employed by the state to perform research on the brain and behavior. With his colleagues, Sandman had developed a series of computerized measures of memory skills, which were useful in assessing brain dysfunction in patients with frank neurological diseases such as Alzheimer's, traumatic head injuries, learning disabilities and stroke, and in patients with psychiatric diagnoses such as schizophrenia and depression.

Sandman had been approached on a number of occasions by Los Angeles CFS expert and U.C. Irvine associate professor Jay Goldstein, who wanted Sandman to administer his new tests to CFS sufferers. For months, Sandman had resisted Goldstein's overtures, pleading prior research commitments. Finally, at the prodding of his wife, a psychologist, he agreed. "I must admit," Sandman recalled later, "I was one of the enemy. I was convinced that the first three or four patients I saw had hysteria or conversion neurosis. I assumed they were giving me psychogenic, nonspecific complaints. And I refused to believe they were actually suffering from anything profound or real. I'll never really forget my total lack of interest in those first patients." After seeing a total of six patients, Sandman reversed his views of the disease, as he "began to see some real consistency in cognitive loss," he recalled.

After several more of Goldstein's patients submitted to Sandman's computerized tests, "we began to ask, 'Are there *specific* memory defects in this disease?' " he said. He decided to undertake a formal study of such patients using depressed patients and normal people as his control groups. By early 1990, his findings— made on 40 people with CFS, 23 depressed patients, and 129 age- and sex-matched healthy controls—were complete. There existed, Sandman stated in his report about his findings, a CFS dementia.

Chronic fatigue syndrome victims' mental scanning time—the time it took them to retrieve long-held or semantic memories from their mental storehouse— was abnormally slow, slower than that of healthy controls and depressives. "Their mental speed is impaired," Sandman said. A more serious problem arose in the realm of short-term memory, however. "The kind of dementia CFS patients exhibit is one in which they have difficulty consolidating information from the environment. If information gets into the sensorium—the nervous system—they can get it out. They just don't get everything in. Even the most simple or brief distraction disrupted the memory trace and the efficiency of information processing deteriorated."*

Sandman was struck, as well, by the mechanisms CFS sufferers employed to compensate for their difficulties. On the object-assembly test, for example, patients were given a childish jigsaw puzzle and told to assemble the pieces into an object, such as an elephant, or a human figure. "These patients get distracted with any extra information," Sandman said. "So here's an array of pieces around them

---

* One of Sandman's tests measured a subject's ability to "make memories" when the opportunity to "rehearse" the information—that is, to actively work at memorizing it—was momentarily interrupted. The performance of CFS sufferers was sevenfold worse than that of either depressed controls or normal controls.

and they have to make an object. And I've seen patients close an eye to solve the test, cock their heads in a funny way to solve the test, posture themselves in some funny ways—strategies that they've learned to minimize distraction."

In his report on his research, published in 1993, Sandman cautioned that his data should be viewed as "preliminary."[2] But, he added, the pattern of intellectual problems signaled "neurological compromise" in the disease. "These results," he continued, "are consonant with lesions of the temporal lobe, hippocampus, and limbic system."

By that winter, Sandman was fully engaged; he had every intention of pursuing his research in the field. "But," he recalled some years later, "I was told that it would hurt my career. Someone in a real position of power warned me that I was making a terrible mistake and that I should disassociate myself from the people studying this disease, that it was a fringe disease. But I ran interference for Jay Goldstein at UC Irvine, and I helped him get other good people involved. I argued, 'We can either accept the politics and the PR that this disease doesn't exist or is a flaky illness, or we can prove or disprove the disease.' "

Sandman, in addition, received support from one unexpected quarter: his boss at the State Developmental Research Institute revealed that his sister was suffering from CFS. The head scientist told Sandman he would give him his full backing to pursue the brain research.

Mayo Clinic, Rochester, Minnesota

In 1990, William Morrow published a 1,300-page compendium, *The Mayo Clinic Family Health Book.* On its book jacket, the publishers claimed the book offered "useful facts on more than 1,000 diseases." In their half-page entry on CFS, the Mayo authors wrote that "emotional and psychological factors may play a role. Usually, there is no underlying viral infection. In most cases, there is no serious underlying disease causing it."

The book, a best-seller, had sold more than 600,000 copies by 1995.

Lyndonville, New York

By the new year, David Bell was in the process of analyzing his own study, and he continued to be impressed with the disease's spread within families. Months before, he had sent a questionnaire to the parents of seventy-four children who were suffering from CFS. Forty-seven children, or nearly 64 percent, Bell discovered, had at least one other family member ill with the same disease; in several families, Bell noted, *every* member of the family had the illness. Curiously, eleven children—15 percent—had an immediate family member who was ill with multiple sclerosis. Bell suspected the high incidence of MS was merely misdiagnosed CFS.

Bell's own practice in the ranch-style house on Lake Street in Lyndonville was crumbling. The majority of his patients now were victims of the epidemic disease; they tended to be either the children of very poor adults, or adults who had been made poor by the circumstances of their ailment. The end result was the same: few of his patients could pay him. Bell's practice had never been a lucrative one; his patients were among the poorest in New York State, but for years Bell hadn't cared. With the epidemic, that had changed. Increasingly he had begun to discourage many of his epidemic patients from seeking his help, not because he didn't want to help them but because he couldn't. He had exhausted his ideas for remedies and therapies. His seriously ill epidemic patients, for whom he could do so little, were depleting his own emotional reserves. Privately, he was infuriated that his peers in medicine were persisting in diagnosing the disease as a depressive syndrome, despite all evidence to the contrary.

"I think doctors make a diagnosis of depression because they're unwilling to admit that they don't have a clue what's going on," Bell said. "And those who say this is depression don't face the critics faced on all fronts by those who say there is a physical source. If I were to make any suggestions for changes in American medical schools," he continued after a moment, "it would be that they train doctors to be more like doctors in the nineteenth century. They were great clinicians, and I think they would have handled chronic fatigue syndrome quite nicely."

Early that spring, Bell sold a portion of his clinic's furniture to raise cash. He also took the unusual step of hiring on as a hospital emergency room doctor in nearby Medina. "I would work in the emergency room all night," Bell remembered later, "and try to get a nap in the morning and work in my clinic in the daytime, or else I would work in the ER on weekends."

To his surprise, he enjoyed the work. He was buoyed by the relative simplicity of the medical problems he encountered in the hospital's emergency room. "It was wonderful!" Bell recalled. "Somebody would come in with a big cut and you sewed them up and they smiled and you got rid of them and you never had to see them again in your whole life! I'm exaggerating—but I enjoyed it. It was very enjoyable to deal with simple problems like that for a while."

Charlotte, North Carolina

At the start of the new year Cheney began to accept the idea that he would need to leave the Nalle Clinic if he was to continue his work in the disease. His immersion in CFS had created insurmountable tensions for him and his staff within the multispecialty clinic. He felt increasingly isolated, and he was frustrated with caring for patients with colds, flus, muscle sprains, and the like that filled so much of an average internist's day. Quietly he began investigating the possibility of starting his own clinic in Charlotte, one in which he would see CFS sufferers exclusively.

"I'm not afraid," the doctor said of the prospect. "I have no lack of patients. Right now we're booked out until May with chronic fatigue syndrome patients. They keep coming out our ears. There are millions of them." Nor was there any indication, the doctor said, that the epidemic was waning. "We're seeing cases here that are just six months old."

Centers for Disease Control, Atlanta, Georgia

By 1990, the CDC was receiving more than two thousand calls a month from the public requesting information about the disease. A year before, when the calls exceeded a thousand a month, they began to outnumber inquiries about AIDS. Larry Schonberger's branch now employed a full-time staff member, Dorothy Knight, whose primary responsibility was to respond to public inquiries about the disease.

To help Knight and other staff members, the agency printed up an information bulletin, which it ultimately sent out by the thousands in response to mail and telephone requests. In it, the CDC assured the public that there existed no "convincing evidence" that CFS was contagious. The bulletin also reported that a "small portion" of patients had been found to have "modest" immune system dysfunction, but that patient support groups' name for the disease, "chronic fatigue and immune dysfunction syndrome," was inappropriate since *most patients do not have these immunologic abnormalities*" (italics added). In fact, every scientific study of patients had turned up immune abnormalities, and the CDC, having failed to conduct research of its own, lacked any data to the contrary.

"It's nothing for us to get two hundred or three hundred calls a day," Knight said that year. Each call was logged into a computer by name, address, city, and country. "We tried having a standard letter, but it didn't work because they kept asking questions." Knight also reported that at least 10 percent of the inquiries were from doctors seeking information.

Knight was impressed with the volume of sufferers—"You just don't *realize* how many people have this!" she exclaimed that winter—but she was struck even more forcefully by a realization that the strange symptoms of which they complained sounded identical to those of a mystery disease she had encountered before. "When I worked at the hospital at Fort Stewart in Hinesville, Georgia," Knight recalled, "we were beginning to see cases there of soldiers and their wives who were always tired. No one knew just what was wrong. They would take sick leave or reduce their training. When you're in the military, you work or you're let go. The hospital had several cases coming in—men and women and even dependents. They complained of a flu that never went away. But what do you do when you run blood tests and they come back normal? Doctors at Fort Stewart hadn't heard of this—it was completely new. But when I transferred here, I said, this is the same thing those people had down at Fort Stewart!"

New York City

On January 28 the *New York Times* syndication service, which fed articles to scores of metropolitan newspapers around the nation, published health correspondent Jane Brody's column headlined "Some Fresh Insights into the Old Problem of Fatigue." Her primary source appeared to be the NIH's Stephen Straus, who told her that he and his collaborators at the agency had "demonstrated that many patients [with CFS] were psychologically 'different' long before they developed the syndrome."

Straus, of course, could only have been referring to the two dozen people in his 1986 acyclovir trial.

National Institutes of Health, Bethesda, Maryland

By January of 1990, NIH researcher Jennie Hunt had prepared a sixteen-page bibliography of medical literature on chronic fatigue syndrome. She found that 285 articles had been published on the subject since January 1980. Reporting on this development in the *CFIDS Chronicle,* lobbyist Barry Sleight wrote, "The National Library of Medicine, the world's largest biomedical information resource, has taken two actions in response to the large demand from biomedical researchers worldwide for information on chronic fatigue syndrome. In January, NLM added a new medical subject heading to all its print and on-line cataloging operations for 'Fatigue Syndrome, Chronic,' with cross-references to a number of other names for the disease. Also, the NLM has prepared a new title on chronic fatigue syndrome in its Current Bibliography paperback book series."

Centers for Disease Control, Atlanta, Georgia

Every Wednesday afternoon the steering committee of the Division of Viral and Rickettsial Diseases met to share information about projects within the division. With Gary Holmes's departure looming, Walter Gunn had stepped into the job of principal investigator of chronic fatigue syndrome, and it fell upon his shoulders to keep his colleagues up to date on the surveillance efforts at these meetings. Unfortunately for Gunn, the disbelieving, dismissive attitude that had prevailed for so many years within the division had yet to dissipate. Privately, Gunn took to calling the weekly sessions the "sneering committee" meetings.

"The orientation of the agency was formed by the Holmes and Kaplan investigation in Tahoe. That's what, quite frankly, I'm trying to overcome—that original investigation," Gunn explained. "There is this perception of the disease that just *hangs* over the place. And they keep moving the target!" he added. "They say, 'Where's the data?' As fast as you *show* them some data, they say, 'It hasn't been confirmed.' "

Gunn by then had crossed over the boundaries of frank disbelief and, more recently, skepticism and embraced the reality of the disease. Now it wasn't merely his telephone conversations with sufferers that were influencing his views. The early results of the surveillance project, which had begun the previous fall, indicated that more than two-thirds of the patients being referred to the agency were free of psychological problems when their disease began. In addition, according to Gunn, the prevalence of depression among these CFS sufferers was about the same as in the general population.

As a result of his transformation, Gunn was experiencing the same censure and humiliation that victims of the disease endured. To suffer from the malady was to be considered a malingerer, a hypochondriac, or a neurotic; to undertake research into the disease as if it were a true medical illness was to be regarded as a dupe of all of the above. "I was trying to do a serious job," Gunn complained some time later, "and there was constant laughter, giggling, snickering."

Gunn's formative years as a naval officer had instilled in him a starched pragmatism. He approached his work with gusto and a sense of mission. "When they give me something to do," he said, "I sit down and I do it." Even so, Gunn was considerably unnerved by his peers' low regard for his new project. After twenty years of distinguished service in the field of public health, he had hoped to bring his career to a more dignified close. In sheer self-defense, he began photocopying everything he came across in the medical literature that suggested an organic basis for the disease. He circulated the copies throughout the agency, even sending one to the director's office. But he found little sympathy for his sober view of the disease.

It was against this background that Gunn made an application, on February 16, to the division's head, Brian W. J. Mahy, for $730,000 to undertake a small case-control study of CFS. The point of the study was to analyze people with the disease and healthy people in an effort to determine what was different about patients. First conceived by Carlos Lopez in 1986, the CFS case-control study had been mired for years in one of the most tortuous development processes ever witnessed at the agency. (Atlanta clinician Richard DuBois, who originally was to supply the patients for the study, had been waiting for four years for the study to commence.) Gary Holmes had written countless drafts of the case-control study proposal. Most of Holmes's proposals focused the investigation on whether the disease was psychiatric in origin; Gunn had reworked the proposal. In his new version, there was more emphasis on organic signs.

Gunn's request was entirely routine; in his years at the agency, he had made similar applications for funds in the multimillions of dollars to undertake studies. Nevertheless, Gunn remembered, "It was an outright decline. I was told the money wasn't there."

The investigator was mystified. Congress had appropriated $1.4 million to the Centers for Disease Control for CFS research that year. Gunn asked for and was granted an appointment to meet with Brian Mahy, Larry Schonberger, Kenneth Herrmann, and Harriet Walls, the division's top four administrators. "I asked them where the money was," Gunn recalled much later. "They said it just wasn't there. This was the first time I was alerted that there might be a problem."

Food and Drug Administration, Rockville, Maryland

Beginning on Monday, February 25, Dan Peterson and a fleet of HEM Pharmaceuticals executives had parleys with officials at the Food and Drug Administration, the National Institute of Mental Health, and the Centers for Disease Control. HEM staff were seeking to fast-track their drug into position for licensing. They were in Washington to present the results of Peterson's Ampligen trial to agency officials and to lobby for enlarging the Ampligen trial to several cities and hundreds of patients. They wanted phase three FDA approval for a second, vastly expanded round of clinical trials (phase three was a final step before legalization). HEM was hoping to avoid phase two categorization, which would require yet another tier of clinical trials after completing the one they proposed. The company believed it could show the same efficacy in larger trials that Peterson had demonstrated in the pilot.

FDA headquarters was the site of the largest of the three meetings. Twelve HEM executives and scientific consultants were present, as were Peterson, Denver researcher James Jones, the University of Seattle's Dedra Buchwald, and a sizable contingent from the FDA. The session lasted ninety tense minutes. "The room was packed," Peterson recalled.

The doctor was attacked by FDA scientist Giovanna Tosato, who had been an author on Straus's 1985 paper about the disease in the *Annals of Internal Medicine*. Tosato told Peterson he must use the CDC's definition of the disease to select his patients. "You can't say they have this disease if they have all the other problems you're describing," she said to the doctor. She was referring to abnormalities such as brain lesions, reduced performance IQ, evidence for active human herpesvirus 6 infection, and sky-high levels of interleukin-2.

"If you use the CDC definition," Peterson retorted, his patience at the breaking point, "then *none* of my patients could be included, because all them have something wrong with them!"

Straus, absent from the FDA meeting, was present at the well-attended meeting at the National Institute of Mental Health, an agency that had recently begun to demonstrate interest in CFS because of the clear signals from Congress that the nation's legislators were in a funding mode on the disease.

"Straus takes the position he doesn't care," Peterson recalled. "He was smug. He got up and left the room several times. He said HHV6 has never been isolated from a single chronic fatigue syndrome patient." Straus seemed particularly disbelieving when Peterson reported the severity of his patients' illness. "When I began to describe some of my patients on Ampligen, he said things like 'I have never seen a single patient like this' and 'Good luck, because it would be a miracle if you're able to prove anything.' "

Peterson took the opportunity to remind Straus that he had concurred in Peterson's CFS diagnosis of two Nevada patients who had also been to the NIH for an evaluation.

Recalling the discouraging two days, Peterson confessed, "I've been getting emotional. It's really getting to me. I predicted this—that things would get worse before they got better. We're getting stonewalled, and I don't know why. I guess it's a typical American bureaucratic disaster."

National Governors Conference, Washington, D.C.

Often it was the illness of a close friend, spouse, or family member that motivated a politician to enter the fray, just as Minnesota governor Rudy Perpich was moved by his son's disability to lobby his fellow governors for support. At the winter meeting of the National Governors Conference, Perpich submitted a policy resolution asking the governors to designate two weeks at the end of February as CFS Awareness Weeks. The resolution also asked the governors to call upon the White House and Congress for better coordination among the federal health agencies on the disease.

Perpich's resolution was passed by the governors—marking only the second time the governors association had passed a resolution pertaining to a specific disease—but not unanimously. California governor George Deukmejian, representing a state of 31 million people with possibly the highest per capita incidence of the disease in the nation, was among the dissenters. Word of Deukmejian's position leaked back to San Francisco, and a letter-writing campaign was launched by the state's support-group network. In a matter of days, Deukmejian's office received five thousand personal letters of protest. San Francisco activist Jan Montgomery described the campaign in the *CFIDS Chronicle,* noting that the letters had "encouraged Governor Deukmejian to change his mind."

Perpich's efforts and the efforts of five thousand Californians had little impact overall, however. Although the resolution passed, the legislative arm of the governors association failed to undertake any lobbying efforts in Washington on behalf of the disease. CFS Awareness Weeks went unremarked upon in the press.

In Perpich's own state, health care institutions were responding to the epidemic with the same disregard and denial as the rest of the nation's health providers. Medica, for example, the largest health maintenance organization in Minnesota, the state that enjoyed the highest HMO membership in the nation, categorically denied membership to anyone carrying a diagnosis of chronic fatigue syndrome. According to Medica's underwriters, the multitude of treatments attempted by CFS sufferers, which ranged from gamma globulin injections to costly antidepressants and other drugs, were so cumulatively expensive they exceeded the HMO's underwriting guidelines.

Charlotte, North Carolina

By February, Paul Cheney had moved from the Nalle Clinic into the sleek new suburban offices of the first private CFS-dedicated clinic—probably in the world. From its lobby with two massive black leather reclining chairs, where patients could lie down while waiting for their appointments, to its sophisticated laboratory with a biocontainment flow hood for working with blood samples and a −70°F. freezer for storing body tissues, the Cheney clinic offered state-of-the-art clinical care for victims of the disease.

It would not be a high-volume practice. Cheney saw just four patients a day. He devoted each morning to a first-time patient; three afternoon appointments were scheduled for repeat visits. For the doctor's Rolls Royce evaluation, which included a multitude of expensive immunologic and neurologic tests, the bill was a hefty $2,500, a sum that would draw fire from Cheney's critics. For those patients who had searched for years for a definitive diagnosis, some of them spending hundreds of thousands of dollars in the effort, however, the doctor's fees seemed bargain basement.

Mammoth–June Lakes Airport, Mammoth, California

In March, the *National Transportation Safety Board Reporter* published a detailed account of a plane crash in northern California. The plane was a Cessna 3200 six-seater equipped with a stall warning system. At the time of the crash, the weather was clear and the runway was dry. Three passengers and the pilot died in the crash.

None of the five eyewitnesses interviewed by the journal reported seeing trailing smoke or any other evidence of fire, and none heard any unusual noises before the plane crashed during its ascent from the runway.

The National Transportation and Safety Board determined the causes of the crash: in-flight planning/decision—improper—pilot in command; (2) procedures/directives—inattentive—pilot in command; (3) airspeed—not maintained—pilot in command; (4) stall—inadvertent—pilot in command.

On autopsy, the pilot was found to be drug- and alcohol-free. According to the *NTSB Reporter,* however, "a letter from a doctor was found in the pilot's personal effects in which it was stated that the pilot complained about chronic headaches, forgetfulness, and disorientation.

"The pilot had recently been treated by a doctor, who reported in a telephone interview that he had been treating the pilot for lack of sex drive, forgetfulness, and confusion," the *Reporter* continued. "The pilot's physical examination was normal in all respects, but his blood tests showed latent Epstein-Barr virus symptoms—[the doctor] advised the pilot not to fly an airplane because of his forgetfulness complaints. The pilot had been referred to another doctor for further cerebral vascular examinations."

Centers for Disease Control, Atlanta, Georgia

Overwhelmed by public inquiries, in March the CDC provided a ten-minute taped message about CFS to run on its disease hot line. Just three other diseases were named on the hot line recording. "For AIDS, dial one, " the recorded voice intoned. "For cancer, dial two. For hepatitis, dial three. For chronic fatigue syndrome, dial four." Using a Touch-Tone phone, callers were able to select from a second menu topics that included a broad description of the disease, information on the "causes" of the disease, diagnostic information, information on support groups, and a general category called "new information on chronic fatigue syndrome." That spring there was "no new information" about the disease, the recorded voice reported. Callers were invited to leave their name and address if they wanted printed material sent to them.

CFS inquiries rapidly outnumbered all others. Dorothy Knight, who managed the hot line, reported that in addition to the two to three hundred calls and one hundred or so letters that poured into the agency every day, the message tape was routinely filled to capacity with calls pertaining to the chronic disease. "Our CFS hot line is always full," she reported. "A lot call in at night—you still get people calling in after nine P.M."

U.S. Senate, Washington, D.C.

On March 28 lobbyist Barry Sleight testified before the Senate Appropriations Subcommittee on Labor, Health & Human Services, and Education, the legislative body with oversight of the federal health agencies. Demonstrating obeisance to the rules of congressional decorum, Sleight repeatedly thanked the subcommittee and its staff for demonstrating a commitment to prodding the health agencies toward investigating CFS. Then the wan young man politely cast doubt on the meager efforts under way by federal scientists. He pointed out, for instance, that the CDC's surveillance plan to determine prevalence was "small" and that the agency's case definition was "narrow."

"It is important to note that there are over twenty other symptoms listed in the medical literature for this disease," he said, symptoms that were missing from the Atlanta agency's definition. "Apparent higher rates of cancers, including deaths, have been documented. Eye, muscle, heart, blood, liver, breathing, brain, neurological, cognitive, and endocrine abnormalities have been documented in CFS patients," he continued. "Some of these abnormalities are similar to those found in patients with multiple sclerosis or AIDS. . . . The summary of current biomedical research is that at least some cases of CFS represent a serious acquired immune dysfunction disorder."

Sleight also pointed out that only three small grants had been made to CFS researchers in as many years, and suggested that inadequately funded researchers outside the agency were undertaking to answer the serious questions about the disease. "We are concerned," Sleight added, "that the activities of the National Institutes of Health and the Centers for Disease Control continue to be less than consistent with a new epidemic of a disease of the immune system."

Ottawa, Ontario, Canada

In March the Canadian federal health department issued an alert to doctors about chronic fatigue syndrome. "We want to let doctors know that this is for real," said Ken Rozee, head of microbiology at the department's Laboratory Center for Disease Control in Ottawa. "These people are really ill. The report will offer doctors a standard way of identifying sufferers. . . . A more stable opinion seems to be developing in the medical community. The views are beginning to consolidate."

Wistar Institute, Philadelphia, Pennsylvania

Elaine DeFreitas, having now invested more than two years in her secret collaboration with Paul Cheney and David Bell, was exquisitely sensitive to rumors and reports of other retrovirology labs that were searching for the same bug. At the start of 1990 she had told Cheney, "I was reluctant to talk about this initially because I wasn't really sure we were right. Now I'm reluctant to talk because I'm afraid someone will steal this from us."

That spring, she tried to calm herself with the thought that confirmation of her work would be helpful not only to her but to patients as well. "If we're first, great. If we're second, great. If we're third, great. I think at this point, *anything* is good," DeFreitas added after a moment. "If two labs come up with the same finding, that will certainly go a long way toward confirming what the first lab found. There's no sense in working against each other now. It's too big a disease. We need some help in this. We need some confirmation. It's good for us."

Nonetheless, she struggled to keep her discoveries under wraps. "I have tried to be very quiet about it. I've told the people in the lab to be very quiet about it. It's been hard on them, too, because they obviously want to talk about their research."

DeFreitas had come light-years beyond her initial observation that retrovirus antibodies were present among a majority of sufferers and a significant number of their contacts. She had identified small portions of the actual gene sequences of the retrovirus. The bug was definitely not the first human retrovirus, HTLV1. Nor was it HIV, the third human retrovirus. However, it shared some but not all sequences with HTLV2. It was, DeFreitas realized, an HTLV2-*like* retrovirus. (HTLV2 had yet to be assigned a disease, although it had been tentatively associated with hairy cell leukemia, a rare cancer. But since retroviruses were known to cause neurologic disease, researchers suspected there were also brain maladies associated with HTLV2.) Additionally, and equally remarkably, there existed the possibility that DeFreitas had discovered the first casually transmitted human retrovirus.

DeFreitas knew she was sitting on top of explosive research, but she continued to have problems with her technology. She and her assistant, Brendan Hilliard, were having difficulty finding the right medium for the virus to thrive in. Solving this problem was critical; the media problems were creating havoc with the test results. The same sample would on some occasions test negative for the virus and on other occasions, positive.

While she was attempting to solve this problem, DeFreitas was seriously injured in an automobile accident. During the month she remained hospitalized, Brendan Hilliard pressed on alone, conducting experiment after experiment to discover the balance of nutrients that would keep the pathogen and its host cells alive.

San Francisco, California

Frustrated by his failure to discover the pathogen, Jay Levy had temporarily put aside the matter of the disease's cause and sought to discover the immunological hallmark of CFS. By that winter, Levy and his collaborators, Alan Landay and Carol Jessop, thought they had found what they were looking for: diagnostic markers in the form of aberrant immunological activity.

Levy began to think about the possibility of publishing their research that spring. He pondered, too, the feasibility of seeking a federal grant. With the luxury of federal money, his team could begin to search once more for the virus causing the disease among this select group of patients, more than half of whom possessed the new immune system markers.

"Our reason for doing this work was not to describe those markers," Levy reiterated at the time. "The reason was to know—who do we look for to find the virus? But we ended up with markers—markers that may tell us the people who are really showing severe symptoms. And at least now we can [look for the virus] in individuals who are actively showing signs of immunologic disorder."

Medical College of Wisconsin, Milwaukee

Remarkably, a third virologist was making scientific strides that would ultimately seriously threaten the hegemony of either of the better-known seekers of CFS retroviruses, DeFreitas and Levy, although neither they nor hardly anyone else, for that matter, was aware of it.

Sidney Grossberg was a mature scientist of sixty years and a world-famous expert in interferons, proteins that are produced by virtually every cell in the human body and that help make cells resistant to viruses. He had been studying the substances for three decades. A graduate of Emory University's medical school, Grossberg had performed his residency at Duke, his fellowship in internal medicine at Johns Hopkins, and had been chairman of the Department of Microbiology at the Medical College of Wisconsin since 1966. He had also undertaken two sabbaticals at the Pasteur Institute, once to work on polio virus, the second time, in 1975, to study interferons with Luc Montaigner, who would later discover HIV.

It was during his third sabbatical, this time at the University of Wisconsin in Madison, that he fell into the study of CFS and retroviruses.

"A patient was admitted to the oncology ward," Grossberg recalled some years later. "She died of a very unusual carcinoma of the lung. I suspected a viral cause and decided to investigate her background." In the course of interviewing the deceased's relatives, Grossberg met a woman, in her sixties, with the initials "J.H.," who "told me about her few years of chronic fatigue syndrome. That's how it all started."

Grossberg studied JH's blood under an electron microscope and observed "budding virus particles" inside the lymphocytes. After expert analysis, Grossberg said, "We were sure it was a retrovirus."

The date was January 1989. At the time, Grossberg was completely naive about the clinical entity known as chronic fatigue syndrome, nor did he have any sense of where his discovery might lead. Nevertheless, he added, "My interest was in identifying the virus—and it was really that which led me on. And, naturally, since I'm a doctor, my real concern was: how is it related to human disease?"

In his effort to isolate the virus and test the serum of CFS patients for it, Grossberg had teamed up with an infectious disease specialist in Milwaukee. By 1990, Grossberg had access to all the CFS blood serum he could ever want.

Cambridge University, Cambridge, England

Rumors about the "Cheney retrovirus" were circulating widely throughout the community of patients and researchers, but Paul Cheney continued to be publicly silent on the subject. Far too many scientific variables remained to be solved before the news could be released (The name of Cheney's collaborator remained unknown as well.) Even so, hopes ran high at a three-day symposium on the disease, convened by Canadian clinician Byron Hyde in Cambridge, England, on April 12, that Cheney would reveal some details of the work. Indeed, in the symposium's official schedule, Hyde listed Cheney's topics as "Retroviruses." But the doctor talked about immune system aberrations instead, capping his presentation with a discussion of fingerprint loss.

Hyde, in his opening comments, called the disease "a major health and economic threat, second only to that of AIDS," and he chastised governments for "turning their backs to this health disaster." He described the Lake Tahoe epidemic as the "truly significant incident" in the history of the disease in North America. "The determination with which Cheney and Peterson have stimulated a group of experts from several major universities, research companies, and both Centers for Disease Control and the National Institutes of Health, in a magnificent and at times frightening voyage of discovery, is truly incredible," he added.

Participants in the Cambridge symposium included the brain imaging experts from the University of California at Irvine; Nevada's Dan Peterson, who described Ampligen treatment results from his cohort of patients, which by 1990 had grown to fifteen and included a Nevada rancher and a Reno newspaper reporter; California neuropsychologists Sheila Bastien and Curt Sandman; and a number of British and Australian researchers. Just one scientist from the NIH, Paul Levine of the cancer epidemiology division of the National Cancer Institute, came to Cambridge. No one from the CDC was present. Hyde sent several invitations to Stephen Straus, who did not attend.

Although Cheney was unable to break the retrovirus news in England, he at last took his former partner, Dan Peterson, into his confidence about the discoveries being made in Philadelphia. Peterson, of course, knew that evidence for a retrovirus had been discovered, but until then he had known few details; and although he had suspected Wistar's Elaine DeFreitas was captaining the bench work, he lacked confirmation. When he returned to Incline Village, Peterson carefully packed and shipped twenty blood samples from his voluminous –70°F. freezer to DeFreitas. In his accompanying letter he asked if she would assay the Tahoe blood for the new virus.

DeFreitas balked. She replied she couldn't possibly undertake the project; she had neither the money nor the time. Privately DeFreitas deemed a collaboration with Peterson to be a betrayal of her relationship with Paul Cheney.

Centers for Disease Control, Atlanta, Georgia

Since becoming principal investigator for CFS, Walter Gunn had begun receiving an average of six press calls every week. He reasoned that his own efforts might be more effective if he could convey to patients and independent researchers a sense that the agency had turned around on the disease—even if, in truth, only he had done so. In the spring of 1990, with surprisingly little effort, Gunn launched a new wave of news coverage. This time the angle was to the agency's advantage.

On April 30, *USA Today* published an article about the CFS surveillance program on its front page; this was the first time the news had been reported. Journalists from United Press International and the Associated Press filed stories about the surveillance study later the same day, casting the CDC in laudatory terms as a public health agency responding aggressively to a significant health threat. Two weeks later *Time* magazine's Linda Williams wrote a short piece headlined "Stalking a Shadowy Assailant." Williams painted the disease as a mysterious, hard-to-diagnose illness that the U.S. government was "finally starting to take seriously."

Ironically, the wave of coverage had a circular effect, crashing back upon the agency and layering new stress upon agency staff. At the end of her *USA Today* story, for instance, Kim Painter listed the agency's disease hot line number as a reference for people seeking more information about the disease. In the next four days, according to Gunn, nine hundred people, most of them patients or doctors treating patients with the disease, called the Atlanta hot line. During the same month the agency received a congressional request for information about the number of people working on the disease in Atlanta. Together, Holmes and Gunn came up with only four people.

"We listed myself, Gary, Dottie Knight, and part of Louisa," Gunn said. Louisa Chapman, an internal medicine specialist just out of her residency, was a newly hired EIS officer assigned to the Division of Viral and Rickettsial Diseases. Among other duties, she was to serve as the medical consultant to Gunn's investigation, since Gunn himself was a psychologist rather than a medical doctor.

"By the time the request left the agency," Gunn recalled, "the list of people working on chronic fatigue syndrome had been mysteriously expanded to eleven. Gary and I had *no* idea who all these people were."

Rochester, New York

By 1990, Skye Dailor had been ill three years. The striae—the purple marks along her forearms—had disappeared, but throughout 1989 she had been, David Bell said, "from an activity level, very severe."

Dailor, now thirteen, had been tutored at home for two years. Since 1988 she had been making trips to Lyndonville every three months for an examination by Bell, and for a blood draw, which the doctor immediately sent to Wistar. The girl's blood had the highest retrovirus count of any of the children Bell had examined. He sustained scant hope that the child would ever recover, given the severity and duration of her disease. That spring, however, Dailor surprised the pediatrician. "She started getting better. As the summer began, she continued improving. It was slow and steady. When I saw her in June, she was really picking up."

21

Waist Deep in Alligators

New York City

In April *Love and Other Infectious Diseases,* a complex and moving book about severe illness within a marriage, was published.[1] The memoir was written by film critic Molly Haskell, who was married to another film critic, Andrew Sarris. Both of them were well-known and well-liked members of New York's literary community. Haskell lucidly chronicled her husband's 1984 attack of viral encephalopathy, which rendered him partially paralyzed and caused a range of alarming cognition disturbances and personality changes before it abated a year later, leaving Sarris in fragile health and suffering from chronic fatigue—a state, Haskell says, that had settled upon both partners some time before Sarris's encephalopathy. "We were tired, exhausted," she wrote. It "was chronic: this business of mutual fatigue, and our inability or unwillingness to distinguish where it came from and to whom it belonged. . . . [T]he rest of the world was furiously in motion; we were at stasis."[2] Most bewildering of all, although Sarris was studied by many of the finest neurologists and infectious disease specialists in New York, the experts were unable to fully comprehend the cause of his brain infection.

After months of investigation, Sarris's doctors came up with a tentative diagnosis of cytomegalovirus encephalitis. Cytomegalovirus was a herpesvirus. The infectious disease specialist who made the diagnosis told Haskell her husband's illness was the first reported case of cytomegalovirus-associated encephalitis and peripheral neuropathy. The doctor wrote up the case for a medical journal as "Cytomegalovirus Encephalitis in an 'Immunologically Normal' Adult." When the astute Haskell asked her husband's doctor whether the herpesvirus infection was new or if it was a reactivated old infection, he was unable to tell her, since Sarris had had positive readings for antibodies to the virus from the very first test. Haskell wrote, "Doubts about whether CMV could be blamed for the entire horror remained." One of Sarris's doctors suggested that cytomegalovirus was a "presumptive diagnosis, perhaps *a piggyback to the real cause*" (italics added), raising a question familiar to any clinician conversant with CFS: what had caused the reactivation, or, more fundamentally, what had caused the immune system perturbation that *allowed* latent herpesvirus reactivation?[3]

In the void left by the federal government's failure to investigate the spread of the new epidemic disease, Haskell and Sarris had been left to consult high-paid world-class experts in infections of the brain, none of whom ever entertained a diagnosis of CFS or, as it was called during the years of Sarris's illness, chronic Epstein-Barr virus syndrome. As time passed, the new government-sponsored name, CFS, militated against incorporating the disease into part of any differential diagnosis in severe neurologic cases. After all, no one as sick as Andrew Sarris had apparently been could possibly be suffering from something as benign-sounding as chronic fatigue syndrome. More problematically, most neurologists continued to believe the federal propaganda about the disease—that it was a psychological condition—because they had been offered little else by way of evidence. By 1990, however, there existed anecdotal evidence that atypical viral encephalopathies had been cropping up in hospitals and neurology practices with increasing frequency in the late 1980s. Some of them may have been the severest cases from the CFS epidemic then under way.

One of Paul Cheney's patients that year was a Boston woman with pronounced temporal lobe damage, and with lesions in other regions of her brain as well. "She's got rather incredible objective findings on MRI and SPECT brain scans," Cheney said. The patient, a twenty-three-year-old former college student, developed the disease suddenly—she could date the onset to the day—and was bedridden. She was unable to stand upright without falling to one side, had abnormal reflexes, and suffered from vision problems, to name a few of her neurological findings. Donald Schomer, director of clinical neurophysiology at Beth Israel Hospital in Boston and an associate professor of neurology at Harvard, had referred the patient to Cheney. Interestingly, Schomer told Cheney that he had a "collection" of patients like the woman, people with incapacitating symptoms of sudden onset for whom he could make no definitive diagnosis other than viral encephalopathy or post-encephalitis syndrome, but who he suspected were CFS cases. Schomer independently confirmed that he had seen a large number of such cases, many of them in his work as director of the epilepsy clinic at Beth Israel.

The neurologist, who often conferred with Harvard's Anthony Komaroff on CFS patients with unusually severe brain disease, believed a virus—possibly a retrovirus—was responsible for the neurological manifestations of the disease. "It's not as fulminant as AIDS, but certainly damaging, nonetheless," Schomer said. He also confirmed that the number of such atypical viral encephalopathies had risen notably in recent years. "I see more and more of these cases," the neurologist said. "And I think it just underscores the likelihood that [CFS] is caused by some kind of viral agent, and is transmissible, because there is a proliferation of these cases very much like what we saw in the early days of AIDS."

Los Angeles, California

Los Angeles General, the largest county hospital in the nation, drew its patients, many of them indigents, from an enormous metropolitan region. Its official name was the L.A. County and University of Southern California Medical Center. With 2,104 beds, it was also the largest teaching hospital in the country.

According to John Martin, chief of L.A. General's molecular pathology labs, hospital neurologists had been making similarly vague diagnoses with increasing frequency in recent years.

Martin had become interested in CFS several years earlier through Los Angeles clinician Jay Goldstein. Perhaps because he had trained as a doctor in his native Australia, Martin was an exceptionally clinically oriented research pathologist who demonstrated more than the usual sensitivity to the medical vagaries of the new syndrome. Beginning in 1988, Martin was a reliable figure at medical conferences on CFS, where he frequently presented suggestive evidence for infection and transmissibility in the disease.*

As early as 1988, Martin had become convinced that CFS was an infectious brain disease covering a wide spectrum of illnesses, starting with extraordinarily severe, perhaps even fatal, cases of encephalitis, and descending to mild, perhaps subclinical disease.

"The first category, the severe forms of chronic fatigue syndrome," Martin said in 1990, "present with a severe neurologic illness that medical science cannot easily catalog. Then there is the larger group of patients whose disease is difficult for practitioners to diagnose because it seems vague to them. Now, there are some very experienced practitioners, people like Paul Cheney and Dan Peterson, who see enough patients that they are starting to see this as an extremely severe illness. But it's easier for us to study the first category through a major medical center, as we have here."

University of Pittsburgh, Pittsburgh, Pennsylvania

Seymour Grufferman had been unable to perform any clinical follow-up of the North Carolina Symphony because of his inability to secure additional funding for his CFS research. That summer, however, one of the members of the orchestra called him. The woman had been a non-case—in other words, she had been symptomless—when Grufferman was doing his early analyses of the orchestra. Even so, she was one of the musicians with immune system damage, characterized by Grufferman as "remarkably low natural killer cell activity and high Epstein-Barr virus antibody titers."

"She was recently hospitalized for an episode of acute confusional state," Grufferman reported. "A neurologist could find nothing wrong except for elevated cerebrospinal fluid protein levels." The finding indicated inflammation and injury somewhere in the brain.

Wistar Institute, Philadelphia, Pennsylvania

Elaine DeFreitas had been consumed by medical problems throughout April as a result of her accident. By the time she was well enough to return to her lab, her

---

* Martin had found patients to be "weakly positive" for a so-far-unidentified virus.

staff had arrived, through trial and error, at the correct concentrations of nutrients to support the cells and the pathogen in them, and the retrovirus research was on track. In fact, now that the kinks had been worked out, many patients who had been flip-flopping between negative and positive were now positive on every attempt. Even some of the persistently negative patients were testing positive. After nearly two and a half years, DeFreitas had to admit the data looked "rock solid." Perhaps she had found the elusive "green dot in the middle of the forehead" as Anthony Komaroff described it, a single definitive marker that united sufferers and distinguished them from everyone else. Publication of the finding could come as soon as the fall, she realized.

The scientist's level of anxiety increased, however, in direct proportion to her inability to *disprove* the evidence for retroviral infection in the disease. She had performed her experiments again and again to be certain the findings were real. She had searched for evidence of retrovirus in hundreds of samples using several techniques—by western blot, in situ hybridization, and polymerase chain reaction. She had gone to elaborate lengths to guard against laboratory contamination, performing crucial phases of her work in three different laboratories at Wistar. She had tested different samples of each patient's blood, drawn on multiple occasions over a period of several months; she had tested single samples repeatedly, as well. When so many exposure controls and patients appeared to be positive for the virus, she wondered if she had in fact detected an endogenous retrovirus gene, that is, one that had been present in host chromosomes for generations. Her experiments with unexposed adults and umbilical cord blood from newborns, the latter sampled within an hour after birth, answered that question. DeFreitas was unable to find evidence of infection with the retrovirus in either newborns or unexposed adults.

"I have spent many a night lying in bed thinking of all the things we could have done wrong," DeFreitas said that spring. "Could someone in the lab have accidentally sprinkled cells into the cultures? What pipettes were used? On and on into the night, night after night, thinking of every possible mistake. And I cannot come up with any systematic error that could account for the results. I can't. The only thing that could account for the results is that those are the results. That's what is there."

Although DeFreitas initially had been unaware of the fierce disputes blanketing the disease, her appreciation of the politics of her work had grown exponentially as she moved closer to publication. "Paul Cheney has filled me in, in great detail, about the controversy," DeFreitas said. "It's started getting to me. What is it— 'Waist deep in alligators, I went in to clean the swamp'? "

Indeed, as she would realize only many years later, DeFreitas was at a pivotal point not only in her research but in her career as well; she could have gone forward—or, at no cost to her reputation, she could have retreated. "When I came back from the accident," she would recall much later, "and Brendan Hilliard laid down the results, I almost fainted. I said, 'This can't possibly be true, because if it were, someone like Jay Levy or Bob Gallo would have found it already. And I sent my entire staff back into the lab to do it all over again. . . . At that point I could have boxed everything up and sent it to Gallo and said, '*You* do this.' But it wasn't like I was operating in a vacuum."

Indeed, when DeFreitas presented her astonishing findings to Wistar chief Hilary Koprowski, the senior scientist's cheerful response was, "Looks good. When are you going to publish?" It was Koprowski's enthusiasm and confidence, filtering down from the administrator's office, that gave her the courage to persist, DeFreitas later remembered.

DeFreitas's resolve was further enhanced by her faith in Paul Cheney. Throughout her two-and-a-half-year collaboration with him, the scientist had been warned by her peers in immunology and virology at Wistar and the NIH to drop the disease and to steer clear of the Charlotte clinician. "My friends told me to get out of this. They said, 'You are ruining your career,' " DeFreitas said later. But in those years when their collaboration was in full swing, DeFreitas believed utterly in the clinician. She defended him on the matter of the Lake Tahoe investigation, for instance, saying, "Paul was there. And documented his findings. Now he goes to Charlotte, and he's got a whole new level of documentation. . . . He's a very intelligent man. Very rational. Very logical. I really don't believe he would be fooled, for instance, by a bunch of hysterical people.

"And I would see exactly the hard proof of what he was talking about," DeFreitas continued. "For instance, he told me about the low sedimentation rates he was getting in patients' blood. When I told a clinician in Philadelphia— who had seen one hundred and sixty CFS patients—about the low sed rate, he went back to his charts. *Ninety* percent of his CFS patients had a low sed rate. So," DeFreitas said, "I was constantly getting objective reassurance that Paul was for real."

On June 8, DeFreitas began breaking the codes on the most recent patient samples from Paul Cheney and David Bell. Sitting in her private office, her burning cigarette unattended in its ashtray, she pressed the telephone receiver to her ear with her shoulder and held her lab notes in both hands as she spoke first with Bell, then with Cheney. The New York clinician's patients were identified as DB, followed by a two-digit number; Cheney's were PC, with a number. When she finished, she knew her work of the previous two years was ready to be published. More profoundly, with the breaking of the code, DeFreitas knew what her paper would suggest: evidence for a casually transmitted retrovirus disease. Four-fifths of Cheney's adult patients had evidence of retrovirus infection: three-quarters of Bell's children demonstrated the same evidence. More frighteningly, 43 percent of healthy adults who had frequent or close contact with someone with the disease—most of the medical personnel in Cheney's or Bell's practice—were positive, too. A third of the healthy playmates of children with the disease were positive as well. None of the healthy nonexposed controls harbored the agent, nor did any of a sample of patients with cutaneous T-cell lymphoma, a fourth constituency in whose blood DeFreitas had searched for virus.

"Once I look at this," DeFreitas said, gesturing at her notes, "I have to admit what my eyes are seeing. And what my eyes are seeing is that there is something in the chronic fatigue syndrome patients and in many of the exposure controls that is not in any of the nonexposed controls or other disease controls. . . . It's frightening to walk the plank on something, which is what we're doing," she continued. "I guess at some point you've got to stand on your own two feet and you've got to make a decision. And we've made it. *I've* made it."

Food and Drug Administration, Washington, D.C.

In June HEM Pharmaceuticals executives alerted doctors in four cities that clinical trials of Ampligen could begin in three weeks. The Food and Drug Administration had given final approval for the drug's experimental use on patients at each of four sites: Houston, Portland, Incline Village, and Charlotte. Cheney's new clinic would be the infusion center in Charlotte; Peterson's Incline Village clinic, now on Tahoe Boulevard, the village's main street, would be the infusion center in Nevada. In Portland, AIDS expert Mark Loveless, a professor of clinical immunology at the Oregon Health Sciences University, would administer the drug to his CFS patients. Another AIDS specialist, Patricia Salvato, would manage the infusions in her clinic in Houston.

This was to be a double-blind study, meaning half of the total of ninety-two patients would receive Ampligen, the other half placebo, for six months. Approximately twenty-four people would be enrolled at each site. It was the assumption of both the doctors and patients that HEM would continue to provide each study subject with Ampligen when the study ended—*if* the study proved that the drug worked—a value reportedly equivalent to between $40,000 and $50,000 per patient per year, including costs of infusion and the drug itself. After all, HEM had continued to provide Ampligen free of charge to patients who had responded well to the drug during the Nevada pilot study. As patients would learn later, however, the promise existed exclusively in the minds of the eager participants and appeared nowhere in HEM's legal documents.

The new study fell short of the large phase three drug trials HEM had sought to fast-track the drug. Yet its completion would position the company to undertake phase three trials, the final hurdle before licensing of the drug. Patients had to meet the CDC's criteria, have the ability to walk on a treadmill, and show signs of intellectual impairment on neuropsychological tests. They also needed to undergo an MRI brain scan to rule out the possibility that they were suffering from a brain tumor. As HEM officials quickly discovered, there was no shortage of qualified test subjects. They learned, too, that all the patients were remarkably debilitated by their disease at the start of the trial. Some required custodial care; several spent much of their time in wheelchairs or in bed. Their average age was forty; a majority had been sick for four to six years; none among the group had been capable of holding a job during the years of their illness.

Everyone entering the trial knew they had only a 50 percent chance of receiving the drug; yet, as might be expected in the case of any severe disease lacking helpful drug therapies, sufferers signed up with few reservations. Still, the rigors of participation were great, requiring first of all that patients stop any and all medicine they were currently taking, even aspirin. The collection of "baseline data," required for participation, was another ordeal. Novelist Floyd Skloot, who entered the trial in Oregon, recalled his own experience: "Baseline required that we walk to the point of collapse on an exercise treadmill. We did this on three separate occasions in order to measure how long it took before collapse and how our bodies responded throughout the physical challenge. It required a lengthy neurocognitive exam, which focused on all the things I could no longer do—jigsaw puzzles, abstract reasoning, memory challenges—and a psychological exam and interview. It required a spinal tap, after which I needed emergency treatment and was immobilized by side effects for nineteen days. There were hours of extensive laboratory work that was lost and had to be redone."

Skloot, it turned out, received the placebo—saline water by intravenous injection twice a week—for the duration of the trial.

Despite the government's decision that summer to allow HEM to proceed with an expanded drug trial, one of the patients in Dan Peterson's original pilot study, a Reno resident named Amy Long who had also consulted the NIH's Stephen Straus for her disease, committed suicide in December. Long had turned down Peterson's offer to continue on the drug.

"Ampligen takes a long time to work—you have to be patient, and she had not had an extremely significant response to the drug in the pilot study," recalled Karen O'Brien, Peterson's research assistant, some years later. "And she was just too depressed and fatigued to get to Incline Village for infusions three times a week."*

University of Miami, Miami, Florida

In spite of money shortages in their lab, by 1988 Nancy Klimas and her Miami colleagues had compiled enough information on the immunologic problems common to CFS sufferers to write a paper. Like Harvard's Anthony Komaroff, however, Klimas had discovered that publishing on the disease was nearly as difficult as securing money to research it. "Our immunology article floundered for eighteen months looking for a home," she recalled later. Finally, early in 1990, Klimas received word that it had been accepted by the *Journal of Clinical Microbiology.*[4] It was published that June.

Klimas reported in the article that the array of immunological defects in the disease "suggest[s] that CFS is a form of acquired immunodeficiency." Her designation was a potential political bombshell since it placed the benign-sounding malady in the same category as the more lethal and indisputably contagious AIDS. In fact, in medical dictionaries, "acquired" describes any condition or dis-

---

* Increasingly, suicide was considered by CFS experts to be the primary cause of death among people with the disease. By 1995, six of Peterson's CFS patients had committed suicide. Between 1990 and 1995, four patients in Paul Cheney's practice had died by their own hand. Virtually any doctor with large numbers of CFS patients in his or her practice could report suicide attempts or successful suicides among their CFS sufferers. Said Marc Iverson, "I have never known a person with this disease who has *not* considered suicide."

ease contracted after birth and unattributable to hereditary causes; in the realm of microbiology, the word fairly screams "infectious microbe."*

"This deficiency," Klimas wrote in her summary, "was present in all the subjects that we studied. It has several manifestations, with natural killer cell dysfunction being the most consistent abnormality."

As for what might have caused the damage, Klimas was unable to say. Her paper went unreported in the lay press.

Duke University Medical Center, Durham, North Carolina

On July 11, Sara Miller, a Ph.D. at Duke University's department of microbiology and immunology, sent Paul Cheney the results of her evaluation of an electron micrograph of a virus-infected B-cell that had been magnified 56,000 times. The cell had once belonged to Pam Butters, who was chief of the diagnostic laboratory in Incline Village, Nevada. According to Robert Gallo's lab, Butters had had some of the highest antibody levels to the newly discovered herpes virus of anyone in Tahoe—even though she wasn't sick. Everyone who had examined the glossy snap in 1986, including Werner Henle, had assumed the virus particles spilling out of Butters's cell were herpesvirus particles.

With the Wistar discovery, Cheney found himself thinking once again about the nature and identity of the virus that had so corroded Butters's cell. On a hunch, he asked his newly hired assistant, Russian immigrant and scientist Irene Rozovsky, to send the photograph to Duke's electron microscopy lab for an analysis by a fully objective scientist—something that had never before been done with the photograph. Cheney and Rozovsky were electrified by Sara Miller's response.

"I have examined your micrograph," she wrote, "and if the magnification is correct, I do not believe these particles are herpesvirus. The virus group that these particles most resembles is retrovirus—both in size and morphology."

At a magnification of 56,000 times, the largest nucleocapsid Miller had found was 70 nanometers; herpesvirus nucleocapsids, she wrote Cheney, are 100 nanometers.

New York City

Also in July, an article about chronic fatigue syndrome by Canadian investigative journalist Nicholas Regush was published in *Spin* magazine. Once dismissed as yuppie flu, Regush wrote, CFS was "now being taken more seriously by doctors and researchers as perhaps a sister illness to AIDS." Regush quoted Cheney's congressional testimony in which the doctor described the disease as an "AIDS

---

* Klimas cited fifty-nine other studies in a review of the literature pertaining to immune dysfunction in CFS. Particularly interesting, however, was her comparison of CFS patients to patients with other immunological diseases, primarily AIDS and multiple sclerosis. In several instances, the immune aberrations in CFS mimicked those that had been documented in these well-studied diseases. More than four-fifths of the CFS patients, for instance, had a depression of their cell-mediated immunity—meaning the responses of their infection-fighting immune system cells were lowered—that resembled AIDS. "The values obtained," Klimas wrote, "were closely similar to those we observed in a group of HIV-positive intravenous drug users." In other ways the immune systems of the patients seemed to be overstimulated, mimicking immunological findings in multiple sclerosis and other autoimmune diseases.

epiphenomenon." The journalist also reported the rumors of a retrovirus finding and described the findings of increased cancer in the North Carolina orchestra.

Regush's article set off a spate of angry correspondence among patient support groups all over the country, but most particularly between a Kansas-based group with national ambitions and the Charlotte organization. The midwesterners condemned links, theoretical or not, with AIDS, but they were incensed, too, over a mention of cancer risks. Kansas president Orvalene Prewitt wrote a letter to Anthony Komaroff, asking him to draft an official statement denying the AIDS and cancer connections. Komaroff agreed, writing that "CFIDS is not a form of AIDS . . . [and] HIV does not cause CFIDS. Similarly," Komaroff continued, "there is no evidence that patients with CFIDS have a higher frequency of cancer than the general population." At Komaroff's behest, Marc Iverson published the retort in the *CFIDS Chronicle,* but Iverson added a disclaimer: "The preceding is published at the request of [Komaroff]. . . . [H]is statement does not have the unanimous support of the Chronic Fatigue Syndrome Advisory Council and was considered 'inappropriate' by several CFIDS researchers we have contacted."

With his statement on cancer, Komaroff roused a formidable opponent: Seymour Grufferman. For some time, the epidemiologist had put his research high on a shelf and turned his back on the disease out of frustration. It was in combination with meeting several new patients at the clinic he had set up at the university's medical school, and a call from Marc Iverson, who offered him an opportunity to rebut Komaroff's statement, that Grufferman's enthusiasm was rekindled. "It occurred to me," Grufferman said later, "that if there's that much controversy about cancer, somebody ought to do something. Let's *test* this hypothesis!"

Centers for Disease Control, Atlanta, Georgia

As Holmes's planned departure became official, Walter Gunn was coming into his own. "The more work I did," he explained later, "the more work I got." That summer, particularly, Gunn was fairly direct in his assessment of his role: "It's not that the Centers for Disease Control itself has changed. The fact is, I have a different view of this. And I'm in charge of it now."

It was, perhaps, folly for one person to believe he could somehow move a sluggish federal bureaucracy off the dime or that he could stem the course of a fast-moving epidemic. But Gunn, in his upbeat fashion, evinced the will to try. He had four daughters, the youngest of whom had two years left in high school. He was fifty-four. For some time, he had been looking forward to a vigorous retirement. His unofficial target retirement date was the summer after his daughter's graduation from high school, which meant he had just two years left at the CDC. His position gave him an element of courage that younger, more ambitious scientists could ill afford in a federal agency.

"They don't really know how to deal with me at CDC," he said. "I keep releasing the surveillance data. . . . I'm kind of a maverick," he continued. "I've never been a standard team player or a company man. I'm staying just within the bounds of what I can get away with. I'm going to keep working on this disease until the case-control study is completed," he added, "at which point I'll retire—that is, unless I'm fired first."

In truth, by the summer of 1990, Gunn had gone completely native. "Have you noticed," Gunn asked that summer, "at CDC, if they know you're a patient, they don't tell you *anything*? And if you're not a patient, they'll try to seem objective. And what they say behind the scenes is that this disease is a joke. When I go to division meetings and present this, Jon Kaplan is usually there snickering. As you go up the line, that's the feeling, except that *now* the feeling is, there's money there—there's funding."

Behind his colleagues' dismissiveness, Gunn realized, a new dynamic was emerging. As a result of the efforts of a few activist patients, Congress was pumping ever-larger packages of money into the agency every year—money that the cash-starved Division of Viral and Rickettsial Diseases could legitimately claim. As far as the scientists in his branch were concerned, the disease was quietly transmogrifying from their personal cross to, as Gunn now characterized it, "the goose that laid the golden egg."

University of Washington, Seattle

The *Journal of the American Medical Association* was the largest of all the medical journals, with a circulation of 660,000 worldwide. On July 3, *JAMA* made a potent contribution to the promulgation of the government's view of the epidemic. Depression, not a virus, was the cause of CFS, according to a press release that *JAMA* mailed to hundreds of print and television journalists. The release was based on a study of twenty-six people by a University of Washington team that included psychiatrists Randy Riggs and Wayne Katon.[5] Riggs had presented a portion of the study findings at a Montreal meeting of the American Psychiatric Association two years before. Larry Corey, a renowned herpesvirus expert in Seattle, was named on the study as well. They based their conclusion on the fact that they had been unable to pin the patients' complaints to Epstein-Barr virus and the fact that half of the patients had experienced an episode of depression at some point before falling ill. But critics raised serious questions as to whether the patients under study were suffering from anything more than common fatigue. The paper's title, "Chronic Fatigue: A Prospective Clinical and Virologic Study," hinted at the problems of definition. The patients had been selected for study before the government's definition of CFS was released, and the researchers admitted that, viewed retrospectively, just six patients met government criteria.

The comments of Deborah Gold, an internal medicine specialist who had launched the study in 1986, shed light on the kinds of biases the researchers involved brought to their investigation. Gold had been a research fellow at the University of Washington's Herpes Clinic at Harborview Medical Center in Seattle when a large influx of patients suffering from the putative Epstein-Barr virus disorder triggered her curiosity. By 1986, in fact, so many patients with the disorder were crowding the medical center's clinic that the clinic's name was changed to the more general Viral Disease Clinic. Gold was interviewed early in 1988, before the study was published but after much of the data had been analyzed. She recalled that a great surge of patients with "chronic fatigue," or "chronic Epstein-Barr virus infection," were referred to the Seattle hospital clinic in 1986, a phenomenon she blamed on "the advent of the publicity surrounding the Lake Tahoe outbreak." Gold was intrigued. "It wasn't just the number of them that was so impressive," she said. "It was the sheer number of their symptoms and the intensity of their symptoms and the absolute lack of physical findings or laboratory abnormalities to explain any of their symptoms.

"Did I believe them? Did I think their symptoms were real?" Gold said in response to a question. "Yes, I thought their symptoms were real. Did I think that they had an infection that was responsible for their symptoms? I lean toward no, since it would be difficult to invoke an infectious agent that might cause symptoms spanning so many years."

Gold was so inundated by people suffering from CFS that she eventually began turning them away from the clinic in order to free up time to finish her research. She interviewed approximately one hundred people with the disorder during her investigation. "It might interest you to know," Gold added, "that when I first proposed this study I had a lot of individuals at the University of Washington who were very willing to help me in terms of laboratory tests and other kinds of evaluations, but there were no individuals who would help me see these patients. None of the others from my cohort, no fellows, no staff people—would see these patients. And that's including Dr. Larry Corey. So if he gave you the impression that he was seeing some of these patients, he did not see them. *He did not see them,*" she emphasized.

(During an interview, herpes expert Corey had portrayed himself as a "physician investigator" whose role was to observe patients through his clinician's eye, then take his observations to the laboratory bench and study the problem in a "systematic way." He also said, "I got Dr. Gold interested to start seeing some of these patients with me.")

Gold's goal was to find other, more established diseases among her patients. "I gave every patient the benefit of the doubt and really assumed there was something else wrong with them that I could diagnose and treat," she recalled. She was able to find just two patients in whom she suspected another disease, however. Significantly, Gold believed both of those patients might have been suffering from MS, though she admitted she had failed to determine the diagnosis with any certainty.

"No question—two patients among all the patients I saw is a small number," Gold continued. "I really have no good explanation for what was causing the symptoms of all the others. Their symptoms were suggestive of vegetative symptoms—sleeping all the time. Now, we did find a very high prevalence of depression." She also noted, "A lot of them were actually quite hostile. I was sometimes the fifth or even tenth physician that they had seen in a span of one or two years. So there's a sense of desperation and also of anger and hostility."*

If anything, lay coverage of the Washington study was more intense even than the coverage of the government-sponsored Stephen Straus paper the year before. The press reported the *JAMA* study—in some cases writing or speaking nearly verba-

---

* By 1988, Gold had completed her fellowship and was a practitioner in San Francisco's Kaiser Permanente system, an enormous health maintenance organization that provided medical care to individuals and companies throughout California. In her new position, Gold said that year, she was seeing more patients with the disorder, and occasionally held noontime conferences for doctors within the Kaiser Permanente system. "There's a lot of interest here," Gold said. "Mainly there's interest in trying to refer these patients to another doctor if at all possible, because they're *very* difficult to take care of."

tim from the journal's press release—in every venue imaginable. "Research Again Finds No Link between Virus, Chronic Fatigue" was the *Washington Post*'s headline on its page-three story by Erin Marcus. In Minneapolis all three network affiliate news stations reported on the story at both 5:00 P.M. and 10:00 P.M., using the story as a teaser to draw viewers into their nightly broadcast. One of the stations pulled the file tape of Rudy Perpich Jr., the governor's son, escorting his sister down the church aisle at her recent wedding. As the wedding film rolled, the voice-over speculated that the younger Perpich, who claimed to have a medical illness, was actually suffering from mental illness. Cable News Network gave the story extensive coverage, although, unlike most news sources, the cable network searched for dissent among patients and doctors; Jay Goldstein, for instance, was asked to present his argument for rejecting the study's conclusions.

Patients were distraught. Some fought back. Letters and telegrams poured into *JAMA*'s offices. CFIDS Association head Marc Iverson called the journal's press officer, Paul Tarini, at the American Medical Association's Chicago headquarters to report the inaccuracies in the release and to seek a retraction. The newly formed National Chronic Fatigue Syndrome Advisory Council issued a dissenting press release on the subject, too.

Three weeks after the nation's press corps had been inundated with *JAMA*'s original release, the American Medical Association issued a new press release to advertise its next issue. Below several unrelated items, the document offered a correction: "A news release in the July 4 packet confused chronic fatigue with chronic fatigue syndrome; the two are not the same. We regret the error and [the] confusion it may have caused."

To this author's knowledge, the correction was not reported anywhere.

[icon]

In a letter to *JAMA,* which was never published, Paul Cheney complained that the Washington study "had little scientific merit and its appearance in your journal says a great deal more about the biopolitics of *JAMA* editors . . . than the real scientific concerns about this pressing clinical issue."

"Medical publishing politics" might have been a more appropriate phrase than "biopolitics," however, since there was some evidence that *JAMA*'s editors were more concerned with attracting readers than with fairly illuminating complex medical problems. *JAMA*'s editors, for instance, had recently changed the journal's publication date to position it more competitively with the *New England Journal of Medicine* for coverage by the lay press. The *Los Angeles Times* reported the unusual news in a piece about a trend among medical journals to seek headlines and saturation coverage in the lay press.

Rhoda Ashley, the associate director of the virology division at the University of Washington, was another investigator named on the *JAMA* study. Interviewed in 1988, Ashley echoed Gold's comments when she said, "There's sort of a universal groan that goes up among clinicians when you mention [CFS] because, to them, [CFS] is a very real, daily occurrence in their practices. But it's interesting to me," Ashley added, "that these patients are ordinarily high achievers. They're *not* loonies. . . . And I think some of the better minds have been saying, 'There's something in this. This isn't just a lot of neurotic, stressed-out people.' Certainly, some of the medical and clinical data on this syndrome matches up with what you would expect from a herpes agent. [Retrovirus infection] is not an illogical notion either."

JAMA's decision, *L.A. Times* reporter Janny Scott suggested, "reflected what critics believe is some journals' growing preoccupation with grabbing the attention of the mainstream media. . . . Newspapers, magazines, television and radio offer the journals not only a pipeline to a public with a seemingly insatiable appetite for health news, but they also are a source of prestige for the journals and for scientists looking for fame as well as funding. . . . *JAMA*'s move comes at a time when more and more journals are supplying reporters with free or advance copies and mailing out news releases and 'tip sheets' translating into English from 'medicalese' the hottest research of the upcoming issue."

Scott quoted Daniel Greenberg, publisher of *Science and Government Report,* a respected independent newsletter on science policy in Washington: "I think the essence is that the editors of the journals have learned brilliantly how to manipulate the science press. And the science press plays the game with them. That's their raw material."

The editors of *JAMA,* in their competitive stance with other major journals, could hardly have failed to notice the way the lay press gobbled up every crumb of information about CFS, no matter how incredible or poorly conceived, when it was presented to them in press-release form. The *JAMA* publishers had latched on to an inferior study undertaken by poorly informed investigators—but one which, as Cheney correctly pointed out, reflected their own biases—and inflated it into their hottest story of the month. The science press, as usual, took the bait.

Wistar Institute, Philadelphia, Pennsylvania

The matter of where the retrovirus paper should be published was hotly debated by Paul Cheney and Elaine DeFreitas. *JAMA* was out, obviously. The collaborators discussed another possibility—the *New England Journal of Medicine*—for less than five minutes. Twice so far the *New England Journal* had held up important CFS studies for nearly two years, then refused to publish them.* Neither DeFreitas nor Cheney wanted to see their valuable research hung up for excruciating months, possibly years, of peer review, only to be rejected.

Cheney argued for the *Annals of Internal Medicine.* That journal had published the CDC's diagnostic criteria, an indication that its editors had a serious interest in elucidating the malady. In addition, Cheney said, a member of the *Annals* editorial board was rumored to be suffering from the disease, an item of speculation that, if true, might better dispose the *Annals* to the subject. Cheney's most heartfelt argument, however, was his belief that the discovery should be disseminated to as wide an audience of internal medicine specialists as possible. Internists, after all, were the specialists most likely to see patients with the disease and as a group they could be influential in forging a better understanding of the epidemic—if they could be persuaded it was real.

DeFreitas, in contrast, ultimately expressed her opposition to submitting the study to an audience of clinicians of any stripe. "This paper should have a very broad readership among scientists rather than clinicians," DeFreitas said. "And I

---

* The first instance had occurred with Richard DuBois's 1984 paper on the disease, ultimately published by the *Southern Medical Journal* ("Chronic Mononucleosis Syndrome," *Southern Medical Journal* 77, no 11. [1984]: 1376–82).

don't want anyone reviewing it who doesn't know anything about technology, and that's a risk you run in *Annals of Internal Medicine.*" Her boss, Hiliary Koprowski, agreed. In what would be the first clash of wills between DeFreitas and her Charlotte collaborator, a decision was made to publish the paper in the *Proceedings of the National Academy of Science*. It was no coincidence that the Wistar chief was one of the most venerable members of the National Academy of Science.

By June 15, DeFreitas was able to report, "It's being written, it's going out. And it's going into a very well respected and very widely read journal, the *Proceedings of the National Academy of Science*."

Harvard University, Boston, Massachusetts

After many months of work, Anthony Komaroff felt the Tahoe manuscript was ready for resubmission to the *Lancet*. The University of Nevada's Berch Henry had fashioned HHV6-specific probes using material supplied by the Gallo laboratory and had proven that all the patients were not only infected with the virus, as were most of the controls, but also that the virus was undergoing active replication inside their immune system cells and causing cell death, a drama for which there was little evidence in healthy controls. The MRI brain scan controls were in order now, too, with unequivocal results. Patients were far more likely than controls to have unidentified bright objects—UBOs—visible on their brain scans.

Komaroff was so pleased with his paper that he decided to show it to another expert at his university who was a renowned disbeliever: infectious disease specialist Elliot Kieff. The latter, of course, was the skeptic who had, in Gary Holmes's words, characterized CFS as a problem of "a lot of neurotic women" and suggested that attempts to define it were "just a bunch of garbage." To Komaroff's immense surprise, Kieff was impressed by the Tahoe research. Struck that the Tahoe data had apparently passed muster with one of the most antagonistic academics around, Komaroff changed his strategy. The Tahoe manuscript, now three years old, landed for the third time in the Boston offices of the *New England Journal of Medicine*.

U.S. House of Representatives, Washington, D.C.

On July 12 the House Committee on Appropriations submitted its annual report, which listed chronic fatigue syndrome as an "area of special concern" in its discussion of the NIH appropriations for the coming fiscal year 1991. "The public health importance of chronic fatigue syndrome cannot be fully assessed without data on the prevalence of the syndrome and knowledge of its natural history," the report stated. The lawmakers urged the National Institute of Allergy and Infectious Diseases to "solicit and fund additional chronic fatigue syndrome grants."* The committee also asked the Social Security Administration to improve its handling of disability claims due to the disease, urging the agency to "do everything necessary to facilitate a consistent national policy for resolving disability claims"

---

* The committee proposed to award to the NIH approximately $950 million for fiscal year 1991. As it turned out, less than $2 million of that sum would be funneled to scientists outside the Bethesda campus in support of their efforts to study CFS in 1991.

filed by sufferers. The agency still had no official listing for chronic fatigue syndrome in its manuals.

Wistar Institute, Philadelphia, Pennsylvania

In early August, Hilary Koprowski made a decision that would have far-reaching consequences for his colleague, Elaine DeFreitas, and her collaborators, David Bell and Paul Cheney. Koprowski had been asked to chair a day-long session on retroviral infection of the central nervous system at a neurology conference in Kyoto on September 4. The redoubtable veteran of countless scientific controversies decided that the Eleventh International Congress of Neuropathology, attended by several thousand neurologists from every corner of the world, would be a fitting setting for the announcement of DeFreitas's retrovirus discovery.

"He's very impulsive," a nervous DeFreitas said of her boss. "That's part of his charm—it really is. He's not at all directorial. He's very relaxed about things." Even so, DeFreitas was uneasy. She would have preferred to remain silent until the study appeared in the *Proceedings of the National Academy of Sciences,* which was unlikely to happen before January. Once the gene sequences of her virus, her viral probes, and all the secret techniques she had honed in the preceding months were published, *then* she would take her news public—and deal with the fallout. It was Koprowski, however, who signed her paychecks.

Koprowski's decision to tantalize the world with a sneak preview in Kyoto reflected an element of mischief and play that was ingrained in his character. Like DeFreitas, he was increasingly cognizant of the potential magnitude of the discovery. It amused him to break the news of the possible etiologic agent for a major epidemic disease, one that mainstream American medicine had treated cavalierly, at a scientific conference of neuropathologists on the other side of the planet. More to the point, however, Koprowski was confident that DeFreitas's data were right and that they would hold up to the most painstaking scrutiny. Still, he made clear to DeFreitas that although she would report her findings, her talk would not be "enabling"—that is, she would not reveal her gene sequences and her methods, without which the finding could never be replicated. Koprowski's admonition to DeFreitas was routine in science: methodologies derived over months and years of trial and error in laboratories were held in confidence prior to their publication in scientific journals to prevent other scientists from, in effect, stealing the work and publishing it first. Nevertheless, Koprowski's request was guaranteed to make DeFreitas's life harder: if the data were presented before the paper was published, she would be in the difficult position of defending her work in a highly controversial field without her full arsenal of proof.

Years afterward, in the course of a conversation about Koprowski's curious insensitivity to his protegée's vulnerability, a government scientist would tender a more cynical interpretation of the ebullient, benign-seeming Koprowski's "impulsive" decision: "He was dangling her out there as the fall-person," postulated Tom Folks, head of the CDC's retrovirus branch. "Koprowski knew what a potential gold mine this thing was," Folks continued in a reference to the monetary value of a diagnostic test, money that would accrue to Wistar coffers. Yet, if the finding didn't pan out, Folks added, it would be DeFreitas, not Koprowski, who would take the fall.

A dispute between the original collaborators, DeFreitas and Cheney, had been simmering below the surface of their scientific discussions as the calendar brought them closer to the release of their discovery. If one believed the data, as they did, then Elaine DeFreitas and her partners had discovered the cause of a worldwide epidemic affecting unknown millions of people. It followed that the trio of collaborators had discovered as well the ultimate diagnostic marker—a marker for which commercial test kits could be fashioned.

Whoever owned the patent on the diagnostic test for chronic fatigue syndrome was destined to become immensely wealthy. Their wealth would accrue not merely because the disease was so common, but because the test would be ordered so frequently as part of a doctor's differential diagnosis. One statistic regularly cited by Anthony Komaroff gave some inkling of the magnitude of the discovery: fatigue was one of the ten most common reasons Americans visited their doctors, according to the National Ambulatory Medical Care Survey. In theory, then, a CFS diagnostic test might be ordered for at least one of every ten patients in a doctor's practice.*

There was yet another business facet to the Wistar finding. The retrovirus discovery might lead to drug treatments for the disease, which would be extraordinarily valuable as well. "What we learn creates concepts about therapy," Cheney noted. "So there are concepts in therapeutics which will derive from this discovery."

Koprowski's move, then, ignited what had been until then an unspoken apprehension between DeFreitas and Cheney. DeFreitas stood to gain little from the discovery aside from the admiration of her peers and a place in medical history. Wistar, not its employees, owned and derived profits from the patented discoveries of its scientists; Wistar scientists themselves were awarded one dollar per patent. Cheney, in contrast, had not only money to gain but also—and in his view, vastly more important—continued high-level involvement with the remarkable scientific process under way. He wanted to be named a co-inventor of the discovery and to become a co-owner of its patent. He would use any profits derived from such an arrangement to support his own research.

"Bench researchers invent, clinicians facilitate—that's the traditional view," Cheney said. "But this is an unusual situation. And being a co-inventor of something of this kind gives you two options: sell the invention and retire, or maintain

---

* If there was any doubt about the size of the fortune to be made, one need only compare the potential of a CFS test to the actual money derived from the AIDS test. After its invention, the U.S. Department of Health and Human Services patented the assay and then sold it to commercial laboratories such as Abbott Laboratories. The patent on the HIV diagnostic test runs for seventeen years. For each of those seventeen years, the government receives 5 percent of the approximately $120 million annual market for the test. National Cancer Institute scientist Robert Gallo, a co-inventor of the assay, has himself received $100,000 every year since December 1986 from the patent. By December 1995, then, Gallo will have earned a million dollars from his share of the patent. After seventeen years, Gallo's ultimate profit will be $1.7 million, and the U.S. government's, an approximate $102 million.

control. And what is life but to do something? I am willing to take less money in order to be a part of this development, to have a say in how things go."

Unfortunately for the stalwart Cheney, the Wistar Institute's lawyers and administrators saw little that was unusual about his contributions. In their ideological universe, Paul Cheney's function had been to supply blood samples, a task he had performed very nicely.

Lyndonville, New York

Bell had continued to see some of his sickest patients, but he was still working on weekends and evenings in the Medina emergency room, too. He faced a difficult decision that summer. "With every month, it was getting harder to be working two jobs," Bell recalled. In August, the pediatrician sent a letter to all of his patients telling them of his decision to close down his practice in the little town. It was a sad event for the doctor, who had spent more than a decade treating the sick in Lyndonville, and perhaps an even sadder one for his patients, who had come to rely on him as their port in the storm of controversy and dissent about their disease. Like Cheney, Bell was by then discouraged about the pace of the retrovirus work.

"I had reached a new low point," Bell recalled later. "I had just closed my practice and given up all hope of this thing ever getting resolved. There had been so many delays over the past year. I was beginning to feel that, although there was clearly something there, it was never going to be published.

"But all of a sudden," Bell said, "Elaine calls and says, 'We're on. We're going to Kyoto, and we're going to present this damn thing.' "

Charlotte, North Carolina

At the end of the second week in August, Paul Cheney called leading biotech patent attorney Leslie Misrock, a famously tough litigator based in New York City. Misrock considered not only the doctor's formidable intellectual contributions to the Wistar project but also the fact that Cheney had arranged for the salary of DeFreitas's postdoc, Brendan Hilliard, to be paid starting in 1988 by Nevada philanthropist Paul Thompson. It was, after all, Hilliard's daily labors in the lab that had ended with the discovery of retroviral gene fragments. When those funds ran out, Cheney had sacrificed his own remaining six months' worth of funding from Thompson, a sum of $18,000, to keep the investigation on track. When in May 1990 that funding also came to an end, Cheney had persuaded the CFIDS Association to support DeFreitas's effort. Most persuasive by far, however, was the fact that Cheney had advanced the concept of retroviral infection in the disease, brought the idea to Wistar, and propelled Wistar's progress by supplying the majority of tissue samples. After consulting with the doctor, Misrock recalled later, "I advised [Cheney] that he was co-inventor with Elaine DeFreitas."

On the Sunday evening following his conversations with Misrock, Cheney called Elaine DeFreitas. Cheney explained his view of the patent issue. DeFreitas seemed to explode with anger.

One point of leverage in the clinician's favor was that DeFreitas had been able to identify only one patient whose spinal fluid produced cells in which she could grow the virus indefinitely, generation after generation. The patient was in Cheney's practice and had signed over the rights to perform experiments on his cells to Cheney, not to the Wistar Institute. If Cheney left the collaboration, in other words, the Wistar scientists would be forced to engage in a scramble to find another such patient before Cheney could forge a second, equally bountiful partnership with another retrovirology team.

Four days later, in a vehement conversation with Marc Iverson, DeFreitas complained she hadn't slept since the doctor's phone call. "This is not the Paul Cheney I've known," she reportedly said. "I wasn't prepared for this. What's he after? Money? Fame? . . . *We* did the work. *We* were in the lab eight and ten hours a day."

Iverson, a Cheney loyalist, retorted, "Paul Cheney's been working on this *sixteen* hours a day since 1985."

According to Iverson, DeFreitas responded, "What matters is *we* found the virus."

That same week, Iverson received a call from Jay Levy. The virologist was seeking grant support from the CFIDS Association, but he was curious, too, about a rumor circulating that Cheney and his collaborators had discovered something. Iverson confirmed for Levy that fragments of an unidentified retrovirus had been discovered in patients. Quite possibly the pathogen was, if not the cause of the disease, closely associated with it. Iverson told the scientist that Elaine DeFreitas would be presenting the data in Japan in two weeks' time.

Levy was silent for a period. When he spoke again, his normally lively affect had turned flat. Six years earlier, working alone, he had discovered HIV in his tiny San Francisco lab. He decided to wait until he had performed several experiments proving the virus was something other than artifact before publishing. Robert Gallo, at roughly the same time, found HIV as well. Gallo, choosing to forgo the same prudent experiments, announced his find at a national press conference, during which Secretary of Health Margaret Heckler virtually anointed him the nation's medical laureate.

Levy, perhaps, had lost the race a second time.

Wistar Institute, Philadelphia, Pennsylvania

On the Wednesday before the principals—David Bell, Elaine DeFreitas, Paul Cheney, and Hilary Koprowski—departed for Japan, Wistar's lawyers filed a patent claim on the retrovirus finding that DeFreitas would be announcing in five days' time. Cheney was not named as a co-inventor in spite of his pivotal role in the discovery. As the days and then hours sped by before the Kyoto conference, the patent dispute erupted into an increasingly ugly conflict fought over the telephone lines and via fax machines between Charlotte and Philadelphia. Third parties were engaged and assigned to advocacy positions by both sides. As the battle escalated, the possibility that reconciliation could occur in Kyoto or elsewhere seemed to recede. The issue of inventorship quickly contaminated every interaction between Cheney and Wistar.

On August 30, two days before his flight to Osaka, Cheney wrote to DeFreitas: "I want you to know I have the utmost respect for you as a scientist and person. . . . It is . . . painful to contemplate the loss of this most stimulating collaboration of almost five years." In closing, he assured DeFreitas, "I will resist being drawn into litigation over this patent. . . . I am willing to accept any fair compromise if it preserves our collaboration. . . . We have much to lose, the patient movement has much to lose, and Wistar has much to lose over what could follow if we cannot resolve this issue."

"Paul is heartbroken," Marc Iverson said later. "He's going to Japan depressed."

David Bell was not a player in the patent rights drama. He remained in Lyndonville, out of the fray, until it was time to leave for Kyoto. The doctor's self-effacing behavior earned him the comradely respect of Elaine DeFreitas. "He asked for *nothing*," DeFreitas would say of Bell admiringly long after Kyoto.

Centers for Disease Control, Atlanta, Georgia

Paul Cheney had halted his dialogue with the CDC upon the publication of Gary Holmes and Jon Kaplan's Tahoe study in *JAMA* in 1987. The day before he left for Japan, however, the doctor took a call from Walter Gunn. Like most people in the field, Gunn had heard the rumors. In fact, he had just heard from *New York Native* publisher Charles Ortleb that Cheney was about to announce the discovery of a CFS-associated retrovirus in Japan. When Cheney came to the phone, Gunn introduced himself and asked if the clinician could relay anything about the announcement. Cheney promised to send him a copy of the Wistar abstract—but only after his return from Japan.

After his conversation with Cheney, Gunn called a meeting with Larry Schonberger and Gary Holmes.

"We started talking about maybe we could replicate this finding," Gunn recalled. "And somehow Gary got talking to Jon Kaplan, and that's how Jon got involved again."

Wistar Institute, Philadelphia, Pennsylvania

An hour before Elaine DeFreitas boarded her plane to Japan, she was telephoned by Howard Streicher, the Robert Gallo associate who had obtained hundreds of Tahoe blood samples from Cheney and Peterson in early 1986.

Streicher asked, "What's going on? We're hearing all sorts of rumors."

"I told him everything," DeFreitas said later.

"Elaine," Streicher responded, "we've looked for retrovirus in chronic fatigue syndrome patients and found nothing."

"It's there," DeFreitas said. "When I get back, I'll send you everything—my probes, the sequences."

At the end of the conversation, Streicher commented, "You're very brave to work on this disease."

Los Angeles International Airport, Los Angeles, California

David Bell and Paul Cheney planned to meet at LAX on September 2, where they would board a Northwest jet to Osaka, Japan, late in the afternoon. Both men were in the airport by noon that day, but before meeting up with his colleague, Bell heard himself being paged. When he picked up the telephone receiver at the Northwest counter in the international terminal, an emergency room doctor from Rochester, New York, gave him the bad news: Skye Dailor had swallowed a lethal dose of tranquilizers. Bell could hear the frantic resuscitation efforts under way on the fourteen-year-old in the background. Those efforts had been in progress for a full hour by the time the emergency staff was able to locate Bell in Los Angeles. "There was no question in our mind that the resuscitation would be unsuccessful," Bell said several months after the event, the first time he could discuss the incident and keep his emotions under control.

The doctor spoke to Dailor's parents, who were at the hospital. They explained that their daughter had been at the mall with her friends that day and that a few of them had begun teasing her about her illness. The teasing escalated when someone joked that Dailor had AIDS.

"As an angry gesture," Bell said, "Skye said she was going to take some pills. So she went and took some Elavil. Twenty-five minutes later she had a heart attack and couldn't be resuscitated."

Skye Dailor was aware of the retrovirus in her blood, but she also knew she did not have AIDS.

"It's inevitable that the University of Rochester people will now think they knew it all the time—that Skye was a psychiatric case," Bell continued. "I've talked to them about looking at teenage suicide victims retrospectively to see what kind of symptoms were involved prior to the suicides, but they've not been interested. . . .

"By law, she had to have an autopsy," Bell remembered. "The ER doc told me it was a coroner's case and asked me if I would like samples saved. I said yes, and they were frozen." Bell asked for samples of his young patient's brain, liver, spleen, and heart.

Paul Cheney and David Bell met in Northwest's first-class lounge at LAX. In the cool, soundproof room with an expansive view of the airport's runways, the doctors spoke in low voices about Dailor's suicide and about the poisoning of Cheney and DeFreitas's relationship. Two hours later it was time to board. Seated directly across the aisle from the clinicians in the first-class cabin was a gray-haired man with bushy eyebrows that formed inverted Vs over pale blue eyes. He wore tortoiseshell half-moon reading glasses and held a magazine in his lap. Although the plane had not moved from the gate, his stocking feet were already cosseted in the slippers provided to first-class passengers. A glass of red wine had been placed on his armrest. Until the jet's hatches were slammed shut and the plane began its runway taxi, his expression conveyed his impatience. Hilary Koprowski's mood would hardly have been surprising in an elderly man facing an eleven-hour flight. In this case, however, it seemed to have been exacerbated by the realization that he was seated in such close proximity to Paul Cheney.

22

Kyoto

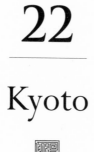

Eleventh International Congress of Neuropathology, Kyoto, Japan

Bell and Cheney arrived at the Takaragaike Prince Hotel just outside Kyoto early on the evening of September 2. DeFreitas arrived later that night. Early the following morning the three met for breakfast. Their discussion focused on the patent rights dispute. Bell immediately assumed a difficult role he would maintain for years to come: that of neutral conciliator. At 10:30, after being politely expelled from the restaurant, which was closing, the trio moved their meeting to the lobby. At noon they broke to change for lunch, at which time DeFreitas and Cheney were, by superficial appearances, on friendly terms.

"There are so many indeterminates about this patent," Cheney revealed later that day. "I've told Elaine that the lawyers will settle the issue and we'll proceed with the science." Still, it was clear that, privately, Cheney had not yet relinquished his intellectual and moral claims to what he believed were his fundamental contributions to DeFreitas's work. He continued to believe that the traditional view—that scientists are the inventors and that clinician-collaborators are merely the suppliers of patient tissue samples—failed to apply in this instance. "This is a disease that can directly influence and affect world economics," he said. "A new dynamic is in place."

Approximately two thousand medical researchers participated in the conference on diseases of the brain, which convened every four years in an exotic setting. That year it was held in a formidable concrete structure in a gracious park on the outskirts of Kyoto.

In the hours leading up to their presentation, DeFreitas, Cheney, and Bell were alternately giddy and somber. Right up to the final moments before ascending the podium, they reviewed their data compulsively, discussing what they should include and what they should eliminate. By three-thirty that afternoon, their appointed hour, their audience had shrunk. Only forty people remained at the all-day session on retrovirus infections of the brain, chaired by Hilary Koprowski. DeFreitas's presentation was mistakenly labeled "Chronic Muscular Fatigue in Retrovirus Infection" in the conference program, which may have explained the small crowd—but perhaps not.

Two American scientists shared a private joke when Koprowski introduced the topic and the speakers; their muffled laughter in the otherwise silent auditorium seemed ominous. Their derision seemed to confirm DeFreitas's worst fears about her involvement in the disease; for months afterward the grinning faces of the two men haunted her. The collaborators shared their own joke as they walked, one behind another, toward the podium. Bell, who was behind DeFreitas, whispered gaily, "We can always get jobs in Fiji!"

Bell began the session by describing the disease in children. Cheney followed with a description of the neurological aspects of the disease. Before he could finish, Koprowski impatiently interrupted the doctor and asked him to summarize his data, a rudeness that threw Cheney off balance. After a moment's hesitation, Cheney folded his notes, uttered a sentence in conclusion, and stepped away from the lectern.

DeFreitas was the last to speak. Koprowski looked upon his protégée, rail-thin and glossy-haired, with something akin to paternal pride. In eight minutes she summarized her work effort of the last two and a half years. "We are not claiming causation," she said in conclusion. "We are not claiming infectiousness. . . . We can't predict how this virus can be transmitted. But we feel this is a fairly strong association with the disease."

When DeFreitas ended, Koprowski opened the meeting to questions. A young Japanese scientist asked DeFreitas an astute question about the percentage of white blood cells that appeared to be infected in the patients she had studied. DeFreitas said she found the virus in about the same quantities researchers found HIV in AIDS patients, or "about one in one thousand or one in five hundred" cells.

The silence in the room seemed to grow loud after DeFreitas's response. Koprowski studied the audience, his grizzled head turning toward one side of the auditorium, then the other, and back again. DeFreitas stood erect behind the lectern as if in a state of suspended animation. As two, then three minutes of torturous silence passed, there were no further questions. At last Koprowski called the day's session to an end.

The audience dispersed quickly, but a handful of American researchers from the NIH and New York City, friends of Koprowski, were invited by the Wistar chief to join him, DeFreitas, Cheney, and Bell for celebratory drinks. Koprowski was expansive and charming, clearly stimulated by the day's proceedings. DeFreitas wore a wary expression as the NIH virologists sparred with her about her finding. Out of range of her hearing, one of them bet fifty dollars that within a year her finding would be discredited. Cheney sat removed from the jovial circle. A day that should have been among the most rewarding of his life had ended in bitterness. In private, he confessed he couldn't wait to leave Japan and join his college-age son for a ski vacation in Idaho.

Later that evening, facsimile copies of the U.S. press coverage of the discovery began to be slipped under the collaborators' doors by hotel staff. Like actors reading their notices on opening night, the three gathered in Cheney's room, passing articles to one another, reading aloud certain passages. Stories had appeared that day in the *Philadelphia Inquirer,* the *Charlotte Observer,* and the *San Francisco Chronicle.* "Medical Sleuth Closes In" was the headline on page one of the *Charlotte Observer;* the story chronicled Paul Cheney's detective work beginning in

Incline Village, Nevada. Veteran science writer Donald Drake's coverage in the Philadelphia paper was the most dramatic. Drake's newspaper announced the story with a bold headline just below the logo: "Chronic Fatigue Syndrome, AIDS-type Virus Linked." The Gulf conflict was worsening that week and the biggest story of the day, just below the *Inquirer*'s CFS news, was Saddam Hussein's decision to bar Western airliners from Iraq. Drake stated flatly that scientists had found evidence that the disease was caused by a virus in the same family of viruses that caused AIDS and a form of leukemia. He also proposed that the finding suggested, but did not prove, that the disease was contagious.

Drake had called Stephen Straus for a comment. The government's expert submitted that what DeFreitas had found was a laboratory contaminant rather than a virus. He told Drake that polymerase chain reaction, one of the techniques DeFreitas had employed to find the actual virus fragments, was notoriously inaccurate because it was ultrasensitive and had been known to pick up "contaminants that are mistaken for the virus." In contrast, Walter Gunn, the only other government investigator quoted by Drake, said DeFreitas's work "was consistent" with other clinical and laboratory evidence for immunological damage in the disease.

When they had digested the coverage, the three retired. By 3:00 A.M., however, they were fully awake, roused by incessant requests from the hotel's desk staff to put through international calls. DeFreitas stayed on the phone for two hours with the *New York Times'* Lawrence Altman. Cheney talked to the wire services. Bell was interviewed by a *Chicago Tribune* reporter, Paul Weingarten, whose wife, a former newspaper reporter, had been wheelchair-bound for two years as a result of the disease and happened to be one of Cheney's patients. At 5:00 A.M., DeFreitas and Bell, unable to sleep, began walking laps through the hotel corridor, a circular hallway in the center of the immense doughnut-shaped hotel. Bell still wore his hotel-supplied cotton kimono. DeFreitas, fully dressed, smoked cigarette after cigarette, frequently gesturing to make her points. Engaged in excited conversation about the next phase of their collaboration, the pair was oblivious to the early-morning hotel staff, all of whom politely averted their gaze and bowed with great solemnity each time the couple passed.

By 6:00 A.M., the triad had their marching orders from Jan Montgomery's group, the CFIDS Foundation in San Francisco, and from the Charlotte patients' organization. They would leave from Osaka that morning for the eleven-hour flight to San Francisco, where they would hold a press conference. Once again DeFreitas felt uneasy about the pace of events. The idea of participating in a press conference about her findings before she had published her paper made her feel exceptionally vulnerable, more vulnerable, even, than having presented them at a scientific conference. Yet Koprowski encouraged her to go. She felt, in addition, a responsibility to the patient associations whose members, after all, had paid for much of the research effort.

The intensity of the collaborators' conversation persisted throughout the forty-minute taxi ride from Kyoto to Osaka and during the wait to board the jet. It wasn't until the plane lifted off and they sighted Mount Fuji from their windows that the talk of gene sequencing finally ceased. Soon afterward, all three fell sound asleep.

As the meeting with the American press loomed, the issue of how they should publicly interpret their data became their first order of concern. Though all three believed the retrovirus, whatever its identity, to be the infectious agent at the heart of the disease, by the time they arrived in San Francisco, they had agreed to interpret the data in the narrowest fashion possible. They had discovered retrovirus fragments in samples from nearly 80 percent of two geographically distinct groups of CFS patients; the virus it most resembled was HTLV2, a pathogen that was not supposed to be in any Americans except perhaps a few intravenous drug abusers and black immigrants from Africa and the Carribbean. They had discovered, too, that a third of the people who had been in contact with those same patients were infected as well. Finally, they had been unable to find any traces of the pathogen in unexposed controls—newborns and healthy adults who were without close contact with CFS victims. Let reporters, other scientists, and the federal health agencies make what they would of the findings. Their job was to point out the association of this virus with the disease, nothing more.

Prince Henry Hospital, Sydney, Australia

By the fall of 1990, there remained little question that the Australians' ability to fund important studies, carry them out, and see them published in the medical literature had outpaced that of researchers in every other nation. In 1989, publishing in the *Medical Journal of Australia,* the team of immunologists and clinicians from New South Wales had proved that immunologic dysfunction was a reliable hallmark of chronic fatigue syndrome.[1] In 1990, they published two more groundbreaking papers. The first of these[2] established that CFS victims were no more depressed or anxious before their illness began than was the general population, thereby contradicting the Stephen Straus–inspired theory upon which the U.S. government's response to the epidemic was based. The authors noted, as had other Straus critics before them, that the "pre-morbid" psychiatric problems Straus described included eight cases of "simple phobia," one case of agoraphobia, and just two cases of depression. They added that Straus had attached "surprising importance . . . to the pre-morbid diagnoses of simple phobia," especially since other researchers had found that rates of simple phobias in the general population varied widely depending on who was doing the interviewing. "The high rate of simple phobia reported . . . is likely to be a result of the interview method and is unlikely to be of psychopathological significance in patients with CFS," the Australians wrote.

The Australians' second paper that year indicated that the disease was at least as common as multiple sclerosis, and likely far more common, in southeast Australia, where they found their study population.[3] Based on doctors' reports and followup exams, the Australians determined that, at a minimum, 37.1 people out of every 100,000 suffered from the disease in mid-1988.* It was the first estimated "point prevalence" study of the disease in Australia and, in fact, anywhere. The paper served to remind American CFS patients that good epidemiology on the dis-

---

* The mean age at onset was 28.6 years; the median duration of symptoms was 30 months. In addition, "The social status of the patients was distributed in accordance with that of the remainder of the population samples, with no bias toward the middle or upper classes."

ease hardly need cost millions of dollars or require what amounted to years of debate among blue-ribbon physician panels over whether a case was a case.

CBS News, New York City

In September, CBS News pronounced chronic fatigue syndrome a real disease. "At first it was derisively called 'yuppie flu,' and it was only this year that the Centers for Disease Control finally recognized chronic fatigue syndrome as a legitimate disease, not just a by-product of stress," Susan Spencer began her four-minute report for the "Evening News." "But what kind of disease? What causes this debilitating problem that can turn an active person into a virtual invalid almost overnight?"

Jay Levy was interviewed. "I think it's a virus," he said. "I think there is a new virus that's causing a great increase of this syndrome in the population."

Spencer reported on immune dysfunction in the disease, citing "[i]mmune system problems that doctors now can measure. . . . The immune system is out of balance, working against an unknown enemy at a frenetic pace. . . . For the patient, that can mean a bewildering array of symptoms." She pointed out that doctors, nonetheless, would still write off many patients as psychological cases.

She quoted Paul Cheney as saying, "In medical school you're often taught that if you cannot define an illness by the technology of the day, the patient must be crazy."

"It's unknown how many people have the disease," Spencer concluded, "but the CDC is getting up to two thousand calls a month, and many of them still start out, 'Please believe me . . . ' "

San Francisco, California

On their arrival in San Francisco after the Kyoto conference, DeFreitas, Bell, and Cheney found that their fears about the repercussions of their research seemed to be coming true. Jan Montgomery informed them that immediately after the news broke in the United States linking the disease to a virus, a local sufferer, a grade-school teacher, was fired out of a concern that she would infect her students. Montgomery's report had a deadening effect on the three. If this was a hint of the hysteria that lay ahead, the future would be grim indeed.

That morning, in a conference room high above Sansome Street in downtown San Francisco, the collaborators held the first press conference on the epidemic disease since Dan Peterson and Paul Cheney had met with the press in Incline Village five years before. Fifteen reporters arrayed themselves around an oval marble table in the room provided by the Genmark company, a fledgling biotech firm whose executives hoped to establish a link with Wistar in the development of a diagnostic test. Representatives from Cable News Network, *Newsweek*, the *San Francisco Chronicle, Medical World News,* the *San Francisco Examiner*, KGO-TV, German Public Radio, Pacifica Radio, and the *Wall Street Journal* attended. A photographer from *Newsweek* arrived to snap DeFreitas and her collaborators for a possible cover photo; the magazine was preparing a lengthy story on the disease. The photographer asked DeFreitas and Cheney to perch casually on the edge of the marble table with their arms folded and their backs to each other; Bell stood behind the two, his hands on their shoulders, smiling beatifically. Curiously, the photographer seemed to have divined the precise nature of the relationship among the three.

The collaborators followed the format they had employed in Japan, with Bell and Cheney laying out the significant clinical aspects of the disease, and De-Freitas, who spoke last, describing her work in the laboratory. Unlike the scientists in Kyoto thirty-six hours before, the San Francisco–based reporters were intensely curious, formulating aggressive queries about contagion and causality. DeFreitas and her collaborators danced around those weighty matters, to the escalating frustration of the journalists. DeFreitas, for instance, stated that she had never made a claim that her virus, or "viral gene," caused the disease. "We are just reporting an association between a relatively rare virus in these two populations—a relatively rare virus that is more closely associated with people who have CFIDS than with non-exposed controls," she said.

A reporter responded, "It's fairly clear that anybody could draw a correlation between the data you've presented and some form of transmission that's not through blood transmission. I'm sure somewhere in your head, scratching and musing over this, you've come up with some kind of notion as to what we're looking at here. Would you be comfortable sharing that?"

Bell stepped into the skirmish, saying that, although evidence from past epidemics and clinical aspects of the disease certainly suggested a pattern of casual transmission, the Wistar data did not "address that issue at all."

"But what do you *think*?" another reporter asked plaintively.

"I don't want to think," Cheney said after a brief pause. "I don't want to think about it because if I think about something on the basis of very small numbers, I could be very, very wrong. Especially in something like this, you don't want to think."

"Then why are we having this press conference?" the reporter asked.

"Because we want to talk about what we *know*," Cheney replied in the pregnant silence, "not what we don't know. . . . We didn't design the study to answer the question you most want answered. All this study was designed to address was whether or not a retrovirus was associated with chronic fatigue syndrome. I think the answer is yes."

That evening, DeFreitas, Bell, and Cheney dined in the Saint Francis Hotel's Edwardian Room. Conversation centered on two subjects: one was their next phase of research, which would be cloning and fully sequencing the gene of the virus using recombinant gene technology, a process that, if successful, would lead De-Freitas to an unequivocal identification of the virus; the other subject was the issue of contagion. The contrast between their conversation over dinner and their comments at the press conference was remarkable. Cheney was fascinated by the moral dilemma the matter presented: he had told the reporter, "We want to talk about what we *know*"—but what about what they *believed*?

"Do we have a duty to tell parents they cannot kiss their child?" Cheney asked his colleagues.

"That would cause more emotional damage to the child than the disease itself," Bell responded.

"Do you really think so?" Cheney said.

"Yes," Bell said with uncharacteristic emphasis.

"I'm not so sure," Cheney parried.

DeFreitas diverted them with a ribald story about one of their patients from whom she had requested a semen sample in an effort to find the virus. "I told him I needed two samples, but I sent him about ten sample tubes, just in case he lost some," DeFreitas said. "A few weeks later I got this *huge* shipment. Every tube was filled to the brim." For a few brief moments the three were consumed with laughter.

Across town three other researchers were dining together, too, but their mood was subdued. Internist Carol Jessop, virologist Jay Levy, and University of Chicago immunologist Alan Landay, who had been collaborating with Levy for several months, had been scooped that day. For Levy it was particularly painful to have the DeFreitas team herald their finding at a press conference in San Francisco, Levy's backyard.

The three spent much of the dinner discussing their grant proposal to the National Institute of Allergy and Infectious Diseases, which they hoped to submit by the November 1 deadline. They had found their own marker: aberrant up-regulation, or hyperactivation, of the immune system in CFS sufferers; it wasn't a virus, but it was a marker nonetheless. They wanted government support to search for the casual pathogen among a group of patients with their marker.

The following morning Cheney and DeFreitas had yet another conversation about the looming patent deal. Cheney advised her he would pursue a lawsuit against Wistar to be named a co-inventor. The conversation left DeFreitas distraught. The patent fight was bad enough, but suddenly a new element, a biotechnology firm in search of a product, had been introduced in the form of Genmark.

"Literally within hours this went from being a scientific finding to becoming a multimillion-dollar business venture," she complained as she folded her clothes into a suitcase in her room at the Saint Francis, her sharp movements communicating a barely controlled fury. "But this is just the beginning. Much more work needs to be done. In science, first there is the discovery, then *years* of work. Then, much, much later, come the biotechnology firms and the million-dollar deals. But this middle step was skipped. We went from the finding to the multimillion-dollar wheeling and dealing—in hours! And long before the scientific paper was even published.

"It's clear Genmark wants to build a biotech company around Cheney's and my discovery," she continued. "I will get no money from a patent—I'll get one dollar. But this is like having my firstborn child stolen from me. . . . Who does Genmark think is going to actually do the work?" she said after a moment. "Cheney seems to think he can get another retrovirologist by thumbing through the yellow pages. . . . What the Genmark directors and Paul Cheney don't realize is that Hil-

ary Koprowski eats people like them for breakfast!" The scientist voiced the possibility that she would withdraw from the collaboration entirely. "H.K. can go
ahead and publish the data, but he can't force me to put my name on the paper."

David Bell, who had tried unsuccesfully to neutralize the conflict that had
erupted like a brushfire between his collaborators, felt peaceful that morning, in
stark contrast to DeFreitas's rage.

"I can back out at any time now, gracefully," Bell said over breakfast, "because
what I set out to do has been done, and that was to see this thing through to the
cause. That's what the first five years were. Now it may take another year or ten
years before that paper gets published. Doesn't matter. I made the commitment to
myself, and to the Pollards [Bell's Lyndonville patients] to find out what was
wrong with them. And I feel I've lived up to that commitment. I feel fairly sure
that this is the cause. In terms of where I go from here, I still don't know. I have
absolutely no idea."

Once the etiological agent of the disease was established, equivocation would
be pushed aside, Bell believed, and a new phase would begin in which discussion
would focus on the pathogen's transmission routes. Throughout academia, understanding the neurological and immunological dysfunction that characterized the
disease would become a priority. In this new phase, Bell believed, doctors like
him were bound to play a minor role.

"There's a big difference between being a stubborn clinician pursuing this disease—because you can be very stupid and still make good contributions—but
from now on, that's not going to count for much, because we're talking high-tech,
now. Overnight the people at the University of Rochester Adolescent Medical
Clinic will get a handle on this disease, because they've been studying it without
knowing it for three years. Overnight they're going to understand the clinical aspects of it. It will just fall into place."

Cheney, too, had a prediction: "I think David's right. This thing will get taken
over by the technocrats, and the mavericks will get shoved away. You don't see
any more mavericks in AIDS."

The same morning Jay Levy was at work in his tiny office on Parnassus Hill writing his federal grant proposal. Since the San Francisco conference, Levy had received a total of $20,000 in philanthropic contributions to his investigations,
mostly from rich patients living in California. The money helped, but it was
hardly enough to do serious science.

"Chronic fatigue syndrome is my pet project," Levy commented brightly that
day. "I'm writing a grant proposal for the National Institutes of Health right
now. . . . If we had more people working on this, we could figure this out in a
year."

Boston, Massachusetts

On September 10 the *Boston Globe* published a surprisingly hard-hitting editorial
on the subject of CFS. It read, in part:

A baffling illness that came to notice in 1984 is a sorry example of how medical scientists can still selectively ignore disorders that do not fit established patterns of illness. . . . It was dismissed as yuppie flu, even though some patients are periodically disabled and develop measurable muscle loss, immune deficiencies, or unexplained lesions in the brain. . . . Last week, three researchers reported that a new and exotic microbe—a member of the same family of retroviruses that cause AIDS—is linked to chronic fatigue syndrome. Beyond providing the first scientific clue in what may cause or spread the disease, the discovery validates that chronic fatigue syndrome is a real and serious disorder.

The research would not have been done were it not for Dr. Paul Cheney, an internist, who in 1984 had nearly 200 patients with the strangely recurring symptoms come into his office in a small resort town near Lake Tahoe, Nevada. Cheney did not accept the idea that these patients, many of them local workers, were not genuinely ill.

Up to five million Americans are already afflicted with chronic fatigue syndrome. Yet a five-year battle had to be fought by doctors like Cheney and the patients themselves to convince the [NIH and the CDC] of the physical basis of this disorder.

As Cheney aptly points out, "The emergence of this disorder has demonstrated a weakness in the medical community's ability to identify and characterize subtle disorders. We stopped listening to patients and started believing in machines."

National Institutes of Health, Bethesda, Maryland

There was no official comment from either the NIH or CDC on Wistar's discovery of retrovirus gene fragments in the cells of four-fifths of chronic fatigue syndrome patients and one-third of asymptomatic people who had been in close contact with sufferers. Although the NIH's public relations officers maintained a public silence, however, the news was resonating inside the brick-and-steel towers of Bethesda. Even outsiders detected the movement. "I sensed that there was quite a bit of scurrying around at the NIH," Cheney recalled later.

Soon after the Wistar announcement, Stephen Straus, who had been silent on the subject of the disease for more than a year, engaged a government neuroimmunologist, Steven Jacobson, to look for HTLV1 and HTLV2 in approximately twenty of Straus's CFS patients. Jacobson, chief of the viral immunology section at the National Institute of Neurologic Disorders and Stroke, employed the resources of his institute's laboratories, using probes for HTLV1 and HTLV2. The results were negative. Straus notified Anthony Fauci, chief of the National Institute of Allergy and Infectious Diseases, and Fauci's deputy, James Hill, of the outcome. Queried later, Jacobson said he decided not to publish the results because "a negative result tells you very little, and I'm not a big believer in publishing negative data." Straus's patients might have had a different disease than the one suffered by the patients DeFreitas had studied, Jacobson continued, and the tests he undertook could well have missed the viral sequences DeFreitas claimed to have found. "All we could say was [that] within Straus's population we could not find HTLV1 or HTLV2."

Some time later Seymour Grufferman was asked why so many scientists tried to replicate DeFreitas's finding using probes for HTLV2 when DeFreitas had taken pains to point out that her virus fragments were not HTLV2, but were HTLV2-*like*. Grufferman answered the question with an old joke: "You've heard about the drunk who stumbles out of the bar late at night and realizes he's lost his car keys? He wanders over to the streetlight and begins to look on the ground. When his friend asks him why he's looking there, he says, 'Because I can *see* over here.'"

Grufferman himself received a call from the Bethesda agency's CFS grant administrator, Ann Schleuderberg, soon after the Wistar finding broke. She reported that William Blattner, chief of the viral epidemiology branch of the division of cancer etiology at the National Cancer Institute, was going to look for antibodies against HTLV retroviruses in chronic fatigue syndrome patients.

Grufferman, happy to have an NIH scientist's ear on the subject of the disease at last, told Blattner he would collaborate. He sent approximately forty blood samples from both the North Carolina Symphony outbreak and the Chillicothe, Ohio, elementary school outbreak to Bethesda. "When you get beat up enough, you're grateful when people are willing to even listen to you," he commented.

Centers for Disease Control, Atlanta, Georgia

In September 1990, Walter Gunn found himself swamped by hundreds of calls every day from people suffering from CFS. "Our phone calls have been averaging one and two thousand calls a month on chronic fatigue syndrome," Gunn reported that September, "although they've run as high as three thousand a month. But we've really begun to hear horror stories since the Wistar announcement." In one family a father suffered from CFS and his daughter from leukemia; because news reports had noted that the newly discovered virus fragments were in the family of viruses that cause leukemia and AIDS, the father was convinced he had infected his daughter with a leukemia virus and caused her disease. "I spent an hour talking him and his wife out of this theory," Gunn said. "He was despondent." Another patient, a man in Chicago, had called to say his friends no longer shook his hand. "The net effect is bad on patients," Gunn insisted.

Nonetheless, it was patently obvious to Gunn and his superiors that the Centers for Disease Control would have to respond to the ball Elaine DeFreitas had just pitched onto the field. After all, how could the federal agency that was created to control the spread of infectious diseases simply ignore a report of an infectious retrovirus finding in chronic fatigue syndrome sufferers, particularly now that the news had filtered through every major news organization in the country and into the public consciousness? There were no options: they needed to do something about this development, and quickly.

Gunn wanted to add DeFreitas's retrovirus assay to the tests that would be performed on patients and healthy controls in the CDC study, and when Marc Iverson called soon after Kyoto to invite him to a medical conference in Charlotte organized by the CFIDS Association, Gunn quickly conceived of a private agenda. He would use the conference to arrange a parley between Tom Folks, the agency's chief of retrovirus research, and Elaine DeFreitas and Hilary Koprowski, who had been invited to the meeting as well. The agency could save considerable time by gaining access to Wistar's gene sequences and viral probes.*

Pasadena, California

Zaki Salahuddin, the discoverer of human herpesvirus 6, had had a very bad year: he had narrowly missed going to prison, and his government career was over. In March of 1989 a grand jury had begun an investigation into Salahuddin's involvement in Pan Data Systems, a small biotech company in Gaithersburg, Maryland, that was developing expertise in HHV6 and in which he and his wife were part owners and officers. A few months later the House committee with oversight of the NIH initiated a separate congressional inquiry. Salahuddin was accused of spiriting valuable biological materials, including HHV6 samples, to Pan Data and of diverting government funds for private use. He had used the money—almost $13,000—to have his house painted and to pay off a second mortgage. Firoza Salahuddin had been a Pan Data founder in 1984; her husband had argued that the payments had been made in compensation for his wife's work.

On April 30, 1990, Salahuddin was suspended without pay. On July 24 he was charged by the Maryland U.S. district attorney with two felony counts: criminal conflict of interest and accepting an unlawful gratuity. And on September 7 he pleaded guilty to two felony counts before a judge in the U.S. District Court in Baltimore. The maximum penalty for each count was two years in jail and a $250,000 fine.

The scientist wept with relief when he was informed that he would be placed on probation for five years and fined $12,000.† But in a gesture that was one of the most telling indications of the status accorded the disease, the judge sentenced Salahuddin to 1,750 hours of unpaid research on chronic fatigue syndrome—the equivalent of a year of forty-hour work weeks—as punishment for his crimes. By the end of the year the disgraced scientist would be ensconced in the corner of a laboratory at the University of Southern California School of Medicine in Pasadena, where an old colleague had offered him space. The experience was

* Gunn's plan was ambitious in the extreme. His immediate superiors, Larry Schonberger and Brian Mahy, had demonstrated on prior occasions an unwillingness to sanction their principal investigator's visits to patient support meetings or medical conferences in which patients played an organizing role. On at least one occasion, congressional pressure was required to empower Gunn to attend a medical conference. Patients in a midwestern state, who had invited Gunn to speak, entreated their senator, who in turn wrote the agency's director after Larry Schonberger refused Gunn's request to attend. The senator's letter won Gunn's freedom. In the case of the Charlotte conference, Gunn advised Marc Iverson to send a carbon copy of the invitation to the new CDC director, William Roper. "I'm reading between the lines here," Iverson said. "Good," replied Gunn.

† According to the *Washington Post,* Dale Kelberman, the prosecutor in the case, reported receiving letters "from throughout the world" praising Salahuddin's contributions to medical science, a phenomenon that apparently ameliorated what Salahuddin had expected would be a far stiffer sentence. Said Salahuddin, "I was looking around the city at halfway houses trying to figure out where I would be washing dishes."

transforming: Salahuddin's dashing good looks and self-deprecating humor had been wiped away; gray had appeared at his temples; unarticulated grief creased his face.

"I would have liked to work on Kaposi's sarcoma," Salahuddin said after the judgment, his bitterness apparent. "My guess is someone suggested chronic fatigue syndrome to the prosecutor. I would say it was a brilliant choice," he added, his eyes conveying the irony of the ruling. As an alternative to prison, what could be more punishing, after all, than for one of the country's top AIDS researchers to be ordered to work on a disease his peers considered a joke? Salahuddin briefly entertained the notion that Anthony Komaroff, who had written a letter to the prosecutor on his behalf, had suggested the punishment. After a pause, he shrugged off the speculation, however, noting that Komaroff would have discussed such a move with him first. (Komaroff, queried much later on the matter, insisted that he "had no memory of suggesting any particular action in the Salahuddin case. I simply indicated that I felt his research on HHV6 had been important.")

Perhaps not surprisingly, Salahuddin's view of his colleagues at NIH had changed as a result of his ordeal, and he was unafraid to speak frankly about the Bethesda institution's handling of the CFS epidemic. "The people who are involved in looking at the disease are all incompetent," he said. "They're not looking at it objectively. Each of them has an ax to grind. The disease is treated rather shabbily. There is no sympathy, no interest at National Institutes of Health."

Salahuddin's position at the university was unfunded. Like every other scientist who was trying to study the disease, the convicted felon and NIH refugee would have to raise grant money if he was to satisfy the judge's sentence. By year's end, he had been unable to secure funding from any source for CFS research.

Wistar Institute, Philadelphia, Pennsylvania

In the weeks following her return to Philadelphia after the Kyoto trip, Elaine DeFreitas was courted by an extraordinary range of researchers and clinicians. Typically, the doctors wanted her to test their patients' blood; the scientists were hungry to collaborate with her.

Anthony Komaroff was among the first to make his move. DeFreitas, noting that the Harvard researcher lacked the capacity to perform polymerase chain reaction, turned down Komaroff's offer of collaboration. When he asked if she would share her gene sequences with him, she demurred.

The CDC's very own Jon Kaplan was another suitor. The epidemiologist proposed to her that she test a group of the agency's surveillance cases for evidence of her retrovirus fragments. DeFreitas was intrigued by the idea of a collaboration with the agency, but she had never heard of Jon Kaplan. When she ran Kaplan's name by Cheney, the Charlotte doctor was outraged; he immediately called Walter Gunn. The latter, who had been enduring Kaplan's disparaging comments about the disease for two years, was similarly enraged that Kaplan had inserted himself into the action without consulting Gunn, who was now, after all, the principal CFS investigator. Gunn was incensed, too, that Kaplan would presume that he had unfettered access to the CDC's surveillance patients. Gunn felt increasingly proprietary about the investigation and even about the patients themselves. "Those are *my* patients," he told Cheney.

Robert Gallo's laboratory reached out to DeFreitas as well. According to the Wistar scientist, Gallo's associate Howard Streicher "offered the assistance of any and all of Gallo's lab." Initially DeFreitas accepted the offer, but the collaboration proved to be ill-fated. Within months, scientists in the Gallo lab were consumed by an in-house investigation of their role in the discovery of HIV.

Yet another scientist, a neurologist from the University of Glasgow named Peter Behan, was pressuring her for her gene sequences. Behan, a physically imposing, opinionated Irishman with an obsession for salmon fishing, had been studying what he preferred to call myalgic encephalomyelitis in the British Isles for fifteen years. He had been a professor of clinical neurology at the University of Glasgow for more than a decade, although he had trained in psychiatry at Harvard and in pathology at Cambridge.* Like many in Britain, Behan disdained the early American obsession with Epstein-Barr virus, adhering instead to the enterovirus theory of the disease. In addition, he and his collaborators in Glasgow had performed hundreds of muscle biopsies on patients. "They are extraordinarily abnormal," Behan said. Since 1988 the neurologist's efforts had been substantially supported by a generous one-million-pound five-year grant from London's Barclay brothers.

In his letters, Behan promised DeFreitas that if she shared her data he would keep her informed of every step of his research and that she would be the first to know the results. He even suggested they might publish a collaborative paper. As the American scientist continued to mull over her options, Behan lost patience. Finally he faxed her that her unwillingness to share her secrets with him was giving him "myocardial infarction."

DeFreitas took pity on the longtime student of the disease and sent Behan a nondisclosure form as a prelude to sharing her protocol with him. "I thought, here's a lab that can obviously do polymerase chain reaction, can obviously find viral sequences, and is looking at the issue of myalgic encephalomyelitis versus chronic fatigue syndrome to finally decide whether this is an artificial distinction—just a geographical distinction—and really the same disease," DeFreitas said.

Cheney, meanwhile, was encouraging DeFreitas to collaborate with another suitor, John Martin, director of the Los Angeles County Hospital's molecular pathology labs, and chief of molecular pathology at the University of Southern California. Martin had been fascinated by the new disease for some years and was himself hunting for microbes in the spinal fluid and blood tissue of a handful of patients with pronounced neurological syndromes he believed were severe cases of CFS. "Let's anoint the good guys," Cheney argued on Martin's behalf.

DeFreitas decided in Martin's favor as well. The latter's large lab at L.A. County Hospital was equipped to perform a range of sophisticated investigative

---

* For many years, he and a score of like-minded researchers met regularly at Behan's Saville Club in London where, over repasts of salmon and fine port, they discussed the disease and read their own papers on the subject, scorning "the shits who've said [the disease] doesn't occur—the neurology establishment in England, which hasn't had an original idea since the turn of the century," as Behan described the opposition.

techniques. Martin, like Komaroff, however, asked for the gene sequences, and ultimately DeFreitas refused. "We want to get official acceptance on this paper first before we start," she said later. Without DeFreitas's cooperation on the gene sequences, the nascent collaboration faltered and eventually dissolved.

Other, more heart-wrenching pressures were exerted upon DeFreitas after Kyoto. For two and a half years she had been working in secrecy, her name unknown to sufferers. Suddenly, as if caught in an ocean undertow, she was being dragged by patients into the very core of their bleak existence. "The letters I'm getting are heartbreaking," the scientist said. "It's the same story over and over— people who sound like they are at the end of their rope. I never really saw this firsthand until now. I only heard about it from Paul and David."

Another class of caller was doctors, many of whom had changed their minds about the disease as a result of her finding. "Some calls are from clinicians I never would have expected to hear from—doctors who three weeks ago didn't believe this disease existed," DeFreitas said. "It was almost a one-hundred-eighty for some people. A psychiatrist called me about a patient who was involuntarily committed to Friends Hospital in Philadelphia by her family.* The admitting diagnosis was hysterical conversion. He told me, 'This woman doesn't have hysterical conversion—she has chronic fatigue syndrome.' "

Eerily, DeFreitas began hearing, too, from patients who told her that before they fell ill they had routinely donated blood to the American Red Cross. Eventually, however, they had been rejected as donors because their blood test results were read as "HIV indeterminate." The ambivalent result could have meant, DeFreitas theorized, that the commercial test kit used by the Red Cross for HIV was sensing the presence of a virus with a genetic structure closely related but not identical to the AIDS virus. An "HIV indeterminate" result could very well signal infection with a related but different retrovirus.

Within a month of her return from Kyoto, DeFreitas again seemed comfortable, for the moment, with her collaborative arrangement with Cheney and Bell. Her rage over Cheney's assertions of co-inventorship before the Kyoto conference seemed to have evaporated. "I've had lots of offers from other clinicians," DeFreitas said, "but why go out for hamburger when you can eat steak at home? I'm getting the best patients. As far as I'm concerned, it's business as usual."

New York City

Late that fall, *Newsweek* published its third story on the disease. The *Time* magazine–fostered phrase "yuppie flu" had been replaced by "the gray plague," wordplay on either the politically incorrect, long-abandoned "gay plague" or the black plague. Indeed, "gray plague" seemed an apt term for a disease that, unlike the fourteenth-century scourge, cast its victims into a gray netherworld of unending illness without killing them. "A debilitating disease afflicts millions—and the cause is still a mystery" was the *Newsweek* subhead. On the magazine's cover was the anguished face of twenty-eight-year-old Gino Olivieri, a former Detroit Lions football star and SWAT team member of the Rochester, New York, police force, who had been disabled by the disease since 1988. Senior writer Geoffrey Cowley,

* Founded by the Quakers, Friends Hospital was America's oldest independent psychiatric hospital.

using supporting research from *Newsweek*'s Mary Hager, estimated that two to five million Americans suffered from the disease. Cowley's report offered no-holds-barred science coverage, describing the evidence for brain damage and infectiousness in the disease and chronicling the highlights of Wistar's retrovirus hunt. Color photographs of Los Angeles radiologist Ismael Mena's SPECT scan images of sufferers' brains appeared at the top of the first page of the seven-page story. The second page was consumed by a striking picture of David Bell, clad in a faded gray sweatshirt and jeans, gazing directly into the camera's lens, a contingent of children crowded behind him, victims of the Lyndonville epidemic.

In his final paragraph, Cowley noted: "The mainstream medical community has been too slow to take the problem seriously. Though federal agencies started funding a handful of chronic fatigue syndrome studies last year, most of the research completed to date has been funded—and published—by patients' groups, or by obscure doctors struggling to get by in one of the least lucrative specialties in medicine. At least one leading researcher has financed his work by selling his office furniture and working graveyard in a hospital emergency room. Telling people they aren't sick is an easier way out when an illness so defies expectations. Unfortunately, it's a lie."

The issue was the hottest-selling *Newsweek* of the year and precipitated an avalanche of work for Dorothy Knight at the CDC in Atlanta. "I'll *never* forget it," she said several months later. "We got over fifteen thousand calls in the space of a few days."

Charlotte, North Carolina

On a map of North America, which Cheney kept in a corridor of his new clinic, clusters of hundreds of yellow and green pins could be found in forty states. Yellow pins signified female patients; green pins, males. "I vacuum," Cheney said as he studied the map that September. Indeed, while he had a large contingent of patients from Orlando, for instance, he had only a few from Miami. "I get patients from cities where there aren't any good CFIDS doctors and from cities where there are strong support groups. In Miami, there's Nancy Klimas, and so she sees most of the chronic fatigue syndrome patients there."

The pins were thickly clustered in the East and Midwest, but they also popped up in places like Four Corners, New Mexico, and Billings, Montana. There were three pins in the Atlantic Ocean. "Those are my patients in Belgium, Saudi Arabia, and Saint Croix," Cheney explained.

One room, "the Ampligen room," had been designed for infusion of the drug. The room held two large "infusion chairs" and a computer provided by HEM to thaw the drug in a precise fashion. In a large freezer in the laboratory, the doctor was storing a multitude of tissues from people with the disease, including a human placenta and breast tissues from women with CFS who had developed breast cancer and undergone mastectomies.

A woman on Cheney's large staff was employed full-time simply to write disability reports and letters to insurance companies explaining the scientific and medical rationale for the sophisticated and frequently costly tests the doctors ordered on most patients. Stored in her computer data bank were the PET, BEAM, and MRI brain scan results on most of the doctor's patients, which could be reproduced and sent along with the neuroradiology report to the Social Security Administration or the patient's insurance company.

Cheney soon would be joined part time by Charles Lapp, a clinical associate professor at Duke University Medical Center with an interest in CFS. In addition, David Bell had agreed to work in Cheney's clinic one week of every four, commuting from Lyndonville. Bell would serve as the clinic's pediatric expert.

University of Pittsburgh, Pittsburgh, Pennsylvania

Seymour Grufferman had revived his CFS project earlier in the year and by the fall was excitedly analyzing new evidence for infectiousness in the disease. "I'm sort of coming to closure on this thing in terms of how to put it all together in a paper," Grufferman said that fall.

The epidemiologist had employed a method of determining the degree of personal contact among cases and non-cases in the North Carolina Symphony. Called Knox's method of all possible pairs, the technique resulted in a complex grid in which every member of the orchestra was named, and next to each name were the names of all other members of the orchestra with whom they'd had contact of any kind. The questions ranged from the general, as in "Do you know this person?" to the more specific, as in "Did you perform in a small chamber group with this person?" to the exquisitely specific, as in "Did you ever have intimate sexual contact with this person?"

As it turned out, the more intimate the contact among the orchestra members—riding together in cars on their way to performances, eating meals together—the more likely they were to have the disease.

"Where we got into our greatest statistically significant difference," Grufferman said, "is the sharing of an eating utensil. Sharing a bed? The numbers got *very* small. . . . Now, these data are hard to interpret. But I think they are the first *hard* data that at least are in support of the notion of person-to-person transmission of some agent."

Centers for Disease Control, Atlanta, Georgia

On September 11, as promised, Paul Cheney sent the abstract letter from the Wistar presentation in Kyoto to Walter Gunn in Atlanta. In an accompanying letter, Cheney reiterated what he called "evidence of a real and present danger to the health and vitality of millions of Americans." Cheney sent a carbon copy of the letter to William Roper, the agency chief, and enclosed a Wistar abstract for Roper as well.

"Probably the most surprising result and surely the most worrisome," the doctor wrote, "is the finding of a large number of sick children showing viral sequences . . . together with a high percentage (30 percent) of exposure controls who are also positive." He ended his letter with the comment "I hope you will come to share my concern and will endeavor to learn more about chronic fatigue syndrome (also known as CFIDS). I welcome any questions that you may have."

As far as Gunn was concerned, Cheney was preaching to the converted. The agency veteran found the concept of a retroviral cause of the disease entirely plausible. To persuade his peers, however, Gunn had to overcome the weight of years of skepticism that CFS was even a medical illness.

Fortunately, Tom Folks, the retrovirology division chief in Atlanta who would shepherd any effort to replicate the Wistar finding, was predisposed to be optimistic about the project because of his respect for Wistar chief Koprowski. "Hilary Koprowski is a legend," Folks said that fall. "When he stands behind one of his people, you've got to believe it."

Folks agreed without hesitation to Gunn's request to look for the Wistar retrovirus, although Gunn predicated the offer on the condition that he could persuade DeFreitas to reveal her gene sequences and her viral probes. Folks also agreed that Kaplan would not be involved in the project, as Cheney had made it clear to Gunn that he would not under any circumstances tolerate a collaboration with Jon Kaplan.

Folks, that September, seemed enthusiastic. "I'm willing to confirm their work in total confidence, just to add credibility and to go forward with the resolution of the disease," he said. First, however, he had to prove to DeFreitas that he could actually reproduce her experiments. To that end, he planned to apply her test to some blinded samples sent to him by David Bell—blood from Lyndonville children. He awaited DeFreitas's unpublished manuscript and viral gene sequences. "If I was able to break the code that some third party had the lock and key to, then we could say, 'Let's go forward,' " Folks said. "I get pretty good vibrations now that resources will be forthcoming to continue to pursue this," he continued. "I don't anticipate anyone will call me and say, 'Don't pursue this for more than thirty days.' . . . If chronic fatigue syndrome can be shown to be a retrovirus disease, research will grow quickly. Believe me, once that's cohesive, the field will explode."

Wistar Institute, Philadelphia, Pennsylvania

In time, Elaine DeFreitas came to regret her decision to collaborate with the Centers for Disease Control. That fall, however, she felt certain she had made the right decision. Walter Gunn's enthusiasm and his apparent commitment to unraveling the mystery of the disease motivated her more than anything else. In fact, the more she listened to Gunn, the more she believed he might be the key to breaching the government's wall of silence on the issue. In addition, Tom Folks had DeFreitas's confidence. "He's got a good reputation as a retrovirologist. He's published in very good journals. I thought he would give it a fair shot," she said later. Her feeling for Gunn and her respect for Folks's scientific acumen softened her view of the entire agency.

Nevertheless, although she agreed to collaborate with the agency, she insisted that the government scientists sign a nondisclosure agreement restraining them from sharing with other scientists any information she provided. In addition, although DeFreitas initially agreed to suppy the federal lab with everything she had, including the gene sequences Tom Folks had been counting on, she later rescinded her offer. Upon hearing that his protégée was about to hand over her gene sequences and her live DNA probes for the virus, Hilary Koprowski stepped in, asking DeFreitas to wait. When she heard from the editors of the *Proceedings of the*

National Academy of Sciences that her manuscript revealing her techniques had been accepted, she could reveal the probes and gene sequences, but not before, Koprowski insisted.

▦

DeFreitas was beginning to feel the sting of having rushed into the public domain with her work before publication. Paul Levine at the National Cancer Institute expressed his skepticism about the finding, and reproved Wistar for using a neuropathology conference on the other side of the world, followed by an American press conference, as its vehicle. But even scientists who believed wholeheartedly in the disease were ready with withering comments about DeFreitas's timing and her seeming willingness to "publish" in the lay press before publishing in the scientific press.

"The way they've handled it is a scientific abomination. It's unconscionable to do something like that, particularly from an established institution like Wistar," Seymour Grufferman complained that fall. "You don't hold press conferences saying you've found the agent when nobody can even figure out what it is you've found or evaluate whether you did it properly. I think if you have a hot finding, you lay it out in front of your peers, not the press."

Of course, DeFreitas had never claimed to have found *the* agent, only *an* agent. Even so, she was unsurprised by the censure. "Koprowski remains totally happy with the timing of the announcement, although he's got much larger accomplishments in his life to stand on," she said that fall, "whereas I felt uncomfortable saying, 'To be published, to be published.'"

DeFreitas was being made increasingly vulnerable, too, by the fact that two investigative teams who had tried to replicate the HTLV1 finding in multiple sclerosis—both of them funded by the Multiple Sclerosis Society, a patient organization that had been cool to the news that an "AIDS-like" virus had been found in MS sufferers—had been unable to do so. Koprowski and DeFreitas were confident of their MS virology, believing they would be vindicated eventually. In the meantime, however, the inability of other scientists to replicate their discovery gave their critics easy and potent ammunition with which to attack the CFS finding.

Centers for Disease Control, Atlanta, Georgia

In September, Walter Gunn made a tour of the agency's surveillance sites in Wichita, Grand Rapids, and Reno. "I want to get a feel from our state health officers how things are going," Gunn said. But he added, "I also want to see how they're handling inquiries from the press. And to talk to patients in support groups."

In Nevada, Gunn made a special effort to smooth the bad feelings of years' duration with Dan Peterson and other Nevadans. "I've had to apologize all over the state of Nevada for Holmes's and Kaplan's behavior [to] the Nevada state health officials and the doctors who say they were treated like country bumpkins," the senior researcher said some time later. He made a special effort with Peterson, who for years had existed for Gunn as merely a name—one his colleagues along the viral epidemiology corridors enjoyed maligning.

Peterson was surprised by Gunn's apparent eagerness to meet with him and struck by the federal epidemiologist's candor. Gunn was clearly a different breed of agency investigator. "He said his higher-ups were very anti-CFS," Peterson said later. "They told him he had to throw a lot of cases out because they were missing only one symptom from the protocol."

Indeed, Gunn noted soon after meeting with the young internist, "The agency's attitude is that there were hardly any cases out there—that's *still* the prevailing view. At CDC there is currently a tendency to throw out cases if anything unusual turns up—say, for instance, lymphoma. At CDC they call it 'undiagnosed lymphoma' and throw out the case. But the CDC doesn't see patients, and if you see patients, you get a different picture."*

Although Gunn himself had yet to see patients in a clinical setting, he was listening to them and observing them in support groups in the cities he visited. In Grand Rapids a group of patients asked him to address a local support group the night before he left. He agreed to do so.

"I thought I was going to be speaking to a small group," Gunn recalled. "I walked into an auditorium filled with more than two hundred people. They were seated in the aisles—it was standing room only. I was stunned. I tried to give an extemporaneous report on our surveillance study. Overall, they were very supportive. But there were some people there—some women and teenagers—who were upset because we couldn't include children in our surveillance study. We can't because there are questions about drugs and sex on the surveillance questionnaire, and the Office of Management and Budget gets edgy when you ask people under eighteen those kinds of questions.

"After my talk," Gunn continued, "they presented me with a huge basket of apples. It stood three feet high. The attached note said that each apple represented a child in Kent County with the disease, and it also said, 'It would take all the apple orchards in Kent County to represent all the children in the United States who have chronic fatigue syndrome.' I told them I was going to take the apples back to William Roper, and I did. I took the basket on the plane, put it in the overhead

---

* It wasn't only CDC investigators who threw out cases when they developed cancer. Stephen Straus at NIH apparently did so, too. During a conversation with Straus that year, Seymour Grufferman learned that Straus had eliminated a handful of CFS patients from his Bethesda cohort because they had cancer. Grufferman pressed Straus on the matter of whether the cancer began before or after the paients' onset of CFS. Straus admitted the cancer had developed *after* the onset of CFS, but he staunchly defended his decision to eject patients from the CFS category when their malignancies were diagnosed. Grufferman, for his part, was equally adamant that it was far too early in the discovery process to rule out the possibility that the CFS led to the development of cancer in some patients and their close contacts. Certainly, a number of other immune dysfunction diseases—most prominently AIDS—lead, to cancer in some patients.

"The contribution our approach makes is that we're dealing with discrete outbreaks of disease," Grufferman said some time later. "Steve Straus and Anthony Komaroff are sampling by symptom. *We're* sampling by outbreak." In other words, classifying and studying people based on their symptoms alone offered little information about whether the disease was spreading, how it was spreading, or whether it was leading to an increased incidence of cancer in patients or in people exposed to patients; the "well" population *around* the patients needed to be studied, too.

bin—it caused quite a commotion. And the next day I sent it up to the director's office with the note. Roper's a pediatrician, you know."

Privately, Gunn hoped he could somehow leapfrog past cynics in the Division of Viral and Rickettsial Diseases and launch a dialogue directly with members of the agency's topmost administrative hierarchy. As would become clear, however, Gunn's message—baskets of apples aside—was failing to penetrate the agency's upper-echelon administrators. In addition, within his own increasingly claustrophobic division, every incidence of unfettered enthusiasm for his investigation only served to harm the senior researcher further.

By September 24 when he returned to Atlanta, Gunn was able to report that the CDC's four-county surveillance system, so far, had been referred a total of 344 patients. Of those patients, he said, 276 had agreed to cooperate with the agency in its investigation, in spite of the fact that the initial interview alone would consume more than four hours. Of those patients, Gunn added, 209 had been screened by surveillance nurses, had fit the agency's criteria for the disease, and were ready to be referred to the Physicians Review Committee, which would further analyze their medical histories. By the end of September, however, just 16 cases had been reviewed.

Among the Physicians Review Committee members that fall were Harvard's Anthony Komaroff, Gunn's colleague Larry Schonberger, University of Massachusetts infectious disease specialist Nelson Gantz, Manhattan immunologist Susan Levine, who had several hundred CFS patients in her practice, and University of Toronto psychiatrist Susan Abbey. Complete files on every patient were sent to two doctors on the committee. If both doctors agreed the patient was a bona fide case, the agency added the patient to its list; if not, the patient's files were sent to all five doctors, who then held a conference call to discuss the case.

"We're finding a significant number of those do meet the case definition," Gunn said. "The majority did not have a psychological problem concurrent with the onset of fatigue. So for anyone who says this is depression in disguise, we can say, 'That's not what the data says.' We're not seeing any rate of depression that's higher than the normal population," Gunn said.

Those simple, innocent-sounding statements wiped out four years of investigation by the government's in-house expert, Stephen Straus. Whether Gunn would be allowed by his superiors in Atlanta to make such statements to the nation's press was yet to be seen.

Wistar Institute, Philadelphia, Pennsylvania

On October 3, David Bell retrieved the frozen samples of Skye Dailor's liver, spleen, heart, and brain from the Rochester hospital where the fourteen-year-old suicide victim had died after suffering a heart attack in the hospital's emergency room. The doctor packed the organs carefully on dry ice inside a protective Styrofoam container that fastened with a strap. He boarded a plane in Rochester and carried the container on his lap during the entire flight to Philadelphia. The driver of Wistar Institute's sleek black station wagon met Bell at the airport and took him and his package directly to the Wistar building on the edge of the University of Pennsylvania campus, passing first between the high wrought-iron security gates on Spruce Street, then into the small courtyard.

Bell thanked the driver and took his precious package through the generous foyer of the Wistar, walking quickly past the silver urns recessed into the marble walls and containing the remains of Wistar's past directors, directly to Elaine De-Freitas's lab. The scientist and her postdoc, Brendan Hilliard, wearing white coats and rubber gloves, were waiting for him.

"David felt it was a kind of closure," DeFreitas remembered later. "He had somehow seen it full circle."

23

Playing Catch-up

U.S. Senate, Washington, D.C.

Patient advocates had been working with congressional aides for nearly four years to impress upon the nation's legislators the need for government support of CFS research within and outside the federal agencies. Congress, in turn, had been increasingly responsive, since 1987 earmarking money in ever-larger increments for the CDC to enable scientists there to measure the breadth of the epidemic and urging the NIH to fund extramural research into the pathogenesis of the disease. Neither agency had demonstrated a commitment to the disease commensurate with legislators' hopes.

On October 10 the Senate Committee on Appropriations addressed the agencies in Atlanta and Bethesda in its strongest language ever. In its report, which was soon to become law, the committee commended the CDC for its surveillance program, but noted that "this illness remains a serious public health concern." Among other requests, the Senate asked the agency to establish a patient registry and to develop a standard method of clinically evaluating people suffering with the disease, one that could be passed on to the "U.S. biomedical community."

"The committee notes with concern," the report stated, "that the number of inquiries at the Centers for Disease Control for information about chronic fatigue syndrome has been as high as several thousand per month and that this has disrupted some [agency] activities." In order to ease the agency's burden, senators went on to award the agency $1.25 million to be used in 1991 to keep the public informed on the disease, to hold conferences on it, and to help train doctors about it.*

Ultimately, the CDC received slightly more than $2 million dollars from Congress for fiscal year 1991, which officially began in October 1990.

The Senate was tougher on the NIH. Four years earlier, Illinois representative John Porter had warned Chicago patient advocate and lobbyist Ted Van Zelst that Congress would never direct the NIH to study any particular disease, nor would it

---

* The agency, of course, had already hired Dorothy Knight to respond to public inquiries. But Knight's annual salary was only $26,970, leaving a balance of $1,223,030. The agency held no conferences on the disease, nor did it make any efforts to educate doctors, aside from its CFS bulletins and its hot line, that year.

earmark money for the study of specific diseases. The research bulwark on the arcadian fringes of the capital was off-limits to political "micromanagement," Porter and his aides insisted. By 1990, however, Congress seemed to have changed its mind. For the first time since lobbyists introduced the disease into the appropriations process early in 1985, the Senate committee earmarked money for CFS research. Most significantly, the committee directed NIAID to fund extramural research. The Senate earmarked "up to" $1 million to "initiate a consortium of research centers for CFS research," and singled out the University of Nevada and the University of Minnesota as "exceptionally well qualified to act as CFS research centers," adding that the committee "expects that the NIH will wish to award such centers to these institutions," since investigators at both schools had already performed considerable research into the disease.* The committee also asked that a "senior agency official" within the NIH be named "to better coordinate" the research effort inside the Bethesda agency.

Centers for Disease Control, Atlanta, Georgia

On October 25, Walter Gunn asked for $80,000 to add children to the agency's surveillance program and $150,000 to expand the surveillance contract with Abt Associates in Cambridge to respond to reports of outbreaks. Brian Mahy, the chief of the Division of Viral and Rickettsial Diseases, turned down both requests. "Mahy said he didn't want to spend any more money on chronic fatigue syndrome until the case-control study proved the disease was organic," Gunn recalled.

Two days after Mahy's refusal, epidemiology chief Larry Schonberger informed Gunn there was to be a meeting of the top administrators of the Center for Infectious Diseases, of which Gunn's division was a major component, to discuss the new CFS budget. The most recent $2 million congressional appropriation to the agency was the biggest yet. Schonberger made it clear to Gunn that he was not invited. The agency's principal investigator of the disease remained in his office, frustrated and concerned, on the day of the high-level meeting.

Hollywood, California

The November issue of *Vanity Fair* reported news of Cher's bout with what interviewer Kevin Sessums called "Epstein-Barr." After a lively stage performance by Cher, reporter Sessums followed the singer to her waiting bus, where an exhausted Cher immediately asked him, "Do you mind if I lie down?"

Sessums wrote: "What sounds like jaded ennui is really Epstein-Barr. Cher discovered she carried the energy-sapping virus during the filming of *The Witches of*

---

* Neither university was awarded money to establish a research center, however. The University of Nevada has yet to be awarded any federal money. In 1994, NIAID awarded a University of Minnesota faculty member, Ph.D. Chunn Chao, $213,205 to investigate mechanisms of fatigue in mice. Chao was a researcher at the forty-three-year-old Minneapolis Medical Research Foundation, the research arm of the Hennepin County Medical Center. The year he was awarded the grant, Chao explained that his success had come only after four successive grant applications. Chao's CFS theory held that the fatigue was caused by excessive amounts of immune system chemicals, or cytokines, in the brain. Chao was systematically creating exhausted mice by dialing up the levels of cytokines in their brains; healthy mice ran two to four miles a day; once Chao "gave" the mice cytokine-induced fatigue, their activity level dropped by as much as 70 percent.

Eastwick in 1986, but she wasn't fully aware of the disease's debilitating force until she began her last film, *Mermaids,* which opens next month. Production had to be shut down while she regained her strength. 'I was so sick I thought I was going to die. I went to doctor after doctor. . . .' "

Most of Sessums's interviews with Cher were conducted at her bedside.

National Cancer Institute, Bethesda, Maryland

In November the National Cancer Institute's epidemiologist Paul Levine sent a nurse-epidemiologist to Incline Village to abstract all the charts of CFS sufferers in Dan Peterson's practice. Levine was looking for an increased rate of cancer. Peterson had by then collected eleven cases of cancer in his practice among CFS victims or their close relatives since the local epidemic of 1984–1985.* Five of the cases were lymphomas. In addition, the doctor now had three cases of brain cancer among CFS patients. Two of the three would die within the next two years; one of those who died was just twenty.†

"We're working on *all* aspects of cancer and chronic fatigue syndrome," Levine said that fall. "We have a nurse out there to see if those lymphoma cases are really unusual. And we're taking blood samples for a retrovirus, which will be analyzed in our Fredericksburg, Maryland, lab. . . . I'm going to ask DeFreitas what her reagents were," Levine added after a moment. (Elaine DeFreitas refused Levine's request.)

Levine had good reason to be curious about Peterson's cancer cluster. According to the American Cancer Society, the incidence of non-Hodgkin's lymphoma among Americans had increased by more than 50 percent in the seventeen years between 1973 and 1990, constituting one of the largest increases of any form of cancer.[1] Indeed, non-Hodgkin's lymphoma was increasingly acknowledged by experts in government and academia to be an emerging epidemic, the third-fastest-rising cancer on the planet, trailing only lung cancer in women and the rapidly escalating skin cancer.‡ The National Cancer Institute estimated that 37,000 cases would be diagnosed in the United States that year alone. For some time, Levine and his colleagues in Bethesda had been attempting to ferret out the reasons for the phenomenal increase in lymphoma. Many cancer researchers suspected a virus was the trigger mechanism for the disease. If the lymphoma cases in north Lake Tahoe constituted a bona fide cluster, it was quite obvious that the

* Approximately half of these patients were CFS sufferers; the others were their first-order relatives—children, siblings, or parents.

† Many of the cancers among Peterson's patients were identical to the rare cancers that occurred among members of the North Carolina Symphony or their close contacts—that is, B-cell non-Hodgkin's lymphoma, carcinoma of the salivary or parotid gland, and glioblastoma multiforme, or brain cancer.

‡ An awareness of the problem began in the late 1980s when non-Hodgkin's lymphoma emerged as a complication in a small number of AIDS cases. Epidemiologists who began tracking lymphoma rates were surprised by the large numbers, at first attributed solely to the AIDS epidemic. As researchers undertook more sophisticated, retrospective methods of tracking the disease, however, they realized that very little of the increase—as little as 3 percent—could be blamed on AIDS. Statistically, the greatest increase in non-Hodgkin's lymphomas has been among people over the age of fifty; well-known American victims have included Jacqueline Onassis, Paul Tsongas, William Casey, and Lewis Thomas. Overall, NHL occurs in men at least twice as often as in women.

agent that caused the Nevada CFS epidemic might be related to the rise in lymphoma cases, too.

Nevertheless, in 1990, the fifth straight year that the Bethesda agency had postured itself in its reports to Congress, the press, and the public as being "in the forefront" of CFS research, Levine was the only epidemiologist at the NIH working on the disease. "I would say I spend ten percent of my time on chronic fatigue syndrome now," Levine said.

Incline Village, Nevada

By that fall, despite Levine's interest, Dan Peterson felt more discouraged than ever. "I will tell you this," he said early in November, "I am considering dropping out of this more strongly than at any time in the last six years." Speaking only half in jest, the doctor momentarily resurrected a childhood fantasy: "Maybe I'll get out of it altogether and go be a forest ranger."

Six years before, Peterson had encountered his first patient with the disease, a wealthy middle-aged Texan, in his examining room. In the intervening years, he had watched literally hundreds of his patients fall ill, he'd been castigated by his colleagues in medicine, and he had crashed financially. He was taxed almost beyond reason, as well, by his patients, who had found in the doctor their sole source of emotional comfort in an otherwise unsympathetic world. And, like Lyndonville's David Bell, he was running out of ways to help those who had been ill for years. Their problems—medical and social—were so grave, their demands so expansive, that Peterson was becoming increasingly exasperated. "I know this is real, I know it's transmissible," he said. "But as far as individual patients go, I'm burned out."

In addition to his Incline clinic, Peterson was running a small one-day-a-month clinic in Los Angeles to accommodate his CFS patients in southern California; when he returned from his day trips to Los Angeles, a corner of his desk was stacked with pink slips—all of them messages from CFS patients. For some time, Peterson had been searching for a partner to help him shoulder the burden, but his practice, he discovered, was "tainted," as he had once described it to Walter Gunn. He was advertising for a full-time partner, but the search was going badly. "As soon as they hear it has anything to do with chronic fatigue syndrome," Peterson said, "they don't call back."

For a year he had been joined by a Reno internist; but that doctor, ill at ease with CFS patients, had left. Now he had a new part-time partner to whom he referred disparagingly as "Rent-a-Doc."

"I saw two new [CFS] patients recently," he continued. "I told them both I had nothing to offer them. There's just no more room inside me. I just don't have the energy. . . . I have about ten AIDS patients and I actually enjoy my AIDS patients more," he continued after a moment. "At least AIDS patients die. And your colleagues, at least they have some sympathy for you rather than censuring you. That disease runs its course. It's not so hard, really, helping people die—not if you're a human being."

Helping people live with a disease that, at its worst, seemed to do everything short of killing them was another matter.

Charlotte, North Carolina

Paul Cheney had begun his own analysis of cancer and its relationship to CFS that year, but Cheney's focus was on close relatives of patients rather than on the patients themselves. By November, Cheney had determined that 32 percent of his CFS patients had first-order relatives—spouses, parents, siblings, or children—who were suffering from cancer. Many uncertainties about that finding had to be examined further before the number could be called excessive, but Cheney's attention was caught immediately by the *kinds* of cancer reported. The most common cancers—lung, colon, and breast cancer, which would be expected to dominate any randomly collected list of cancers—seemed to be overshadowed by rare cancers. There were, for instance, six hematologic malignancies (blood cancers), three lymphomas, two leukemias, and even a myeloma (cancer of the bone marrow). And, interestingly, he'd found five brain cancers, including two glioblastomas, the most malignant form of brain cancer and the same cancer that had killed one of the North Carolina Symphony cancer victims. There were almost as many brain cancers as breast cancers among first-order relatives of CFS sufferers. In the general population, such a high incidence was unheard of; brain cancer accounts for just 1.5 percent of all malignancies, whereas breast cancer is surpassed only by lung cancer as the leading cause of cancer deaths in the United States.

Cheney was particularly struck by the brain cancers in this population. In spite of the relatively low incidence of brain cancer compared to other forms of cancer, he also knew that cancer epidemiologists were studying a dramatic surge in brain cancers in the U.S. population, a surge they were unable to explain by better diagnostic methods or more accurate reporting techniques. Interestingly, the incidence of brain malignancies caused by lymphoma, which accounted for less than 5 percent of all brain cancers, had risen 300 percent in recent years. Some cancer experts attributed the rise to AIDS, a disease in which immune deficiency created heightened vulnerability to lymphoma; others speculated that the rise could be blamed on Epstein-Barr virus.* Two years before, Epstein-Barr virus experts at Harvard had reported that patients suffering from non-Hodgkin's lymphoma had undergone apparent reactivations of EBV infection years before their lymphoma announced itself; significantly, the EBV antibody patterns in these patients were similar to the pattern typical of many CFS sufferers. The Harvard researchers wrote that their data supported "the role of Epstein-Barr virus either in the pathogenesis of non-Hodgkin's lymphoma or as an important marker of immune function."[2]

Centers for Disease Control, Atlanta, Georgia

On November 14, Walter Gunn and Larry Schonberger met with Walter Dowdle, the second-in-command at the CDC, to discuss the early surveillance results. The

*In July of that year, the *New York Times* reported on the "stunning" rise in brain cancers in recent years, most particularly central nervous system lymphomas. The surge of rare brain cancers was occurring not only in the U.S. but also in Japan, France, West Germany, England, and Italy (Natalie Angier, "Rising Incidence of Brain Tumors Is Drawing Attention and Concern," *New York Times,* July 31, 1990).

government scientists' search for sufferers already had turned up between three and six times more qualified cases than most people at the agency had anticipated. Against predictions that less than 5 or 10 percent of all cases reported to Abt Associates would actually qualify, the figure was nearly 30 percent of all cases reported. "It would be closer to forty-five percent if they would include people who may be lacking only one symptom," Gunn said.

Another issue the men discussed was Gunn's attendance at the CFIDS Association–sponsored conference in Charlotte. Schonberger was against it, arguing that the scientists who planned to attend the conference—they included Anthony Komaroff, Nancy Klimas, Elaine DeFreitas, and Hilary Koprowski—"weren't real researchers," according to Gunn, and that the presence of agency investigators would lend them "credibility." Gunn successfully persuaded Schonberger that the trip would have value if a summit meeting was held between the Wistar team and the CDC's retrovirology expert, Tom Folks. In a memo, Gunn also explained that agency staff members would have an opportunity to meet their counterparts in the private sector in order to "obtain important unpublished information." He sought to focus his agency's efforts on attempting to replicate those data in government laboratories.

Privately, however, Gunn was most concerned that Wistar team members open their minds and hearts to Tom Folks. "I'm hoping they'll trust us and open up," Gunn said the night before the meeting was to occur. "We'll offer them complete security. If they do, Tom Folks could start [attempting to duplicate the Wistar finding] that day. Otherwise, it's going to cost us months."

Charlotte, North Carolina

On the afternoon of November 15, a Friday, Paul Cheney performed a lumbar puncture on his sister-in-law, a former teacher who had been disabled with CFS for five years. He inserted a long spinal needle, or syringe, into the woman's spinal column in order to draw spinal fluid. It was a "clean" tap, meaning there was no blood in the fluid.

Everyone in the doctor's clinic was under orders to wear two pairs of protective gloves when handling tissue samples from patients, and Cheney took that precaution too. Whether because he was distracted by thoughts of the medical conference beginning that evening or because he was tired and recovering from a cold, he accidentally stuck his thumb with the needle as he was preparing to discard it. The needle penetrated both pairs of gloves and pierced his skin. That evening over dinner he told his wife, Jean, what had happened, breaking the news in as casual a manner as possible, even making a joke of it.

Jean, an English literature teacher at a private day school in Charlotte, was shaken. She put her fork down beside her plate and was momentarily speechless. "Paul!" she said finally, cutting through her husband's forced levity. "Isn't there something you can do right now? Some antidote, some drug—something?"

Cheney shrugged. Unfortunately there was absolutely nothing he could do. Privately, he was reassured that there had been no apparent blood in the fluid; in addition, he was recovering from a cold, which meant his immunological response mechanism was stimulated and might better quell any nascent infection. Two years earlier he had offered a sample of his blood to DeFreitas for a western blot assay; the test was negative. He did not have his blood tested again after the needle stick. Although he has subsequently not developed the disease, he has admitted that fear of acquiring the disease is a little-discussed but powerful element of patient care in his chosen field. "Those of us who take care of large numbers of patients with this disease," he explained, "are sensitive to all the varied symptoms, and whenever we experience one of them, even in mild form, we wonder, Could this be the beginning?"

On the weekend of November 16 and 17, the Omni Hotel in Charlotte was the site of the seventh patient-organized medical conference on CFS in three years. Hilary Koprowski addressed the gathering of five hundred doctors, scientists, and patients, disclosing that two more of the exposed controls in the Wistar study had fallen ill in the two months since the retrovirus finding was presented in Kyoto. The Wistar chief also stated flatly that CFS was an "infectious disease of the brain." "When a virus reaches the central nervous system, the brain, it usually will not be attacked by the immune system," Koprowski said, "so it can stay there forever. . . . The large number of individuals in contact with the patients who have the retrovirus gene sequence, as compared with normal controls, would indicate that there is a contagious factor in this disease," he added. Koprowski concluded with a discussion of the feasibility of engineering a CFS vaccine, one that could be administered to the population en masse, much like polio or smallpox vaccines.

New scientific data was presented in Charlotte—most strikingly virologist Jay Levy's news of a potentially diagnostic immunologic marker for the disease—but the scientific progress was made, as usual, in the private conference rooms, lounges, and bars of the hotel. Walter Gunn's summit was held at 5:00 P.M. on Saturday when his handpicked invitees gathered in a hermetic meeting room and arrayed themselves around a long conference table. The hotel had opened for business the day before, and the air was heavy with fumes from the newly laid carpet. As the scientists drifted into the room, Gunn stood at the head of the table, shifting from one foot to another like a patriarch waiting for his unruly children to settle themselves. Although he did not smile, his eyes sparkled with pleasure as the group assembled.

The manner in which people positioned themselves spoke volumes about the medical politics of the previous five years: virtually all of the government scientists drifted to one side of the table; the private sector researchers sat opposite them. One of the defectors was Anthony Komaroff, who sat among the goverment scientists, next to grant administrator Ann Schleuderberg. Another was the National Cancer Institute's herpesvirus expert Dharam Ablashi, who sat with the independents, sandwiching himself between Paul Cheney and David Bell. There were two notable absences: Stephen Straus and Gary Holmes. Straus had made a habit of avoiding all medical conferences in which patients played a role as organizers or participants. Holmes had wanted to attend, but out of deference to Paul Cheney, Gunn had asked him to stay away. Gunn's obeisant nod to the man who had, with Dan Peterson, struggled to bring the federal agency to some understanding of the Tahoe epidemic, was telling. If doubt remained that at least one person at the CDC was trying to make amends, Gunn's gesture erased it.

Eventually all eyes looked expectantly in Gunn's direction. "We're starting our case-control study on Monday," he told the independents. "We will try to replicate all your studies. . . . I've asked you to be here to get together with your counterparts from Centers for Disease Control."

It was the first time government scientists had met face-to-face with the private sector. They had come to the meeting to learn the techniques being used by immunologists Nancy Klimas and Elaine DeFreitas. By doing so, the government scientists fairly admitted they were being outpaced by researchers outside the federal health agencies. Gunn, of course, was convinced that government researchers would reproduce these scientists' findings upon learning their scientific protocols.

Quickly the Wistar team and Tom Folks retired to a smaller conference room across the hall, with Gunn following. Nancy Klimas and Anthony Komaroff were left behind to confer with the NIH's Ann Schleuderberg, Dharam Ablashi, and others.

In the smaller room, at a rectangular table, Bell and Cheney sat across from Koprowski and DeFreitas. Tom Folks, a boyish-looking scientist with dark hair and freckles who wore a herringbone tweed sport coat, sat at the head of the table. The forty-two-year-old retrovirologist was deferential and soft-spoken, his inflections conjuring a youth lived in Texas. Gunn and Louisa Chapman, the agency's CFS project medical adviser, sat near the other end of the table, telegraphing their view that this was Folks's meeting.

DeFreitas and Koprowski quickly agreed to send blood from Bell's and Cheney's patients and controls to Folks to enable him to replicate the finding. "The critical piece," Folks said gingerly, "will be the region where you feel like we can exchange sequences."*

"Okay," DeFreitas said, inhaling sharply. She agreed to Folks's request for the precious gene sequences of the virus—the sequences from which she had fashioned probes to identify its presence in cells.

Koprowski interrupted their negotiation with a comment to Folks: "I suggest we send you some of our positive control, the patient who was positive for us." He was referring to one of David Bell's patients, a fifteen-year-old from Lyndonville's Duncanson family, whose spinal fluid and blood were consistently and floridly positive for the retrovirus.

DeFreitas looked directly at Bell. "Is that okay?" she asked.

"Sure," Bell responded. "Fresh from the patient? Or do you want both?" He was referring to the blood taken on serial draws over the course of two years and stored in his freezer.

Folks turned to DeFreitas. "You're isolating from whole blood?" he asked, clearly surprised.

"Yes."

"We don't do that."

---

* Folks was referring to the HTLV2 "gag" gene sequences that DeFreitas had identified using polymerase chain reaction and in situ hybridization.

"We choose to do that," DeFreitas replied. "It's more than just theoretical." She explained that she found important differences in testing fresh and frozen blood. Although it seemed a minor issue at the moment, the agency's routine of testing blood that, for the sake of convenience, had been spun in a centrifuge into an amber-colored serum free of cellular debris, then frozen, and DeFreitas's insistence upon running her experiments on fresh whole blood, would take on much broader implications as the impending collaboration unfolded.

"How many samples do you want?" Bell asked Folks.

"I would prefer to have a negative for every positive," Folks answered.

"So Elaine will send the stored series, and I'll send the fresh."

Folks nodded in assent. "Mark on the vials that this is not to be refrigerated," Folks said. "We have some people at CDC who like to freeze everything."

In five minutes the deal was struck; the government was taking the first step toward isolating a possible agent of the disease.

"So . . . that's it," DeFreitas said brightly. "This was very efficient."

Cheney, however, was uneasy. Folks was going to test not only his own and David Bell's patients for the virus, but also patients in the Atlanta case-control study. He wondered if the agency really had the expertise to identify a true case of the disease. If not, Folks was unlikely to find the Wistar retrovirus in such patients. Cheney was equally concerned about CDC's method for selecting controls. Were the controls friends or relatives of the patients? If the agency's controls had been exposed to the agent, a portion of them would test positive, Cheney knew, giving in-house skeptics an opportunity to declare the Wistar pathogen a harmless endogenous retrovirus, one carried normally in the genes.

"Are the CDC's controls *non-exposed* controls?" Cheney asked Folks.

The latter shrugged; he had no idea. He turned to medical adviser Louisa Chapman, who looked uncertain. "The patients are bringing in their own controls," she told Cheney.

Cheney's shoulders sagged. If the agency's scientists understood the degree of infectiousness of the disease, they would never allow patients to choose their own controls from among their friends, families, and neighbors.

Cheney's anxiety was spreading to DeFreitas. She too was worrying about potential pitfalls. One of the things she had learned in her two and a half years of work on the problem was that there existed a pattern, one she did not yet entirely understand, in which patients were consistently negative, then consistently positive, depending on variables like the length and severity of their disease. Eleven-year sufferer Marc Iverson, for instance, tested consistently negative when he was most ill. When he was feeling better, his tests turned positive. Other patients, however, who had been ill for shorter periods and failed to manifest the severe symptoms from which Iverson suffered, had turned out to be the most spectacularly positive patients of all. Lastly, there was the specter of virus-positive but symptomless people who had been in close contact with patients, some of whom were just now coming down with the disease, as much as two or three years after their exposure began. Based on experience, DeFreitas fully expected these new victims to reach a plateau in their disease when they might turn temporarily negative on her tests.

"Is there a special selection for *acuteness* of disease?" DeFreitas asked Folks.

Louisa Chapman, who was a young doctor new to the agency and the disease, responded, "Gary Holmes and Walt Gunn are working on that with the surveillance nurses."

Cheney felt a frisson of dread. "The CDC's case definition is biased in favor of mono-like patients because of the diagnostic criteria's emphasis on fever and lymphadenopathy," he said finally. "Those patients are usually negative. I worry about the CDC's selection bias. You may be pitching out some who will be positive."

"That will resolve itself," Folks said, clearly nervous. "Once we're sure where your positives came from and where ours came from, that will get worked out. And then we can start redefining our selection process."

"A lot of our patients are being misdiagnosed as multiple sclerosis," Cheney persisted in an effort to drive his point home about the neurologic aspect of the disease, an aspect that was virtually absent from the government's case definition. "The moment these patients become ill, it's like mono. Later, the neurocognitive problems emerge. They start developing dementia."

"Would it be appropriate to mention," Bell said, looking at DeFreitas, "that patient A.L., who was eleven years old in 1988, had the strongest evidence of retrovirus infection, but he was *not* sick?" Bell was referring to a child he had chosen originally as a healthy control.

"It drove us crazy!" DeFreitas said.

"He's had gradual onset of disease over the last two years," Bell continued.

"When David told me that A.L. was the *control*," DeFreitas added, "I couldn't believe my eyes!"

"My clinical judgment of his becoming sick," Bell added, "was without my knowing that he had a high signal."

"It's *sky* high," DeFreitas emphasized.

"Well," Koprowski said, seeking to bring the meeting to its conclusion, "you all know retrovirology is not easy. These viruses sit in our body. They sit because they have nowhere to go. We'll help you all we can," he added after a moment, looking directly at Folks, thirty-one years his junior. After an exchange of phone numbers, Koprowski smiled at the government virologist. "You're on!" he said brightly, and the meeting was over.

Years later, Folks's most vivid remaining impression of the meeting was Koprowski's subtle way of silencing DeFreitas whenever she began to reveal singular, enabling details of her work to Folks: "Here she was—this was a scientist who was *ready*. She knew she was destined to crash if she couldn't get this confirmed—and quickly. She wanted to share, but every time she tried, Koprowski cut her off."

The Charlotte conference was notable for the remarkably high profile assumed by Jay Levy. One might have expected the retrovirus finding to continue to dominate any stories about CFS. Instead, the national press focused almost entirely on Levy's announcement of a new assay he and University of Chicago immunologist Alan Landay had devised, which he said might function as a diagnostic test. A three-page news release prepared by the University of California was headlined

"UC San Francisco Doctors Find Way to Identify Patients with Chronic Fatigue Syndrome." The release stated that "with viral infections such as a cold or influenza, the immune system typically reacts vigorously, but then quiets down after the attack. With CFIDS, Levy says, the immune system remains activated for months to years, showing chronically elevated levels of one type of white blood cell in particular, the CD8+ cytotoxic T-cell."

A difficulty with Levy's work, as Cheney and other clinicians present were quick to point out in their private conversations, was that the immune systems of most CIAS patients—or "chronic immune activation syndrome," as Levy recommended renaming the disease—was frequently in overdrive, but some were also in "underdrive." Cheney had noticed, in fact, that the longer the disease lasted, the more likely the patient was to go from overdrive into a markedly anergic state—that is, lacking any immune response at all. The doctor had noted that by the fifth year of illness, many patients exhibited anergy. In addition, as Cheney frequently pointed out, the human immune system "has many different parameters, and one could have destruction of one component and tremendous up-regulation in others. It's a mixed bag. In early HIV infection you see a similar picture."

Nevertheless, during a press conference held on Sunday morning, which was covered by CNN, *USA Today,* the *Wall Street Journal,* the *Philadelphia Inquirer,* the *Charlotte Observer,* and several other news organizations, questions directed at Levy consumed the lion's share of reporters' time. Not a single question was posed to Dan Peterson, Paul Cheney, or Elaine DeFreitas.

When Peterson returned to Incline Village, he sent a batch of blood samples to Immuno Sciences laboratory in California with a request that the laboratory perform a test looking for the markers Levy had said were potentially diagnostic for the disease. Mixed in with CFS samples were several drawn from children with colds and other mild, self-limiting viral diseases. The samples were coded. Two weeks later Immuno Sciences mailed Peterson the results: the children with colds were positive for the same constellation of immunologic abnormalities Levy had declared was a diagnostic marker for "CIAS."

"It's just another immunological marker," Peterson said. "It is true that the vast majority of CFS patients have those particular markers, but I just don't think it's specific to chronic fatigue syndrome."

Ann Schleuderberg, the government's CFS grant program director, continued to draw flak from researchers. She had come to Charlotte with potentially good news: her agency was going to fund a center grant, meaning money would be supplied to an academic institution where study would be undertaken to elucidate several facets of the disease. Schleuderberg's behavior in the southern city won her few friends, however. One grant hopeful recalled that Schleuderberg befriended him at dinner one night and informed him that her institute would be funding a CFS research center. Although he was pleased to know an opportunity existed for his university to become a center grant recipient, the scientist was struck by Schleuderberg's perspective on the matter. She seemed almost apologetic, he recalled, her tone suggesting that the impetus for establishing such a grant had not come from her or her peers at NIAID, but from "higher up." Indeed, Congress had legislated that the NIH fund one or more research centers by 1991; Schleuderberg and her associates had been offered little choice in the matter.

Elaine DeFreitas, meeting Schleuderberg for the first time, was shocked by her conversation with the bureaucrat. "She told me, 'If you want a study section to look favorably on this grant, you will not be able to use Paul Cheney and David Bell's patients. They don't have'—and I quote—'the CDC's stamp of approval,'" DeFreitas recalled. "She said, 'The only way to study this disease is with bona fide patients, and only the Centers for Disease Control have bona fide patients.'" DeFreitas was angry. She reported her conversation to Koprowski. "He was *hopping* mad," DeFreitas said. "He said it's actually unethical for Schleuderberg to have said that. It's not the role of an administrator to dictate what is in the grant."

The Charlotte press conference generated articles in the *Wall Street Journal, USA Today,* and the *Charlotte Observer.* Ron Winslow, writing in the *Wall Street Journal* on November 19, seized on the fact that the CDC was undertaking a case-control study of the disease: "CDC to Study Illness Derided as 'Yuppie Flu'" was the *Journal* article's headline. The research presented in Charlotte, Winslow wrote, "is already lending credibility to CFIDS patients and researchers who often confront skeptical doctors when seeking treatment and reluctant policy-makers when battling for recognition of what is increasingly viewed as an important public health problem. The research could lead to a blood test to help doctors diagnose the illness, and perhaps to new effective drugs to combat it. And it could increase pressure on insurance companies, many of which refuse to recognize the disease on grounds that it can't be diagnosed, to pay for diagnosis or treatment."

Winslow concluded: "Plenty of other hurdles lie ahead. Despite an emerging broad consensus among scientists over the cause and implications of CFIDS, there is sharp disagreement over details. Research funds are scarce, as they were in the early years of AIDS study, and scientists lament, among other things, the inability to conduct adequate controlled trials to test drug treatments. Nor is it known how CFIDS spreads—and thus how to prevent its dissemination. Until the cause is determined, treatment is by trial and error and intuition.

" 'Nobody is going to really believe the disease is real until we know the cause,' says David S. Bell, a pediatrician in Rochester, N.Y."

On December 4, *New York Times* medical correspondent Lawrence Altman had the lead piece in the newspaper's weekly science section; it was headlined "Chronic Fatigue Syndrome Finally Gets Some Respect." Altman pointed out that the CDC's surveillance study had found that only 33 percent of patients with the disease were suffering from depression when they came down with the disease, a statistic that was compatible with many estimates of the rate of depression in the general population and which was supported by the Australian study of psychiatric aspects of the disease reported that year in the *British Journal of Psychiatry.* The CDC was also attempting to confirm the Wistar retrovirus finding, Altman reported, "and has taken the unusual step of sharing critical substances to speed the experiments. The step is unusual," he added, "because when researchers in one laboratory report a discovery, those elsewhere generally try to confirm the findings using their own techniques. Sometimes the confirmation comes quickly. Other times it may take years to resolve differences that reflect minor but critical differences in the technique."

In the third paragraph of his story, Altman reported that although the new research was providing "tantalizing clues, experts like Dr. Stephen E. Straus . . . cautioned that the clues could join a list of leads that evaporated after more extensive research."

Centers for Disease Control, Atlanta, Georgia

On Monday, November 19, the long-promised case-control study got under way, five years after it was first proposed by long-departed CDC scientist Carlos Lopez. Walter Gunn had written the protocol, the seventh such protocol in four years. That morning, the first patient, an Atlanta resident, came to the agency and provided 125 milliliters of blood—the equivalent of four and a half liquid ounces—as did a healthy control who had been selected by the patient. Some of the blood was to be frozen; some of it was stored at room temperature. A lab technologist divided the blood into tiny vials, which were then distributed to an array of labs around the agency, from the AIDS lab to the retrovirus lab to the herpes and enterovirus labs. "There are about twenty-five different Centers for Disease Control labs involved in this," Gunn said.

In Gunn's ambitious plan, eighteen experiments would be conducted on the samples. These tests included an attempt to grow retrovirus in cell cultures from people with the disease, and assays for reverse transcriptase (an indicator of retroviral infection), interleukin-2, and heavy metals. Controls and patients would be subjected to identical tests, except that the controls would not be tested for retroviruses. Gunn was concerned that if controls were told they were going to be tested for retroviruses, particularly HIV, they might refuse to participate.

The "logistical nightmare" Gunn had been dreading never materialized. Instead, he reported, "it was like worker bees!" Dorothy Knight, Gunn's assistant, served as the "runner," dodging white-coated lab techs and scientists in the corridors of the agency's several buildings as she carried blood samples from lab to lab. "The blood is drawn in the sperm bank in Building Four," Knight said. "Then I have to go to Building Fifteen. They need the blood right away—I get it there within five minutes. They're poised—they're ready and waiting. Then I go to Building One, then Four, then Seven—I have to go to three different floors in Building Seven. All this must be done right away. It's done in less than twenty minutes—because you're movin'!"

At Gunn's insistence, Knight wore rubber gloves. "I wear a single layer," Knight said, "but thick—very, very thick."

When Gunn introduced Larry Schonberger to a lab tech who was working with the CFS blood samples, the lab tech reached out to shake Schonberger's hand. Upon taking her hand, Schonberger seemed to recoil in fear when he realized she was wearing gloves. "That's okay, Larry," Gunn quipped. "It's all psychological, isn't it?"

The agency planned to follow the same routine every Monday for the next twenty weeks, when they would have a total of twenty controls and twenty cases. The final data, Gunn anticipated, would be ready by June. "This is a really dangerous field," Gunn confided that mouth. "And I'm taking a lot of flak for my involvement. But it's always in the back of my mind that it's only seven months until the case-control data come in. Then let the chips fall where they may."

Agency scientists were ignoring just one problem: What if the controls—who were, after all, either friends or neighbors of the patients—were also infected with the retrovirus? "Gary [Holmes] wrote the original protocol for the study a long time ago," Gunn recalled later. "He was trying to get *easy* controls—friends and neighbors. But if you believe the Wistar data, you don't want controls who have that kind of contact with the patients. But nobody *here* really believed that data. They said, 'That's ridiculous,' because they didn't believe the disease was infectious!"

Retrovirology chief Tom Folks seemed to be the only CDC scientist to share Gunn's concern about the potentially exposed controls. Even Folks, however, was insufficiently concerned about the problem to demand that the agency set about finding new, unexposed controls.

University of Southern California, Los Angeles

In December a San Fernando Valley infectious disease specialist referred to pathologist John Martin an encephalopathic patient whose case had turned into a legal imbroglio. When the patient's doctors began to suspect the nineteen-year-old was suffering from herpes encephalitis, they started him on intravenous acyclovir, the only treatment for the devastating, usually fatal disease, but by then it was too late; the patient survived but he sustained tremendous brain damage. Martin was asked to help clarify the diagnostic dilemma.

In his laboratory at USC, Martin studied samples of the boy's cerebrospinal fluid using a test designed to detect herpesviruses. He observed an extremely strong positive signal for virus. Curiously, however, the specific virus did not appear to be herpes simplex, the cause of the rare encephalitis for which his doctors, some insisted, had belatedly treated him.

By the end of the year, Martin had collected a number of atypical encephalopathy cases that he suspected might bear some relationship to the CFS epidemic. Two of them were adults: a grade-school teacher from Palm Springs who had suddenly developed bizarre spelling and language problems in 1989, and a counselor in a doctor's practice who had fallen ill in July 1990 with presumed meningitis but had been released from the hospital after seven days, only to develop classic CFS in the following weeks. From the blood of these patients he began to develop cell cultures in which he was able to cause the mysterious virus to reproduce.

Wistar Institute, Philadelphia, Pennsylvania

For two and a half years DeFreitas had been afforded the luxury of a secret collaboration. Now, having relinquished her anonymity, she assumed that the NIH, 88 percent of whose annual research budget was funneled to independent scientists, would provide her with funds to pursue her work, thus freeing her from her reliance upon small monthly sums from patient charities. The agency had, after all, funded 100 percent of her research in multiple sclerosis and cutaneous T-cell lymphoma, neither of which appeared to be as widespread as CFS. Her eagerness for that funding was such that a week after Kyoto, she and Hilary Koprowski wrote Ann Schleuderberg to alert her that Wistar intended to submit a grant proposal.

Not long after the Charlotte conference, however, DeFreitas learned that her work had been discussed in a derogatory fashion by an NIH scientist during a meeting of the recently formed CFS Advisory Council, a development DeFreitas believed constituted a damaging bias against her within the Bethesda agency, especially since Ann Schleuderberg had been present at the meeting. Along with Schleuderberg, council members Anthony Komaroff, Paul Cheney, Ed Taylor, Paul Levine, and a handful of others, had listened while Stephen Straus's collaborator, Steven Jacobson, a neuroimmunologist from the National Institute of Neurological Disorders and Stroke, made his damning comments. At Straus's request, shortly after DeFreitas's annoucement in Kyoto, Jacobson tested twenty patient samples for HTLV1 and HTLV2, with negative results.

"What went on behind that closed door session was an absolute scandal," the hot-tempered DeFreitas said later. "Steve Jacobson actually said that our Swedish collaborator on the multiple sclerosis paper had spiked the patient samples with HTLV-one!" Jacobson, in addition, seemed to question DeFreitas's slides of her western blot assays for retrovirus antibodies in CFS. Cheney, who realized Jacobson was coming perilously close to accusing DeFreitas of scientific fraud, stepped into the fray in his collaborator's defense.

"Ann Schleuderberg was in that room," DeFreitas continued, "and afterward she came up to Jacobson and asked him to be on the study section—the retrovirus section that would review our grant! This was an absolutely premeditated attempt to sink this grant!"

DeFreitas was beside herself, as was her boss, Hilary Koprowski, when she described the meeting to him. "[Koprowski] called Jacobson's boss at the National Institutes of Health and asked to have Jacobson fired," DeFreitas said. "I thought Koprowski was going to have a heart attack."*

DeFreitas's real concern was not Jacobson, however, but Schleuderberg, who, in DeFreitas's view, had grossly overstepped her role.

"Schleuderberg is not the person who should be making these decisions about the composition of the study groups," DeFreitas added. "They are supposed to consider grants prima facie. It should be a panel of your peers! I can think of six retrovirologists around the country I would like to propose to review our grant, and Steve Jacobson would not be among them.

"But if they don't get me on the retrovirology, they'll get me on the diagnosis," she said after a moment, in a reference to her affiliation with Cheney and Bell—

---

* Jacobson, when queried about the incident some years later, recalled that Schleuderberg had asked him to "assess the data somewhat objectively. I said DeFreitas's [retroviral gene fragments] needed to be verified and sequenced. I think Elaine is a very conscientious scientist," he added. "I always have. Her work is valid and it should be followed up on."

an affiliation that Schleuderberg had warned her would destroy her prospects for being funded. "David and Paul are being punished, for the very reason that they are bright and they recognized the disease."

DeFreitas ruminated for a minute about the possibility of walking away from CFS and turning full-time to cutaneous T-cell lymphoma instead. Fewer than five hundred people in the country suffered from the rare disease. "I can get all the money I want to study it," DeFreitas said. In fact, she had no fewer than three NIH grants to pursue her investigations of cutaneous T-cell lymphoma.

DeFreitas was unable to abandon her CFS project, however, perhaps against her better judgment. "I made a pledge with myself that as soon as I didn't believe it anymore, I would walk away from it. Until that evaporates, I can't walk away. It would be like walking away from my child."

Centers for Disease Control, Atlanta, Georgia

In early December, Gary Holmes worked his last day at the CDC. His colleagues along the rambunctious corridor presided over by Larry Schonberger held a party for the ungainly Texan who would soon return with his wife and young children to his home state. The festivity had a muted quality. Holmes's tenure had been marked by perhaps one of the most controversial public health issues in the agency's history, and the unprepared Holmes had found himself at the torrential center of the controversy, a position he had never sought. While others around him had been rewarded for their efforts with promotions, Holmes had languished with just two publications in five years to his credit, both of them having to do with the greatly disdained disease. That his name would be forever attached to the government's definition of CFS, as in "the Holmes criteria," had failed to enhance his position with his superiors.

According to Walter Gunn, who was among those present at Holmes's farewell party, Jon Kaplan stood to give a farewell speech. "You should have heard it," Gunn said. "After five years, all Jon said was the following: 'I worked with Gary for five years. The first time I went out with him, it was to Tahoe—and it was bizarre. The patients were bizarre. The doctors were bizarre. The whole situation was bizarre.' And that's all he said, and then he sat down!"

Charlotte, North Carolina

On December 6, Walter Gunn and Dave Connell of Abt Associates flew to Charlotte to discuss Paul Cheney's diagnostic criteria with the doctor. Gunn had been quietly impressed at the Charlotte summit by Cheney's concern about the agency's criteria for selecting patients. The doctor's anxiety, Gunn reasoned, was legitimate: the CDC's attempt to reproduce the Wistar results likely would fail unless the patients undergoing the test at the agency were selected using the same criteria Cheney and David Bell had used to select Elaine DeFreitas's test subjects. Gunn's move, too, reflected his perceptual evolution in matters relating to the disease. He was increasingly cognizant that investigators like Cheney, Bell, and others outside the agency knew more about the disease than his colleagues inside the agency.

During their half-day conference, Gunn's intuition about the doctor was confirmed: it was clear to both Gunn and Connell that Cheney had a greatly more complex and subtle means of evaluating the disease than did the CDC. In the years since Tahoe, Cheney had learned to stage the disease much the way other severe and progressive diseases are medically staged. Cheney was not terribly interested in a patient's degree of fatigue. He graded the disease, instead, by its progressive phases, which he believed began with a mononucleosis-like illness and an "up-regulated," or hyperactive, immune system. Then, over the years, it progressed to a neurologic, multiple sclerosis–like illness, with mild to severe dementia and an AIDS-like, or down-regulated, immune system. And because DeFreitas was looking for retroviruses, known drivers of chronic neurological disease, Cheney selected his Wistar patients based on their neurological signs and symptoms. All of this was a departure from the CDC's criteria, which essentially looked for one thing—disabling, un-explained fatigue—and excluded patients who exhibited unambiguous signs of disease.

Gunn's faith in Cheney was further enhanced when the clinician began to dis-cuss the fingerprint phenomenon. Gunn had heard the doctor talk about his pa-tients' lost fingerprints at the Charlotte conference, and he had witnessed his own colleagues in Atlanta scoffing at the notion.

"The people at CDC found this hysterically funny," Gunn recalled later. "But when I sat down with Cheney, he showed me photographs of the fingerprints as well as a number of fingerprint charts that had been created at the local sheriff's department, and by God, they're gone! Thirty percent of his patients had lost fin-gerprints. Now, people at CDC will sit and pontificate about this stuff for years and never bother to look at the evidence."

Malibu, California

On December 16, the microbe hunters became Hollywood's pitchmen for the evening. Would the Dream Factory back a production called *Cell Wars*?

Blake Edwards and Julie Andrews's house was on a high bluff overlooking the Pacific Ocean. That evening their cathedral-sized dining hall, a separate room constructed nearest the cliffs, was filled with linen-draped tables. Ap-proximately forty guests stood in small groups around the room as uniformed waiters served drinks. Most of those present were middle-level Hollywood, a majority of them friends that Edwards had acquired during his thirty-year career in the film industry. Nearly everyone in the room suffered from CFS, or was close to someone who did. There were agents, a few actors, screenwriters, pro-ducers, and production people. Only one industry heavyweight, Mike Medavoy, chairman of Tri-Star Pictures, attended; clad in jeans, he was escorting his wife, Patricia, who had been hit with the disease the year before. Edwards himself be-gan the evening at the far end of the room near the sea, just outside the French doors that were opened onto a tiled floor cut into the smooth grass. In the cen-ter of the tile, a gas-fueled flame rose a foot into the air from a round pit. Ed-wards stood near the flame as it warmed the air, his narrow, handsome face overtanned. His featherweight handshake and bloodshot eyes communicated a profound world-weariness.

Edwards had invited a number of Hollywood celebrities to the event, among them his friends James Garner and Mrs. Garner, both of whom were sick, as well as Cher and Morgan Fairchild. The actresses and Garners were no-shows. Instead, Herb Tanney, Edwards' and James Garner's doctor who was the first to diagnose them with the disease, attended, as did a handful of interested internists from Los Angeles. Minnesota governor Rudy Perpich and his wife, Lola, flew from the Midwest to attend. Jan Montgomery was there from San Francisco representing the CFIDS Foundation, the nonprofit organization she had helped found the year before. Hilary Koprowski, Anthony Komaroff, and Max Palevsky dined at a table for four with Julie Andrews.

After dinner, Marc Iverson stood before the draped tables and made the first pitch. "This gathering could not be more timely," Iverson—who seemed ready to faint—began. He briefly described the Wistar discovery, adding, "The federal government's response to this disease is just disgraceful. The Centers for Disease Control are now playing catch-up, but at the National Institute of Allergy and Infectious Diseases, more than a third of all calls coming into that institution are from people with CFIDS. Even so, their budget for this disease, for 1991, is approximately $500,000. We can't wait for the National Institute of Allergy and Infectious Diseases to catch up. Too many lives are being erased. We need everyone who has this disease, or cares about someone with this disease, to help."

The scientists, used to addressing other scientists, were palpably nervous, and a little giddy. As Komaroff began his talk, he joked that this was the first time he had flown three thousand miles for dinner. DeFreitas and Cheney, in turn, described their detective work. DeFreitas explained that for two years the research that led to the discovery of the retrovirus in CFS had been supported by patients. Paul Thompson, of Incline Village, and Marc Iverson's association, had paid the salaries of her postdocs, who performed the expensive assays on hundreds of CFS patients, she explained. Cheney projected slides of the retrovirus in human lymphocytes on a screen that stood in front of the glass wall overlooking the ocean. Outside, soft lights could be seen lining thirty miles of coastline.

Koprowski alone seemed utterly at home in the role of explaining retrovirology to Julie Andrews and Mike Medavoy. His mind was on the dollar, however, as he focused his audience's attention on Wistar's potential role in creating a diagnostic test for the virus causing the disease. He began by reminding the Hollywood audience of the polio epidemic fifty years ago: "We are dealing today with a different type of virology," he said. "Retroviruses are weak viruses. They cannot destroy the cells of the host, so they do not remain as a complete virus; they break apart. This is why this is such a sly and difficult virus to study. We have to use very different tools. It is very difficult, and the average practitioner cannot produce a sophisticated kit for chronic fatigue syndrome diagnosis. It is very expensive. Treatment, too, is very difficult, because you actually have to enter the cell to prevent damage. . . .

"I come now to one of the most important aspects of chronic fatigue syndrome. We need money. It is not sufficient to pressure the government to support chronic fatigue syndrome research. Propaganda is not enough. We have five, six, eight, or ten million people with chronic fatigue syndrome. *That* will convince the government. This disease is as important as AIDS. It doesn't kill, but it immobilizes millions of people for years, perhaps for life.

"We need to convince the federal government to do what Nixon did in 1973—he funded the National Cancer Act. George Bush must be convinced that chronic neurological disease is as important as cancer. We need to put pressure on the government to give money for research—not small grants from National Institute of Allergy and Infectious Diseases or the Centers for Disease Control, but big grants, comparable to the war on cancer."

After Rock Hudson's death from AIDS, members of the rich and celebrated Hollywood community participated in lavish fund-raising galas and donned red ribbons for the TV cameras at the Academy Awards. Mirroring the indifference of the larger society, however, Hollywood was apparently unwilling or unprepared to finance research into a second new infectious disease of immune dysfunction. The fond hopes of Hilary Koprowski and other researchers who had come to Malibu in search of cash were crushed when it became apparent, some weeks later, that none of Edwards's guests had chosen to contribute money to their cause.

Wistar Institute, Philadelphia, Pennsylvania

By year's end, Elaine DeFreitas and her lab associates, using polymerase chain reaction, had been able to study fourteen-year-old Skye Dailor's liver and spleen for evidence of retroviral sequences. All of the samples were positive for the Wistar retroviral fragments, DeFreitas reported. As with seemingly every aspect of her difficult investigation, however, there was a caveat: "Liver and spleen have blood in them, so one could argue that the signal is coming from blood instead of the organ itself, which I can't disprove. The signal could be coming from the blood that's sitting in the tissue. The only thing that would argue against that is if we find a negative organ. Because blood is everywhere. And so if an organ turns out to be negative, then we can say the virus is organ-specific."

Of course, the most pressing question was whether this virus made its way into the brain. That question had gone unanswered until now because brain samples from CFS sufferers were next to impossible to come by. DeFreitas had not yet examined the teenager's brain sample for the infection, nor had she tested a second brain sample that had been sent to her by Byron Hyde. The Ottawa clinician had obtained the brain sample at the autopsy of one of his CFS patients who, like Dailor, had committed suicide.

"We haven't looked at either piece of brain," DeFreitas explained, "because we have such a small piece of both that we want to wait until we have primers and probes that are *very* specific for this agent and will not cross-react with HTLV-two. When we do use those samples, we have to be sure we'll be getting the longest slide for the shortest run."

DeFreitas had found novel retrovirus particles in semen from two of Paul Cheney's patients, however, a discovery which, if duplicated by other scientists, would suggest that an infected man could transmit the pathogen to a partner during sex.

Harvard School of Medicine, Boston, Massachusetts

Just before Christmas, the *New England Journal of Medicine* rejected Anthony Komaroff's Tahoe manuscript for the third time in three years. According to Paul Cheney, the comments from the reviewers were "horrendous." Cheney found it difficult to believe that, after the announcement of the retrovirus findings in September, followed by a seven-page cover story in *Newsweek* portraying the disease as a chronic brain infection of two to five million Americans, the Boston medical journal could turn the Tahoe manuscript down yet another time. Normally, reviewers' identities were protected by the publication's editors, but Canadian Byron Hyde had been told by someone he deemed to be reliable that Stephen Straus, along with the Salk Institute's Alexis Shelokov, who had collaborated on studies of "epidemic neuromyasthenia" published in the *New England Journal* in 1959, were two of three reviewers.

After his initial shock, Cheney seemed resigned to the rejection that winter. "It's interesting, despite the fact that the paper's never been published, how much of the Tahoe epidemic is in people's *minds,*" the doctor said. "It's out there. It's just that the whole story has yet to be told."

Other researchers were less sanguine. Byron Hyde fulminated against the *New England Journal* in his newsletter the following summer. Hyde left little doubt that he blamed Straus, in particular, for the Tahoe manuscript's ill fortune. He wrote:

> Why was it rejected? . . . At the *New England Journal,* there were three supposedly secret external examiners for this paper. I believe I know two of the three. . . . The paper was refused by one examiner simply because, as far as I can judge, this unfortunate reviewer had spent five years of his life looking at [chronic fatigue syndrome] from the wrong perspective. After his own work was discredited it was difficult for him to judge anyone else's work objectively. He just turned around and kicked the disease, a bit like kicking the cat after a bad day at the office. . . . Suppression of this important work constituted a major error of judgment and has delayed recognition of some of the important diagnostic features of [CFS].

Hyde also railed against the scientific literary establishment in general for what he believed was its tendency to give greater credence to negative studies that set out to disprove the existence of the disease than to studies that proved the opposite, even though the negative studies typically had serious scientific flaws. "In the fear of making an error, many editors will not comment positively on subjects that have not gained wide public acceptability. Many editors are so apprehensive that they believe that if they publish a serious article on [CFS], their friends and colleagues will ridicule them. However, they *do* accept negative papers that are not well researched and are not based upon the careful examination of [CFS] patients. Are these editors simply following the time-honoured tradition of ridiculing the less fortunate?"

1991
BLACK
DIAMONDS

One of the most striking contributions of Hippocrates is the recognition that diseases are only part of the processes of nature, that there is nothing divine or sacred about them. . . . [H]e remarks that each disease has its own nature, and that no one arises without a natural cause.

—Sir William Osler, *The Evolution of Modern Medicine*

24

Malfeasance and Nonfeasance

Centers for Disease Control, Atlanta Georgia

Staff at the CDC were the recipients each year of more than 170,000 blood samples from all over the world, most of which were host to organisms requiring identification. Over the years, a system had emerged to grade organisms by virtue of the risk they posed to the people who worked with them. Biosafety levels corresponded with a rigid scheme of containment and safety measures. Organisms without apparent ability to cause disease rated a biosafety level of one. "Moderate-risk" pathogens, like cold viruses and diarrhea-inducing bacteria, earned a biosafety level of two. Bugs that caused serious disease, but for which effective vaccines or antibiotics existed, like rabies virus and the rickettsial pathogen responsible for Rocky Mountain spotted fever, were rated level three. Level-four organisms, according to one agency definition, were those that "pose a high risk of life-threatening disease" and for which vaccines and antibiotics were nonexistent. They included the hemorrhagic fever viruses discovered in 1969. Members of this grisly genus bore evocative names like Marburg, Ebola, Lassa, Junin, Congo-Crimean, and Machupo, but their toll was deadly, and not only in the Third World. Because of what epidemiologists call "jet spread," exotic ailments were being imported to industrialized countries with increasing frequency.* Perhaps surprisingly, HIV was frequently handled as a level-two organism in many labs in the agency. A dab of Clorox was enough to kill a fragile retrovirus like HIV a thousand times over, nor could it be transmitted through the air; HIV was not a hardy virus. Wherever lab technicians grew and manipulated large quantities of HIV, however, the laboratory's biosafety level was bumped up to three.

Level-four viruses landed in Building 15, the newest addition to the agency's infrastructure. The $20 million edifice housed a state-of-the-art maximum-containment laboratory, one of two in the nation and a monument to the lavish federal money that began to flow to Atlanta once AIDS was perceived as an epi-

---

* In February 1989 a Chicagoan who had recently been in Africa died of Lassa fever, the first known case in the United States. His physician failed to identify the disease before it advanced to an untreatable state.

444

demic threat.* Within its six stories, three of them underground, microbiologists in biosafety-level-four laboratories wore pressurized space suits and inhaled oxygen piped to them from steel tanks. They entered labs through air-lock chambers; the doors were secured with pneumatic rubber seals. Inside, they observed their deadly menagerie in negative-air-pressure biological safety cabinets. Upon exiting a lab, researchers showered, and their space suits were decontaminated; the building's incoming air was filtered once; its outgoing air was filtered twice. Most of the agency's AIDS laboratories relocated to Building 15 when its biosafety-level-three labs opened in late 1988. The colossal scientific prestige of the disease was such that its researchers could lay claim to more and better space without argument.

Tom Folks, the youthful-looking chief of the Retrovirus Diseases Branch, ruled the second of the three aboveground floors of Building 15. The laboratories where Folks and his staff of thirty worked were rated at a biosafety level of three. Folks's branch existed for the purpose of studying non-AIDS human retroviruses, specifically the human retroviruses HTLV1 and HTLV2. Its offices ran along the structure's periphery; laboratories occupied the center. The latter consisted of an enclosed anteroom that led to any of four smaller rooms, or containment labs. Scientists and lab techs donned their gowns and gloves in the anteroom before entering the containment labs; they de-gloved and de-gowned there upon departing. Although Building 15 had been in use for only three years, Folks's staff was already overpopulating their state-of-the-art space; by 1991, desks and chairs had been set up in the corridors, part of the overflow from cramped offices.

Walter Gunn had requested that David Bell send blood samples from Lyndonville children who had been repeatedly positive on Elaine DeFreitas's tests. In theory, this first step would allow Folks and his staff to fine-tune their tests to match DeFreitas's in both sensitivity and specificity; afterward they would test for the agent in a mix of unidentified samples from controls and cases. On January 4, in anticipation of the arrival of the blood from Lyndonville, Gunn went to Folks's fiefdom to discuss his concerns about contamination. Gunn knew Folks to be a professional who would respect the biosafety-level-three protocol appropriate to the disease, but he was concerned that the years of jokes and asides at the agency about CFS might induce laxity among retrovirology staff members, who would underestimate the risks. "I was worried because of the positive [exposed] controls among David Bell's kids and the fact that of two positive [exposed] controls of a prominent researcher, one had become ill," Gunn said. (In the latter case, Gunn was referring to a nurse in Paul Cheney's practice who had become disabled by the disease four months after accidentally pricking her finger with a contaminated needle.) "I recommended to *everyone* that masks and goggles be used by all lab techs working on the CFS study."

Though uncertain whether he had successfully conveyed the seriousness of the situation to anyone, Gunn was satisfied that he had done his best. A week later, during the second week in January, the Lyndonville blood arrived. Bell had cho-

---

* A second, older germ fortress was operated by military scientists at Fort Diedrich, Maryland. There were just three other "maximum containment" labs in the world, located in Australia, South Africa, and Japan.

sen children who were now thirteen and fourteen, but they had been eight and nine when they fell ill. Soon after the samples arrived, Folks posted a sign on one of the laboratory doors leading to a series of containment rooms. It read: "This room is for chronic fatigue syndrome isolation work only."

Folks's crew had drawn from the world of sports to name each of the containment cubicles off the anterooms—"Super Bowl," "World Series," and "Wimbledon" were typical. "It was a little government-ish to call them by their numbers," Tom Folks explained that winter as he showed a visitor around. The tiny containment lab where a bench researcher prepared the children's blood for study was called Black Diamonds—formerly 210–2101-D. Black Diamonds was the international rating for the steepest, most difficult ski runs in the world.

National Institute of Allergy and Infectious Diseases, Bethesda, Maryland

On January 10, the *Medical Tribune,* a clinician-oriented journal with a circulation of 130,000, published an article about the accelerated pace of CFS research, citing the launch of the Ampligen clinical trials and Jay Levy's immunological research. Stephen Straus, who was interviewed by reporter John Carpi, predicted that the coming year would result in "a lot of anecdotal information bombarding patients and physicians, only a fraction of which will prove to be valid and not misleading."

University of California, San Francisco

By the new year, microbiologist Jay Levy had learned that his grant proposal to the NIH—the one that he had begun writing the day after Elaine DeFreitas made her retrovirus announcement in Kyoto—had been turned down by Ann Schleuderberg's government panel. "They felt we could not prove that the individuals in our proposed study group had CFIDS," Levy said. "It's a Catch-Twenty-two," he added, pointing out that unassailable scientific certainty about diagnosis would exist only when the causative agent of the disease was identified and could be found in every sufferer's blood. In his grant request, Levy had proposed to search for that agent in patients who had demonstrated the aberrant immunological markers he and his collaborators had identified the year before. Further, unlike members of the NIH study section who reviewed his grant, Levy was confident that his collaborating clinician, internist Carol Jessop, who had more than 1,500 sufferers in her practice, knew a case when she saw one.

Like other grant applicants before him, notably Seymour Grufferman, Levy vented his frustration with NIH officials. "I got angry," Levy said. "I told them that it will take two and a half million dollars to *prove* to them that these patients have chronic fatigue syndrome, because you need a good clinical trial with controls." In the end, however, Levy concluded, "We aren't happy about the proposal's rejection, but there's nothing we can do about it."

Levy returned full-time to his AIDS research.

National Cancer Institute, Bethesda, Maryland

In January, Seymour Grufferman, at the invitation of the National Cancer Institute's Paul Levine, described the history of his investigations of the North Carolina Symphony and the Chillicothe, Ohio, elementary school to approximately thirty scientists in the Division of Cancer Etiology, a branch of the NCI. The Pittsburgh epidemiologist spoke for nearly two hours. His audience included the administrator of the perpetually becalmed CFS grant program, Ann Schleuderberg.

Levine had asked Grufferman to describe his cluster investigations as well as to talk about the preliminary results of the retrovirus investigation undertaken by William Blattner, the viral epidemiology branch chief of the Division of Cancer Etiology. By the new year, Blattner had completed his analysis of blood samples from both of Grufferman's cluster populations. Afterward, Grufferman confirmed, "We have some very puzzling results that may implicate a novel retrovirus." According to Grufferman, 20 to 30 percent of the people in each cluster had suggestive evidence of a retrovirus infection; researchers had used probes for both HTLV1 and HTLV2 to test for the presence of retrovirus.*

Grufferman was delighted by the response from National Cancer Institute scientists who gathered to hear him talk. He seized the opportunity to propose a study to evaluate the risk of cancer in two thousand CFS sufferers and their families. He would do so, he explained, by surveying the patients in a collection of what Grufferman called "mainstream" CFS practices, which would include Anthony Komaroff's general medicine clinic at the Brigham, James Jones's clinic in Denver, Dedra Buchwald's clinic at the University of Washington, and of course, Stephen Straus's patient cohort in Bethesda. He would also survey patients being referred into the CDC's surveillance system. Most of those present, Grufferman recalled, evinced enthusiasm for the cancer study. Afterward, relieved to have had his day in court, the epidemiologist attributed his hosts' nonpartisan interest to what he viewed as the intrinsically superior scientific acumen of the National Cancer Institute investigators as compared to those at NIAID. "These are real scientists," he commented.

Grufferman planned to try once more to obtain a federal grant to support the cancer study. "I've been told by my sources at the NIH that it will be very difficult, very chancy," Grufferman said. "But we're going to take our patients from Komaroff, Straus, and Jones. We'll go with the mainstream investigators."

Like everyone else in the field, Grufferman had heard that the NIH had rejected Jay Levy's proposal to search for the cause of CFS. "To drive Jay Levy from this field is criminal," Grufferman commented. "I suspect he's sorry he ever got involved. But the mainstream scientists are being scared away from this, and we're left with amateur researchers. . . . The only thing that will really change this will be the identification of the virus. Then we will see what in essence was a conspir-

---

* Blattner, queried about the results some time later, said, "There might have been some western blots that had stray bands that were positive, but it was not our perception that there was anything suggestive of HTLV2 infection. I pointed out to Seymour that if he wanted to pursue this from Elaine DeFreitas's approach, which was molecular, he should contact her." (DeFreitas, of course, had long since moved on from looking for antibodies using western blot to the more specific polymerase chain reaction.)

acy by very rigid people who didn't have the imagination to believe this disease exists. They didn't *decide* to do this. It wasn't people sitting around a table," Grufferman added. "It's been institutional sabotage in the broadest sense."

Centers for Disease Control, Atlanta, Georgia

By January 1991, Walter Gunn had taken himself off every other project at the CDC. For the first time ever, the agency had someone working full-time on CFS. Within weeks, however, he was running into serious problems with the Atlanta-based case-control study. Several patients had been unable to keep their appointments for a blood draw at the agency because they were too ill to come in on the appointed day. "It's been catch as catch can," Gunn said. He was disappointed, too, that DeFreitas had yet to reveal her DNA probes and gene sequences to Tom Folks. DeFreitas was following the orders of Hilary Koprowski, who advised her to wait until the *Proceedings of the National Academy of Sciences* alerted her to whether and when her article would appear.

Also that winter, the intellectual conflicts between Gunn and his colleagues were becoming increasingly sharp. The investigator's self-restraint began unraveling during a January 14 meeting with his supervisor, Larry Schonberger, and the CDC's second-in-command, Walter Dowdle.

Dowdle, a small, energetic white-haired man of sixty-one, listened as Gunn vociferously disagreed with Schonberger about the essential nature of the disease. Schonberger, Gunn recalled later, had just said to Dowdle, "This disease is overblown—these people are all crazy. Schonberger said he thought CFS was just depressed people—complainers," Gunn added. "And I said, 'I have to disagree. We're not getting any evidence of that.' " When Dowdle evinced interest in his comments, Gunn jumped at the opportunity to elaborate. He explained that the surveillance data suggested that, prior to the onset of their disease, CFS victims lacked evidence for any higher incidence of psychiatric problems than the general population. Gunn further explained that the psychological profiles of CFS patients closely resembled those of people suffering from multiple sclerosis and other debilitating chronic diseases; more significantly, their psychological profiles failed to resemble those of people suffering exclusively from depression.

As Dowdle pressed Gunn for more details, conversation among the three segued into the discrepancies between the annual sums Congress was appropriating to the agency to investigate the disease and the money Gunn had been able to shake loose from Brian Mahy, the director of the viral diseases division, to finance his studies. Mahy had told Gunn the money simply "wasn't there," suggesting that other divisions and branches within the agency were cutting slices from the pie.

"It was at that meeting that it came up for the first time with Dowdle that our division wasn't getting all the chronic fatigue syndrome money," Gunn said. "Schonberger and I knew there was money at the CDC—money that was earmarked for chronic fatigue syndrome—that wasn't coming to us."

Schonberger, for once, appeared to take Gunn's side. "We told Dowdle, 'We are the people in the trenches—we're doing the research. Why aren't *we* getting the money?' " Gunn said.

Gunn was encouraged by Dowdle's apparent responsiveness, although he was loath to reveal the full extent of his suspicions in Schonberger's presence. He felt certain that someone in his branch or division was quietly and irrevocably diverting money meant for CFS research to extraneous agency projects, but he doubted his concern would get a fair hearing within his own corner of the agency. He would have to go outside the division and higher up.

The next day, Gunn returned to Dowdle's office for a second meeting, this time without Schonberger. For nearly two years he had watched and listened as his colleagues ridiculed CFS, its victims, and the doctors who took their complaints seriously. He arrived in Dowdle's office driven by a sense of mission. "I knew it was a huge personal risk to take this to Dowdle," Gunn remembered later.

If his accusations led to his dismissal, he would lose his retirement pension and medical insurance for his wife, who had been battling cancer for eight years. However, closeted with Dowdle, the senior researcher skipped pleasantries: "I told Dowdle that I suspected there was gross misappropriation of money going on. I told him I couldn't live with it.'"

By Gunn's report, the administrator responded evenhandedly. Dowdle replied that he had been intending for some time to "look into the money situation" because he had been troubled by the agency's slow progress.

"Dowdle said he had watched two million dollars come into the agency for the disease, and yet all we had going was this little surveillance program," Gunn said. "He wasn't buying Schonberger's argument about the disease. He said, 'I think this is a very serious illness, and it needs to be studied seriously.' I said, 'What kind of progress do you expect? We're not getting enough money.'"

Near the end of their conversation, Gunn expressed his fear that, having relayed his suspicions about misappropriation of funds to an administrator outside his own division, he would be shut out of his division's activities or fired. The agency's second-in-command reassured Gunn: "Dowdle said, 'Oh, no, don't worry about that.' He promised he would 'investigate,' and he told me to—quote—'hang in there.' He said, 'I'll check it out.'"

Gunn had long admired Dowdle. "[He] was the most outstanding public administrator I've ever known," Gunn said some time later. Nevertheless, four days later Gunn was taken aside by Larry Schonberger, who told him he had learned that Dowdle had placed a call to Carmine Bozzi, the assistant director for management of the Center for Infectious Diseases, the largest center at the agency and the parent center to Gunn's division. According to Schonberger, Dowdle had expressed to Bozzi his belief that neither Gunn nor Schonberger should be functioning as press spokesperson or principal investigator for CFS. For some days, Gunn's future as principal investigator remained in limbo.

"Schonberger balked," Gunn recalled. "He asked Bozzi and Dowdle to wait a week on any decision."

Gunn was particularly unnerved by the news that Dowdle had sought Carmine Bozzi's counsel on the subject of the CFS appropriations. "I'll bet Dowdle said, 'Make sure you can account for every damn penny,'" Gunn said later. In fact, Gunn had begun to suspect that Bozzi might be part of the problem.

Carmine Bozzi was a career bureaucrat with a master's degree in public health. When it came to CFS, he was a shadowy figure at the agency, unlikely to be consulted on the subject by either journalists or scientists. Among other duties, he played a powerful role in the management of the division's finances. By virtue of his post, Bozzi (who declined an interview request) had been monitoring the flow of CFS money into the agency since 1988, the first year Congress was awarded such funds. In December 1988, for instance, when Illinois congressman John Porter wrote to agency head James Mason to inquire specifically about the agency's use of the funds, Bozzi had prepared the agency's response, which was sent out over agency chief James Mason's signature. Typical of the letters being drafted by the federal health agencies in response to congressional inquiries on the controversial disease, Bozzi's letter was marked by hyperbole and half-truths.

"We are conducting case-control studies to . . . evaluate the role of potential etiologic agents," Bozzi wrote, even though the agency was then more than three years away from such studies. "[We] intend to expand the surveillance . . . by adding additional sites," he went on. There existed no such intention, in spite of a 1987 congressional mandate to perform *national* surveillance; indeed, the agency had to be strong-armed by Congress into adding Reno to its three-city surveillance that year, and in 1993, six years later, the agency had not expanded its surveillance beyond the original four sites, nor did it have plans to do so.

"We also plan to investigate clusters of CFS in order to delineate the illness," Bozzi continued. The agency had no such plan, however—again in defiance of a congressional mandate to investigate clusters. In fact, the Division of Viral and Rickettsial Diseases had an unofficial policy to avoid such investigations. Until 1993, eight years after the Tahoe outbreak, the division's epidemiologists failed to undertake *any* full-scale investigations of clusters despite the scores that were reported to them by medical professionals and citizens in the intervening years.

Bozzi avoided linking any of these putative projects with dollar sums in his letter to the congressman. Significantly, however, he revealed to Porter that equipment was being purchased for agency laboratories with CFS funds. To some extent, then, Bozzi's revelation clarified the uses to which the money was being applied. He wrote: "Much needed laboratory equipment is being purchased in order to support the increased laboratory studies focused on the development of better diagnostic tests and techniques."

Until a modest case-control study was started late in 1990, the agency was doing nothing in its laboratories to investigate *any* aspect of CFS, much less working to develop either "diagnostic tests" or "techniques."* Yet, by Bozzi's account, agency scientists were using the appropriated funds to buy lab equipment. How, then, could these purchases be justified? Despite repeated assertions by agency scientists, beginning in 1988 and in years to come, that CFS was extremely unlikely to be caused by or related in any significant way to the newly discovered herpesvirus, HHV6, it appears likely that at least some CFS funds were being used to help cash-starved laboratories in the Atlanta complex pursue their HHV6 investigations. A multitude of "initiatives" generated by agency scientists at the

---

* In addition, three months after it began, the tardy effort to conduct a case-control study was halted after only a few samples were obtained.

time repeatedly, and disingenuously, linked CFS with the new virus when proposing expensive schemes for studying HHV6. In fact, there was and remains a far greater scientific curiosity about the role of HHV6 in AIDS.

Tracking the flow of federal dollars into a bureaucracy-laden research agency like the CDC was a formidable undertaking, as Walter Gunn was learning that year. Others had tried from outside the agency—notably advocates like CFS lobbyists Barry Sleight and Ted Van Zelst—and failed. Even congressional staff had found the effort daunting. The same year Congressman John Porter sought the information from Carmine Bozzi, Senator Claiborne Pell's administrative aide, Lauren Gross, had tried to extract figures from both the NIH and the CDC. Gross had been similarly thwarted and, in fact, had concluded, "There's really no way of being absolutely positive what the numbers are."

From inside, Gunn was equally stymied in his effort to understand exactly how or by whom the money was being siphoned from its true target. "The way the money works at the Centers for Disease Control," Gunn explained that year, "is that Congress can send money to the agency marked for a certain disease. The agency itself can take twenty percent right off the top for overhead—that's legal. The Center for Infectious Diseases [of which the Division of Viral and Rickettsial Diseases was a part] takes another twelve to eighteen percent for overhead. After that, the money gets very fuzzy."

Short of a congressional investigation of the problem, the best that might be done was to measure what the agency charged to its CFS fund against its progress in the disease.

By the time the fiscal year 1989 congressional allocation—$1.2 million—filtered down to the Division of Viral and Rickettsial Diseases in fall of 1988, for instance, it was, according to agency documents, $740,759. (Nearly $445,000 had been removed from the original sum by administrative branches of the agency for "overhead" costs.) The agency paid about half of that sum—$375,493—to Abt Associates in 1989 to continue the four-city surveillance program.*

A more surprising expenditure was charged off to the fund that year as well: $275,421 worth of laboratory supplies. When Walter Gunn was apprised of the supplies expenditure some years later, he responded, "What the hell was *that* for? We didn't do *anything* that needed supplies that year." Certainly there is no public record, in the form of published research papers or reports of findings, of any laboratory research on the disease that year. According to Gunn, Gary Holmes had collected a total of five patients by 1989 whom he intended to enroll in the agency's case-control study, should it ever get off the ground; but, noted Gunn, agency scientists performed no laboratory work on samples from those five patients, or any other CFS patients, during 1989.

Another expenditure, one that arose for the first time that year, was a $20,000 travel charge. In successive years, as well, the agency would routinely debit the

---

* The agency's practice of subtracting lavish overhead sums from the CFS appropriation—17.3 percent in 1989 and 12 percent in succeeding years—was questionable. Abt Associates in Cambridge was conducting the day-to-day surveillance activities and was charging the agency for its own overhead.

CFS fund $20,000 for travel. Gunn, however, the agency's principal investigator, insisted he had not spent more than "five to eight thousand dollars in any given year" on travel related to CFS. If Gunn, who traveled for the disease more than anyone at the agency by virtue of his need to visit surveillance sites on a quarterly or half-year basis, spent only $5,000 to $8,000 on travel, it is difficult to imagine that other agency staff, far less embroiled in CFS research than Gunn, cumulatively spent another $12,000 to $15,000 dollars each year on CFS-related travel.

In 1990, the second year of the agency's surveillance, Congress awarded its biggest amount ever to the agency for the purpose of investigating the epidemic: $1,232,500. That sum was reduced to $867,680 by the time the agency and the Center for Infectious Diseases subtracted, respectively, 20 and 12 percent for overhead. That same year, according to the CDC's formal record, Atlanta scientists purchased $150,000 worth of supplies for their laboratories—a curiously even denomination—and charged the cost to the CFS appropriation. Since the agency performed laboratory research on the disease only in the final month of the year, when scientists in different laboratories analyzed blood samples from fewer than eleven patients and eleven controls, one might conclude that a substantial portion of this money went for laboratory supplies that were unrelated to CFS. According to Gunn, who was probably in the best position to know, very little money was spent in 1990 on equipment directly related to the CFS project. "I don't recall *any* equipment being purchased in 1990 other than a few desktop computers," Gunn said.

The year 1990 saw a radical jump in personnel charges to the fund. The agency claimed that year that twelve people were working full-time on the disease. In truth, Gary Holmes was devoting a portion, but not all, of his time to the problem in 1990; Dorothy Knight was devoting perhaps 80 percent of her time by responding to public inquiries about the disease; a second secretary in the same division was devoting about 50 percent of her time to helping Knight. Gunn estimated he was working on the disease 50 to 75 percent of the time.

By 1991, Congress was fully engaged on the subject of CFS and awarded the agency $2.1 million dollars to investigate the disease during that fiscal year. Given 1991's inauspicious beginning, Gunn suspected, the odds that the lion's share of the money would be used on projects directly related to CFS were poor.

Late in January, Brian Mahy, chief of the Division of Viral and Rickettsial Diseases, proposed that rather than remove either Walter Gunn or Larry Schonberger from authority over the disease, an official chronic fatigue syndrome steering committee be established within the division, with himself as chairman. This committee, Mahy suggested, could steer the CFS project along its bumpy course while Gunn continued to shepherd the surveillance and any in-house research, such as the case-control study and the Wistar replication project. More significantly, as Gunn later realized, Mahy noted that the committee could also make decisions about how to spend the CFS money.

Although the committee's formation initially struck Gunn as a promising sign, he soon saw it as another component of what he once called the agency's "smoke screen" research program on the chronic disease. The committee, Gunn came to believe, was a body of people united in one goal: to thwart an aggressive, cash-intensive investigation of the epidemic.

On February 4, retrovirology chief Tom Folks reported that all of David Bell's children were negative for HTLV2 in his laboratory's studies. On February 6, Walter Gunn called Elaine DeFreitas with the bad news. It quickly transpired that Folks had not used the same method DeFreitas had used. In fact, Gunn recalled later, "This was the first time that we realized that Elaine was using a procedure that the CDC never used." DeFreitas looked for the virus's DNA only after employing a machine called a DNA extractor, which dissolved the protein in cells and left the DNA exclusively, or "total" DNA. The government scientists had never followed that procedure, primarily because they didn't have the machine, but also because they believed the procedure to be superfluous. "People here were all saying it didn't matter, that if the retrovirus was there, they would find it," Gunn recalled. "But Elaine was very definite about this."*

The test could not be run again on the Lyndonville samples, since agency scientists had prepared them inappropriately the first time. David Bell would have to round up his young patients once more, draw more blood, and send more samples to Atlanta.

The same day, Gunn suffered a second defeat when he abruptly halted the agency's case-control study. The plan wasn't working on several fronts. The most elemental problem was a lack of cases. Only nine Atlanta patients had managed to squeak through the government's elaborate screening process. Nine people would hardly provide a base large enough from which to derive statistically significant data.

Lastly, the Wistar finding had moved the agency sufficiently off center that Gunn and Tom Folks, at least, were beginning to be uneasy with the CDC's lab protocol, which had included a test for generic retrovirus but had not included the sophisticated methods for finding retrovirus employed by Elaine DeFreitas.† "The cumulative feeling was," Gunn recalled, "let's stop and rethink this. . . . Our retrovirus lab here wasn't up to speed on the new finding, and we wanted to wait."

That same month, a private citizen whose wife suffered from the disease, Ed Taylor of Tulsa, donated $15,000 to the agency to enable it to pursue one avenue of its case-control study: the matter of natural killer cell dysfunction in the disease. Seeking to replicate the natural killer cell abnormalities Miami immunologist Nancy Klimas had reported, agency staff had asked Klimas to send blood samples from her Miami cases.

At the previous fall's "summit" with researchers in the private sector, Folks had cautioned that when blood samples are shipped by jet from south to north, they

---

* Much later, Folks explained, "We didn't feel we had to do this. Of course, we were looking for classic HTLV-two at the time, and we were not then using her probes and primers."

† "I wanted to be able to use *her* reagents, exactly as she described them," Folks noted later. "So we did not want to start the case-control study until we knew we had the same specificity and sensitivity as Elaine."

frequently freeze. And just as Folks had warned, the Miami samples froze in the cargo hold of the Atlanta-bound jet, and the cells died. "Freezing is particularly damaging to natural killer cells," Gunn said.

Although Congress had awarded the agency $2.1 million that year to investigate the disease, Walter Gunn was unable to dislodge funds from his agency to pay for the new reagents and other supplies required to test a new batch of samples from Miami. He called Marc Iverson to ask if the CFIDS Association would make a contribution. Gunn told Iverson the agency needed $15,000. Iverson, in turn, called Ed Taylor. The Tulsa entrepreneur complained bitterly. "The government should be paying for this!" he fumed. Nevertheless, Taylor sent a check.

Gunn had been told that he would have $683,000 to pay Abt Associates for the surveillance project in 1991, but he was acutely aware that the sum constituted only a portion of the year's congressional allocation for the disease. After deducting the CDC's 20 percent overhead, and the 12 percent overhead of the Center for Infectious Diseases, Gunn knew that $1.5 million remained. Even after subtracting surveillance costs, the balance remaining was *still* approximately $800,000. On February 7, he was pondering these sums when he heard from retrovirology chief Tom Folks. "Tom told me that his lab was not getting *any* money for chronic fatigue syndrome that year," Gunn said later. "He said he would have to stop work after analyzing the nine case-control samples for retrovirus." Gunn was astounded by Folks's news. Among other things, it suggested that further efforts to replicate the Wistar finding would be canceled.

Gunn called Walter Dowdle. "I told Dowdle that we were getting only $683,000 of the two million. I said, 'Where's the rest?' " Dowdle advised Gunn to ask the chief of the Division of Viral and Rickettsial Diseases, Brian Mahy, for an explanation of the division's CFS budget.

In a tense meeting on February 14, attended by Gunn and his immediate boss, Larry Schonberger, Mahy revealed a stark truth about the financial practices of the Division of Viral and Rickettsial Diseases.

Gunn, who kept careful notes of the meeting, recalled that Mahy had explained, "Chronic fatigue syndrome money is simply added to the pot of money that the Division runs on, and the fact that there is a handout indicating that $110,000 is supposed to be devoted to retroviral studies is no guarantee that $110,000 is actually going to be *used* for retroviral research." Mahy further explained that money from the CFS appropriation might be used to shore up a particular project or lab; after all, Mahy reasoned, he couldn't fire a scientist simply because the scientist's funds had run out. "He said that the money is diluted and used as the division pleases," Gunn continued, "but he assured me that I would have whatever money I needed. He said, 'Don't worry about it. Whatever money you need, we will provide.' I said, 'That's great, except Tom [Folks] is telling me his lab can't do any more research!' "

"There are serious problems with the agency's system," Gunn said some months later. "But these problems might never have surfaced without the emergence of this controversial illness. If everyone was in agreement on how to approach this disease, then their way of doing things could have continued indefinitely. And until they brought me in on this project, they *were* in agreement—that people with chronic fatigue syndrome are mentally ill and that Congress was forcing them to perform research on a non-disease. As a result, CFS became the division's golden goose.

"But—my feeling is," Gunn added, his consternation evident, "if you don't believe this is an illness, *then don't accept the money!*"

Washington, D.C.

Suspicions about fiscal bad faith inside the federal agencies were spreading among patient activists as well. In spite of the congressional allotment of several million dollars to investigate the disease, the CDC had contributed nothing to the public understanding of the disease since publishing its 1987 working case definition. Administrators at the NIH, too, for all their braggadocio before Congress, had little to point to, aside from Stephen Straus's psychiatric assessment of two dozen longtime CFS sufferers, as evidence of progress toward understanding the disease. Incredibly, Straus's in-house research program at the National Institute of Allergy and Infectious Diseases was by 1991 costing taxpayers close to $1 million a year. Because Congress had failed, until 1991, to earmark money for the disease in its NIH appropriations, however, CFS money inside the Bethesda agency was even harder to track than money in Atlanta.

That winter, volunteer lobbyist Barry Sleight, who was monitoring as best he could what he privately called the "malfeasance and nonfeasance" at both agencies, composed a three-page memo about the history of the CFS research agenda of the National Institutes of Health for a well-known Washington lobbyist, Tom Sheridan of the Sheridan Group. The memo was, in effect, Sleight's swan song. A newly formed conglomerate of members of the Charlotte-based patient association and the San Francisco–based foundation, as well as assorted activist-minded patient association leaders around the nation, had hired Sheridan for $2,500 a month, a sum scrounged from the new organization's modest coffers. The organization called itself the CFIDS Action Campaign for the United States, or CAC-TUS. Its members, particularly the politically oriented patient leaders in northern California, increasingly believed the disease required a professional lobbying effort, and the Sheridan Group was among the best-known health lobbyists in the capital. Sheridan himself was a polished thirty-one-year-old who had been active in both the Mondale and Clinton presidential campaigns; one of his clients was Elizabeth Taylor, who had taken up the cause of AIDS two years before. In return for their $2,500, the poised and savvy Sheridan promised the activists expert navigation through the corridors of Washington power.

Sleight was unable to provide Sheridan with a paper trail of the NIH's financial activities, but he tried to acquaint the lobbyist with the gloomy history of the disease in Bethesda and to provide what he considered suggestive evidence of that agency's mishandling of research money:

> The National Institutes of Health still has only two grants out directly related to CFS. At times in the past, they have claimed that a variety of virology or immunology-related grants totaling into the hundreds of millions of

dollars were CFS-related grants. The dollars total only about $1 million annually. . . .

Since the mid-1980s, there has been one small intramural research program at NIAID, under S. E. Straus, M.D. Some patients and, privately, some non-NIH researchers, feel that this program is due criticism on these bases:

1. There is a lack of agency commitment. The number of patients followed has consistently declined, and attrition has been encouraged by unprofessional staff conduct and extremely willing assignment of other-than-CFS diagnoses to patients.
2. Straus has a bias against women, shown via comments in person, via public presentations, and in publication. This puts him at odds with an illness that is believed to affect mostly women.

   Also, Straus has taken a blame-the-victim approach to the illness by excessively emphasizing the possible role of psychiatric factors and emotional stress in CFS, an illness that is generally understood to involve infection by a virus.
3. Needlessly invasive and/or high-risk test procedures have been used on patients.
4. The program does little. Only one potential therapeutic, acyclovir, has been both tested in a controlled trial upon these patients and reported in the scientific literature.
5. Straus has undue influence upon the granting process related to CFS. This has included one reported incident of unprofessional conduct.
6. Straus has undue influence on NIH intramural research outside of the National Institute of Allergy and Infectious Diseases.
7. Straus has actively tried to reduce congressional focus on this issue. He and Director [Anthony] Fauci asked for and were granted a meeting with a member involved in leadership on this issue. Also, Straus gave a presentation in the Rayburn Building on CFS. In both cases, an underlying theme was that NIAID had everything under control and no congressional attention to CFS was needed.

"I hope this material is of use to you in your work," Sleight concluded in his deadpan style.

Hollywood, California

The grocery store tabloids' free-for-all with Cher's "mystery disease" continued into 1992, as did the actress's disease. On February 12 she was featured on the front page of the *Star* next to an eye-catching cover line: "Mystery Disease Wrecks Cher's Sex Life. She's Been Without a Man for Months." Cher had declared a moratorium on sex, an unnamed source explained, because "it's simply too exhausting." She continued to be so weak, the source said, that "she could barely lift her head from her pillow. . . . She's always tired." The actress's publicist, Lois Smith, had at last confirmed for the *Star* that Cher suffered from CFS. "She first realized she had it at the beginning of 1989," Smith said. "It's something that comes and goes. It's never been completely cured."

Centers for Disease Control, Atlanta, Georgia

On February 20, David Bell sent a second batch of samples from the Lyndonville children to Building 15. Tom Folks assured Walter Gunn that his lab would have results by March 5.

The following day Gunn received a document he had been waiting for since the previous August: the manuscript of Elaine DeFreitas's paper detailing her discovery, which would be published in the *Proceedings of the National Academy of Sciences* on April 1. The scientist's paper contained information regarding the viral probes she had developed during the preceding three years, information crucial to enabling the agency to reproduce her work. Gunn made a copy for himself and Tom Folks, and gave the chief of the Division of Viral and Rickettsial Diseases, Brian Mahy, the original to read overnight.

National Institute of Allergy and Infectious Diseases, Bethesda, Maryland

As a direct result of patient advocacy efforts with legislators, administrators at the Bethesda agency were forced by legislation that winter to provide grants to independent scientists seeking funding in the CFS field. Congress had failed to mandate a dollar sum, however, and as a result, the amount the NIH settled upon turned out to be $488,000, a relatively small figure by biomedical research standards, particularly since the money would be used to fund one or more "cooperative research centers." To qualify for a center grant, researchers needed to include *four* independently standing project grants in their proposals, all of them supported by a core facility such as a university or research institute. Normally, center grants were among the most far-reaching and expensive offered by the NIH. By those measures, then, the budget for CFS research was grossly inadequate.

"This budget was capped at [under] $500,000, including indirect costs!" Miami researcher Nancy Klimas said that spring. Indirect costs were the university's administration and overhead charges, which, according to Klimas, could amount to 40 or 50 percent of the total. "So you really had $250,000 to $300,000 to do four projects—I mean, you're getting down to $50,000 a project," she added. "It was untenable. You couldn't even *begin* a center for that kind of money. They wanted clinical and epidemiologic-based science, in-depth virology, immunology—you name it. It all had to be a part of that center grant, any *one* of which would have tied up the whole budget."

In addition, there were strings attached: the NIH would play a controlling role in decisions about the direction of the research, acting in essence as a partner in the cooperative investigation. Given the bias of the federal agency's scientists and administrators, the research agendas of the cooperative centers by necessity would reflect that bias to an unknown degree. Still, money was money, and the new legislation meant that dollars *had* to be appropriated to someone—a significant departure from earlier prospects.

Because the NIH's stance for so long had been to avoid funding, the congressional order caught agency officials off guard. By congressional order, the money had to be committed to researchers by the end of fiscal year 1991: September 30. But grant program officer Ann Schleuderberg failed to issue the formal announcement of the centers grant in the Federal Register until early February. Proposals had to be submitted by April 1.

Many researchers, watching the process like children with their noses pressed against the candy store window, complained that the agency had imposed an impossible deadline. One researcher, who failed to receive a copy of Schleuderberg's request for proposals until March, said later, "I called everyone in the lab together and I said, 'Do we want to try—in two weeks—to put a center together?' And everyone wanted to, and finally I said, 'I think we better not. Let's not shoot ourselves in the foot.' "

Other researchers scoffed at the proposal once they saw its budget. San Francisco virologist Jay Levy deemed the sum to be insultingly small. "It was a stupid thing," he said dismissively when asked about it later. "The money was a pittance." Seymour Grufferman described it as "a crumb." He also noted the importance of the word "cooperative" in the plan: "That means the NIAID will have control . . . they want to make sure that their dollars are used in a plan that fits in with the institution's ideas, and what NIAID thinks is that this is all psychoneurosis. . . . It's tokenism—a cynical gesture in response to congressional pressure."

Elaine DeFreitas and Hilary Koprowski learned only in late February, when they read the request for proposals, that the grant would be structured as a cooperative center. "If for some suicidal, masochistic reason I were to apply for this grant, it would take me working on it full-time for the next six months," DeFreitas said that February. "Instead, we have five weeks."

If Elaine DeFreitas once had lacked a "global perspective" on the disease, as Paul Cheney had said two years earlier, she was now as sensitive as her former collaborator to the bizarre twists and turns of the medical politics in which the disease was enmeshed.

"A doctor called me the other day," DeFreitas said that winter. "He's in his fifties. His wife has this disease. He said, 'In all my years of medical practice, I've never experienced anything like this. It's almost as if there is an underground comprised of doctors and scientists, and they're all being *kept* underground by the incredible arrogance of mainstream medicine. He cited a comment made during a medical grand rounds he had attended on the disease. Someone stood up and asked, 'Come, now—do you really *believe* in CFS?'

"Are we talking medicine or are we talking *theology*?" DeFreitas asked.

She had been asked to speak about her work at several medical meetings in Philadelphia and elsewhere since Kyoto. "These doctors come up to me afterward and take me aside," she said. " 'I'm a clinician in Oxnard, California, and I've got hundreds of these patients!' 'I'm a clinician in Clearwater, Florida, and I've got three hundred cases!' It's a secret society!"

University of Glasgow, Glasgow, Scotland

In late February word came from Britain that neurologist Peter Behan, using the gene sequences Elaine DeFreitas had sent him in October, had confirmed the Wistar retrovirus finding in a number of Scottish myalgic encephalomyelitis patients.

"I just wish the bastard had told me first," DeFreitas said. "I had to hear it from the English support-group people. But I'm thrilled. He's going to be besieged, just like we were, the poor darling. But the ball is rolling."

In fact, Behan and his associates had found something very different, something that ultimately would elicit a vastly different response from DeFreitas.

Changuinola, Panama

During the years that Gary Holmes had sat in his narrow windowless office under siege from members of the press and from patients suffering from the notorious Tahoe malady, Jon Kaplan had been studying the Guayami Indians of Changuinola, Panama. There were indications that a retrovirus, HTLV2, was carried in the blood of this Spanish-speaking population, but none of them were actually ill. Kaplan had made one field trip to Panama and interviewed members of the Guayami tribe, drawn samples of their blood, and performed physical examinations of the healthy Indians.

On February 21 the results of his investigation appeared in a letter to the *New England Journal.*[1] He and six other authors reported that HTLV2 was spreading among the Guayamis, but the route of transmission was mysterious, unlike any traditional patterns attributed to retroviruses, such as sex or blood contamination.

25

A Conspiracy of Dunces

American Medical Association, Chicago, Illinois

Medical authority, social prestige, and a large income hardly conferred immunity from the disease. Most doctors who contracted CFS, however, refrained from discussing their ordeal in any public forum out of concern for their livelihood and dignity. By 1991 a few doctors who had abandoned hope of returning to their practices decided to speak out; having faced the bedrock certainty of permanent disability, they were free to bring their personal crises to bear on their profession's inadequacies.

Thomas English, a fifty-two-year-old Asheville, North Carolina, surgeon was a patient of Paul Cheney's who had fallen ill in 1987. On February 27 the *Journal of the American Medical Association* published English's carefully reasoned plea to his colleagues to open their minds to the possibility that CFS was a real disease. English conceded that a mind-set of skepticism "permeated" the medical profession and was widely perceived as "the prudent, conservative way to deal with ambiguous situations," particularly during times when even the experts were confounded. "Healthy skepticism," English added, "is the 'in' attitude for intelligent, discriminating physicians. But," he asked, "healthy for whom? Four years ago," he continued, "I was diagnosed as having chronic fatigue syndrome. The experience has given me a new perspective on my profession, one that is not always flattering. In one early report, the average CFS patient had previously consulted sixteen different physicians. Most were told that they were in perfect health, that they were depressed, or that they were under too much stress. Many were sent to psychiatrists. . . . Is chronic fatigue syndrome a real disease?" he asked. "I believe it is, but I cannot settle that here. I would only plant this seed in the mind of skeptics: *What if you are wrong?* What are the consequences for your patients?"

The surgeon asked his colleagues to imagine for a moment that they were the "subjective patient" rather than the "objective physician":

> You catch a "cold," and thereafter the quality of your life is indelibly altered. You can't think clearly. Sometimes it's all you can do to read the newspaper. . . . Jet lag without end. You inch along the fog-shrouded precipice of patient care where you once walked with confidence. . . . Myalgias wander

about your body with no apparent pattern. Symptoms come and go. . . . What is true today may be partially true tomorrow or totally false next week. You know that sounds flaky, but, dammit, it's happening to you.

You are exhausted, yet you sleep only two or three hours a night. You were a jogger who ran three miles regularly; now a walk around the block depletes your stamina. Strenuous exercise precipitates relapses that last weeks.

English described the sensations of the disease in a manner that he believed might stimulate empathy in his colleagues. *"There is nothing in your experience in medical school, residency, or practice with its grueling hours and sleep deprivation that even approaches the fatigue you feel with this illness,"* he wrote (italics his). "Fatigue is the most pathetically inadequate term.

"You, too, might wonder about some of your symptoms had you not talked to other patients with similar experiences . . . or talked with physicians who have seen hundreds of similar cases. With experience, a pattern emerges: the bizarre and implausible become commonplace and credible."

And he quoted clinician and medical educator Sir William Osler: "To comprehend this illness, one must heed Osler's advice to study the patient firsthand: 'Learning medicine without books is like going to sea without charts. Learning medicine without patients is like not going to sea at all.' . . .

"I have talked with scores of fellow patients who went to our profession for help," English continued, "but who came away humiliated, angry and afraid. Their bodies told them they were physically ill, but the psychospeculation of their physicians was only frightening and infuriating—not reassuring."

English concluded his letter with an understated plea to his colleagues for patience:

My career is but a faint memory. There is little demand for absent minded surgeons, even if I had the stamina. Too, I harbor the lingering fear that I might transmit my illness to a patient. So I wait. I hope. I pray. . . . Internists have long prided themselves on incisive intellects and superior diagnostic skills. It is time for those skills to focus on the complex subtleties of this illness. I ask for your patience. CFS is sufficient indignity by itself; do not compound it. It takes considerable time and infinite patience to take an accurate history from a frail patient with impaired memory and concentration. . . . But if you take that time, you can do a world of good. CFS may frustrate you, but it is equally fascinating and rewarding. Resist the temptation of hurried, superficial evaluation. This is no illness for cookbook doctors. It is a disease for medical intellectuals with supple and open minds.

Privately, English was more outraged by his peers in medicine than his calm prose suggested. "I was working at the Veterans Administration Hospital when I got this disease," he recalled some years later. "I was put through the equivalent of a Salem witch trial. The medical profession is like a quasi-military system— there is a childlike faith in authority. Everyone parades around in white coats pretending to be scientists, but what really changes most doctors' minds is herd mentality."

Looking back on his own surgical training at Duke University, English remembered, "So much of medical education relies upon proverbs, and one common one is 'If you hear hoofbeats, think of horses, not zebras.' " His fellow students quickly learned, English continued, "if you think you've found anything rare or unusual, prepare to be laughed at. But that ignores the obvious fact that there are *lots* of rare things. And it took me a long time to realize that people *were* seeing rare things; they were just squeezing round objects into square holes. Of course, the greatest zebra of all is something *new*. And, you know, how *dare* someone like Paul Cheney, someone who is not working at one of the great tertiary referral centers, discover something new? But the people at the cutting edge in this disease are *not* working in those prestigious centers, because, in order to take care of people with this disease," he added, "you run the risk of being ridiculed."

The former surgeon's bitterest words were reserved for Stephen Straus, however, whom he had consulted in the earliest days of his illness, a call that resulted in, English said, "one of the most degrading conversations I've ever had."

"He's an empathic retard," the doctor said of the nation's CFS expert. "I think of empathy as a different kind of intelligence, one not measured on IQ tests. It's a right brain skill, and it probably can't be learned. Straus is a left-brain computer-model thinker. In a way, all this is not his fault. He simply doesn't have the capacity to understand what other people are going through."

Long Island, New York

Not long after English's essay appeared, the *New York Native* published an interview with a Long Island internal medicine specialist who was now disabled. The lively tabloid's CFS reporter Neenyah Ostrom was the interviewer. Internist Paul Lavenger, she wrote, had practiced medicine for twenty-five years when, in December 1989, he became ill. His diagnosis came relatively quickly, since Lavenger's wife had been suffering from the identical symptoms since September 1987. According to Ostrom, in Lavenger's "extended household," which included adult children and their spouses, "five people now have been diagnosed with or are starting to display symptoms of CFS."

In his comments to the *Native,* Lavenger revealed himself to be an angry man who felt betrayed by his profession and his government. He called the failure of the American medical establishment to comprehend and investigate the CFS epidemic a "conspiracy of dunces." Members of that conspiracy, Lavenger said, included health authorities who had adopted a "blame the victim" strategy to deflect public concern about the disease; public and private disability insurance providers, "whose payment schedules and actuarial tables would be devastated by a widespread epidemic"; and doctors who are unable to help sufferers and, as a consequence, dismiss them. Interestingly, addressing a subject that was rarely aired in public, Lavenger also fingered victims' immediate families, many of whom, he said, followed the government's lead in blaming the patient as a means of avoiding responsibility for the CFS sufferer's care. "The only reason the public tolerates the government's behavior," he said, "is because they've been told *and* they believe the patient is the cause of the illness and they can't catch it—you see, you can't catch depression; you can't catch yuppie burnout."

Lavenger also said he found it "absolutely ironic" that in spite of the fact that many CFS patients tended to be sicker than virtually any other patients doctors see, including people suffering from "end-stage chronic obstructive pulmonary disease," cancer, and heart disease, most doctors turned them away as malingerers, or "crocks." One reason doctors rarely considered the disease in their diagnostic musings, Lavenger added, had to do with the government's subtle persuasion that the disease was bogus: "I recently spoke to a doctor friend who's been sick with this disease for six years. He continues to practice. He tells me his friends say, and I quote, 'You have that bullshit disease.' And this is from *colleagues.*"

Reporter Ostrom asked Lavenger if he expected the federal health agencies to soon right the wrongs of the past several years. His response was unhesitating:

It seems they're going to adhere to this line—that the public is not at risk—until hell freezes over. Nobody's willing to take a fresh look at what's going on. . . .

The government is doing nothing, and there is an organized conspiracy to take the patients and use the old divide-and-conquer method. They isolate them, they cut them off from everything. They cut them off from funds, so they can't get insurance. They tell doctors not to believe them, so they get no medical care. Their families don't believe them, so they get no compassion. It's very hard to fight back when you can't get into a cohesive group, when all you are is a bunch of isolated people with nothing to grab on to. It's very, very difficult. They've got the patients where they want them—they're winning this war.

Centers for Disease Control, Atlanta, Georgia

Walter Gunn had heard via letter or telephone from so many doctors and medical researchers who claimed to be suffering from the disease that he began keeping a tally. He stored their letters in a legal-size folder, obliterating their names to protect their privacy, and he began routinely sending copies of the letters to William Roper, head of the CDC.

"I'm hearing from more and more doctors and doctors' wives who have chronic fatigue syndrome," Gunn said during the winter of 1991. "I'm uncovering this whole underground of doctors and health care workers who have the disease and who are afraid to admit it because they'll lose their jobs. My folder of letters from physicians is currently about four inches thick. But there are thousands of nurses—*thousands.* We've stopped *counting* the number of nurses who have called in saying they have this disease."

Recently Gunn had been quietly approached by a doctor newly employed by the agency who claimed he had contracted the disease two years earlier but had eventually recovered. The doctor told Gunn he suspected he had acquired the disease in his own clinical practice after examining a number of patients who had recently come down with the illness. Two other doctors in the same practice had fallen ill with the disease as well.

Without revealing his correspondents' identities, Gunn read aloud short portions from a sampling of doctors' letters from his file late that winter. "Here's a surgeon who says he's stopped surgery because he was afraid of killing someone when he wasn't thinking straight," Gunn said. Another letter was from an internal medicine specialist who had fallen ill in November of 1987. The internist reported he had stopped working, primarily because he was unable to handle the intellectual aspects of his work. One letter from a disabled psychiatrist was five pages long, single-spaced: "The impact is overwhelming," the psychiatrist wrote of his ordeal. Yet another letter was from a doctor who had been working at the National Institutes of Health on a fellowship when he fell ill. "I was struck down on December 6, 1986," the doctor wrote Gunn. "I have been a bedridden invalid ever since. I have experienced a total loss of income from my household. Now my wife is ill."

There were more sad missives: a Harvard Medical School Ph.D. candidate in neurobiology reported that he had been bedridden since his illness began in January 1990; a Ph.D. scientist working on the development of an artificial heart who had fallen ill in 1990 wrote that "my ability to support my wife and children is endangered"; an internal medicine specialist and the chairman of the intensive care unit of his hospital who reported he had worked sixty to eighty hours each week for the last twenty years without ill effect had become suddenly and wholly disabled by CFS eighteen months earlier.

Brian Mahy, the director of Gunn's division, cautioned Gunn against sending the letters to Roper, suggesting he was at risk of losing his job. Gunn ignored Mahy's admonition.

Gunn began to develop the idea, gleaned entirely from his voluminous correspondence from medical workers, that the disease was flourishing disproportionately in the health care field. His intuition, in fact, echoed more scientifically based observations made by researchers in the 1950s. If one considered the medical literature of an earlier generation, the preponderance of hospital workers with the disease provided the most powerful evidence that the malady was, indeed, a highly infectious illness in its earliest, or acute, stages.

In their seminal 1959 *New England Journal of Medicine* article about "epidemic neuromyasthenia"—a disease that was remarkably similar and perhaps identical to CFS—American epidemiologists Donald A. Henderson and Alexis Shelokov reviewed the documentation of twenty-three cluster outbreaks that had occurred between 1934 and 1958.[1] Close to half of the clusters—ten of twenty-three—had afflicted hospital staffs particularly. Nurses and doctors, in fact, were "the most notably susceptible" to the disease in both the hospital-based epidemics and the community-wide outbreaks. And those doctors and nurses who had the most intimate contact with patients were the most likely to have fallen ill; hospital workers whose jobs kept them distant from patients were the least likely to suffer the same fate. In the 1934 outbreak at the Los Angeles County Hospital, for instance, "analysis of cases among nurses by place of work . . . demonstrated that cases occurred considerably earlier and four times more frequently among those working on the communicable-disease wards in the main admitting office than among those working elsewhere in the hospital."*

But *all* the scientific literature suggested that contact with patients was a determining factor in the rate of disease among health care workers. As Henderson commented to *New Yorker* reporter Berton Roueche in the late 1950s, "It is now perfectly clear that medical and hospital people are especially vulnerable to epidemic neuromyasthenia, so we'll concentrate on them. We'll get to them as early as possible, and we'll keep them under the closest possible observation."

Henderson and Shelokov had made their important observations decades before and then moved on, leaving epidemic neuromyasthenia behind as little more than a hobby. Walter Gunn, a member of the new generation of investigators faced with an epidemic of massive proportions, remained in the thick of it, however. Unfortunately, Gunn lacked resources to pursue his hunch about the epidemic's virulence in the health and science professions, nor was he aware of Henderson and Shelokov's observations on the subject. He had only his steadily expanding file of correspondence and his gut feeling: if the disease was infectious, it was reasonable to assume that doctors, nurses, and anyone else who repeatedly came in contact with either sufferers or their tissue samples was more vulnerable to the disease than the population as a whole.

Wistar Institute, Philadelphia, Pennsylvania

In late February word went out that the National Institute of Allergy and Infectious Diseases, in collaboration with the National Institute of Mental Health, would host its second workshop on CFS the following month. (The first had been a by-invitation-only affair three years earlier.) Elaine DeFreitas was not invited. In fact, NIH administrator Ann Schleuderberg, who was organizing the meeting, called DeFreitas and suggested she not attend. Schleuderberg told the Wistar scientist that the purpose of the conference was to better define the disease. Viruses would not be discussed, Schleuderberg assured DeFreitas. In fact, no discussion at all would be devoted to matters of causation and transmissibility, issues which,

---

* According to the Henderson and Shelokov chronology, the Los Angeles County Hospital epidemic of 1934, investigated by the U.S. Public Health Service's A. G. "Sandy" Gilliam, was followed by a hospital cluster in Harefield, England, in 1936. Fourteen years later, in 1950, an epidemic occurred among student nurses in Louisville, Kentucky. In 1952, a third such epidemic broke out among student nurses at London's Middlesex Hospital. The following year a hospital staff in Coventry, England, constituted the core victims of an epidemic that also spread, though less intensely, throughout the city of Coventry. In 1953, Shelokov was invited by his superiors at the NIH to investigate an epidemic among the nursing staff at the Chestnut Lodge Hospital in Rockville, Maryland. Two years later, perhaps the most famous hospital-based epidemic of all broke out at London's Royal Free Hospital, claiming at least three hundred victims among the staff. (The legitimacy of the epidemic neuromyasthenia diagnosis at Royal Free was discredited by a psychiatrist and his student in 1970 as mass hysteria in a paper that gained wide currency in England and, in Shelokov's view, set progress on the disease back by twenty years.) A hospital in Durban, South Africa, was the site of another 1953 epidemic cited by Shelokov and Henderson. Three years later, a second, smaller outbreak of the disease occurred among nurses at the Royal Free Hospital. In 1958, the last outbreak that Shelokov and Henderson were aware of in 1959 when they published their article, occurred in Athens, Greece.

for DeFreitas, as well as for patients and for the nation's expert CFS clinicians, were paramount.

"This will be a clinically oriented workshop," DeFreitas recalled Schleuderberg telling her. "You wouldn't be interested. Maybe someday," Schleuderberg had added, "we'll put together a conference on etiology."

One week before Schleuderberg's call, the CDC's Jon Kaplan had introduced himself to DeFreitas at the Third International Conference on Human Retrovirology: HTLV, a meeting among retrovirologists in that field, held that year in Jamaica.

"I asked him what he thought about Tahoe," DeFreitas recalled. "He said, 'What I thought was that Cheney and Peterson had a lot of very tired patients. But the skiing was wonderful!' "

DeFreitas was annoyed by Kaplan's specific disregard for the medical acumen of her primary clinical collaborator and by his more general disdain for the legitimacy of the event. Moreover, she couldn't imagine what purpose it served to study viruses in South American Indians who had no demonstrable disease, while ignoring hundreds of thousands of severely ill Americans. "You have lab after lab talking about the HTLV-two-like viruses that they're cloning out of these obscure Indian tribes—who aren't even sick!" DeFreitas said, exasperated.

Privately, Kaplan was equally dismissive of DeFreitas's work in CFS, expressing doubt that the Wistar finding would stand up to scrutiny. He made it clear, however, that if the CDC did replicate Elaine DeFreitas's retroviral discovery, Kaplan himself would be put in charge of the ensuing national epidemiological investigation of CFS. "That's my job," he said, smiling. "To investigate retroviruses. But we haven't gotten to the point where that's an issue, and I suspect we won't."

University of Southern California, Los Angeles

Six years into the epidemic the reality of CFS—manifested by hundreds of thousands if not millions of sufferers, a discrete constellation of signs and symptoms, and objectively documented evidence of multi-system damage—had yet to win the biomedical community's respect. Many of those who were trapped in the quicksand of the disease now believed their salvation lay exclusively in the identification of the pathogen that had launched their slide. Only then, they reasoned, would the powerful, technology-rich research establishment turn its head in their direction. As a result, Elaine DeFreitas's discovery of retrovirus fragments in four-fifths of CFS victims and in a third of their close contacts had ignited a profound degree of hope among patients. As odd as it might seem to the detached bystander, an unknown but presumably sizable number of Americans were now longing for confirmation of the news that they harbored a disease-causing retrovirus in their immune system. After all, the worst had already happened; nothing would alter the fact of their disease. Confirmation might, however, change its course by ushering in therapies or even a cure.

It was in this spirit that patient advocacy associations began monitoring the work of John Martin, director of the molecular pathology labs at USC and Los Angeles County Hospital. Of the handful of bench researchers working on the disease, Martin was the most sensitive to its clinical aspects. As a result, he inferred a connection between severely encephalopathic hospital patients who were virtually comatose and CFS patients who were merely housebound by their illness. Most infectious diseases demonstrated a spectrum of severity, Martin reasoned. Why should CFS be any different? Martin, in addition, was convinced, like his clinician-collaborators, that the essential nature of the illness, its core disorder, was brain dysfunction of viral origin.

For some time, Martin had been struggling to find unequivocal evidence for viruses of any stripe in a series of patients who ranged from the virtually brain-dead to the mid-level range of severity for CFS. Three years before he had found positive signals for the presence of an unusual virus in some patients using probes to detect herpesviruses. More recently, he had come up with positive signals for both herpes and retroviral "tax" genes in two CFS patients. Each patient was a woman with classic CFS; one had begun her illness with encephalopathy requiring hospitalization. Using spinal fluid from these patients, he had been able to develop living cell cultures in which the unusual microbe began reproducing.

That winter, Martin's efforts began to pay off. With an electron microscope, he was able to see particles of virus in these cultures and to observe cytopathic effect, or cell destruction. Excitement ran high among patients and doctors privy to Martin's work, all of whom wondered whether he was onto the same virus DeFreitas had found. CFIDS Association president Marc Iverson guaranteed Martin $8,000 a month for the ensuing six months to pursue the work.

Martin's findings were as confusing as they were intriguing. After all, he was getting signals for a virus that seemed to have genetic links to both herpesvirus and retrovirus. More remarkably, Martin's genetic analysis of the retroviral portions of the virus were suggestive of a family of retroviruses not deemed to cause human disease.

So far, molecular biologists had identified three subclasses or families of retroviruses. The first human retroviruses to be discovered, the HTLVs, were called oncoviruses, or tumor viruses, because they were considered capable of causing cancer. A second subfamily were lentiviruses, into which HIV had been placed after initial inclusion in the oncovirus family. Lentiviruses were so-called slow viruses that targeted the host's central nervous system. Spuma retroviruses, a third subfamily, had been described by one scientist as the "Cinderella group," because they were viewed as microbes lacking a definitive association with any known human or animal disease.[2] Such viruses caused the cells they infected to expand and stick to each other in foamy clusters. Because of the microbe's distinctive effect on the host cells, spuma viruses were commonly known as foamy viruses. Spuma viruses abounded in apes, monkeys, hamsters, cats, and cattle, but researchers had yet to prove that any particular disease state in these animals was associated with spuma virus infection. So far, just one human spuma virus had been identified, and it had yet to be linked to a disease. In addition, although spuma viruses seemed to be contagious among animals, no one had yet proved that the lone human spuma virus could be passed among humans.

The viral particles Martin observed in electron micrographs showed a definite foamy cell cytopathic effect. The appearance of the virus itself matched every known description of a foamy virus: its spherical outer coat and its habitation of the cell's vacuoles—liquid cavities within the cell—were identical to the foamy viruses already categorized. But the virus's dual reactivity with herpesviral and retroviral gene primers on PCR testing led Martin to suspect he had discovered an unusual recombinant virus—a virus that had somehow originated from a genetic merger of two distinct families of virus. (As Martin, only half joking, noted some years later, "It didn't surprise me when we had a very funny-looking virus—this is what you might expect with a funny disease.") Nevertheless, it was to the spuma group that Martin initially assigned his novel virus, a conclusion that was bound to be controversial: Martin's virus did not react to probes for the only known human spuma virus. Still, the virus reacted with probes made from simian foamy virus, which bore a close genetic relationship to human foamy virus.

"We have the virus out," Martin noted that winter. "We have amplified a fragment of the virus's gene. Right now we've got three hundred cultures going. It just grows everywhere!"

In a late-night conversation with Marc Iverson, the scientist expressed his view that the novel agent he was studying was responsible for a panoply of illness in the population, much of it being written off as idiopathic, or atypical, in the case of the acute, devastating encephalopathies cropping up at L.A. County Hospital and elsewhere, or psychiatric, in the cases of CFS. "The public health ramifications of this are *horrendous*," Martin told Iverson. "CFS is the tip of the iceberg. There are all *kinds* of misdiagnoses going on. . . . I've got a moral obligation to get this out."

In July, Martin submitted his discovery to the *Annals of Internal Medicine, Lancet,* and the *Journal of the American Medical Association.* All three articles were rejected. He also presented his work at a symposium on myalgic encephalomyelitis in Cambridge, England, organized by the Canadian doctor Byron Hyde.

Meanwhile, the CFS network was such that several other researchers were becoming increasingly aware of the activity in Martin's lab. Dan Peterson sent scores of additional samples from Nevada to the scientist, as did Paul Cheney from Charlotte. Three of the samples Cheney sent were from patients who had consistently tested positive for the retrovirus in the Wistar study and who had been included on the paper Elaine DeFreitas had delivered in Kyoto. Martin infected cell cultures with these samples; within seven to fourteen days the cultures flourished with what Martin and his lab associates took, based on its appearance and behavior, to be an atypical foamy cell–inducing virus. In fact, Martin was able to infect new cell cultures with the foamy virus nearly every time he injected them with tissue samples from CFS sufferers. Cheney began to suspect that Elaine DeFreitas and John Martin were looking at different parts of the same virus.

Marc Iverson, too, was encouraged. "Wistar is plodding along in a very traditional way, but Martin's got the throttle all the way down to the floor," Iverson mused. So far, the CFIDS Foundation's scientific board had awarded Martin $40,000, a Lilliputian sum in the Brobdingnagian economics of biomedical research. The former banker, who in his early wunderkind-style career had processed millions of dollars' worth of transactions every month, clearly believed the sum had been a good investment. "Forty grand to buy agent X," Iverson said, marveling.

In early March, Paul Cheney flew to Los Angeles to meet with John Martin. The two men huddled for hours in Martin's university lab, with Martin showing the Charlotte clinician cell culture after cell culture, each one infected with the new virus.

"I'm not convinced this thing is spuma, although that would explain the disease's infectiousness," Cheney said, referring to the casual transmission of spuma viruses among animals. "But I think it could be a new retrovirus family. Why not? It will be either a spuma or its own. I'm going to guess that it's something between HTLV and a spuma. Because we have an enigma here of a virus that doesn't quite seem to match the epidemiology of the disease."

Martin, however, was so convinced of the legitimacy of his finding that he proposed to Cheney a new scientific name for the disease based on the virus and its ability to cause central nervous system disease: spuma-associated myalgic encephalopathy, or SAME.

Charlotte, North Carolina

The March issue of the *CFIDS Chronicle* reprinted guidelines that Cheney and his new partner, internist Charles Lapp, issued to their patients in their effort to counsel CFS victims on the transmissibility of their disease. Included in the guidelines were the following suggestions:

- Do not share food, glasses, cups, or utensils.
- Do not kiss others on the mouth.
- Do not feed table scraps to pets.
- Do not donate your blood.
- Remind lab personnel to use precautions when drawing your blood or handling body fluids.
- Consider using a condom during sexual intercourse.

Harvard School of Medicine, Boston, Massachusetts

In March, having rebounded from his disappointment over his rejection by the *New England Journal of Medicine,* Anthony Komaroff submitted the Tahoe manuscript to the *Annals of Internal Medicine* for review. The *Annals* sent the paper to three reviewer's; at least one of them was sympathetic to the subject matter.

"I said it was one of the most important papers ever," the reviewer said later. "There's so much good data out there about this disease that has never been published. It's sad—my heart breaks. That's what has hurt this field."

The reviewer's only criticism of the paper had to do with its title: instead of calling the disease chronic fatigue syndrome, the journal's editors were insisting on "chronic idiopathic syndrome." The name quite appropriately suggested that the syndrome's cause was unknown, but it undermined the paper's strength, which was to synthesize an extraordinary wealth of new information about a pandemic disease, by implying that the syndrome was an obscure phenomenon seen exclusively in northern Nevada.

Lyndonville, New York

By early March, David Bell and Elaine DeFreitas had uncovered findings that Bell described as "ominous." Since they had announced their original findings in Kyoto the previous fall, 15 percent of the retrovirus-positive controls in Lyndonville—all of them children—had come down with the disease.

"This means that the virus is latent and asymptomatic—for a while," Bell said. "This is really a very ominous finding. This is *not* the power of suggestion in these children. What this implies, if you extrapolate it to the population of Lyndonville," he continued, "is that fifteen percent of the population of Lyndonville is eventually going to come down with this. This data would also imply that the disease is quite contagious."

Bell was commuting to Charlotte once each month to evaluate children suffering from the disease in Cheney's clinic. The doctor had seen ten pediatric cases so far. Increasingly, however, he was worried that the simmering feud between DeFreitas and Cheney over patent rights would end his professional ties, perhaps even his friendship, with the Charlotte doctor.

"We have an agreement to go until May," Bell said. "But I've told Cheney I don't want to be caught in an unpleasant thing between him and Elaine. And I kind of don't think it's going to be resolved."

Reno, Nevada

Early in March, Paul Levine of the National Cancer Institute flew to Nevada to study the state's cancer registry. He wanted to see for himself whether the cancers Dan Peterson had identified among his CFS patients and their close relatives really were uncommon and, if so, to what degree.

"Nevada has an excellent cancer registry," Levine said. "We're looking at cancer statewide."

Centers for Disease Control, Atlanta, Georgia

Out of a conviction that extracting total DNA was a superfluous task, agency microbiologist Walid Heneine had prepared the new samples from Lyndonville using the agency's standard techniques. Heneine's method, in common use throughout CDC labs, was a less labor-intensive and time-consuming process than total DNA extraction, the method DeFreitas had told Gunn was "absolutely critical" in the effort to duplicate her work.

By March 11, using these samples, Heneine was able to produce little that he considered a positive result. Walter Gunn stepped into the retrovirology lab to look at the results that day and noted that one of Bell's children seemed to have signs of infection. Heneine insisted the chemical reaction Gunn spotted meant nothing, but Tom Folks wasn't as certain. "It *could* be something," Gunn remembered Folks saying. But because Heneine had failed to run any healthy control samples with the Lyndonville samples, there was little that was conclusive about the results.

"That was *so* stupid!" Gunn complained later in a reference to the absence of controls. As a result, the work would have to be done a third time using controls.

Gunn worried that Heneine would run out of Lyndonville tissues if any more mistakes were made. In his office journal that week, Gunn wrote: "They keep using
up my DNA!"

Gunn set about securing control blood samples for Heneine, eventually coming
up with nine normal samples of agency employees' blood that had been stored in
the CDC's blood bank. Nevertheless, Gunn's early optimism about the Wistar
project and the depth of his agency's commitment to it was beginning to crack.
"So far, they hadn't used the total DNA technique *or* included controls," he would
recall later.

Along with the copy of her final manuscript, DeFreitas had sent the CDC a disclosure agreement for signature. The statement committed the agency to keeping
DeFreitas abreast of all developments in their efforts to duplicate her work and to
sharing their final conclusions well in advance of publishing them in a scientific
journal. In addition, the document asked the agency to keep its progress and its results confidential during the course of their work. The agreement also stipulated
that the agency could disclose no results unless they were disclosed jointly with
Wistar.

National Institutes of Health, Bethesda, Maryland

Anthony Fauci, director of the National Institute of Allergy and Infectious Diseases, refused requests for an interview in the spring of 1991. According to a
member of the Institute's public relations staff, Laurie Doepel, Fauci didn't feel
he "had followed chronic fatigue syndrome" closely enough to be interviewed on
the subject. Fauci's deputy assistant, James Hill, would be happy to talk about it,
however, Doepel said. During an interview, the lean, silver-haired Hill assured his
interviewer he could speak for Anthony Fauci on the disease. When pressed for
his boss's scientific views of the disease, Hill said, "Fauci wonders why the patients are so upset about being labeled with a psychiatric problem. I remember he
said to me, 'Haven't we come far enough along in our society that mental illness
needn't carry a stigma?' "

When asked how much clinical experience with actual patients he felt resided
within his institute, Hill reported that NIAID relied on the clinical acumen of one
person, Stephen Straus, for its understanding of the disease. And although Straus
was the "only person that we have in our institute who is interested in this particular area," Hill added, the disease ranked "number two in time consumption, at
least, in terms of our responses politically and to the public—mailings, et cetera,"
after AIDS.

NIAID would be willing to fund any worthy CFS research outside the agency,
Hill added, but he proposed that the "state of the science" continued to be too
murky to result in sizable grant support. "We do not feel that it's very clear exactly
what the status of the science is," Hill explained. "The disease itself, the diagnosis—there are a lot of questions that you really need to answer before you can
home in on something into which you could probably pour a lot of money. The

state of the science in CFS right now would probably not absorb a ten-billion-dollar effort and still make good use of the money."

If his agency learned that the disease was in fact an infectious viral illness similar, in many ways, to AIDS, would Hill and his colleagues retract the psychiatric conclusions drawn by Straus and promoted by the institute with such vigor through the conduit of the lay press?

A surprised "No!" was Hill's initial response. But he quickly amended his remark: "I think that we are scientists. Now, let's say—hypothetical situation—if, in fact, the evidence is clearly there that this is a single viral etiology—I mean, we're scientists—I think we would be big enough to admit that we have discovered the cause."

On March 18, a damp, overcast day in the capital, NIAID held its second workshop on CFS in three years. The approximately fifty scientists and researchers attending the second meeting, according to its organizers, would examine the CDC's diagnostic criteria with an eye toward fine-tuning them. On paper, their goal was a noble one. Yet, from the opening remarks of the very first speakers, the scientific bias of the meeting was resoundingly apparent.

University of Minnesota infectious disease specialist Philip Peterson, whom grant administrator Ann Schleuderberg had designated chairman of the workshop, cautioned participants that efforts to define the etiology, pathophysiology, or natural history of the disease were well beyond the scope of the meeting. Given the rigid agenda set by Stephen Straus and Ann Schleuderberg, what remained on the table, then, consisted of the ongoing debate over whether CFS was, in fact, depression.

The preponderance of that debate during the course of one and a half days focused on techniques for quantifying and qualifying the degree of psychiatric suffering in the disease. Clearly, rather than broadening its approach, the NIH was walling off its adversaries and digging in for the long haul. The agency's commitment to a belief that CFS was a vague, wastebasket diagnosis embracing innumerable disparate conditions, that it was not infectious, and that a sizable portion of its victims were plagued more seriously by neuroses than by anything else seemed more resolute than ever.

The serious investigators who participated in the NIH workshop were dismayed. "That meeting was just a sham," complained Temple University immunologist and biochemist Robert Suhadolnik some months later. Suhadolnik was studying the impact of Ampligen on the immune systems of people with CFS and AIDS. Another immunologist, Nancy Klimas, was only slightly less damning. "They were really highlighting the more negative data that's coming strictly from psychiatry- and psychology-based protocols in a *very* cynical mode," Klimas said afterward. "The immunology part, which was the reason I went, turned out to be a little side meeting, and the side meeting was supposed to come to some consensus that couldn't possibly be obtained in an hour of discussion."

No mention was made of the strides that brain-imaging experts had made in comprehending the origins of brain dysfunction in the disease. Ann Schleuderberg's reason for going out of her way to discourage Elaine DeFreitas's participation was readily apparent, too: DeFreitas's evidence for transmission of a novel retrovirus and for the infectious nature of the disease seemed to be the most forbidden topic of all. Participants hewed to the Bethesda agency's line, and by meeting's end a consensus emerged: immunologic and virologic tests, as well as brain scans of any variety, were experimental and therefore unworthy diagnostic tools in CFS. In fact, according to the majority of the participants, aside from routine blood tests—helpful for ruling out other diseases—there existed absolutely no laboratory test of value in confirming a case of CFS. Later, when the agency published the workshop's consensus conclusions in the medical literature, that was the take-home message.

Paul Cheney, who had been invited to describe his own methods for diagnosing the disease and to enumerate the characteristics of his patient population, was typically sanguine when the meeting ended, despite two days of institutionalized savaging of his ideas and observations. His thoughts, instead, were on Stephen Straus, whose presence at the conference had been an oppressive, inquisitor-style challenge to open discussion.

Straus's theory about the psychoneurotic origins of the disease had gained so much ground in the years since his acyclovir trial, Cheney believed, that mainstream medicine now considered mental illness to be virtually axiomatic in a diagnosis of CFS. "Straus has imposed his view of the disease by lining up an unbelievable number of psychiatrists and psychologists to inflict the view of the day. It's almost assumed now that you can't have CFS without having a psychiatric problem.

"I think there are some personality traits that may make the disease more severe," Cheney continued. "If a guy who is obsessive-compulsive catches this agent, [his obsessive-compulsiveness] becomes a marker for *severity,* but not for illness. I have plenty of type B people in my practice. One of them worked for the fire department. He liked to drink beer and jaw with the boys. A few months after resuscitating someone mouth-to-mouth he developed this disease and was destroyed. How can obsessive-compulsive personality explain this disease? Personality may *modulate* the disease. But it's like the Heisenberg uncertainty principle—the very act of a personality interacting with this disease changes the personality.

"I did get one thing out of the meeting," the doctor said after a moment. "I really do believe that there is a variety of ways by which this pathophysiology can be maintained, and in that sense, I believe that CFS is a heterogeneous illness that can be produced by a variety of triggers. But there was some *new* triggering agent in the 1970s. Now, today, we're seeing millions of people suffering disablement without end. And *that's* a change."

26

Smoke and Mirrors

Centers for Disease Control, Atlanta, Georgia

The CFS steering committee meetings were the most unpleasant two hours of Gunn's workweek. "I'm someone who has always been in charge of my own projects," Gunn said in the spring of 1991. "I'm not used to fifteen snarling, laughing people deciding if my ideas are workable. I think the reason the steering committee was set up, in fact, was to say no to spending money on the disease without making it *seem* like a money issue. They've amply demonstrated they can stop me in my tracks. If they functioned as a team that wanted to solve the problem, that would be one thing. But they don't. They function as a filter, or a sieve."

In the previous seven months Gunn had written no fewer than seven different protocols for a new, improved case-control study. All of them had been vetoed by the committee. The basic proposal crafted in 1985 by Gary Holmes and Carlos Lopez—to carefully study twenty or so patients and compare the results with twenty or so healthy people—was now six years old. With each new protocol Gunn submitted, the committee members would launch assaults; every member but Gunn seemed to harbor veto power.

Gunn's colleagues on the committee confirmed that year that the sessions were contentious, although they unanimously defended the style of the dialogue. "The committee has a personality all its own," commented Jim Dobbins, a demographer in the Viral Exanthems and Herpesvirus Branch who sat on the committee. "We have these terribly acrimonious meetings. [But] given what little we know about CFS, there is a variety of ways to approach it. It produces heated interactions." John Stewart, chief of the Clinical Virology Section, laughed when the phrase "tough audience" arose in reference to the committee. "I think you hit *that* on the head," he said. Mark Pallansch, the agency's enterovirus chief and a steering committee member, called the committee "not a timid group." Division chief Brian Mahy, Pallansch added, "functions as a referee." Another member, epidemiologist Scott Schmidt, said, "I don't think they're by any means uncivilized," then added, "certainly not by some of the standards I've seen in academia. No one calls anyone names or anything like that."

Matters of decorum aside, Gunn's complaint that the hypercritical committee failed to function as a "team that wanted to solve the problem" seemed to have some validity. Solving the problem was going to require epidemiologists and other scientists with, as North Carolina surgeon Thomas English had written, "supple and open minds," plus at least *some* familiarity with the disease. As it happened, nearly all of the members of the steering committee were operating under a similar and dubious hypothesis in their consideration of CFS.

"Easily the most prevalent if not the universal view [of steering committee members] is that the causes are multifactorial," enterovirus expert and committee member Mark Pallansch said. He was obviously not speaking for Walter Gunn when he added, "I don't think there's anyone on the committee who thinks it's just one agent. I can't think of *anyone* who is convinced it's a single hit. I think it's still an open issue whether this is even infectious. The possibilities are greater than fifty-fifty, but not much more than that."*

Multifactorial explanations for mysterious diseases were hardly new, but they nearly always arose as a means to explain the inexplicable when the cause of a disease was unknown. The notion of multifactorial agents being operative in cancer had long been presumed. Cancer, scientific theory went, was the end result of many events, many constituents, including genetic makeup, immune suppression, exposures to toxic substances or viruses, all culminating in the denouement. Before government researchers declared the cause of AIDS to be HIV in 1984, multifactorial theories that blamed the illness on two or more agents arose again and again in the struggle to understand transmission and physiologic pathways of the disease. There were also a number of respected "experts" who stated as categorical fact the unlikelihood that "a virus alone is inducing AIDS."[1]

Susan Sontag, in her 1979 essay *Illness as Metaphor*, described with transporting clarity the romantic and ultimately punishing meanings cultures attach to inscrutable diseases, most particularly cancer and, in the nineteenth century, tuberculosis. In theorizing about the causes and pathways of unsolved diseases, Sontag wrote, scientific and popular thought tended to fashion complex scenarios in which several factors were suspected of causing an illness. But, argued Sontag, "all the diseases for which the issue of causation has been settled, and which can be prevented and cured, have turned out to have a simple physical cause—like the pneumococcus for pneumonia, the tubercle bacillus for tuberculosis, a single vitamin deficiency for pellagra—and it is far from unlikely that something comparable will eventually be isolated for cancer. The notion that a disease can be explained only by a variety of causes is precisely characteristic of thinking about diseases whose causation is not understood."[2] This view had been seconded by at least one august member of the medical fraternity. The late Lewis Thomas, the doctor and medical philosopher, was paraphrased on the topic by National Cancer Institute scientist Robert Gallo in his 1991 book *Virus Hunting*. "[M]ultifactorial," Thomas believed, "is multi-ignorance."[3]

That spring, Gunn began to feel repercussions from his activist style. On March 29 the chief of the Division of Viral and Rickettsial Diseases, Brian Mahy, ordered

* Gunn was persistently frustrated by his colleagues' inflexibility on this point. "You keep hearing people say there are probably many causes of this disease," he said, "but the data don't support that. When you look for other diseases, they're just not there!"

him to cease providing Elaine DeFreitas with results of the agency's efforts to replicate her finding. Mahy's policy of secrecy soon applied to Gunn himself: Mahy ordered Folks to withhold from Gunn entirely the vicissitudes of the Wistar replication project.

Gunn, by now convinced that the Wistar finding was real, was increasingly concerned about the quality of the work being performed by CDC microbiologist Walid Heneine. Elaine DeFreitas had told Gunn during a conversation several weeks earlier that the exposure for the autoradiograph—a clear plastic negative approximately twelve inches by fifteen inches on which genetic matches between the PCR probes and the DNA of the virus could be visualized as dark bands—needed to be at least seven days. "Elaine said there weren't enough copies of the virus per cell to do a short exposure," Gunn recalled.

Although he harbored suspicions that the effort to reproduce DeFreitas's work was getting short shrift, Gunn was not himself a virologist and was thus in a difficult position. On April 5 he had noted in his office journal: "The auto-rad shows that two of six of Bell's kids are now positive. None of the [nine] controls lit up on the auto-rads. . . . They will now do a four-day exposure."

During a large, interbranch meeting on the Wistar project on the afternoon of April 4, Brian Mahy announced that Folks's HTLV2 findings in the Lyndonville children's blood were "all negative." Gunn had looked at the autoradiographs, however. Two out of six samples tested had displayed suggestive evidence of retrovirus infection, and the results of the four-day exposure remained unknown.

Gunn spoke up: "I said, '*I* see bands there, and Tom Folks thinks it's something.' "

Mahy contradicted Gunn, who, in turn, issued an invitation to the members of the steering committee and others present: "I said, 'As principal investigator on this project, I invite everyone here to the lab to look at these autorads!' " Afterward, according to Gunn, one agency virologist caught Gunn in the hallway and confirmed that the results of the experiment had suggested at least two positives. Nevertheless, Gunn had pounded a nail in his own coffin by confronting Mahy. "If they weren't scared of me," Gunn said later of his face-off with Mahy, "I would have been fired on the spot." Three days later Gunn called Walid Heneine to get the results on the four-day autoradiograms. Heneine told the senior investigator that the results were "inconclusive."

Progress proceeded at a snail's pace that spring. At steering committee meetings, Tom Folks was beginning to express doubt about his lab's ability to replicate the Wistar findings. Heneine had been unable to achieve the same sensitivity—an ability to find the same number of viral copies per cell—that Elaine had achieved in her assays.

"It got to the point where Folks told me he couldn't do much more for me," Gunn remembered.

On April 11, Folks told Gunn that his lab would be unable to support any further study of CFS blood after completing tests on just seven more samples. Folks explained to Gunn that he simply was without funds to pursue the research; in addition, Folks complained, the project was taking up all of Walid Heneine's time—time that Heneine, and evidently Folks, believed could be better spent on other diseases. Finally Folks told Gunn that in order to effectively reproduce De-

Freitas's work, his laboratory would require a sophisticated machine called a beta scanner. With this $65,000 piece of equipment, Folks told Gunn, he could get results in forty-five minutes that were equivalent to results provided by a seven-day autoradiograph.

The senior investigator scrambled to help Folks, whose work, Gunn believed, was the key to unlocking the agency's cache of expertise and enthusiasm. If the Wistar finding was confirmed in an agency lab, likely the resources of the entire agency would become available to pursue the disease. The next day Gunn wrote a long memo to Brian Mahy. "It was personal—me to him. I wanted to be manly about this. I handed it to him and I said, 'I think we're having a problem with communication.' "

Gunn's three-page single-spaced memo was a passionate statement in which he reminded Mahy of the potential weight of the Wistar finding in the public health realm and the agency's responsibility to fairly replicate DeFreitas's work, "using comparable specimens, techniques, equipment, and procedures."

Gunn wrote, "There are three problems that stand in the way of accomplishing our goals in this respect. Possible loss of continued retrovirus lab support, lack of critical up-to-date equipment, and an almost paranoid atmosphere of distrust of non-CDC scientists." He told Mahy that although the division chief had promised him "adequate lab support" and $110,000 specifically for retrovirology studies, "Dr. Folks informed me yesterday that all such support will cease as soon as the specimens delivered to him this week have been studied."

Gunn asked Mahy to "provide additional person power" to the Wistar project in Folks's lab. He asked, too, that CFS money be applied to the purchase of a beta scanner for Folks's lab, complaining that the delays caused by the agency's outdated technology were costing the investigation "valuable time and money."

"It seems to me that since [the agency] has been given $2,000,000 this year for the study of the causes of CFS," Gunn wrote, "you should be able to provide the perhaps $65,000 necessary for the scanner and possibly other equipment necessary for the completion of this important study."

Other excerpts from Gunn's memo of April 12 reveal the depth of Gunn's distress as well as the extraordinary tone of his colleagues' jocular disparagement of both the disease and the independent scientists studying it:

> I am concerned that the suspicion, distrust, and lack of respect for non-CDC researchers which I have observed in every DVRD meeting I have attended over the past four years is interfering with the progress of the proper study of this illness. I would like to ask that you, personally, see to it that future meetings be conducted in a professional manner with the focus on data and techniques rather than personalities. I am appalled at the vicious attacks I have heard made on Dr. Nancy Klimas, Dr. Elaine DeFreitas, Berch Henry, Dr. Komaroff, and others. . . . Although I, personally, have (so far) been able to endure the frivolous way in which the study of chronic fatigue syndrome is treated here at CDC, it is clear that the negativism of the past has hurt morale and is evident in the current lack of interest in chronic fatigue syndrome on the part of the lab people. I think that it is high time that CDC begin to treat the study of this syndrome with the same degree of concern which would be afforded to any other serious illness.

Gunn further protested Mahy's ruling that Elaine DeFreitas be kept innocent of the developments in the agency's attempts to reproduce her work:

> I wish to communicate freely with Dr. DeFreitas during our attempted replication of her study so that we will not make critical mistakes. Past communication with Dr. DeFreitas has not only prevented serious errors but has resulted in the implementation by the retrovirus lab of the use of the whole blood technique in *all* of their retrovirus polymerase chain reaction studies, because this technique, suggested by Dr. DeFreitas, has turned out to be better than the technique [nuclear DNA] previously used by our lab. I therefore request that you rescind your directive that I not discuss our results with Dr. DeFreitas as we proceed. We need her input.

Gunn concluded his memo with a request that in the future he be included in every division meeting held to determine how money appropriated for research was to be spent, "so that the resources can be focused in an organized way on the study of chronic fatigue syndrome."

On April 17, Gunn received from Mahy a written response to his memo of the week before. Unlike Gunn, who had kept his communication with Mahy private, Mahy sent copies of his memo to Gunn to members of the CFS steering committee and to Fred Murphy, the director of the Center of Infectious Diseases, who was Mahy's boss.

"My memo threatened him—right to his bones," Gunn recalled. "He must have thought I had distributed it to the whole steering committee, or that it would get out to them, because he carbon-copied *his* memo to everyone on the committee."

Division chief Mahy's lean missive instructed the principal investigator to stay out of the business of the retrovirology lab entirely; it also communicated a barely suppressed rage at what Mahy clearly viewed as Gunn's insubordination:

> You state that long delays have been caused by the less-than-state-of-the-art equipment used by the retrovirus laboratory to produce PCR results on autoradiograms. This is nonsense, and your comments indicate a considerable lack of understanding of the scientific procedures necessary for this study. In future, you must not involve yourself in the laboratory studies under way in Building 15. These are not within your area of competence. Dr. Folks and I will ensure that all CFS-related samples are processed as quickly and efficiently as possible.

Mahy, in addition, strove to diminish Gunn's authority by insisting that, in the future, any "actions or decisions of [the steering committee] must be communicated [to the public] through Dr. Schonberger or myself," a move that amounted to muzzling the agency's principal investigator from keeping patient organizations and the press abreast of the agency's progress on the disease. Mahy also reiterated his directive to Gunn to refrain from keeping DeFreitas abreast of in-house attempts to replicate her work: "You must not communicate experimental results obtained at the CDC to Dr. DeFreitas or any other investigator without my express permission."

Gunn's superior ended his memo with a particularly caustic paragraph in which he alerted Gunn to a spelling error in a letter Gunn had recently sent to Los Angeles pathologist John Martin. The spelling error, Mahy said, "gives a poor impression of the CDC. In such a sensitive area as this, we need to give the very best impression to our scientific colleagues who work on CFS. In future, all such communications must be approved by your supervisor, Dr. Schonberger, or myself before they are sent out." Mahy's seemingly petty outrage over a spelling error more subtly conveyed a truth about his division's effort in the disease: the agency's CFS project was a show of smoke and mirrors, an inquiry driven more by public relations concerns than by science, in which "impressions" created for people on the outside counted for everything. CFS itself was less a disease than it was a "sensitive area" requiring scrupulous political management.

On the day Mahy distributed this memo to steering committee members, Gunn discovered that his card key no longer unlocked the doors of Building 15. Someone had reprogrammed the agency's security system computer to deny him entry. (Retrovirology chief Tom Folks immediately reprogrammed Gunn's card key to allow him access to the building. Gunn was once more able to reach the outer administrative offices in the maximum-containment facility; Folks did not renew the senior researcher's access to the retrovirology laboratories, however.)* An intellectual renegade on the subject, clearly out of sync with his colleagues, Gunn needed to be both censured and demoted.

On April 18—for the third time that year—Gunn went to see Walter Dowdle, the second-ranking administrator in the agency. He complained to Dowdle that he was being virtually muzzled by his immediate superiors. A week later, Mahy clarified Gunn's new status. By default, Gunn would be allowed to continue talking to reporters; no one else wanted the job. But, Gunn recalled, "Mahy told me he didn't want me in direct communication with the patient activists."

Gunn's internist diagnosed him with a duodenal ulcer that spring; in addition, the senior investigator began to have heart palpitations several times a day. His blood pressure, he discovered, was climbing, too.

In July, Tom Folks got his beta scanner. The machine speeded up the work of the retrovirology lab by at least thirtyfold, Folks said later.

Philadelphia, Pennsylvania

On April 1, Elaine DeFreitas's paper on an HTLV2-like retrovirus in patients with CFS and their asymptomatic contacts appeared in the *Proceedings of the National Academy of Sciences.*[4] Several weeks before the paper came out, the scientist sent her gene sequence data in the form of journal preprints to Anthony Komaroff, John Martin, Jay Levy, and, of course, Tom Folks.

DeFreitas was getting closer, she believed, to identifying the virus. The more she evaluated it, the less it seemed to resemble HTLV2. She was also beginning a

---

* Years later, asked about the event, Folks merely said, "No comment," but he went on to describe an unpleasant "tension" that had been created by the escalating conflict between Gunn and Mahy, tension that spilled into his own laboratory and dampened the morale of his staff.

crucial part of any effort to identify a virus: mapping the pathogen's genetic structure, a process known as cloning and sequencing. In an effort to learn if the virus resembled any other known virus, she was entering descriptions of portions of the virus's nucleic acid into a computer that was programmed with the genetic structures of every known plant and animal virus.

"I'm going mad!" DeFreitas said. "It's just interim confusion, but we're getting partial matches with everything from dengue fever to cucumber necrosis virus to hog cholera to cymbidium ring spot virus to cauliflower mosaic virus. We're getting there," she added, "but, at every level, it keeps us excited."

For once, the scientist was placid about the years of damaging politics that had so harmed the reputations of CFS researches and turned the disease into a laughingstock. "That is all going to be swept away," she said. "Since Kyoto, I have not seen a single piece of data that has convinced me we are wrong. The virus is there, it's real, it's alive, it's not a lab contaminant, it's not my imagination, and I don't care what Steve Straus tries to do, he can't make it go away."

University of Southern California, Los Angeles

On April 13, Walter Gunn, having heard about John Martin's progress, from CFIDS Association head Marc Iverson, decided to call Martin. The pathologist was pleased to know that the CDC was curious: "I thought, Fantastic." He described his work to Gunn, saying he had isolated a virus from the spinal fluid and blood tissues of CFS patients and that the bug induced a foamy-cell cytopathic effect similar to that described for spuma viruses.

University of California, Irvine

By springtime, clinical neuropsychologist Curt Sandman had studied eighty-five patients with CFS, a figure that was double his patient cohort of the year before. "We haven't deviated a bit from our original inquiry," Sandman said. "We're still asking the same questions: Is there a CFS dementia? Are there *specific* memory deficits?" With twice the number of patients, Sandman was more confident than ever that the answer to both questions was a resounding yes. "The cognitive profile we initially described has remained steady."

Sandman's early profile had confirmed neuropsychologist Sheila Bastien's 1986 finding that people with the disease were highly dysfunctional in the realm of short-term memory: they had difficulty, Sandman said, "making" memories. Patients suffered, in addition, from serious attention deficits; virtually anything, however minor, could irretrievably derail their mental focus, as in novelist and sufferer Floyd Skloot's example: "If I see you scratch your head while I'm talking to you, chances are I'll forget what I'm trying to say." Given these findings, it was easy to understand why children with the disease experienced such profound difficulty in school. During the months and years following the onset of their illness, most children dropped at least two grade points below their previous average; failing one or more grades was hardly uncommon.

Another intellectual deficit suggested by Sandman's original research had become more prominent, however, with the addition of forty-five more patients to his study. "These people always expect to do better than they actually do on these tests," Sandman said. "That metacognitive deficit is so consistent that it is a very pathognomonic [specific] sign for these patients. The only other syndrome in which we see this deficit is in learning-disabled adults."

Sandman further suggested that a significant component of CFS victims' overt, often powerfully expressed distress—which had caused skeptics to dismiss the malady as hysteria or major depression—might actually be attributable to the experience of consistently performing in a fashion that fell so far beneath their expectations. The investigator's hunch was a deceptively simple-sounding postulate with profound resonance for sufferers. Healthy people might only begin to imagine the potent emotions CFS sufferers experienced as they struggled to maneuver within a world that had become complicated and demanding beyond all reason. For the trial lawyer who had misplaced his wallet in the freezer, for the real estate saleswoman who tried to make a phone call at a parking meter, both early patients of Anthony Komaroff's, for the college professor who couldn't hold a thought long enough to deliver a coherent lecture, and for the pilot who was unable to complete even a cockpit preflight check, the transformations wrought by onset of CFS signified a trauma beyond words.

Although Sheila Bastien and Curt Sandman each had found significant loss of short-term memory function in the disease, Sandman was beginning to see a pattern having to do with long-term memory that was both unique to the disease and distinct from Bastien's observations: sufferers were remarkably vulnerable to losing long-term memories typically assumed to be of lifelong duration. "The stuff that's supposed to stay around forever seems to be unraveling," Sandman said.

Like many researchers who worked with victims of the disease, Sandman had heard patients complain of disorientation as a result of their altered perception of time. The disease seemed to fling its victims into a new dimension where time was bowed and stretched into a shape lacking recognizable dimensions. He wondered if the problem had to do with the disappearance of old memories in CFS sufferers, and he further questioned why "remote" memory was harmed in this way. "There's definitely some kind of telescoping of time, some perturbation in the *sense* of time in this disease," Sandman said. "The organs of the brain that keep track of time are the frontal lobes, and it may be that that is where the problem resides. We know there are processing deficits and abnormalities."

By 1992 Sandman was of the opinion that the mild-sounding, nonspecific neuropsychological symptoms included in the CDC's case definition of the disease—which included forgetfulness, confusion, difficulty thinking, and inability to concentrate—failed to capture the profundity of the disease's cognitive devastation. Like Marshall Handleman, the Los Angeles neurologist and brain-mapping expert, Sandman increasingly viewed the disease as a serious brain injury, comparable in many ways to a number of other severe brain diseases such as Huntington's chorea and herpes encephalitis.

In sum, a former skeptic who had written off the first three CFS patients he examined as suffering from hysterical neurosis, Sandman was now thoroughly on the side of the believers. Nevertheless, he explained, "We've been working piecemeal. I don't have grant support for this."

University of Southern California, Los Angeles

Before the end of April, pathologist John Martin had three conference calls with Walter Gunn, Tom Folks, Brian Mahy, and Walid Heneine at the CDC. Retrovirology chief Folks and his colleague Heneine complained bitterly that Martin was either unable or unwilling to describe his discoveries and techniques to them in sufficient and therefore persuasive detail. They noted, too, that spuma viruses were notorious for contaminating laboratory cultures, a fact that only added to their skepticism about the importance of Martin's discovery.

Privately, Martin was disappointed with Gunn, who he said "couldn't hold his own with these cynical people"—the CDC scientists, in other words, who seemed unwilling even to admit CFS was a disease, let alone a neurological one.

In the meantime, Martin sent a case history of one of the encephalopathic patients from whom he had obtained a viral isolate—a patient who was officially brain-dead but who was being maintained at the Los Angeles County Hospital—to *Lancet*. "It was rejected," Martin reported later. "They said spuma viruses are common contaminants in cultures." *Lancet*'s editors also told Martin that in the past they had regretted publishing reports of atypical viruses in patients with unusual diseases, since such reports frequently could not be confirmed in other labs. "Lancet said they'd been burned in the past by publishing new findings," Martin lamented some years later. "But my feeling is, medical journals have a *responsibility* to publish new findings!" Indeed, how else was medical knowledge to be advanced?

Martin was frustrated by the response of the medical press to his work. His impulse was to take his news public, but he was strongly advised by the CFIDS Association and by his colleagues to refrain from doing so. There was tremendous fear that the discovery would be discredited if it was unveiled in the lay press before publication in a scientific journal. His confidants reminded him of the prejudice the Wistar discovery had suffered as a result of its release prior to publication in the literature.

Senate Office Building, Washington, D.C.

In April, participating in an annual ritual, administrators of the federal health agencies testified before the House Appropriations Subcommittee on the Department of Labor, Health and Human Services, Education, and Related Agencies. Cardiologist Bernadine Healy, in her new role as director of the NIH, appeared before the committee for the first time that spring; Anthony Fauci, the director of the National Institute of Allergy and Infectious Diseases, and William Raub, her predecessor, were at her side.

During the hearing, Congressman John Porter asked the directors this question: "I wonder if you can tell us where NIH is in respect to chronic fatigue syndrome and what kind of priority you place on research?"

By his response, Fauci, the Bethesda institute's AIDS expert, revealed that six years after the Tahoe epidemic, his agency still didn't know what constellation of signs and symptoms constituted a case of CFS: "I think we are having some slow success in tracking them down. One of the most difficult issues is really understanding the definition of what this is, what are the diagnostic criteria, which have really not been defined. . . . We are making progress, but it remains a very perplexing and elusive problem."

As for the priority assigned to the disease inside the agency, the assembled administrators informed the subcommittee that not even one Bethesda scientist was working on CFS full-time. "This is one of the many diseases that is the responsibility of our extramural program," Fauci said, meaning the institute expected research on the disease to be conducted outside the agency with agency support. (Fauci failed to mention that his agency had rejected nearly every grant proposal submitted on the subject.) Nevertheless, Fauci told Porter, the NIH was requesting $2,651,000 for CFS research.

Lying to Congress is a crime subject to prosecution under the Federal Perjury Statute of Title 18, U.S. section 1621, and carries a punishment of five years' imprisonment or a $2,000 fine, or both. That's if you're under oath. Fortunately for the director of the CDC, William Roper, who appeared before the committee the following day, he swore no oaths before giving his testimony.

"I have served on this committee ten years," Congressman Porter said to Roper. "Ten years ago, nobody knew anything about [CFS], and we have gone quite a long way to understanding this syndrome better. So I wonder if you could tell me where we are, and if you could focus on . . . the amount of money—$2,000,000—that we put in. Is that all spent? And how is it being spent? What about the apparent clusters of chronic fatigue syndrome? And the case-control study? Where are we in regard to that? What about preliminary reports that link a retrovirus to chronic fatigue syndrome, and finally, how many FTEs [full-time equivalents] do you have working in this area?"

Roper told Porter he would "expand on our laboratory breakthroughs or our laboratory findings" in a written report, but he reassured the congressman that "we have between ten to twelve FTEs working on CFS."

Medical College of Wisconsin, Milwaukee

By that spring, Sidney Grossberg had given a temporary name to the novel retrovirus he had isolated from a CFS sufferer in 1989. Grossberg took his inspiration from the patient in whom he had isolated the virus, a sixtyish woman whose initials were "JH," and the healthy person's cells in which the virus, harbored in JH's lymphocytes, flourished, "K." Thus, "Human JHK Virus" became the third retroviral discovery in the disease by an American.

In mid-April, the scientist requested $150,000 from the CFIDS Association to pursue his research. His timing was impeccable. The North Carolina organization's leadership, following with dismay the sluggish Wistar-CDC collaboration, had begun to wonder if perhaps they had put too many eggs in one basket. Impressed with Grossberg's credentials, the association's scientific advisory board voted unanimously to fund. Grossberg made one request of the patient advocacy group: he asked that they assign his project the lowest profile they could possibly manage, given that they were compelled to reveal to their membership the identities of their major scientific grant recipients. His request was granted.

University of California, San Francisco

Soon after receiving the primer and sequencing data from Elaine DeFreitas, Jay Levy set to work in an effort to duplicate the Wistar finding. "We have tried to confirm their work, and failed," Levy said some months later. "The primers are *very* bizarre." Unlike Larry Schonberger at the CDC several months earlier, however, Levy had no impulse to publish his failure to confirm the Wistar finding. By then he knew too much about the disease to reject the retrovirus theory out of hand simply because he had been unable, in a matter of days, to confirm a finding that DeFreitas and her lab associates had worked for three years to achieve.

Levy did not linger over the problem, however. His focus that spring was on the immune system marker he had announced in Charlotte the previous November. He was preparing the finding for publication in *Lancet.* After composing the manuscript, Levy sent it to no fewer than ten clinician-epidemiologists in San Francisco for their opinion. "I wanted to be sure this paper would stand up to scrutiny," Levy said, "because the grant proposal that we sent into the NIH in this area was rejected with a very high score—meaning *real* high." (Study review sections in Bethesda scored grant proposals like golf: the higher the number, the worse the score.) His colleagues' comments were followed by what Levy called a "tough review" by *Lancet*'s reviewers, three scientists in London. Because the paper had passed muster with his San Francisco colleagues and the London reviewers, Levy was confident of publication. "I hope this paper is going to be a classic," he said.

Interestingly, an immune system abnormality that Levy and his coauthors Carol Jessop and Alan Landay described was remarkably similar to one of the primary immune aberrations frequently seen in one stage of AIDS. It was a T-cell hyperactivity that typically precedes the sudden loss of T-cells, an event that usually presages the fatal stages of the disease.

Centers for Disease Control, Atlanta, Georgia

In an effort to improve his lab's ability to replicate the Wistar results, CDC retrovirology chief Tom Folks invited Elaine DeFreitas to his lab in Atlanta to advise his staff on her techniques firsthand. She suggested instead that Folks send Walid Heneine to her lab at Wistar. "I said, 'Stay for three days,' " DeFreitas recalled later. " 'See the experiment through!' " It was senseless for her to travel to Atlanta, the scientist continued. "I told them that was . . . a waste of their money and my time. They have to see the setup here and work side by side with the people who do the work. If I went down there, I would work with *their* stuff, which is suspect."

On May 15, Gunn and Larry Schonberger, impatient with the rate of progress in Tom Folks's laboratory, asked DeFreitas to test the blood specimens taken from Atlanta patients referred to the agency by local doctors through the surveillance project. They promised they would send her samples from patients and from controls, mixed together in such a way that she would be innocent of the differences. DeFreitas did not welcome the request. She had too little help in her lab as it was, and she was working toward the next milestone, identifying the virus. This new request would cost her precious money, manpower, and time. Nevertheless, she speculated, perhaps Gunn was right: maybe this was a way to leapfrog over the government lab and get confirmation. Reluctantly she agreed to undertake the work.

Having secured DeFreitas's cooperation, Gunn posed what he assumed was a mundane question: should he ship the samples to her on dry ice?

DeFreitas was alarmed. Samples must *never* be frozen, she told Gunn. Freezing caused the strands of DNA to fragment; when the strands were fragmented, proper binding, or hybridization, of strands was prevented.* It had been her experience that freezing blood samples greatly reduced the chances for binding to occur during the PCR process.

"In order for a strand of DNA to serve as a template," DeFreitas explained later, "it must be whole. The ideal thing is to preserve the DNA as close to its original configuration—full-length DNA—as possible. When you repeatedly freeze and thaw it, the water crystals, as they form and melt, break the DNA into tiny pieces. If that piece is broken, the PCR won't work—there will be nothing for the primers to cling to."†

In defiance of division chief Brian Mahy's orders, Gunn felt compelled to reveal to DeFreitas a fact of life in the agency's retrovirology lab: staff people in Tom Folks's lab had been freezing all the CFS samples to −20°C. as a matter of routine since the Wistar replication project began in February.

---

* To fully comprehend Defreitas's criticism, it is necessary to understand the daunting intricacies of searching for novel viruses using the polymerase chain reaction technique. PCR is a powerful tool for finding viruses in tiny amounts. But to accomplish this feat the scientist must know the genetic code of the virus. Obviously the genetic code of a novel virus is unknown. In such cases, scientists are essentially feeling their way in the dark when undertaking PCR. To begin, the scientist assumes that at least some portion of the new virus's DNA will be similar to that of a known virus. The investigator therefore constructs a probe, a piece of DNA material for which the code is known. During the amplification period, a bonding or binding of the two complementary strands of DNA, the one manufactured by the investigator and the virus's own DNA material, occurs.

PCR may be both exquisitely sensitive (able to detect virus in small numbers) and exquisitely specific (able to detect the virus under investigation), but it is exactly these qualities that complicate such experiments beyond the wildest imagination of most mortals. As the investigator experiments with different stringency conditions to optimize the binding of viral probe and viral DNA, the specificity may be altered. For instance, when stringency conditions are relaxed, the probe may bind to similar but not identical strands of viral DNA; if the stringency is profoundly relaxed, the probe will bind to virtually any DNA in its presence, rendering any positive result meaningless. In contrast, if stringency is too high, there will be no binding at all. Stringency and specificity, then, are intimately linked in PCR. Ideally, the goal is to maintain high stringency to encourage specificity. But when a scientist is trying to identify a new virus, the stringency must be kept relatively low to allow binding to occur. Computing precise stringency conditions, then, is a worrisome task. The greatest challenge when virus hunting, however, lies in achieving the same results at each experiment. When results are difficult to reproduce on multiple attempts, the finding is rarely considered legitimate. Once the code of the new virus is determined, however, these difficulties fade. With the full code, a scientist can fashion a probe that will allow him or her to run PCR under high-stringency conditions, producing the same result each time.

† "I agree," Folks commented when told of DeFreitas's reasoning, but he added that such concerns were legitimate only when viral copies in cells were "extremely low," lower than DeFreitas claimed she was finding in her own patient samples. "If a single freeze-thaw were eliminating that copy, then she might have had some grounds to stand on, but we eventually tried the assay on unfrozen [CFS] blood, with the same results. We tried everything she said," Folks continued. "She stood on the edge of credibility when she made suggestions and we tried them and they actually worked!"

DeFreitas, stunned by Gunn's revelation, explained this was an especially significant problem because Tom Folks's PCR test was 15,000 times less sensitive than hers. The two scientists had already compared sensitivity and discovered the discrepancy.

According to Gunn, Folks viewed DeFreitas's complaint as evidence that the Wistar scientist was deliberately changing and complicating the game plan as the project proceeded. "His comment was 'Oh, there she goes—another wrinkle,' " Gunn said.

Gunn, in contrast, was profoundly disturbed by these revelations. "At that point, as far as I was concerned," he said later, "I believed none of Folks's tests had been valid because they weren't sensitive enough and because he had been working with DNA that had been frozen. . . .* Of course, Brian Mahy and Walid Heneine disagreed."

The day Schonberger and Gunn called DeFreitas to propose that she run her tests on CDC patients, Gunn received a call from John Martin in Los Angeles. In his office that day, Gunn wrote, "Martin's clamming up."

Gunn and Folks had asked Martin to call the agency again when he had a manuscript and data in hand. Martin, in turn, was suspicious of the federal scientists. By late spring he had begun to suspect that they might be audacious enough to steal his ideas and his methods and claim the discovery as their own. Inevitably, Martin's reticence was interpreted by the Atlanta staff as evidence of the flimsy nature of his claims.

Santa Monica, California

As news of John Martin's discovery percolated through the patient activist community, hopes were raised. A pervasive longing for rapid resolution of the dilemma coalesced into one fond desire: proof that the Wistar virus and the pathogen in Martin's lab were one and the same. Confirmation would be followed, this desperate community imagined, by diagnostic tests; drug therapy might be close behind.

Unfortunately, Martin was running out of money. On May 15 a CFS sufferer and former stockbroker, Richard Carson, organized a second Hollywood fundraiser, this time at Lowe's Santa Monica Beach Hotel, to raise funds for Martin and his staff. Julie Andrews, Blake Edwards, and rock singer Rod Stewart's former wife, Alana, were there, as were approximately thirty other film and television industry people. Blake Edwards had pledged to match anyone's donation of $25,000. John Martin and Paul Cheney addressed the group, which had gathered in a suite overlooking the ocean.

---

* In the minutes for the June 26 steering committee meeting, Walter Gunn recorded Folks's explanation: "[T]here may be a real problem with the CDC-produced primers and probes, severe enough to have made it impossible to detect the retrovirus particles reported by the Wistar Institute if they did in fact exist in the peripheral blood of the participants in the pilot phase of the case-control study." Gunn added that, as a result, DeFreitas had agreed to send Folks her actual probes and primers.

Carson had pitched the event to his guests as an opportunity to hear about cutting-edge research from a scientist who had isolated a virus that might well be the cause of the disease. Martin, with his low-key delivery and his tendency to be brutally clinical in his discussion, was not well received by the Hollywood crowd, however. He showed pictures of doctors performing a brain biopsy; he talked about finding the virus in six encephalopathic patients, one of whom was comatose.

"No one present wanted to think they had the disease Martin was talking about," Marc Iverson recalled.

For a second time, an effort to engage the Hollywood community in the problem failed. Blake Edwards's $25,000 offer went unmatched.

Paris, France

On May 23 the lay press in France officially recognized CFS as a serious health problem in that nation. *L'Express,* France's equivalent of *Time* or *Newsweek,* carried a cover story about CFS.

"Fatigue: Une Vraie Maladie" (Fatigue: A Real Disease) was the cover line. Inside, editors devoted nine pages to the subject, five of them focused on the "chase for the virus" in America. Paul Cheney was featured in a photograph; he was sitting in his Charlotte clinic, studying a series of MRI brain scans.

Cambridge, Massachusetts

David and Karen Bell moved away from tiny Lyndonville to Boston in the summer of 1991. Twelve years after it had begun, their adventure in rural living and small-town doctoring had come to a quiet end, to Karen's substantial relief. Both of the doctors had secured new jobs, David as a pediatric specialist at Harvard's Cambridge Hospital, Karen as the associate medical director of a Harvard-affiliated health maintenance organization. David, in addition, was named school physician for the city of Cambridge. Years before, he had hoped his affiliations with academic medicine were permanently severed. Now he found himself practicing in the nation's most prestigious academic medical center with five other pediatric specialists.

The epidemic disease that had so dwarfed other aspects of his life in Lyndonville continued to haunt him in academe. Unable to expunge it from his thoughts, Bell struggled to suppress his knowledge of the topic in the presence of his colleagues, who had made it clear to him that they considered CFS "a passing fad." His partners, he added, were "the cream of the crop—the best Harvard pediatricians." Yet they were wholly uninterested in his singular expertise: the manifestations of CFS in children. Moreover, his colleagues, he said, "made it very clear that they don't want me to see CFS patients in our group practice." Bell sensed that his regard for the disease was tolerated by his associates as a harmless peccadillo. "I'm like some guy who ties flies for a hobby," Bell said, but substantive discussions about the disease were unwelcome. "I'm not allowed to talk about anything I know about—things like T-four cells and other immune aberrations in the disease. They view that as *very* weird stuff." Like a muzzled Cassandra, Bell struggled with his conscience. The effort left him feeling alienated, even bewildered.

Yet, however much the doctor tried to suppress his thoughts on the subject, CFS refused to vanish from his world. As Cambridge school physician, for instance, Bell had been called in for meetings between parents and the administrators of a grade school where a number of children had fallen ill with what was presumed to be "sick-building syndrome," a malaise caused by toxins leaching from building materials or other environmental sources. "The parents are saying the school is poisonous," Bell said. "But ... *sixteen* air-quality experts [have] looked, and they've found nothing. What probably is going on is an outbreak of chronic fatigue syndrome."

When Bell broached the possibility of performing a sign-symptom complex history for CFS on all the sick children, the response from parents and administrators alike was, he said, " 'No way!' That's so threatening."

In August the medical journal *Pediatrics* published a study of teenagers suffering from CFS by Mark Scott Smith, head of a clinic for adolescents with psychosomatic illnesses at the University of Washington in Seattle, and a handful of other Seattle specialists, including virologist Larry Corey and internal medicine specialist Deborah Gold.[5] (In 1990, Corey and Gold had collaborated on a widely publicized paper that suggested CFS was a manifestation of depression.) More research was needed, Smith concluded, to learn whether the problem was depression, "a discrete psychosomatic condition, or an infectious immunologic disorder that mimics depression."

Smith had studied fifteen teenagers. Although one third met his psychiatric criteria for "major depression," ten "showed little evidence of a psychiatric disorder." A majority had fallen ill quite suddenly with an acute infection and gone on to develop chronic disease. After fatigue and headache, Smith wrote, the third most common and debilitating symptom among this group was "concentration problems." Three children were so impaired by their condition that they were being tutored at home. There were, in addition, "significant family problems in four subjects and isolation from peers in six others."

Interviewed three years before, Smith, a medical doctor, had expressed a belief that CFS sufferers, including children and teenagers, were ill advised to worry themselves with "left brain" concerns like whether a virus had caused their disease. Instead, he suggested, they should look inward, examining their personal role in the acquisition of their disease. "I'm more interested in what piece of this problem can you *own*?" Smith explained, "so that you can deal with it and get back and involved with life somehow. And the sense I get with the handful of adolescent CFS patients who I've seen so far is that that's a problem for them. They really do get stagnated. They really do get dead in the water."

Lyndonville, New York

Medical journal articles about teenagers suffering from CFS were devoid of subjective information about the anguish of being simultaneously on the cusp of adulthood and debilitated by an incurable brain disease with an insidiously benign name. Real children living in real households who had fallen ill during the middle 1980s were now well into their adolescent years. Many of them had passed through adolescence and become young adults without knowing a day of good health. For those who had fallen ill in their earliest years, good health was just an idea, an elusive abstraction that for unfathomable reasons had been denied them, something, in fact, they would have been unable to describe, having long ago lost their memory of it.

In Lyndonville, the epidemic that had begun six years before continued to inflict torment upon nearly two hundred young lives. In one grand old house on Main Street, every family member was sick. Hannah, Megan, and Libby Pollard had been in grade school in the impoverished town on the Lake Ontario shore when they fell ill in 1985. Alison, the eldest Pollard child, had been the last to succumb at age fifteen in 1987, the same year her parents began to exhibit symptoms of the disease. Now twenty, Alison was about to enter her second year of college; her younger sisters were in high school. None of them had recovered. The girls' precious formative years had been ravaged by illness and their future was clouded by uncertainty. As they moved toward adulthood, their mother, Jean, said, a recurring sadness burdened their conversations with her and with each other: "They wonder, What if I *hadn't* been sick? What could I have accomplished?"

Each child had tested in the upper ninetieth percentile and, seemingly effortlessly, carried high averages before developing CFS. Afterward, their relationship with school and the process of learning changed dramatically. In fact, their academic progress had been achieved with effort and sacrifice unimaginable to most teenagers. Alison learned to tape-record her classes; at home in the evening she painstakingly transcribed the lessons, then fashioned flash cards with which to drill herself over and over. As her younger siblings moved along in school, they adopted Alison's system. There was little time or energy left for anything else. "All of the kids had to give up musical instruments," Jean Pollard said. "You start instruments in fourth grade, but all three younger girls got sick when they were in fifth grade, and after the fifth grade they didn't have the memory capability to learn music." The once shiny new instruments, stored in their cases, had become small monuments to her daughters' thwarted potential over the years; their sale had precipitated a bout of quiet grieving in the Pollard household.

All of the sick children of Lyndonville had fared better than most stricken children elsewhere because of David Bell's presence, Pollard noted. In an effort to diminish the school trauma experienced by such children, for instance, Bell had developed an educational literature on the brain impairment caused by CFS and had distributed it to Lyndonville teachers. Often, the teachers provided remedial classes and after-school tutorials for children of the epidemic, nursing them along in their studies. As late as 1989, some in rural Lyndonville were unaware that CFS could strike adults as well as children; they viewed the disease as an affliction of childhood, like chicken pox or measles, if vastly more consequential. As years passed, however, it was both impossible and impractical to hold these young sufferers within the village's protective cocoon. "We've had tremendous medical support from David, and from the Lyndonville schools *because* of David," Jean Pollard said. "But my kids still have been tremendously affected because they've had to go out in the world and deal with people who don't believe they're sick."

The Pollards' youngest daughter, Hannah, who was ten when she fell ill six years before, had undergone the most hospitalizations for her disease and had suffered the most pronounced neurological symptoms. Some of her most dramatic symptoms, such as sudden extreme abdominal pain and partial limb paralysis, were also the most impregnable to emergency-room diagnostic procedures in Medina, New York, site of the nearest hospital. "She's had many hospital trips where people did not believe her—they thought she was faking," Jean Pollard said. "And of all my children, Hannah has had the most trouble with issues of identity and with depression." Pollard recalled that when Hannah was very young she would crawl into her mother's lap and cry. "She would say, 'I don't see myself in the future.' But—*all* my children have been deeply affected by chronic illness. It wasn't just Hannah," Pollard said. "Throughout their adolescence, they had no sense of their future. They couldn't say, 'What will I be doing in ten years?' They didn't have that luxury. It was just, 'Let's survive today.' "

Tragically, as the years passed, their recall of an era when their intellectual and physical suppleness matched or superseded that of any other child's had faded entirely. "With the exception of Alison," their mother said, "none of them have a memory of ever feeling well."

27

Heartsink

New York, New York

In the May 30 issue of *Patient Care,* a journal distributed to 115,000 clinicians, an article informing doctors how to "manage" CFS patients appeared under the by-line of Seattle's Dedra Buchwald, Boston's Nelson Gantz, University of Washington psychiatrist Wayne Katon, and University of Connecticut internist Peter Manu.* The article encouraged doctors to perform a "thorough psychiatric workup" of their CFS cases *"even if the history does not suggest a psychiatric disorder"* (italics added). Interaction with support groups should be discouraged, the doctors cautioned, since "chronic fatigue syndrome groups may be dominated by people who have the most severe illness (and a tenacious commitment to being sick). . . . And most groups are heavily invested in believing that chronic fatigue syndrome is a distinct postviral disease."

The article also offered advice for dealing with "difficult" patients: "Despite your attempts to persuade her otherwise, [the difficult patient] may continue to insist that she has CFS. She may become the sort the British call heartsink patients—those who exasperate, defeat and overwhelm their doctors by their behavior."

Further, the authors suggested that CFS patients be urged to take antidepressant medications and to exercise—reckless advice in both cases. Due to an apparent metabolic disorder which developed after the disease's onset, CFS sufferers were exquisitely drug-sensitive. When given antidepressant medications in amounts typically prescribed for depression, they often became more ill. Exercise, of course, was the great pillar of the Mayo Clinic's prescribed regime for sufferers. Those doctors who maintained a consistent relationship with their CFS patients, however, knew exercise to be among the most predictably devastating events, second only, perhaps, to the physical trauma of a car accident or surgery, in the lives of such patients; increased severity of symptoms usually began twenty-four to

---

* Immediately after the article was published, Dedra Buchwald, who headed a clinic for five hundred CFS sufferers in Seattle, and Nelson Gantz, clinical director of infectious diseases at the University of Massachusetts, wrote to the officers of the CFIDS Action Campaign for the United States (CACTUS) to explain that, although they had been interviewed for the article by a *Patient Care* writer, contrary to appearances, they, themselves, had not "written" the article.

forty-eight hours after even a minor workout. Vigorous exercise, in fact, frequently moved people who were only partially disabled into the category of fully disabled for an indefinite period of time.

By 1991, Los Angeles clinician Jay Goldstein had suggested that monitoring the CFS victim's response to exercise was among the simplest ways for doctors to distinguish the disease from major depression. "Exercise or exertion of any sort can cause the CFS patient to relapse in virtually every respect," Goldstein wrote in his second book on the disease.[1] That same year, responding to misguided exhortations to exercise, Canadian clinician Byron Hyde stated bluntly that anyone who *improved* with exercise likely did not have CFS. And in 1995, Cheney remarked, "It is my opinion that patients with this disease cannot be trained aerobically unless their disease has improved. . . . One cannot train what is broken or dysfunctional."*

University of Nevada School of Medicine, Reno

Even though the Wistar's retrovirus theory remained, as researcher Seymour Grufferman said that summer, "where the action is," there continued to be credible CFS researchers who were committed to studying the role of human herpesvirus 6 in the disease, either as the causative agent or as a contributing player in the development and symptoms of the disease.

---

* Over the years, researchers had advanced numerous hypotheses to explain the disastrous impact of exercise on the disease. Investigators who theorized that the fault lay in the muscles amply demonstrated muscle fiber abnormalities that could not be attributed to mere disuse (Peter Behan et al., "Post Viral Fatigue Syndrome," *CRC Critical Reviews in Neurobiology* 4, no. 2 [1988]: 157–78). Another study revealed that the muscles of inactive CFS sufferers resembled the fatigued muscles of post-race marathon runners, exhibiting acidosis and other by-products of physical duress (D. L. Arnold et al., "Excessive Intracellular Acidosis of Skeletal Muscle on Exercise in a Patient with a Post-Viral Exhaustion Fatigue Syndrome," *Lancet* 1, 8391 [1984]: 1367–1369). There were indications, too, that the mechanism cells used to metabolize oxygen were flawed, a defect linked to the mitochondria, which are related to cellular energy levels (observations by Peter Behan, Elaine DeFreitas, et al.). It was also known by 1991 that people with CFS exhibited abnormally low oxygen uptake during exercise; although the cause remained mysterious, blood oxygen levels rose to normal levels among Ampligen "responders" but returned to subnormal levels when the drug was withdrawn. Red blood cell malformation, first noted in CFS patients by scientists in Australia and New Zealand and later confirmed in the United States by Anthony Komaroff's Harvard collaborators, was yet another pathological condition that might affect muscle functioning and energy, since one consequence of deformed red cells might be inadequate oxygen and nutrient delivery. One such investigator suggested that "a pathogenesis is proposed which envisions that when the number of [deformed red cells] exceeds some unknown threshold value they may impair capillary blood flow sufficiently for stasis to develop in the smallest capillaries." The most famous symptom of the disease—fatigue—this researcher added, "may be an inappropriate term in such circumstances." (L. O. Simpson, "The Role of Nondisocytic Erythrocytes in the Pathogenesis of Myalgic Encephalomyelitis/Chronic Fatigue Syndrome," *The Clinical and Scientific Basis of M.E./CFS* [Ottawa, Ontario: The Nightingale Research Foundation, 1992], p. 597.) For many investigators, however, the brain itself seemed the organ most likely to reveal the reasons for the ravaging impact of exercise on victims. Indeed, research that year suggested that, among CFS sufferers, blood flow to the brain decreased significantly during exercise and remained abnormally low for at least twenty four hours; in normal people, blood flow to the brain remains steady or increases slightly during exercise.

On June 1, for example, *Lancet* published a letter signed by Gallo lab virologist Steve Josephs, the University of Nevada's Berch Henry, HEM Pharmaceuticals adviser and medical oncologist David Strayer, Incline Village's Dan Peterson, the National Cancer Institute's Dharam Ablashi, and Harvard's Anthony Komaroff.[2] In their letter the collaborators presented evidence for active replication of the herpesvirus in CFS patients and suggested that it contributed to the pathogenesis, or the development of the disease.

Centers for Disease Control, Atlanta, Georgia

On June 4, Brian Mahy, chief of the Division of Viral and Rickettsial Diseases, informed Walter Gunn and other members of the CFS steering committee that Walter Dowdle, the agency administrator, had decided to initiate an internal review of the division's CFS studies and its plans for future studies. The internal review would be headed by Claire Broome, the CDC's assistant director for science, a post previously held by Mary Guinan, the herpes expert who had responded to Dan Peterson's request for federal help during the 1984–1985 outbreak.

Privately, Gunn welcomed the news. Given the steering committee's intractability, he was convinced that a comprehensive, unbiased investigation of CFS would never occur as long as the disease was mired in the Division of Viral and Rickettsial Diseases under the supervision of Brian Mahy and Larry Schonberger.

Mahy asked committee members to submit questions to him that might be addressed by Broome and her colleagues. Over the next twenty-four hours, Gunn prepared a two-page memo for Mahy. Virtually all of his suggestions had one goal: to break the death-grip the division had held on the disease since 1985.

"Would it not be appropriate for CDC to institute a centers-wide advisory committee to ensure that such a complicated illness is not studied from the rather narrow perspective of just one science discipline?" Gunn wrote. Farther on, he added, "Would it not be desirable and feasible to involve researchers from a wide range of scientific and medical disciplines from a number of different centers in a comprehensive study of this illness?" Gunn also proposed that the CDC establish its own grant program to support "well-qualified non-CDC researchers [who] have some good ideas but lack funds to conduct research."

Pretenses that the CFS epidemic of the middle to late 1980s was a figment of the lay press's imagination or the hysterical fantasies of sufferers, themselves, were being contradicted by the agency's own surveillance data that summer. On June 24, Abt Associates, the Cambridge, Massachusetts, firm that had contracted to perform surveillance for the CDC, sent a fax to Walter Gunn, updating him on statistics regarding the "year of illness onset" among patients being recruited into the surveillance project. In the 1970s, approximately one patient a year in any one of the four cities under surveillance claimed to have fallen ill with the disease during that decade. In the middle 1980s, however, the numbers began expanding rapidly. In 1981, for instance, two Atlanta surveillance patients came down with CFS; by

1987 thirteen had fallen ill; in 1988 there were twenty-five new cases; and in 1989 twenty-eight.

Houston, Texas

During the first week in June the CFS network was riveted by news that Elaine DeFreitas's retrovirus discovery had been confirmed in a commercial diagnostic laboratory in Texas. The molecular biologist who performed the test, C. V. Herst, had never spoken to the Wistar immunologist; he had worked exclusively from her paper in the *Proceedings of the National Academy of Sciences.*

Herst was a PCR expert who worked at a small commercial lab in Houston, Oncore Analytics, Inc. Established in 1989, Oncore had evolved exclusively as a resource for local AIDS doctors who needed sophisticated white blood cell analyses and viral diagnostic capability. "The real focus here in the beginning was on AIDS," Herst explained. "Then we got interested in cancer." Herst had gained his PCR expertise while at Cetus, now known as Chiron, the biotechnology firm in northern California where PCR technology was developed in the early 1980s.

Paul Cheney, impressed by Herst's reputation, had encouraged him to try to replicate DeFreitas's finding by following the procedures described in her *PNAS* article.

Once Herst revealed he had been able to differentiate between blood samples from Cheney's CFS patients and those from healthy controls using the Wistar protocol, Cheney and several other CFS clinicians began sending Herst coded blood samples, some of them from controls and the rest from patients.

Dan Peterson soon became the greatest provider of CFS blood to Herst. "The test," Peterson pointed out, "only costs fifty-five dollars." Given the remarkably high cost of medical care, that did seem like a small sum for a test that might ultimately identify the cause of a patient's shattered health. By the end of June, Oncore had processed 150 patient samples.

"I cannot tell you whether we're looking at a new or old retrovirus," Herst said that summer. "All I can say is that we're looking at a DNA retrovirus sequence. I don't even know what it is. I can say for sure it is not endogenous—that is, it is not normally in the genome—because not every cell has it, and not every patient has it. About seventy percent do seem to have it."

Centers for Disease Control, Atlanta, Georgia

On June 3, Paul Cheney called Walter Gunn with word that Oncore Analytics in Houston was reproducing the Wistar findings en masse using the techniques DeFreitas described in her April 1 paper. Gunn was described by one eyewitness as "livid" at the news that the government's lab was being outpaced by a commercial lab. He told Cheney that his colleagues in retrovirology were dragging their feet and that they had refused DeFreitas's invitation to come to Philadelphia to learn her techniques.

Speculation that a government cover-up of the disease was occurring, always close to the surface, began circulating among patients and clinicians when they heard about Herst's accomplishment. It was beginning to seem to outsiders that the federal scientists in Atlanta, even with Elaine DeFreitas's tutelage, were floundering like scientific Keystone Kops, while a commercial firm had replicated her finding from the literature. "The government is getting *inside information*," CFIDS Association president Marc Iverson complained, "and they *still* can't find it. They've got to be either covering it up, or—they're just boobs!"

Inside Building 15, not surprisingly, a different view prevailed. Tom Folks and his colleague Walid Heneine had been unable to differentiate between HTLV2-infected cell lines and uninfected cell lines using probes and primers that had been manufactured at CDC as soon as they received DeFreitas's article containing what, in lay terms, might best be described as the "recipes." Something was wrong; the CDC's test just didn't seem to discriminate. In the face of Heneine's increasing distaste for the project, Folks, mindful of the congressional mandate to investigate the disease, pressed Heneine to continue.

"We were really worried about sensitivity," Folks recalled later. "Why was Elaine able to get such a stronger band? We made a whole bunch of changes in our temperatures, our buffers, and so on. But all the experts we talked to just said she was running us crazy."

Wistar Institute, Philadelphia, Pennsylvania

During the first week in June, DeFreitas wrote to Tom Folks and Walid Heneine in response to a photograph of an autoradiograph they had sent her. The letter, a complex document for its highly technical discussion of molecular biology, enumerated a number of methodological and technical errors she believed the agency scientists were making in their efforts to reproduce her work.

Near the end of her letter she referred to the problem that had so distressed Walter Gunn: "[W]e don't routinely freeze-thaw DNA used for PCR. After extraction, we aliquot it, thaw two or three times maximum, then discard, *or* we store at 4 degrees centigrade. Freeze-thaw can degrade high molecular weight DNA down to oligonucleotides . . . which often can't be amplified under these conditions."

In an apparent effort to salve the egos of her male counterparts in Atlanta, DeFreitas pointed out that she was merely trying to save them from making the same mistakes that she had made early on. "We are most happy to share these insights with you, having been through these same stages ourselves," she wrote. In her postscript she once again invited them to Wistar: "Our invitation to you both to bring your samples and run some of ours with a fellow in our lab still stands. You could use CDC's and Wistar's primers and probes, perform Mo-T titrations, etc., which I believe will be most helpful in our quest."*

She enclosed her protocol for extracting DNA from specimens and quantitating it, a lengthy document she had typed herself. She also sent a copy to Walter Gunn, as requested.

"At that point they knew *exactly* what she had done," Gunn recalled much later. "To this day they haven't followed her protocol."

On the very day DeFreitas wrote her letter, in fact, the CFS steering committee fell into a heated debate about the importance of following her protocol. Gunn,

---

* "Mo-T" was the name of a human, HTLV2-infected cell line, commonly employed in molecular biology labs.

who routinely kept the meeting's minutes, wrote, "While some believe that if a finding is valid, it shouldn't matter which accepted technique is used in replication, others feel that when one is working near the threshold of sensitivity, as is the case with the Wistar study, following the exact procedures of the original investigator can be critical to the success of the endeavor."

By mid-June, DeFreitas was mystified by the reluctance of the CDC retrovirologists to come to her lab at the Wistar to learn her techniques. "I don't know *why* they won't come," she said that summer. "I repeated the invitation a number of times. Then, I was asked at one point if I would *pay* for them to come. I was absolutely flabbergasted at that suggestion. I said, 'You have to be kidding!' I heard they had millions for this study."

In fact, the agency had received $2 million to support its CFS research that year, and before the fiscal year ended in September, the Division of Viral and Rickettsial Diseases had charged off a flat $20,000 for travel expenses related to the CFS investigation. For unknown reasons, however, there was not enough money to pay for either Walid Heneine's or Tom Folks's airfare to Philadelphia.

DeFreitas, meanwhile, had moved light-years beyond her initial findings. Having found an HTLV2-like viral sequence in CFS sufferers, she went on to attempt to isolate a "complete, living virus" from the blood of those same patients. By that summer, her lab associate, Hiroshi Terunuma, had discovered a unique human cell line that, when mixed with blood cells from CFS patients, produced two types of virus particles. One type, examined under an electron microscope, looked precisely like a retrovirus in size, shape, and density, according to DeFreitas. It also contained the identical viral gene sequences DeFreitas had found in the CFS patients included in her *PNAS* paper. This virus was uniformly seen outside the cells. But there were other, smaller viral particles visible inside the cell, most frequently in the cells' mitochondria, that served to heighten the mystery.

DeFreitas and her associates had also identified the virus in the cells of several different kinds of human tissues, including liver and semen. Her efforts to clone and sequence the pathogen continued. Frustratingly, however, she was increasingly sidetracked by the CDC's requests. The government's demands upon her were accruing in proportion to its alternately stalled or failed attempts to duplicate her findings; the less successful the government scientists, the heavier the burden shouldered by DeFreitas.

National Institutes of Health, Bethesda, Maryland

On June 12, CFS victim Meghan Shannon, a former respiratory therapist at Children's Hospital in San Diego, grabbed the attention of participants at a workshop held by the agency's new Office of Research on Women's Health when she proposed a new name for her disease: acquired immune deficiency syndrome, non-HIV.

"We must recognize that 'chronic fatigue syndrome' and other obfuscatory labels need to be scrapped," Shannon said.

She suggested that hospital staff members, in particular, needed to be better protected from the severely ill victims of the disease who came to hospitals early in their search for a diagnosis. Shannon, herself, had been one among several employees at the San Diego hospital who fell ill years before. "There is a growing problem in protecting health care workers," she said, "especially . . . women. Women are dying from the complications of this disease," Shannon continued. "Not only physical complications, but emotional, financial, and social. Suicide is high on the list of causes of death. . . . Although I have a large support system, I still live on the edge. I wonder when I will finally end up on the streets because I cannot take care of myself any longer."

Centers for Disease Control, Atlanta, Georgia

Folks had been struggling for months to achieve identical sensitivities to Elaine DeFreitas's assay. In July, Folks believed he had achieved his goal. He proposed sending DeFreitas samples of a widely used human cell line containing HTLV2, called Mo-T, to test his newfound sensitivity against hers. DeFreitas agreed to the collaboration; Folks's staff notified her that the samples would be shipped on Monday, July 8, and would arrive at the Wistar on July 9.

DeFreitas ran her test on the DNA samples and sent her results to Folks. "He said the data looked the same as his," DeFreitas said, meaning Folks had at last achieved a sensitivity equivalent to hers.

At the July 17 meeting of the CFS steering committee, Folks announced that he had stepped up his virus-hunting abilities considerably and might be close to being able to duplicate the Wistar work. The news seemed to make several people uncomfortable, Gunn recalled. "It's heartwarming to me to watch the faces," Gunn said, his delight obvious. "Brian Mahy's face, particularly—it was kind of a sputtering, red-faced expression."

Gunn, meanwhile, continued to worry about his division's use of that year's $2 million congressional appropriation for CFS. "I hear rumors that we have seventeen people working on CFS. Who are these people? Why don't I know them?"

American Cancer Society, Atlanta, Georgia

During the second week of July, John Martin flew from Los Angeles to Atlanta, where he was to spend the week reviewing grant proposals at the American Cancer Society. Martin had a second item on his agenda. The cancer society's solemn, gray stone building stood approximately three hundred feet from the Centers for Disease Control on the other side of Clifton Road. On Thursday, June 20, Martin arranged a lunch with the agency staff he had been telling about the virus he was culturing in his Los Angeles laboratories from CFS patients' brains, spinal fluid, and free-circulating blood.

Walter Gunn, Larry Schonberger, Brian Mahy, Kenneth Herrmann, assistant chief of the Division of Viral and Ricksettsial Diseases, and Walid Heneine met Martin in the agency's stark, noisy cafeteria. Retrovirology branch chief Tom Folks was unable to attend. Descriptions of the event by agency participants and by Martin were in diametric opposition to each other, although both sides pronounced the meeting a major disappointment.

According to Walid Heneine, "The problem with John Martin is that he never revealed any data. He sat and talked generalities—nonspecific things that could apply to anything."

Gunn, too,was critical. "We've talked to him four times now, and so far nobody has enough information to make a judgment. In order to duplicate his work, you have to know what he did, and he's not telling anybody."

"The only comment I would have," Martin said, when asked about the lunch, "was that I had gone through several of these phone calls telling them that they should respond to this simply from a public health consideration. The Centers for Disease Control has an obligation to investigate." The agency owed it to the public, he said, to at least acknowledge the virological phenomenon he was observing in Los Angeles among severely ill encephalopathic patients and to explain why there had been a decision against using public funds to investigate it. "If you have an individual with a major illness and you're *not* going to investigate," Martin said, "the Centers for Disease Control has an obligation to come clean, to say, 'We're not going to investigate this. There is a failure to investigate.' " (Folks revealed some years later that his lab did actively search, without success, for spuma viruses among CFS sufferers as a result of Martin's lobbying.)

Two weeks after the meeting with Martin, Gunn announced he had received permission to hold the National CFS Advisory Council meeting at the Centers for Disease Control. The meeting was scheduled for September 21. Elaine DeFreitas was to present her latest work on her novel retrovirus, and University of Glasgow neurologist Peter Behan would discuss his recent investigation into retroviral infection in the disease. John Martin was invited for the same purpose. A number of agency staff, including members of the CFS steering committee and scientists from the retrovirology laboratory, were also invited to attend.

Wistar Institute, Philadelphia, Pennsylvania

During the summer of 1991 the CFIDS Association in Charlotte made a difficult decision. The philanthropy's coffers were nearly empty. After much discussion, the board agreed it would have to cut off DeFreitas's funding of $11,000 a month, at least temporarily. Somehow no one from the association told DeFreitas of the decision, however. On the evening of June 25 she received a call from David Bell, who was in his hotel room in Charlotte. He had spent the week evaluating children in Paul Cheney's clinic. He reported that the CFIDS Association had ended her funding.

DeFreitas was devastated. "I never in a million years would have expected this," she said soon afterward. "I am totally and completely numb. We've *got* this thing. It's beautiful, it's everywhere, and we're sequencing it. I was just saying to the people in my lab [that] we're over the hump. We're on the other side of the mountain now, and we're flying down at ninety miles an hour. We'll be there in two to three months.

"I was getting calls from people in Gallo's lab telling me Cheney was a schizophrenic," she continued, "and I walked farther and farther into the quicksand.

My colleagues were telling me the patients were crazy and malingerers, and I *still* kept going. I had no money, my colleagues were laughing at me behind my back, and I persisted in the midst of that.

"We could have stopped when those first five samples were negative in 1986. We could have published that, and that would have ended all investigation of this as a retroviral disease. No retrovirologist would have pursued it further. We could have put a lid on this forever.

"I have to believe that what doesn't destroy us makes us stronger. We'll do what we can with the last pipette, the last ounce of media, and then we'll publish what we have. Whatever happens in the future," she continued, "the only thing that keeps me in this is the fact that someday there will be a test, and a vaccine, and a drug, and fewer people are going to have to suffer with this."

Harvard Medical School, Boston, Massachusetts

Also on June 25, Anthony Komaroff sent a memorandum to the coauthors of the Tahoe manuscript.

> The *Annals* has had our manuscript reviewed by three external referees and an internal statistical consultant. Each of these reviewers had extensive comments to make. The editors have asked us to submit a revised manuscript that responds to the comments of the reviewers, of course making no guarantees that they will accept the revision.
>
> In my judgment, one of the external reviewers was very sympathetic, one was positively inclined, and one was quite hostile. The statistical reviewer misunderstood some of our methodology, but found no errors.

The doctor then warned his collaborators that he would need their help in responding to some of the reviewer's questions. He ended by saying, "In summary, I do not believe any major flaws were found in the study. I am cautiously optimistic that the editors will find our revision satisfactory, but you never know. I will keep you posted regarding their decision."

Hennepin County Medical Center, Minneapolis, Minnesota

In early July, five years after the Tahoe epidemic, a remarkable event occurred: two staff members from the Centers for Disease Control visited infectious disease specialist Philip Peterson's clinic for CFS sufferers in Minneapolis and actually met and interviewed a handful of patients. Louisa Chapman, now in her fourth year in Atlanta, and her boss, Larry Schonberger, went to Minneapolis at Chapman's request. Schonberger, who by 1991 had been promoted to assistant director of the Division of Viral and Rickettsial Diseases, had hired Chapman to replace Gary Holmes the year before. During her job interview with Schonberger, the young doctor, trained in internal medicine and infectious disease, had told him she "needed to go and see patients," Chapman recalled later. Her job description, after all, called for her to provide medical expertise to psychologist Walter Gunn. Now, having been medical director on the CFS project for more than a year, she arranged to meet "about seven or ten" patients over the course of two days. Schonberger, who like Chapman and the vast majority of their colleagues in the division, had never met or examined a CFS patient, went along for the first day.

When she arrived in Minneapolis, Chapman asked Philip Peterson to select those patients he felt were "classic and who could give a good history." Chapman said, "We allowed a good bit of time for each patient. My interest was in letting them tell their story. These people described to me how they felt when they suffered a major loss because of their disease. Usually it had to do with how they felt when they realized that they were never going to be able to go back to their job or their career again," Chapman recalled. "A couple of people mentioned a depression so severe that they lost interest in everything around them. They were really describing a clinical depression. But when I said, 'Are you depressed?' I was struck that there was a tremendous amount of defensiveness about discussing the issue of depression."

The disquieting hostility to her questions about depression seems only to have focused Chapman's mind more solidly on patients' moods rather than on the pathophysiology of a disease that struck overnight and disabled formerly healthy adults in their prime years. "CFS," Chapman said, "raises an interesting issue of psychological and psychiatric illness in our society. We don't deal with psychiatric disease very well. If you suggest that psychiatric problems may play a role in illness, people get defensive. . . . Actually," she continued in response to a question, "there's been very little energy expended by our scientists into studying whether in fact CFS is a mental illness. None of our scientists is looking into that.

"Basically, when I began here, I had no experience with chronic fatigue syndrome, negative or positive," Chapman continued. "I knew of people who had been productive role models for me who were now disabled by what was *said* to be CFS, but no one has yet produced convincing data for me that it is an infectious illness. And what astonishes me," she added after a moment, her eyes wide with indignation, "is the real lack of legitimacy that is accorded mental illness in this country."

∎

Chapman's failure to comprehend CFS as an organic illness, even after meeting sufferers, might have been predicted by any of an earlier generation of investigators, each of whom expressed a conviction that the malady was extraordinarily difficult to recognize or diagnose in small numbers, particularly for neophytes. Anthony Komaroff, when told that someone from the CDC had finally made an effort to meet patients in a clinical setting, was dubious about Chapman's inroad in Minneapolis: "I don't think interviewing ten patients does it," the Boston researcher said. "You have to see [the disease] again and again."

Donald Henderson, who had investigated the Punta Gorda, Florida, outbreak of 1956 during his tenure as head of the Epidemic Intelligence Service at the CDC, insisted on the name "epidemic neuromyasthenia" in part, he explained in a 1959 article, because it "emphasizes the need for epidemiologic as well as clinical appraisal of cases." In other words, diagnosing people whose disease appeared outside the context of an obvious cluster was extremely problematic.

By 1991, of course, there were doctors who were able to diagnose CFS in its sporadic form; they had derived their expertise from years of experience with hundreds of patients. Unfortunately, no one in the federal health agencies seemed terribly interested in or respectful of their erudition.

Wistar Institute, Philadelphia, Pennsylvania

Before the end of July, Tom Folks let Elaine DeFreitas know that Walid Heneine had been taken off the CFS project because, Folks said, Heneine was not taking it seriously enough. According to Walter Gunn, Heneine thought the retrovirology lab's project to replicate the Wistar finding was a waste of his time.

DeFreitas was relieved to know she would no longer have to struggle with the skeptical Heneine over the phone. But she was uncertain whether to believe Folks's reason for Heneine's departure from the project. Maybe, she mused, the agency was retreating from its commitment to the work. "Tom has this real sweet southern accent, and he's always very up and positive on the phone. But you don't really know what's being said when the phone gets hung up."

In fact, once Folks hung up the phone, he was forced to continue his struggle with Heneine. Some years later, Folks recalled, "Walid basically said, 'Look, how much of my time, my career, do I have to put into this?' I had to tell him that he *would do this*—it became an order. It was no longer a request. He kept saying, 'I don't *care* if I achieve the same sensitivity, because it's going to be *endogenous.'* Now," Folks continued, "I don't think I would have fired him if he refused to go on, because, deep down, I agreed with him. And I don't run my lab like the army, where you tell people to charge the hill and die."

In a masterful understatement, Folks also conceded that the Middle Eastern scientist in his lab and the outspoken Brooklyn native "did not get along."

Centers for Disease Control, Atlanta, Georgia

Toward the end of July, Gunn began to revamp the case-control study, which he hoped to begin anew the following fall. It was Gunn's seventh major overhaul of the study in as many months. The new plan called for the establishment of a pool of controls selected randomly from the community and screened to be sure they'd had no contact with anyone suffering from CFS or, as Gunn ominously expressed it, "at least, no more contact than anyone else." Six years after Tahoe, the federal scientists were at last starting to investigate the disease as if they suspected there was at least a *possibility* of an infectious agent at its heart. Nevertheless, the issue of psychiatric health continued to be a prominent element of the investigation; twenty-five sets of patients and controls would have to endure an extensive psychiatric interview. In addition, both groups would need to donate a lot of blood— enough for twenty-five different laboratories at the agency. Unlike patients, the controls would be paid for their trouble.

Gunn said the agency planned to run two sets each week, beginning on October 1. "By the time the study is underway," he said, "our retrovirus lab will be able to find DeFreitas's virus. His projected date of completion was February 1992. "I don't have a doubt in my mind that this is real," he said, adding, "And it will be so much more earth-shattering than anyone ever would expect."

Gunn was planning to take a two-week vacation beginning the second week in August. He was going to Phoenix to see his daughter and his newborn grand-daughter. He was unusually serene. "I'm fairly realistic about my role in this," he mused. "I'm not a virologist or an immunologist. I'm an unlikely person to be running something that is going to turn out to be an infectious illness. It's *so* controversial in medicine, but in my case, it doesn't bother me at all that half of the M.D.'s out there don't believe this is real. I don't have a medical reputation to lose in this."

The Division of Viral and Rickettsial Diseases was divided among three buildings bridged by catwalks; in the course of a day, most of the division members saw one another at least once on these outdoor steel-and-concrete bridges. On July 30 the catwalks were alive with news emanating from Tom Folks's virology empire on the second floor of Building 15. Using his new techniques, supplied by Elaine DeFreitas, Folks had performed a retrovirus assay on old DNA samples from six Lyndonville children and six local cases. All six children were positive, as were four of the six cases from Atlanta. None of the nine healthy controls Folks tested were positive.

Because the experiments had been performed using low-stringency PCR, which is more likely to pick up false positives, Folks ran the samples again at high stringency on August 1. This time all six children remained positive; two of the five Atlanta patients remained positive, and the controls remained negative.

Folks called DeFreitas on July 30 to tell her the good news. Gunn called De-Freitas on August 2. "I'm happier today about this project than I've been in three years," the agency veteran told DeFreitas.

That same day, Gunn decided to postpone his long-awaited vacation. "The sneering committee is no longer sneering," he said. "No one is laughing at chronic fatigue syndrome anymore. The attitudes have changed, thank God. The attitudes are never going to be the same." Gunn hadn't experienced any stomach pain in two days.

Tom Folks's finding galvanized Larry Schonberger: the investigation he had tried to scuttle for so long had suddenly acquired a more attractive cast. On Monday, August 5, Schonberger outlined to Gunn his plan for a collaborative effort with the state of Georgia's health department. Typically, these agreements, called "epidemiological study aids," or "epi-aids," are drawn up when a state seeks the CDC's help in investigating a disease outbreak. Sometimes, the CDC instigates an epi-aid with a state when the agency itself wants to investigate a disease outbreak. In such cases, the agency asks the state to extend an invitation to investigate, which is what Schonberger proposed doing now. Epi-aid agreements are attractive to the agency because they are a relatively painless way to gain access to patients in an outbreak without first obtaining clearance from the federal Office of Management and Budget to conduct a federal study. As Gunn eventually explained, "It makes it a lot easier if the formal invitation comes from the state." Thus, the epi-aid Schonberger was now proposing would allow the agency rapid access to CFS patients in Atlanta—and, most critically, their blood—without having to go through layers of federal red tape.

Schonberger explained to administrators in the Georgia State Health Department that agency scientists would invite twenty-five patients who had been clearly defined as cases in the Atlanta surveillance program to come to the agency for a blood draw. Controls would be chosen from the CDC's own staff. Folks's new retrovirus assay would be the first test. Later on, the agency would undertake in-depth interviewing of the cases and controls to determine what, if any, other toxins or pathogens people had been exposed to.

Gunn felt buoyed—in fact, nearly euphoric—at his boss's about-face. For the first time in two years he felt stirrings of renewed pride in his colleagues and in the agency. "These are good scientists here," Gunn said. "They just had to be shown that CFS was real. It was mostly getting people past this *perception*. . . . The thing that's amusing to me is that people have begun approaching me privately. Several have commented, 'I always knew this was a transmissible illness.' One scientist here said he believes it's transmissible from humans to animals and vice versa! There will be some wrestling around to see who gets to work on this now," Gunn added. "Chronic fatigue syndrome will be a major program at the CDC. Things are never going to be the same."

On Wednesday, August 7, Schonberger's epi-aid plan was approved by the state of Georgia. Two days later Walter Dowdle received a briefing on the retrovirus findings and epi-aid from Schonberger and Gunn. "There were no chronic fatigue syndrome jokes," Gunn recalled. "Dowdle's comment was 'This is very exciting. This is what Centers for Disease Control does best. Let's get the lab on it.' "

Dowdle advised the scientists gathered in his office to keep the news a secret. The tests needed to be repeated at least once to confirm the first finding. Gunn was in sympathy with Dowdle's request. "There's no point in getting patients excited," the investigator said, "if we fail to confirm."

Some years later, Folks remembered events differently. He had been, he said, less enthusiastic than Gunn and had cautioned Dowdle that although DeFreitas's probes and primers seemed to work on her own patients, they failed to identify HTLV2 in the Mo-T cell line. "I was very concerned we were jumping the gun," Folks recalled. "I told Dowdle, 'I'm not going to say I've confirmed *anything* yet.' In fact, we really didn't feel like we were in the game until we had her primers working at the same sensitivity on Mo-T," the scientist added in reference to an event that would not occur until late that year.

In spite of Folks's reservations, Gunn immediately made arrangements for two dozen Atlanta CFS patients who had been referred into the agency's surveillance program to present themselves at the Clifton Road headquarters for a blood draw. All of the patients were classed as group one patients—people who had no previous history of major depression or any other psychiatric symptoms prior to the onset of their disease and no abnormal results on standard lab tests. Larry Schonberger and others at the agency considered group one patients to be the purest, cleanest cases within a four-tiered classification system devised to stratify surveillance cases. From among agency staff, Gunn rounded up controls, each of them matched for age (plus or minus five years), gender, and race, with the Atlanta patients. In a matter of days, the blood was drawn.

In spite of the fact that Walid Heneine had expressed overt hostility to the research and to Elaine DeFreitas, Folks reassigned the Lebanese scientist to the CFS project for the next phase of work. Shortly before the blood was drawn, however, Folks honored Heneine's request to fly to Beirut for two weeks' vacation. Thus, when this latest batch of samples arrived in Building 15, lab techs were forced to preserve the blood samples from both cases and controls by treating them with lysate and freezing them—in defiance of the detailed protocol DeFreitas had written and mailed to the agency the previous month. When queried about his decision afterward, Folks said, "I thought the vacation was worth more for Walid's piece of mind [than following DeFreitas's protocol], just because Elaine said, 'You *have* to do it this way.' "

Würzburg, Germany

On August 2, *Science* magazine published an article by a team of German scientists that seemed to answer a number of perplexities facing John Martin's questions about the nature of spuma, or foamy, retroviruses.[3] The paper not only suggested a disease-causing role for human foamy virus (HFV), it also suggested how that disease might manifest itself: in massive central nervous system destruction. The German researchers believed that the pathologies they observed in HFV-infected mice were "reminiscent of human retroviral disease of the central nervous system." In addition, the authors pointed out, one of the original isolates of HFV had come from the brain of a woman suffering from encephalopathy, whose "neurodegenerative" disease, they wrote, exhibited "features reminiscent of the lesions in the HFV mice. These unexpected findings," they concluded, "call for a reevaluation of the pathogenic potential of [human foamy virus] in humans."

Within days of reading the paper, Cheney had called the lead author at the University of Würzburg. The researcher invited Cheney to send blood samples from his patients to Würzburg, where the researcher promised to test them for human foamy virus.

The results were negative.

Harvard Medical School, Boston, Massachusetts

In early August, Anthony Komaroff sent a revised version of his five-year-old Tahoe manuscript back to the *Annals of Internal Medicine*. His revision included a lengthy response to the criticisms raised by two of the three reviewers. "The . . . response was bigger than the paper itself," Komaroff said. "In my view, there was not a single serious challenge of the work. However," Komaroff added, "if even one highly placed person at the *Annals* has an ax to grind, the paper won't be published."

At least one of his collaborators, Dan Peterson, was increasingly frustrated by the Tahoe manuscript's ill fortunes. "Even the *supportive* doctors out here are asking, 'Why can't you get published?' " Peterson said that summer. "It's easy to publish a negative study in this disease," he added. "I could publish tomorrow in the *New England Journal* saying, 'After seven years I've reached the conclusion this is a psychiatric disease.' I could say, 'I've seen twelve hundred people, and I've done [natural killer] cell studies and EBV studies and CD-four studies and MRI studies, and in my opinion these people have a psychiatric disorder,' and I promise you they would take that.

"My model for that is AIDS," he continued. "When I was first in practice, when that disease was being disputed, it was the *same* kind of argument. It just happens that people with AIDS die, and so the scientific world was *stuck* addressing the issue. I swear, if AIDS weren't a fatal disease, we would still be having the same argument about it."

Komaroff also took notice of the August 2 *Science* article about foamy virus infection in transgenic mice. The Boston doctor, like Cheney, called the German scientists and sent them samples of CFS blood from his New England practice. Two weeks later, however, Komaroff learned by telephone that the German investigators had been unable to find evidence of spuma virus in the American CFS victims.

In Glasgow, neurologist Peter Behan, having heard about Los Angeles researcher John Martin's results, had also sent some patient and control serum to the Germans, and the outcome was similar: no evidence of any spuma virus could be found.

28

The "Charly" Syndrome

Philadelphia, Pennsylvania

Much as Paul Cheney had been at the center of a nexus of scientists and clinicians searching for the pathogen at the heart of the disease, his former partner Dan Peterson had been struggling to find its cure. Since his first successful experiment with Albuquerque housewife and golf enthusiast Nancy Kaiser, Peterson had made numerous trips east to discuss issues of Ampligen therapy with executives and scientists at the HEM Pharmaceuticals offices at One Penn Plaza in downtown Philadelphia. On his early forays Peterson had talked about Kaiser's response to the drug; on later ones, he talked about the responses of fourteen more patients from Nevada and Idaho, several of whom had moved to Incline Village. Those fourteen people were participants in an open-label study, so called because the patients, as well as Peterson, knew they were receiving Ampligen.

On March 19, 1991, Paul Charlap, the company's flamboyant founder and chief executive, had died of cancer, leaving his thirty-five-year-old widow, Maryann, and William Carter, the scientist and oncologist who had developed Ampligen, in charge of the closely held company and its biggest shareholders. Charlap's death had been a blow to Peterson and, Peterson clearly believed, to humanitarian efforts to resolve the disease. "Although he was difficult, I enjoyed him," Peterson said. "He was a clinician at heart—he'd gone to medical school. He *believed* patients. His death was very untimely for this disease. It really was."

The mother of a young girl bedridden with CFS, who had written to Charlap for help in the form of Ampligen and received it, echoed Peterson's conviction. Had Charlap lived, Texan Bobbi Ravicz told a magazine journalist in 1994, "things would have turned out differently."[1]

In the months since Charlap's death, activity at HEM had centered almost exclusively around the CFS trials in Incline Village, Charlotte, Houston, and Portland, which had begun the previous summer. Of the ninety-two patients enrolled in the study, forty-seven had received placebo, a saline solution. Few placebo recipients demonstrated improvement; in fact, several deteriorated during the six months of the trial.* The forty-five people who received Ampligen were demonstrably better. The outcome was so dramatic, in fact, that HEM decided to end the trial after just twenty-four weeks rather than the forty-eight weeks it had first planned.

By spring, HEM's investigators in Philadelphia had begun breaking the codes and analyzing the data. Carter was convinced the results would persuade the government to arrange a fast-track limited approval for the drug; after all, he insisted, he had seen at least one AIDS drug win similar approval with far less supporting data. Not surprisingly, HEM's decision devastated patients, not only because the trial was cut short but because they had believed HEM would continue to provide them with the drug until it won government approval. With the trial's end, however, free infusions of the drug also ended.

Carter has denied such a promise was ever made, and the matter has been bitterly contested by trial participants in any number of forums.

HEM's was the first major double-blind clinical trial in CFS, meaning that neither patients nor doctors knew for certain who was getting the drug, although a few patients later noted that clues emerged as the weeks passed. Ampligen had a fairly distinct scent; harder to ignore was the fact that approximately half the patients in the trial began to improve markedly during the first twelve to fourteen weeks and those remaining began to deteriorate.

Carter declared it to be "a study of unprecedented scope," a statement federal scientists could hardly deny. Irrespective of the drug's efficacy, the expansive nature of the investigations had created an abundance of hard scientific data about the disease. For instance, there had emerged strong evidence that interleukin-1, a substance manufactured by the immune system in response to viral infection, might be a marker of disease severity. Patients who received Ampligen experienced a reduction in interleukin-1 as well as a reduction in symptoms. In addition, in 1994, Temple University School of Medicine biochemist Robert Suhadolnik and other clinicians and scientists who collaborated on the trial published a study reporting that the drug ameliorated a defective antiviral pathway common to CFS patients.[2] Before treatment with Ampligen, the molecular indicators for damage to this pathway were "significantly elevated" compared to those of controls. (This finding was yet another link between CFS and AIDS; victims of AIDS suffered an identical defect.) After treatment, these molecular indicators were vastly improved in CFS sufferers, as they had been in AIDS patients after Ampligen treatment, and Suhadolnik and his coauthors noted that they corresponded with "clinical and neuropsychological improvements."

The drug itself was not without side effects, but its toxicity was minor compared to that of the disease. Dan Peterson hospitalized an Ampligen recipient in the Incline Village trial after the patient developed spinal pain, heart palpitations, and elevated liver enzymes. The patient, Cynthia Modica-Gaines, who had been a ballet teacher at Sacramento State University when she had fallen ill five years

---

* Their deterioration may have been due to the fact that they were required to stop taking all other medications in order to participate in the trial. In addition, simply getting to and from the infusion site two or three times a week (frequency was determined by dose; not all patients received identical dosages) amounted to tremendous exertion for CFS sufferers and may have exacerbated their disease.

earlier, pleaded to be reinstated in the trial. When, after temporary withdrawal from Ampligen, Modica-Gaines's liver enzymes returned to normal, Peterson acquiesced, but kept her on a half dose. She suffered no further ill effects. In fact, she improved significantly. None of the patients at the other sites asked to stop the trial, nor did their doctors deem the side effects sufficient to discontinue the therapy or even reduce the dosage for any of their patients.

Still, there was little reason to believe, at this stage, that Ampligen was a cure, that it was universally effective, or that its beneficial effects were equal in all sufferers. Among patients in the first open-label pilot study who had responded well to the drug, none had been restored to a degree of health that had allowed them to return to their jobs. Even more problematically, among those who were taken off the drug temporarily, for whatever reason, the disease had become significantly worse, suggesting that to derive benefit patients needed to be maintained on Ampligen indefinitely and that withdrawal from the drug could actually exacerbate symptoms.

Early in August, HEM officials shipped the data to analysts at the Food and Drug Administration in Rockville, Maryland, enabling agency investigators to begin their review. It was the first time FDA scientists had focused on Ampligen as a treatment for CFS. The drug agency, in turn, sent auditors to all four sites to study the methods by which the data was collected and to certify that all patients had met the criteria for inclusion. HEM had demanded that patients have a Karnofsky score no higher than 60; as a result, virtually all of the ninety-two patients in the trial were confined to bed or to a wheelchair when the trial began.

Until his colleagues began to analyze the data from the four-city trial, HEM chief and Ampligen co-inventor Carter's interest in the disease had been minimal. Now his interest was keen. CFS caused anatomical holes to develop in its victims' brains and lowered their IQs, among other problems; his drug restored the sufferers' IQs and returned them to some semblance of normal functioning.

During the week of August 19, Carter held a series of meetings with FDA staff in an attempt to persuade the government to approve use of the drug in an even larger trial with 350 patients lasting one year. HEM was seeking a treatment IND—shorthand for "treatment investigational new drug"—exemption, one of several ways drugs could be fast-tracked into the American marketplace. To qualify, the manufacturer had to have already conducted phase two clinical trials using from ten to three hundred patients, and those trials had to have provided powerful evidence of the drug's safety and efficacy. The agency ruled in favor of treatment INDs in cases where the drug in question seemed "promising" and the patients for whom the drug was intended suffered from a "serious and life-threatening disease for which no alternative therapies [were] available." Historically, drugs exempted in this fashion went on to win the agency's approval.

Carter made his case for Ampligen on the basis of the severity of the illness, citing brain damage and immune system dysfunction, and what the company believed was the drug's demonstrated ability to moderate the disease, based on the trials completed that summer.

The new trial, he told FDA officials, would be structured as a double-blind crossover study that would relegate 100 percent of the patients to at least six months of saline infusions as well as six months of Ampligen infusions. There was a significant catch: the patients themselves would be required to pay for the phenomenally expensive infusion cost—approximately $25,000 a year for each patient—in addition to the cost of the drug—approximately $25,000 for a half year's supply. Simultaneously, HEM executives were consulting with Blue Cross/Blue Shield to learn whether the company might be willing to pay for either the infusions or the drug during the trial.

"This is going to be the first controlled drug trial among 350 millionaires in this country," Paul Cheney wryly observed. "I have no doubt," he added, "that there are at least 350 millionaires in this country with this disease. It's a very smart move on HEM's part. I can't think of a better way to put pressure on the Food and Drug Administration. The FDA has created a situation where only the rich can get treatment, and Americans aren't going to like that."

HEM executives were discussing, too, a less expensive oral form of the drug, but they estimated a three- to five-year development period. Everything—the new trial, the development of an Ampligen pill, the formal establishment of the drug as a bona fide CFS therapy—hung for the moment on the FDA's appraisal of the four-city trial, however.

With the premature end of the trial, the forty-five victims of the disease who had received the drug were cut adrift. Many of them had been restored from total disability to a degree of ability that had eluded them for years, and when the Ampligen was withdrawn, they noticed their intellectual clarity and physical strength slipping after as few as ten days. By the third and fourth week off the drug, patients who had been confined to wheelchairs before they entered the trial were returned to their wheelchairs; almost everyone was again housebound. For these patients, who had been raised momentarily out of their zombie existence, the slide back down was excruciating. One such sufferer told a journalist, "It's like somebody turned on a light and I could see, and then they turned it off again."[3] Another compared the rapid loss of intellectual acuity to that described in Daniel Keyes's 1966 novel *Flowers for Algernon,* the story of Charly, a severely retarded man who is given brain surgery that temporarily raises his IQ to genius level. As the surgery's good effect wears off and his IQ falls to its previous depressed state, he watches in horror as the accoutrements of intelligence—discourse, society, material comforts—drift out of reach. CFS was among the few brain diseases that left its victims witness to their own intellectual deterioration; withdrawal of Ampligen caused them to experience the anguish a second time.*

---

* Patients who had suffered a different fate, that of having a saline solution injected into their veins two to three times a week, were hardly better off than their counterparts who had received Ampligen but were now without it. During the trial, four of the patients in the placebo arm of the study—8 percent—attempted suicide. HEM later reported that "a significant number of placebo patients clinically deteriorated during the course of the clinical test." Floyd Skloot, the novelist, had entered the trial in Oregon under infectious disease specialist Mark Loveless's supervision. Although Skloot eventually divined he was a placebo recipient—("I knew this the way I'm told a woman knows she's pregnant")—he decided to "just hang in there," in spite of the collapsing veins in his arms, because of an assumption, common to all participants in the trial, that HEM would provide the drug to placebo recipients, just as the company had provided the drug indefinitely to participants in the small open-label study in Incline Village.

In Charlotte, one of Cheney's patients, a thirty-five-year-old former civil engineer who had been an invalid since 1988, made violent threats when he was denied additional infusions of the drug. Cheney hired a plainclothes policeman to stand guard in his clinic for the next three months. Other patients talked about suicide. "Every day now," said one, "I can't remember the day before. When you were normal just two weeks ago, it's really a blow to be this sick."

"I don't think people appreciate the desperateness of these patients," Cheney said later. "To have this drug pulled from you is to watch your IQ fall by ten points a month."

Houston, Texas

By August, C. V. Herst had performed the Wistar PCR test, as it was described in the April issue of *Proceedings of the National Academy of Sciences,* on five hundred blood samples. The positivity rate remained at 70 percent. All of Herst's five hundred samples had come from four sources: Dan Peterson, Jay Goldstein, Paul Cheney, and Patricia Salvato, the Houston AIDS specialist. In recent weeks, however, as the news spread, Herst said, "We've been contacted by about twenty other doctors. I figure we could handle about one hundred patients' tests a day.

"As far as possible viral etiology for this disease goes," he added, "there's no stigma about that here. I'm a scientist—I *have* to listen to the patient. *He's* the one with the problem, not the doctor. I know tons of pompous doctors—I could hand you a whole *directory* of people who don't believe in this disease, *but they don't have the problem.*"

Wistar Institute, Philadelphia, Pennsylvania

As a direct result of her successful effort to grow the virus in cell cultures, "X," as Elaine DeFreitas called the mystery bug, was coming into clearer definition now. By carefully measuring its weight, she had determined definitively that the virus was not HTLV2. In fact, based on its size and shape, she and her lab associates were increasingly convinced she had discovered a completely new microbe, perhaps even a new family of retroviruses.

Viewed under the electron microscope, it was apparent that "X" had properties of both foamy and lenti, although it was not a hybrid in the traditional sense.* "I don't mean necessarily half and half," DeFreitas explained. "It's not Mendelian genetics, where you cross a red rose with a white rose and get a pink rose. It's more like mutation, recombination, selection, over maybe scores of years."

DeFreitas admitted, however, that her original enthusiasm of the previous fall, which had led her to predict that she would be able to identify the bug within six months, had fallen by the wayside. Complexity upon complexity was being layered into the laboratory work. The more she and her lab associates learned about "X," the more enigmatic it became.

Larger viral particles were routinely found outside the cells, but there were frequently intracellular viral fragments as well. Whether these extra- and intracellular

* Lentiviruses such as HIV destroy cells. Foamy viruses are less well understood because they have been less well studied; they have yet to be firmly associated with disease, even in animals.

particles were the same virus remained unclear. From a clinical perspective, perhaps the most remarkable aspect was that electron microscopy revealed the smaller particles to be frequently harbored in the mitochondria of patients' white blood cells. Mitochondria are tiny granular or threadlike bodies found in the cytoplasm of every cell in the body. They play a crucial role in cell metabolism, particularly the cell's utilization of oxygen; they are sometimes called "energy-producing factories." At least two researchers—Glasgow neurologist Peter Behan and New Zealand microbiologist Michael Holmes, who found evidence for retroviral infection in CFS sufferers in 1986—had previously reported abnormally large and misshapen mitochondria in CFS sufferers. Many presumed these mitochondrial abnormalities, of unknown origin, contributed to the symptoms of profound weakness in the muscles and brain fatigue, but no one had yet reported finding a virus within mitochondria.*

The location of viral particles in mitochondria, therefore, was highly significant because it suggested a pathogenesis for the organism—in other words, an explanation of how the virus actually caused disease. Although DeFreitas cautioned that a great deal of work remained to be done before she could conclusively make such connections—work that included studying the pathogenic processes in animals injected with "X"—the finding had the potential to vault her research forward phenomenally. "Look at how much they know about HIV," she said. "I mean, they've got that thing sequenced up and down and they know *everything* about it, but they are *still* arguing about the mechanisms of the pathogenesis."

After making these critical discoveries, DeFreitas had prepared a paper in which she discussed the viral findings in three of David Bell's patients from Lyndonville, all of them children. Her paper was limited to children, she said, only because Paul Cheney had not sent her any additional patient tissue samples since the Kyoto conference. The divisive issue of inventorship remained paramount in the relationship between the former collaborators, and Cheney obviously had decided to withhold his contributions to DeFreitas's work until the matter was resolved.

DeFreitas submitted her paper describing extra- and intracellular retrovirus particles in three chronically ill children for internal review by her Wistar colleagues that month, a preliminary step before publishing the data. She hoped to find a home for the article in a scientific journal that would publish it quickly. "I'm really interested in a fast turnaround, because I know other people are working on this, and while they may not be doing the same experiments, they may be coming to the same conclusions. I'm going to take the journal with the shortest turnaround."

In the meantime, she was determined to keep her head down, avoid the press, and ignore the still-simmering controversy over her initial observations reported in Kyoto. "I'm just doing what I've been doing for eleven years," she said. "This is the only route I know. It's what scientists do. It's worked for one hundred and fifty years. I'll talk to Hilary Koprowski and the people in my lab. And that's it! I don't talk to anybody else, and I don't want to." Above all, there would be no pub-

---

* There had been just one paper in the medical literature in which scientists reported finding a virus in a cell's mitochondria. Published in the 1960s, it was a report of a tobacco mosaic virus that had hybridized inside the mitochondria of a plant cell. The presence of a virus had never been reported in human mitochondria.

lic discussion of her remarkable observations until their publication: "I'm not going to make the same mistake twice."

Berkeley, California

George Rutherford, an infectious disease specialist and epidemiologist, had served as chief of AIDS epidemiology for the city of San Francisco during the first years of the AIDS epidemic. He grew interested in CFS when he was appointed chief of infectious disease for the state of California in 1990. On any given day at least one-quarter of the calls to his Berkeley office from the public and from members of the medical profession pertained to CFS.

"One of the things I'm trying to do," he explained, "is to mainstream, or de-peripheralize, chronic fatigue syndrome among infectious disease physicians, to move it onto the front burner. AIDS is absorbing huge amounts of resources, and it doesn't leave much for anything else. . . . To put something on the public health agenda, there really have to be bodies."

Evidence for infectiousness was probably the only way to get a disease onto that agenda. Rutherford indicated that he was looking for outbreaks of the disease, which offered the best demonstration of transmissibility.

Rutherford, in fact, was among a group of public health officials in the Bay Area who were increasingly concerned about the public health ramifications of CFS. "I think the city's experience with AIDS made people highly sensitive to making a big mistake with regard to another infectious disease," Rutherford said. "The climate was that we were going to pursue this aggressively because this is a problem for many, many people in this city."

Working with patient activist Jan Montgomery, Rutherford had formed a local committee that included Ray Baxter, the director of the San Francisco Health Department, and Richard Fein, chief of medicine at San Francisco General Hospital. The group had videotaped a grand rounds on the subject for the clinical staff at California's Kaiser Permanente, the largest HMO in the country. In addition, health department head Baxter pondered whether CFS should be, like AIDS, anthrax, plague, syphilis, tuberculosis, and several other infectious diseases, a reportable disease in California.

Charlotte, North Carolina

By the end of August, Walter Gunn and Anthony Komaroff had formally announced that the fall meeting of the National CFS Advisory Council would be held at the Centers for Disease Control in Atlanta on the third Saturday in September. Since the retrovirus debate was at the top of the agenda, John Martin, the University of Glasgow's Peter Behan, and Elaine DeFreitas were invited to attend. Tulsa multimillionaire Ed Taylor agreed to the pay the expenses of all non-agency personnel who attended, including Behan and his microbiologist, a young Scot named John Gow.

The San Francisco–based lobbying organization, CACTUS, had scheduled its own meeting on retroviruses for the first Saturday in September in San Francisco, inviting not only several major researchers in the disease but also a handful of

California public health officials, including Rutherford. The CACTUS meeting would be the smaller and, predicted Paul Cheney, who would attend both meetings, the "more progressive" and more important of the two. Its purpose was twofold: to discuss ways to bring the disease from the shadows into the limelight, placing it at the heart of the nation's public health agenda, and to allow researchers like Cheney, Elaine DeFreitas, Jay Levy, John Martin, C. V. Herst, and Nancy Klimas, who were on the trail of viruses and other crucial keys to the disease, to sit in one room and candidly discuss their work, something they had yet to do.

Centers for Disease Control, Atlanta, Georgia

Walid Heneine returned from his vacation in Beirut to find an even larger CFS project awaiting him. Blood samples from "twenty-four card-carrying CFS cases"—as Gunn characterized the blood that had been drawn from cases picked up in the agency's own surveillance program—were stored in a freezer in Building 15, ready for Heneine's experiments.

In spite of division chief Brian Mahy's interdiction, Gunn was following the retrovirus lab's progress on the CFS project as best he could. By August 27, it was apparent to him that the success of late July, when Tom Folks, using Elaine DeFreitas's primers, had found evidence of retrovirus in Lyndonville and Atlanta patients, had given way to further complexities. Unfortunately, Heneine had been unable to perform PCR on any of the new samples because, Gunn said, "[he] had received a couple bad batches of probes and primers from our core facility."

Philadelphia, Pennsylvania

According to one estimate, it took twelve years and $200 million, on average, to bring a new drug from the chemist's laboratory to the patient.[4] Of every five thousand compounds tested, only five made it through the scientific and legal maze to Food and Drug Administration approval. On September 3 HEM Pharmaceuticals tried to speed the process along when it made formal application to the FDA for permission to supply Ampligen to CFS sufferers under a treatment IND, a special exemption from the agency's normally lengthy approval routine. The agency had exactly thirty days to respond to the request.

In the meantime, HEM's scientific advisers and its president, William Carter, continued their analysis of the data from the completed four-city clinical trial. So convincing were the statistics that they discussed the possibility of presenting a paper on the trials at the Thirty-first Interscience Conference on Antimicrobial Agents and Chemotherapy meeting in one month in Chicago. This annual meeting was the largest North American gathering of microbiologists, clinicians, pharmacologists, pathologists, and other specialists interested in infectious diseases and new drugs to treat them. Submissions were to have been made months in advance, but Carter wondered if the news value of the trial and its findings might persuade the organizers to add HEM's presentation to the schedule at the eleventh hour.

Wistar Institute, Philadelphia, Pennsylvania

By September, Elaine DeFreitas had begun to regret her involvement with Glasgow neurologist Peter Behan. In spite of his promise to sustain close communication with her while he worked to confirm her retrovirus finding, the Irishman, according to DeFreitas, had ceased all contact upon receiving her gene sequences the previous March. By fall it appeared that, although he had found retroviral gene sequences in his patients using the PCR technique, he believed it to be an endogenous virus. Behan's conclusion was a damaging one, since endogenous retroviruses are presumed to be harmless pieces of genetic substance that have resided in the human chromosomes for millennia, having been passed from generation to generation in the wake of a single ancient contamination.

In addition, in spite of the optimistic spin Walter Gunn was putting on CDC lab affairs, DeFreitas continued to be frustrated by the agency's virologists and their methods. "They're sloppy when they shouldn't be, and they're nitpicking when they shouldn't be," she said. "Koprowski is so fed up with them, he says, 'To hell with them! Don't talk to them!' He says, 'Drop it. Forget it. Spend your time doing the sequencing. We don't need the Centers for Disease Control doing Freshman Biology.' "

Hilary Koprowski's cavalier dismissal of the federal agency was a posture DeFreitas might have strived to adopt, but her credibility and expertise were on the line, not Koprowski's. Though she avoided any expression of concern, she could not have been other than acutely aware of the damage likely to accrue to her career, at least in the short term, should the CDC fail to confirm her work. There was every reason to believe the agency would step into the public arena, just as she had done, and proclaim its negative findings. She was certain she was correct: the virus was there, and all evidence she had found so far pointed to it as the etiological agent. But it might take two years or more for her to establish that fact in a major international forum like *Science*. In spite of her growing frustration with the virologists in Atlanta, therefore, DeFreitas pursued the collaboration.

University of California, San Francisco

Although mainstream medicine failed to reflect the change, tremendous progress had been made in understanding the disease since the first days of the Tahoe epidemic. CFS was, at minimum, an infectious chronic disease of the immune system in which latent DNA viruses like human herpesvirus 6 and Epstein-Barr were reactivated and virulently high levels of immunological chemicals or hormones such as interleukin-1 and -2 circulated in sufferers' tissues. In addition, the most knowledgeable students of the disease knew it to be a devastating affliction of the brain, as demonstrated by findings of lowered IQ, brain lesions, and more recently, abnormal brain metabolism and reduced blood flow to the brain. That fall, Philip Lee, a former assistant secretary of health who was then on the faculty of the University of California in San Francisco, predicted that the "critical mass" of scientific knowledge developing around the disease would result in dramatic medical advances in the very near future.

For sufferers, however, progress seemed to be stalled. No matter how persuasive the physical evidence, the federal research establishment—and frequently the patients' own doctors—simply refused to respond. In San Francisco, patient activists like Jan Montgomery and others had watched, their hopes raised with each new scientific revelation; surely now, they had assumed at every turn in the discovery process, the health agencies would marshal their money and technology to fight the disease, whether out of conscience or as a result of public outcry. Their expectations had probably never been higher than after Elaine DeFreitas released her evidence for retroviral infection. Yet, like a bomb that somehow failed to detonate, the discovery had languished, its alarming portent all but forgotten one year later.

The situation seemed to be deteriorating, in fact. Stephen Straus and Ann Schleuderberg's Bethesda workshop the previous March had impressed the major researchers in the disease and patient advocates, alike, that the government was determined to hew to its psychoneurotic theory of the disease, even in the face of powerful evidence contradicting that theory. More ominously, the government's authority in all matters medical and scientific appeared to be inviolate in the public sphere, its officials able to blot out important advances with bland reassurances and subtle disparagement of independent researchers' work. Stephen Straus's comments a year before to *New York Times* medical writer Lawrence Altman, that the Wistar findings and any future breakthroughs could well "evaporate" upon more thorough investigation, were typical—and difficult for the targets of such comments to dispute publicly without abandoning hope of federal grant support. The independents, virtually all of whom were seeking financial support for their CFS research from Straus's institute, were hardly in a position to suggest to *New York Times* writers that Straus's research findings might lack authenticity or "evaporate" under scrutiny.

Faced with these seemingly impenetrable barriers to progress, the San Francisco patient advocates began reevaluating their tactics. Instead of looking to each new scientific breakthrough to advance their cause with the federal health agencies or to gain public support, they increasingly believed the politics of the disease needed to be uncoupled from the science of the disease. Patients simply couldn't wait any longer for the cause of the disease to be conclusively resolved in order to receive the medical care and social services accorded victims of other serious illnesses. Efforts needed to be redirected toward developing a coherent public health policy for CFS in California and elsewhere. The activists envisioned a statewide medical education campaign to teach clinicians how to provide, at minimum, compassionate, intelligent care for sufferers. They imagined, too, the establishment of social services for fully disabled indigent patients. Finally, in the face of the CDC's unwillingness to perform epidemiology at a national level, they conceived of a California-based epidemiology program to track the spread of the disease inside their state. All of these programs, they hoped, might serve as models for other states.

The activists looked to the history of the AIDS epidemic in their city for their inspiration: "We saw a similar evolution in AIDS," Jan Montgomery said that fall, "whereby, although the science was still coming in, we had to start working on risk factors, prevention strategies, and really looking hard at public health issues."

During the first week in September, Montgomery and members of the patient advocacy organization CACTUS took a step toward their goal of creating a responsive public health system when they invited a handful of CFS researchers to San Francisco to meet with a group of state and local health officials. CACTUS members charged their guests with one task: to plot a strategy for propelling the CFS epidemic to the fore at the federal, state, and local agencies responsible for guarding the public's health. "We have good core researchers," Montgomery explained, "but they don't have the clout to move this disease out of their labs into the public health arena. That's what this meeting is about."

Early in the morning on September 7, a Saturday, Montgomery's guests gathered in a windowless library at the medical school on Parnassus Hill. Several of them rolled up their shirtsleeves and loosened their ties. Paul Cheney, Nancy Klimas, John Martin, C. V. Herst, and Ann Butcher, a PCR specialist from Roche Diagnostic Systems in Chicago, were introduced to the state's infectious disease chief, George Rutherford; the city's health department head, Ray Baxter; the head of the state's Viral and Rickettsial Disease Laboratory in Berkeley, Michael Ascher; and Philip Lee, who would soon be appointed assistant secretary of health in the Clinton administration. Virologist Jay Levy, well known among local health officials, was present, as was Mark Hurt, a scientist with the university's Centers for AIDS Research PCR core facility. Levy, Hurt, Butcher, Herst, and Martin were all looking for the Wistar retrovirus in CFS patients; Elaine DeFreitas, who was unable to attend, would be available by speakerphone later in the day.

All of the California health officials who were present either knew people with the disease or, like state epidemiologist George Rutherford, had watched from their vantage as public health officers as the disease mushroomed. The epidemic was, for many of them, a nearly tactile experience. Philip Lee, for instance, had witnessed the deterioration of a close friend, a board member of an international philanthropy, who apparently acquired the disease during a short stay in San Francisco. Initially, Lee thought she had fallen victim to hepatitis. "In following the course of her illness, not as her personal physician but as a friend," Lee said, "I've observed the evolution of this syndrome."

The public health officials demonstrated a refreshing humility as they encountered, many for the first time, scientists with expertise in the field of CFS research. Health department head Ray Baxter graciously presented himself and his agency to researchers as "a partner in the knowledge-seeking around this disease and as an organization that has a critical role to play in terms of bringing attention to all the issues here." In a comment that likely took the embattled researchers by surprise, Baxter added, "My role, and our role here today, is receptive—that is, to learn from all of you." For once, the epidemic's reality and the urgency of the crisis were above debate.

Most of the San Franciscans present had lived through the drama of that city's AIDS epidemic, and in the morning sessions they drew analogies from their experiences in bringing a poorly understood infectious disease to the reluctant attention of the federal health bureaucracy.

"I think it's important to look back and try to see what made AIDS research gel in 1983 and 1984," state epidemiologist Rutherford said, "because within the paradigm of what AIDS taught us, we're sort of in 1983 and 1984—if this disease were AIDS. The most important thing then was the isolation of an etiologic agent. . . . But the other thing that really kick-started AIDS research was the first international conference and, even more important, the second international conference on AIDS." Rutherford proposed an international conference on CFS.

Phil Lee suggested leapfrogging over middle-level health officials and taking the matter directly to either Walter Sullivan, then the secretary of health and human services, or James Mason, Sullivan's assistant secretary and former CDC head.

Joan Iten-Sutherland, executive director of CACTUS, told Lee her group had been unable to penetrate even the senior-level administrators at the CDC or NIH. "We have no idea where [CDC head] Roper stands on this—none," she said.

"I could tell you where they stand," countered Rutherford. "They don't want to be wrong. They want to cover their bases as long as it doesn't cost them a lot of money."

Michael Ascher said of the Atlanta agency staff, "They will not lead—they will follow. The people there who are working on the problem are going to be mavericks who are putting their careers on the line. They're not in the mainstream."

Eventually the group agreed to send a letter to the assistant secretary of health, James Mason, asking that the Public Health Service sponsor an international research conference on CFS.*

Conflicts erupted among the scientists that afternoon when Levy chaired a meeting from which all but hands-on researchers were barred. Elaine DeFreitas was present as a disembodied voice on a speakerphone placed in the center of the conference table.

Jan Montgomery, who had conceived of the meeting, recalled, "I wanted to provide these people with a true scientific session of confidentiality." That idea seemed sound enough. After all, DeFreitas, Herst, and Martin, three researchers who claimed to have evidence for retroviral infection, had yet to sit in a room together and discuss their techniques or their findings with each other or with scientists who had tried to duplicate their work. Perhaps naively, patient organizers hoped researchers would share all and tell all, resulting in a consensus on the virus causing the disease and ways to test for it. It was soon apparent, however, that the scientists' circumspection dominated the proceedings.

By reports, DeFreitas, who had been criticized in the past for withholding important details of her virus-finding protocol, was direct and explicit. Speaking the dense language of molecular biology, she satisfied her colleagues by describing in detail the techniques that had brought her to her original discovery. Not surprisingly, she commanded the full attention of her audience, whose members stared silently at the speaker box from which her voice emanated. "This is like no virus ever reported," DeFreitas said, as she described the appearance of the virus under the electron microscope. Still, she did not offer details of her current work, nor did any of her colleagues press her on the matter.

John Martin, whose work held equal fascination for these researchers, proved to be less accommodating and was treated less delicately. Unlike DeFreitas, Martin was present in the flesh and unable to deflect inquiries, although he tried and,

---

* By 1995, the Public Health Service had yet to sponsor such a conference.

in at least one case, flat out refused to reveal information. "John got asked the really tough questions," Cheney recalled. "People dealt with him more brutally. He *looked* bad, compared to other people, but he was the only one who really had something that could be profoundly helpful to other people, and he didn't divulge it."

By several accounts, Martin skated over a succession of direct questions about his work. Jay Levy found Martin's reticence merely annoying at first, but as the meeting wore on, Levy lost his temper. Among other things, he had demanded to know which cells Martin was finding his spuma virus in. That question was hardly trivial; the information could make or break an effort to reproduce the finding. But Martin ignored the question until finally Levy banged his fist on the table and asked, "Are you or are you not going to tell?"

"I'm *not* going to tell," Martin said, a response that could not have been more contrary to the meeting's stated goal.

"Do you think we're going to try to scoop you on this?" Levy asked, outraged.

Martin deflected the question, but his failure to provide Levy with enabling information about his discovery communicated the Los Angeles scientist's increasingly strong proprietary attitude toward his work.

To complicate matters further, two profoundly different conceptions of the disease emerged as the afternoon wore on. One faction was inclined to view CFS as an immune system problem, a disorder that could be provoked by perhaps several different pathogens or inciting incidents, in which the major symptoms were caused by an excess of poisonous cytokines, such as interleukins and interferons, generated by the immune system in response to the trigger or triggers. Another faction conceptualized the disease as a viral infection of the central nervous system.

For John Martin especially, CFS was an infectious brain disease, pure and simple; to view it as anything less was naive. "Nancy Klimas and Jay Levy want to see chronic fatigue syndrome as immune dysregulation," Martin said later. "Paul Cheney fits just halfway into that camp. I say no—the presence of an infectious agent overrides the immune dysfunction issues. The biggest implication of this is how do you *treat*? Klimas would say immune modulate. I say use an antiviral." Martin added, "Have we convinced people other than Paul Cheney that spuma virus can cause chronic fatigue syndrome? I think the answer is, Cheney, yes. Martin, yes. The rest of the world, no."

In spite of little appreciable conciliation, the immune dysregulation theory prevailed.

Significantly, Martin had described his discovery to state health officials earlier in the day. He had avoided specifics, but he did tell them forthrightly that he had cultured a peculiar new virus from CFS patients. He had done so at the urging of Marc Iverson of the CFIDS Association, Martin's sole benefactor in his CFS research, and Jan Montgomery, who represented CACTUS. In part, the activists believed the move would afford the state scientists an opportunity to attempt replication, and Martin agreed to the request. But Montgomery and Iverson wanted a second favor from Martin: his permission to disseminate a national press release about his spuma virus discovery at meeting's end. Martin was reluctant to grant that request; after all, he had yet to publish his work in a scientific journal.

Montgomery argued that a press release might prod the CDC into moving forward with its own spuma virus investigation.

"That's what we've seen in this illness, and [in] the early days of AIDS, too," Montgomery said later. "The press forces the discussion. It's the reporter at the *L.A. Times* who calls the CDC and says, 'Have you seen Martin's work? What do you think about it?' "

After some thought, Martin agreed to Montgomery's request, for only one reason: to avoid being scooped by CDC scientists who, Martin worried, might already have reproduced his work. A press release would at least establish his ownership of the discovery; at best, it would inspire the public to exert pressure on the federal agency to follow up. He gave Montgomery permission to prepare the statement. While the scientists held their meeting, Montgomery composed a three-page draft for Martin's approval.

On Monday, September 9, Jan Montgomery issued her press release touting Martin's discovery: "Virus Not Previously Known to Cause Human Disease Linked to Severe Cases of Chronic Fatigue Syndrome."

University of Southern California, Los Angeles

On September 9, Paul Cheney flew from San Francisco to Los Angeles, where he spent the day with John Martin in the pathology laboratories Martin directed. The experience was a revelation for Cheney, who quickly realized that Martin's weak replies to the rough questions posed to him in San Francisco had been contrived. "It turned out Martin had just *chosen* not to defend himself," Cheney recalled. He was not *unable* to defend himself.

"The pictures he showed in San Francisco were the *least* revealing," Cheney said later. "He showed pictures with one virion breaking out of a cell," the doctor added, referring to the virus particles that bud from cells in search of new cells to infect. "But now I've seen pictures where he's got *hundreds* of virions pouring out. He did not play his strong hand in San Francisco, which I didn't understand until later."

Martin enfolded the Charlotte clinician in the swirl of scientific activity around the virus discovery, instructing him in each aspect of the research under way, beginning with the effort to grow the virus in cell cultures seeded with the blood serum of CFS victims. In the morning, Martin took Cheney into the long, narrow viral culture room of his laboratory at the university, where Martin was the head of the infectious disease and molecular pathology labs. There, four lab techs, supervised by the senior scientist, Ahmed Kahleed, were engaged in seeding and tending the viral cultures in hundreds of test tubes plugged with rubber stoppers. The team kept a running tally of the positives and negatives on a board in the laboratory. By September 9 they had tested 368 CFS sufferers for the virus; slightly less than half—170—had been positive by the culture assay.

In the afternoon, Martin and Cheney drove from the university to the L.A. County Hospital, a massive, crumbling Art Deco structure not far from downtown Los Angeles. The hospital had been the site of a 1934 "atypical polio" epidemic that many suspected was actually the first documented outbreak of CFS. Martin oversaw several laboratories, but he took Cheney to the one where efforts were being made to sequence the genetic code of the new virus. "The sequencing is not going as well as the culturing," Cheney said later. "That's where Elaine DeFreitas is ahead of Martin."

New York City

Jan Montgomery's press release generated results. On September 16, exactly one week after it was issued, the *Wall Street Journal* weighed in on the spuma virus discovery, the first national publication to do so. Reporter Ron Winslow's story about John Martin's work was followed on September 17 by an article in *USA Today* by health writer Kim Painter. *Newsweek*'s Geoffrey Cowley and Mary Hager were preparing a story that would run on September 30. All four journalists, who had been assiduously cultivated by the San Francisco activists, had a demonstrated interest in new developments in the disease. Reports of the spuma sighting also appeared in the *San Francisco Chronicle,* the *Philadelphia Inquirer,* the *Boston Globe,* and the *Chicago Tribune.*

The *Journal*'s Winslow noted that other scientists were likely to question whether Martin really had discovered a microbe associated with CFS because the original patients in his study were people with severe brain disease. These patients, Winslow wrote, "had been suspected of having such diseases as multiple sclerosis, lupus, and encephalitis, but their symptoms didn't clearly fit the classic definition of any of them." CFS patients "aren't usually thought to be so sick," Winslow added.

Winslow quoted Martin: "It's not a trivial illness. We are dealing with something much more serious and complex than the name implies."

Winslow also noted that the disease continued to be controversial within the medical establishment, in spite of a growing body of evidence in favor of a viral cause. He wrote that "in medical research, just looking for a cause of the ailment is extraordinarily controversial. Indeed, Dr. Martin acknowledges that three prominent medical journals have declined to publish his current data, even as a letter to the editor."

Charlotte, North Carolina

Few involved in the struggle to bring Ampligen into the marketplace failed to appreciate the larger political issue that had emerged along with the promising results of the clinical trial. One arm of the nation's federal health establishment, the Food and Drug Administration, was being asked to rule on the use of a potent antiviral drug for a disease the Centers for Disease Control and the National Institutes of Health had dismissed for years as a psychiatric condition. The ramifications of the FDA'S decision were hardly lost on patient advocacy groups.

"If Ampligen is approved for treatment of CFIDS," the CFIDS Association in Charlotte had told its 25,000 members in a special mailing that summer, "this will be a monumental step toward gaining credibility and focusing more attention *and research* [italics theirs] on CFIDS."

At the same time, Paul Cheney noted, "The FDA is *really* in a bind. If the agency approves the treatment IND application, they will, in one swoop, destroy the credibility of two government agencies."

In the case of drug approvals, the FDA's mandate was generally straightforward. The agency was required to answer just two questions: was the drug safe, and did it do what its manufacturer claimed it did? On the matter of Ampligen as a therapy for CFS, however, the FDA's decision acquired significance reaching far beyond matters of Ampligen's safety and usefulness in the disease. Unfairly, the drug agency's impending decision was shaping into a referendum on the existence of the disease itself.

As the October 3 deadline for the FDA's decision neared, patients began applying pressure on both the FDA and HEM Pharmaceuticals. An appeal by the CFIDS Association of Charlotte to its national membership in late June had generated a write-in campaign to members of Congress alerting them to the recent Ampligen trial and urging their support for increased research into treatments for CFS. While the FDA remained mute on the subject, patient support groups and doctors monitoring the approval process sensed that the pressure on critical members of both houses of Congress was significant, coming primarily in the form of constituent mail and phone calls. Participants in the Ampligen trial were particularly desperate that fall as they embraced the reality of their situation: should the FDA withhold its approval, Ampligen might never again be available to them.

Nevada patients who had participated in the Ampligen trial—among them a newspaper reporter, a rancher, a computer software programmer, and a neurologist, all of whom had been disabled for several years—turned to the state's civil courts for help when the drug was withdrawn. Neurologist Kristine Dahl, who began to suffer from the disease while a resident at Duke University's medical center, was the first to hire an attorney. Soon she was joined by several co-plaintiffs. By early fall, U.S. District Judge Edward C. Reed in Reno had heard testimony from several local CFS sufferers about the ill effects of being removed from the drug. Having heard of Dan Peterson's patients' lawsuit against HEM, a handful of Paul Cheney's Ampligen trial participants, among them a female Baptist minister, decided to file suit against the firm as well. Ultimately seventeen patients joined the suit to force HEM to continue to provide the drug.

Officers at HEM Pharmaceuticals were hardly displeased with these developments. A passionate display by patients might constitute enough pressure to sway the government, and although patients looked upon the FDA's decision as a life-or-death issue, the consequences of that decision were equally dire for HEM. The company was struggling for its economic survival that year. Should the agency approve HEM's application for expanded clinical trials among chronic fatigue syndrome patients, cash backers could be expected to flock to the little firm.

Centers for Disease Control, Atlanta, Georgia

Dorothy Knight might not have been contributing to the agency's scientific progress on the disease, but she was performing a yeomanly humanitarian service. Once a missile repair worker, later a military police investigator at Fort Stewart, Georgia, and now a program assistant at the Atlanta health agency, Knight spent her days responding to hundreds of telephone calls and letters from CFS victims who called or wrote the Centers for Disease Control for help. One hundred calls a day, Knight said, was "very low" volume. More commonly, two to three hundred sufferers telephoned, leaving their names and numbers on the agency's CFS hot line. In the summer of 1991 the agency had hired another woman to help Knight manage the task. Both women worked full-time at computers and telephones, logging the name and address of every caller and correspondent. Between July 15 and September 24, 2,619 people had called Knight directly. The calls came from all over: Passaic, Fort Leavenworth, Tucson, Dallas, Boise. Knight's empathy for these patients, many of whom described their illness in long, anguished letters, had grown during her eighteen months at the agency. "You stay on the phone, you listen to people cry . . . By the time you get home, you're depressed, too," Knight said late that September.

Little affected Knight more, however, than the victims of the disease who actually came to the agency's Atlanta headquarters—usually two or three of them each week—seeking an explanation for their devastation. Instead, they were met in the agency's lobby on Clifton Road by Knight. Under the indifferent gaze of the agency's uniformed security guards, who had grown accustomed to the spectacle, these despondent visitors frequently wept.

"I went down to the lobby yesterday and spent an hour with a patient who came here all the way from Vermont," Knight said that fall. "He's sixty-four. He cried, poor thing. This was his last resort. He's been tested for every disease imaginable." The medical establishment refugee had been a forester before developing the disease. He had been unable to work for fourteen months. "His doctor told him it was all in his head," Knight said.

Staff in the Division of Viral and Rickettsial Diseases were aware of the remarkable number of calls to the agency from the public; division head Brian Mahy, in particular, frequently asked Knight for a tally.* Still, Knight rarely discussed her interactions with patients with others at the agency unless she heard them making jokes about the disease. "They wonder if this really exists," Knight said. "I tell them yes—and it's a *terrible* thing to have this every day, all day long, year after year."

In recent weeks, as the possibility that CFS was a retroviral illness—one that could be passed casually from person to person—began to penetrate the agency's scientific rank and file, Knight added, the jokes about CFS that she routinely heard from co-workers had ceased abruptly. "Nobody's laughing anymore," she commented.

* At this writing, no one at the agency has investigated whether the calls suggest geographic clustering, nor have there been efforts to analyze any other demographic aspects of the calls.

29

The Retrovirus Caper

Centers for Disease Control, Atlanta, Georgia

The CFS Advisory Council's meetings were erratic, floating affairs, held wherever and whenever a quorum could be obtained, usually in a hotel suite during CFS medical conferences. Since its formation in 1989, the self-appointed body of fourteen that included a multimillionaire entrepreneur, a former governor, clinicians, scientists, two National Cancer Institute investigators and, more recently, the CDC's own Walter Gunn, had met six times in places like Milwaukee and Los Angeles. Soul-searching over the council's purpose was ongoing. Members grappled with sticky questions: should the council serve as an advisory board to patient organizations struggling to decide which independent research proposals to fund? Some members wondered whether the council had a right to exist at all. "By whose authority do we serve?" Paul Cheney once had asked his associates on the council. In spite of collective doubt, the council had demonstrated little inclination to dissolve itself, and on September 21 its members gathered for the seventh time. The Centers for Disease Control in Atlanta was the site. Their stated task: to consider the divisive, politically charged question of retrovirus infection in chronic fatigue syndrome.

Anthony Komaroff, who was the council's chairman, and Walter Gunn, the council's newest member as of that fall, had deemed the CDC a practically and symbolically appropriate venue. John Martin of L.A. and Peter Behan of Glasgow, the independent scientists actually performing retrovirus research, had agreed to present their evidence to the council and to all interested agency personnel. Gunn, who viewed the meeting as an opportunity to ease suspicions between government scientists and independent researchers, invited his fellow steering committee members to attend.

On the evening of September 20 invitees converged on the Emory Inn on Clifton Road in Atlanta, opposite the agency's Building 1. Rudy Perpich, the former governor of Minnesota, was among the first to arrive. Peter Behan and his collaborator, molecular biologist John Gow, had come from Glasgow. Paul Cheney, Jay Levy, Dharam Ablashi, Paul Levine, Nancy Klimas, Mark Loveless, and James Jones also checked into the inn that night. John Martin would arrive early in the morning after taking a red-eye from Los Angeles.

Unfortunately, developments in DeFreitas's family life were intruding into her professional world, and her attendance at this critical event was in some doubt. Her marriage to internist John Woodward was over, and DeFreitas was involved in a custody battle for her teenage son. Her attorney had strongly advised De-Freitas to remain in Philadelphia until the custody hearing on September 23. "My son comes first," DeFreitas said. "I'm not going to risk losing my son over a one-day meeting at the Centers for Disease Control."

That evening, Behan and Gow reported they had not confirmed Elaine De-Freitas's work. "The retrovirus stuff is finished! Over!" Behan announced while nursing his red wine in the inn's cozy bar. The "retrovirus caper," as he called the Wistar find, soon would be revealed for the fraud that it was. "We're going to blow them out of the water. Permanently. Her claim is spurious," he added in reference to DeFreitas, avoiding her name. "How she *ever* got that published in the *Proceedings of the National Academy of Sciences* I don't know. But one has to be allowed one's say, and tomorrow we shall have our say."

Gow, a lithe, moon-faced young Scot, was more temperate than the neurologist who was his boss. He explained that he had little personal interest in the disease; to him it was a medical problem, like any other. "We have spent many months and many thousands of pounds trying to reproduce those results," he reported. "And to date we cannot detect any sign of an exogenous [acquired] retrovirus."

Atlanta-based CNN sent a TV crew to film the council members leaving the Emory Inn and filing into the CDC the following morning, but by the council's majority rule the press was banned from the deliberations. Council members assembled in a windowless conference room, seating themselves at long tables arranged in a rectangle. Only a few of Gunn's colleagues from the notorious "sneering committee" chose to attend; they lined the edges of the room as they were introduced, most of them for the first time, to the "players," as agency immunologist Alison Mawle later called them—researchers like Komaroff, Cheney, Klimas, Martin, and Levy. At the rectangle's center, a small table supported a slide projector and a speakerphone, the sole material evidence of Elaine DeFreitas's participation.

Tom Folks launched the proceedings with a brief description of his lab's efforts to replicate the Wistar findings. Folks said his colleague Walid Heneine planned to use the identical methods and genetic probes to search for fragments of the virus in patients of their own: Atlanta sufferers who had been referred to the agency through its surveillance system.

DeFreitas spoke next. Her speakerphone-relayed voice was forceful; after being assured that there were no reporters present (save this one), she began by saying, "Clearly this virus is not HTLV-two. We now have additional data that verifies that point." She went on to describe a series of experiments that had clarified that matter. "Unfortunately," she said, "when you take [the genetic sequence of a portion of the virus] and put it in the various computer databases and ask if it's homologous to anything, the answer is no. It's clearly different, but not different enough to be named something *else* in the computer's database."

DeFreitas added that in the past five months she and her staff had struggled to grow the virus in several human cell lines. Tissue samples from five patients— three children from the study presented in Kyoto and two adults—had resulted in thriving viral colonies when added to these cell lines. "We feel we have a culture system," DeFreitas added. "It's not ideal. It's certainly not the H-nine of HIV," she said in a reference to the premier human immunodeficiency virus culture system developed in Robert Gallo's Bethesda lab. "But we can make genomic libraries."

Then DeFreitas moved on to the most interesting aspect of her work: the virus's appearance. "We've looked at four of these five cell lines. We can see particles by electron microscope, but not extracellular virus," she said. "We are not looking at a C-type retrovirus." The significance of DeFreitas's comment likely was appreciated by most present: every *known* human retrovirus was a C type. "I do not feel we can make an absolute identification of this virus, but my conclusion is that it is not an endogenous [inherited] virus, but is an acquired retrovirus. We would like to reserve our judgment as to what kind of virus this is."

In response to a question, DeFreitas responded, "Certainly, there's a possibility John Martin and we are looking at the same thing. But I would not be willing to go on record with the subfamily of retrovirus. We're not ready to say this is a foamy or that it isn't."

AIDS specialist Mark Loveless tried to pin DeFreitas down further. "Have you tried any neurologic cell lines?" he asked, obviously curious to know if De-Freitas's virus might be a cause of CFS brain damage.

"We haven't gotten to those studies yet," DeFreitas said.

John Martin, who had sat quietly while Folks and DeFreitas talked, now described how he had cultured a virus from a range of patients, all of them suffering either from severe brain diseases like encephalitis—even, in one case, coma—or from "classic" CFS. Telling his audience he would "cut to the meat," Martin showed slides of the virus itself. The magnified image revealed a swollen, misshapen cell with hundreds of tiny virions clustering just inside its membrane. The isolate had come from the counselor in a doctor's office who had been hospitalized in Los Angeles General the previous August.

"Her admitting diagnosis was encephalitis-slash-meningitis bacteremia," Martin said. "She was treated with antibiotics and discharged. Since then, this lady constitutes a classic CFS patient. One of the most telling aspects of her disease is that items have no names—she cannot name things. She has some very real, clear cognitive debilitation. From this lady," Martin added, "we have now seven positive cell cultures which we have obtained every month for the last six months. It is the same virus every time."

Martin described how another patient, the Palm Springs grade-school teacher who had originally seemed normal to her doctor on examination, also had tested positive for the virus, providing the first link for the pathologist between the encephalitis cases and CFS cases. "She tested positive, and I wondered why," Martin said. "But as one sees more and more of these patients, the cognitive impairment becomes more and more apparent. This woman cannot draw a clock face. . . .

"Now, probably because we offer polymerase chain reaction in our lab, we are getting referrals from doctors with very interesting patients. These patients are bouncing from specialist to specialist. They come to us with diagnoses like 'multiple sclerosis-slash-lupus with pseudo-tumor cerebri.' If this infection is not specifically looked for, we won't see it. . . . I consider this to have some public health implications," Martin concluded.

In the afternoon, Peter Behan and John Gow were at last given their opportunity to blast DeFreitas, a task they embraced with relish. The government scientists arrayed around the edges of the room watched with interest as the large, peppery professor stood to launch what everyone present by now knew was to be a refutation of the Wistar scientists' work.

"When people make spurious claims and go to the press," Behan began, setting the tone for his challenge, "the poor bloke who suffers is the patient." He went on to summarize the status of CFS in England and its clinical parameters. When he was finished, Behan gave microbiologist John Gow the floor. In contrast to Behan, Gow spoke rapidly in a soft, high voice, his rich Scottish burr at times rendering his words unintelligible to the American ear. Based on his research, Gow believed the retrovirus fragments DeFreitas had reported a year earlier were merely an "endogenous sequence," a piece of retrovirus that had been in cells for generation upon generation and that could hardly be blamed for a disease. Most interesting was Gow's proof: he had found the virus fragment in people with CFS *and* in controls.

Even before Gow had finished, Nancy Klimas looked at the little black speakerphone. "Elaine, can you hear all this?" she asked.

There was no answer.

Jay Levy asked a question of Gow, then directed his powerful baritone at the speakerphone: "Elaine, they've taken your primers, gone into patients, amplified the sequence, probed it with radioactive probes, and they find [the virus] represented in lots of endogenous cellular activity."

"Okay," DeFreitas responded, clearly trying to collect her thoughts. But before she could proceed, Tom Folks and Walid Heneine showered Gow with more questions.

When they were through, Levy endeavored to engage DeFreitas in the conversation once again: "Elaine, we don't know the techniques they were using, but essentially this is the first group that has presented work that is unable to replicate your findings. They find endogenous retrovirus."

For a moment the room in which thirty people sat was dead silent.

Realizing that DeFreitas had been unable to understand anything Gow had said, Levy now assumed the role of interpreter, putting DeFreitas's questions to the Scot and relaying Gow's response to her. "What they did, Elaine, was come back with your band . . . but maybe they didn't make the band correctly."

"Ours was four-forty," Gow said. "It's a very specific band."

"Is it possible," Levy asked him, "that you just missed making the DeFreitas four-oh-nine band?"

"It's possible we missed it, but unlikely," Gow replied.

"Do you test sensitivity?" Tom Folks asked Gow. "When we don't get the correct sensitivity, we do not see any bands in patients and controls."

Before Gow could respond, DeFreitas, who obviously could understand Folks, interrupted. "There are two very crucial factors in your ability to amplify the bands you're interested in," she said to Gow. "Number one is the concentration of magnesium. Number two is taq-polymerase [an enzyme]. We use the lowest concentrate of magnesium and taq-polymerase. If you do it with excess magnesium or taq-polymerase, those bands can come up and just swamp your reaction."

DeFreitas offered Gow the precise concentrations of these substances used by her team in their experiments, but she cautioned that taq-polymerase varied in quality and concentrations even from lot to lot.

Gow, in turn, mentioned that instead of taq-polymerase he had used an enzyme called Replinase.

"Replinase?" DeFreitas asked, clearly alarmed. "We have found that to be absolutely worthless! It's *always* proved inferior."

Levy jumped in again, this time in an effort to moderate rather than interpret. "Now we'll have to use both systems," he said.

But DeFreitas continued: "I've been in contact with Dr. Behan by fax on a number of occasions and these faxes went into great detail about this. In terms of resolving this issue, we need the perfect matched primers and probes in order to identify this virus."

Behan interposed with a gracious comment: "As it stands, [the Glasgow project] has to be done over—and done properly."

A fifth scientist who had looked for evidence of retrovirus in CFS sufferers, C. V. Herst of Oncore Analytics in Houston, was not present that day, but he had designated Paul Cheney to describe his results to the assembled group. Cheney told his audience that he had given DeFreitas's *Proceedings of the National Academy of Sciences* paper to Herst and asked him to attempt replication using the methods she described in the article. Herst had found a positivity rate of 83 percent among patient samples. Just two of fifteen healthy controls were positive using the same method.

Faced with five uncertain and conflicting results from as many retroviral inquiries, few in the room knew exactly what to do or say next.

"So, Paul . . . what do you think?" Komaroff asked Cheney.

"I think we're standing between a system that's of suspect specificity," Cheney said, referring to polymerase chain reaction, "and a system that has superior specificity but less sensitivity." The latter reference was to the system of growing viruses in cell cultures. "The virus needs to be sequenced, but the culture system might be the ideal system, not PCR."

Jay Levy proposed that in the future retroviral investigators use only umbilical cord blood from newborn babies, the purest blood available, to compare with blood samples from patients. The possibility that the virus was by now prevalent in the population was too great. "The *only* control is cord blood," Levy said. "We have to be concerned that whatever causes this disease is widespread, so it's carried. Herst should be sent cord blood."

Interestingly, the name Sidney Grossberg and his discovery of evidence for retroviral infection in CFS sufferers went unmentioned by government and independent scientists alike on this day; Grossberg's work in Wisconsin was being undertaken in such deft isolation it was as if the researcher and his finding didn't exist.

Perhaps the most poignant moment of the day occurred at the end of the discussion when Komaroff, in his capacity as council chairman, told the assembled scientists that Cheney wanted to play a videotape of four CFS patients who suffered from the central nervous system abnormalities Cheney believed were typical of the gravest form of the disease. The doctor had prepared the film especially for this occasion. "I think this tape will shatter any myths that this disease is not a serious illness of the brain and will demonstrate that this disease has an evolution like AIDS encephalopathy," Cheney had said before his Atlanta trip.

The doctor had ordered the four patients on a scale of progressive disability. One of them, an extraordinarily beautiful twenty-nine-year-old M.B.A., was acutely ataxic, with shaky movements and an unsteady gait. Cheney included her SPECT scan on the film; it revealed that the former business manager had no blood flow at all to her temporal lobe. Another patient, a secretary in her mid-thirties, suffered bouts of encephalopathy during which she would be hospitalized; her pupils would "blow," Cheney said, becoming fully dilated, and she would become incoherent; she also suffered from frequent bouts of pneumonia and staph infection. All four patients suffered extreme head pain, one to such a degree that she was prescribed I.V. morphine.

"I would like to play this for some people who have never really seen a sick CFIDS patient," the doctor said, his voice quiet in the room lined with federal scientists.

Immediately, vehement protest erupted from several government scientists who insisted such a film was an inappropriately clinical adjunct to a session devoted to molecular biology. The debate raged for a full twelve minutes. Komaroff, seeking to avert an all-out conflagration, put the matter to a vote. With the exception of retrovirology chief Tom Folks, all of the agency staff present, including Louisa Chapman, the agency's CFS medical officer, whose task was to provide clinical expertise in the disease to her colleagues, voted against screening the video. Komaroff proposed that only a portion of the film be screened. With a tiny majority won from his colleagues on the council, Cheney gained the right to show a truncated version of his film.

Shaken but determined, the doctor rose and inserted the tape into the VCR. As the film commenced, several scientists ostentatiously stood and departed; others began to talk loudly among themselves. Of the government scientists, only virologist Tom Folks gave the piece his full attention.

On the screen, Cheney, standing in a hospital room, interviewed the former business manager. Speaking over the sound track, Cheney noted that she had fallen abruptly ill after a blood transfusion, that she had been hospitalized three times with an "encephalopathic illness," and that she now suffered from CFS. "I misjudge door frames and walls," she told Cheney. "It's hard for me to stand without a wall nearby. . . . My head always aches." While agency scientists drifted from the room, Cheney pressed on, noting that her right temporal lobe was atrophied. She had been this way for two years. The screen displayed her MRI brain scans, which revealed multiple UBOs, and her SPECT scan. When the film excerpt ended a few minutes later, virtually all of the meeting's participants except for John Martin, Jay Levy, Anthony Komaroff, and Tom Folks were gone.

Some days later, Jim Dobbins, an agency demographer and CFS steering committee member, was asked why he had objected so strenuously to viewing the tape. "We don't need to see a film of someone with polio to study polio," he replied.

Glasgow neurologist Peter Behan, who had watched the film for a few moments before leaving the room, later insisted that the patient was merely "hysterical" and that Cheney himself was "depressed." (This patient died two years later, when she was thirty-one.)

The government scientists' extraordinary belligerence toward the opportunity to witness—all of them for the first time—a series of gravely ill CFS sufferers undergoing neurological examinations in a starkly clinical setting, was a pivotal event in Cheney's life. It was as if a door swung closed in his mind. He would continue seeing patients and studying the disease with whatever means were available to him. But his endeavor to lead federal investigators toward an understanding of the clinical manifestations of CFS, an effort that had consumed him for six years, was finished.

Reno, Nevada

Participants in the Ampligen trial who had joined neurologist Kristine Dahl in her lawsuit against HEM Pharmaceuticals were provided a short-term solution that fall: a court injunction against the company, requiring it to provide the drug to patients for a year, or until the legal issues could be worked out. On November 7 and December 2, U.S. District Judge Edward C. Reed in Reno issued interim rulings until the case could be tried in court. He ordered HEM to provide Ampligen to the plaintiffs for at least twelve more months, "or until the motion for permanent injunction is decided on the merits, whichever comes first." He stated that the "potential harm faced by the plaintiffs outweighed any harm to defendants that could result from granting such an injunction." HEM's defense for removing patients from the drug was that the government had yet to rule on its efficacy. In addition, in the absence of federal approval for HEM's recently proposed expanded trial, a precursor to full approval, the company had no income with which to manufacture, distribute, and administer the drug.

"If the new trial is approved," Cheney said, "HEM will reactivate their compassionate care program, because they would then have money to pay for the drug and projected large moneys in the future. Maryann Charlap feels very strongly about that. But if it's not approved," he added, "then all bets are off. Because they'll have no income. The proof of efficacy is not what HEM says but what the Food and Drug Administration says. The FDA action is their litmus test. And patients don't quite understand that little distinction. And patients could get screwed, and the way they'll get screwed is by the FDA—that is, the drug did work, but the FDA didn't approve it—and then it won't be HEM's fault."

Atlanta, Georgia

In the aftermath of the CFS Advisory Council's meeting, Peter Behan and John Gow were livid. Immediately following the day-long session, Behan, who had expected to meet his scientific adversary face-to-face, suggested, "Elaine DeFreitas is not here because she knew she was going to be blown out of the water. . . . To sit back and not come when your whole scientific reputation is on the line! That was an affront. That was the first indication I had that there's something seriously wrong."

Behan's colleague, microbiologist John Gow, saw DeFreitas's insistence upon the use of Replinase in the experiment as mere eccentricity. "The enzyme doesn't *matter*," Gow insisted. "I've worked with Replinase for six years—it makes *no* difference."

Behan seconded Gow's comment with characteristic fervor: "Let's be honest here," Behan interjected. "You often find that when someone is caught behind the eight ball and they've made a mistake, they say, 'Oh, you didn't use the technique that I used.' We used *exactly* the same technique. An enzyme is an enzyme."

Yet, both Behan and Gow admitted they lacked information that might have been crucial to their effort to replicate the Wistar work, a deficit they blamed on DeFreitas, whom they portrayed as a recalcitrant, withholding collaborator. "Actually, I personally telephoned Elaine DeFreitas's office last December. I spoke to her secretary and I said, 'Look, I will personally come to the Wistar Institute—let me see your data and your conditions.' " According to Behan and Gow, DeFreitas failed to respond to their overture. In the meantime, the Glasgow scientists were eager to see their retroviral experiments published. They had, in fact, already written their paper. Behan hoped to send his report contradicting DeFreitas's discovery in the form of a letter to an American journal like *Science*.*

Several days later, after having spent time huddled with Tom Folks in Building 15, Gow acknowledged, "There's obviously a lot of politics involved in this. Lots of people are under pressure from different sources to solve this thing one way or another, and many people seem to have a vested interest in either finding a retrovirus or not finding a retrovirus. . . . *We* have no political ax to grind," Gow continued. "We're working at a university. No one says to me, 'It would be better if you did find a virus or you didn't.' To be fair to Elaine, the thing may be there and we just haven't found it. But we need hard scientific data published in reputable journals."

In the days following the council's meeting, agency staff seemed pleased with the Scottish team's conclusions and ever more suspicious of Elaine DeFreitas. Tom Folks, although he avoided accusing DeFreitas of lying, found it "worrisome" that the Wistar scientist had remained in Philadelphia. "This is very critical to her career and to Wistar's reputation," he said, "and even though she couldn't be here, she didn't even send a representative." He confirmed that he had found "basically the same thing that the Scottish group finds—that is, amplification of endogenous material." And Folks, like Gow, was unimpressed by DeFreitas's concern about enzymes. "The idea [that one should] reproduce something exactly by the letter that someone else has done, it's just nonscientific," Folks said. "If it's reproducible and it's real, then based on the publication, some other laboratory that tries it should be able to find it."

Miami immunologist Nancy Klimas disagreed. Peter Behan and John Gow, she said, "didn't use [DeFreitas's] method, and then they said they couldn't confirm her findings. They had to follow her protocol to the letter, no matter whether they

* The paper was never published.

agreed with it or disagreed with it. At this point, confirmation means using some-one's precise method, without variation, and reconfirming on *their* blood sam-ples—the *same* samples.

"I'm hopeful that someone will confirm Elaine's work," Klimas added. "I think that she really deserves a lot of credit for sticking her neck out and trying to name that tune."

Paul Cheney had a different view of the controversy. He felt that patent issues were very much involved in the current debate over DeFreitas's findings. The doc-tor, in fact, suspected that DeFreitas had stayed in Philadelphia for reasons having to do with patent rights issues rather than family affairs. "I personally think she wasn't there because the Wistar's patent attorneys did not want her cornered. As I understand it, if she inadvertently releases information that hasn't been patented, then the patent is destroyed. It's called 'prior disclosure.' "

In actual fact, neither John Martin nor Elaine DeFreitas stood to gain significant financial rewards from their discovery; proceeds from a patented diagnostic test for their viruses would accrue to their institutions, although the scientists likely would derive a percentage of royalties on the patents. Their scientific reputations, however, would enjoy enormous enrichment should they prove to have discov-ered the cause of a worldwide scourge.

Wistar Institute, Philadelphia, Pennsylvania

Miami immunologist Nancy Klimas was increasingly concerned about Elaine De-Freitas, who was, after all, the only other bench scientist working in the field who was also a woman.

"Look at the position she's in. She's made an enormous investment of her time. And she's *still* not funded. Now, at Wistar she must have to defend every day to her boss all the energy she's putting into this. And if someone says, 'I can't con-firm your findings . . .' "

In fact, the ground was shifting under DeFreitas that summer as a result of dra-matic developments in the Wistar's director suite. Her mentor Hilary Koprowski, who had headed the institute since 1957 and captained its most remarkable con-tributions to medicine, including rubella and rabies vaccines and monoclonal an-tibody technology for cancer therapies, had been fired by the board of directors. The seventy-five-year-old Koprowski's reputation for freewheeling scientific bril-liance remained intact; in the board's view, however, his freewheeling adminis-trative skills had failed him at last. For the first time in its one-hundred-year history the institute had needed to dip into its endowment to pay the bills.

Unfortunately for DeFreitas, Koprowski's successor failed to share Koprowski's ardent fascination with the relationship between retroviruses and chronic neuro-logic disease in general and his interest in CFS in particular. The new director, Gio-vanni Rovera, who had been appointed for his professed commitment to fiscal conservatism, was aware only that for two years DeFreitas's immunology lab had focused most of its brainpower on a virtually unfunded search for a retrovirus in CFS. He was puzzled by the immunologist's failure to secure grant support from the NIH, and he was concerned that the CDC had yet to confirm her finding. De-Freitas increasingly found herself without internal support.

In August, a Wistar accountant had told DeFreitas she would have to fire two people in her lab; she suggested their salaries be taken out of her own instead. More ominously, DeFreitas learned that Rovera had begun a private correspondence with Atlanta retrovirologists Tom Folks and Walid Heneine.

Centers for Disease Control, Atlanta, Georgia

In mid-September, Walter Gunn told his superiors, Larry Schonberger and Kenneth Herrmann, that he planned to retire the following June. According to Gunn, Schonberger in particular worried that if Gunn left, patient support organizations would suspect he had been fired, thus creating a public relations nightmare for the agency.

On September 24, Walter Gunn received a direct call from James Mason, the assistant secretary of the Department of Health and Human Services and the former CDC head, who was also a bishop in the Mormon church. He told Gunn he was concerned about a number of young Mormon missionary trainees enrolled in a Mormon training center in California: there had been an apparent outbreak of CFS among the missionaries affiliated with the center. After years of indifference to the disease, the nation's second-ranking health administrator posed a question: was CFS contagious?

"I told him ten to fifteen percent of our surveillance patients have someone in their household who also has the disease," Gunn said later. "I thought this [phone call] was meaningful. This problem was now touching the Health and Human Services' deputy secretary."

Gunn referred Mason to George Rutherford, the California state epidemiologist. Rutherford called Gunn two days later to report that most of the afflicted Mormon trainees had left the state for home, but he gave Gunn the name and phone number of the epidemiologist with jurisdiction over the county in California where the young missionaries had lived with their host families. Gunn passed the information on to Ali Kahn, the division's new Epidemic Intelligence Service officer, and suggested he follow up, but, according to Gunn, Schonberger seemed to want the investigation quashed. "They never investigated," Gunn said later. "It was killed."

State University of New York, Stony Brook

In September a study appeared in the *Journal of Clinical Psychiatry* indicating that CFS was significantly more debilitating than multiple sclerosis, lupus, or Lyme disease and that, although there appeared to be "a high coincidence of major depression in CFS," a "substantial portion" of sufferers lacked any identifiable psychiatric disorder.[1] The authors, a neurologist and two psychiatrists at New York State University, had reached their conclusions after a review of the large body of CFS medical literature of the last decade and after performing their own research.

Their report contradicted the position Stephen Straus had taken in the same publication three years earlier and cast doubt on his methods. Straus's 1988 study, the authors wrote, was "hampered by its reliance on the DIS"—the Diagnostic Interview Schedule, a psychiatric assessment of depression. They doubted the DIS was an "appropriate means of assessment" of CFS sufferers because the test "was not designed for medically ill patients. Hence, its use [in assessing CFS sufferers] must be interpreted with extreme caution." The New York researchers suggested as well that physical problems such as pain and cognitive deficits described by such patients could cause "confounding effects" on the DIS, again because the test was designed for people who were free of organic disease.

Centers for Disease Control, Atlanta, Georgia

On September 16, having received better probes and primers from the agency's core facility, Tom Folks and his lab associate Walid Heneine were ready once more to begin performing PCR on the Atlanta cases and healthy controls. A week later, however, Folks admitted to Gunn that he was not processing the blood in the fashion Elaine DeFreitas had requested because he had been turned down in his request for a DNA extractor and he didn't have time to extract the DNA by hand, a procedure that took approximately three hours per sample. In addition, he acknowledged that the retrovirology lab technicians were using the patient samples that had been treated with lysate and frozen.*

"It's Murphy's law of science," DeFreitas complained when she learned of the development. "There's never enough time to do it right, but there's always enough time to do it again and again and again."

Folks and Heneine were as frustrated as DeFreitas that week, their faces and voices conveying a harried weariness. Folks, in particular, was unable to disguise his resentment of the magnitude of his lab's investment in the project to replicate the Wistar finding, especially given its so-far-bleak results. Even so, unlike his more skeptical colleagues at the agency, Folks had never been heard to express conspicuous doubts that the disease in question was anything other than an organic, or medical, condition, and one that was affecting disturbingly large numbers of people. He was, in fact, impressed with the retroviral postulate and, like Wistar chief Hilary Koprowski, eager to explore the hypothesis that retroviruses caused any number of central nervous system and autoimmune diseases. "If anything, it was Koprowski who convinced me to pursue this," Folks said. "His theories are sound. It makes sense that these viruses hide out in the brain, that they come out periodically to cause disease."

Folks defended his snub of DeFreitas's multiple invitations to come to Philadelphia on the grounds that a scientist's published work should be reproducible from the literature without additional hands-on instruction in the scientist's laboratory. Now that she had sent a written protocol that was more detailed than her published techniques, Folks said he wanted to attempt to replicate the study based on the protocol and the paper exclusively, without going to Wistar.

---

* "No, there wasn't perfect compliance [with Elaine DeFreitas's techniques]," Folks admitted some years later. "We weren't going to do exactly as Elaine DeFreitas said simply because it was coming from Elaine DeFreitas. We did as much as we could that was within the limits of scientific logic."

He held out the possibility that he might yet travel to Philadelphia, however, if DeFreitas could demonstrate her ability to differentiate between the Atlanta cases and controls using her test. "Now that we have her sensitivity," Folks said, "we want to test the epi-aid [blood]. If we can distinguish between patients and controls based on our assay, then I think we've reproduced her work . . . and we'll stand by it. If we cannot and we send the samples up to her and *she* can pick them out, then *we're* wrong. And we'll go up there and learn how to do it, and come back here and test it again.

"We've spent hundreds of thousands of dollars—maybe half a million dollars—in attempting to reproduce her work," Folks said. "And this is the taxpayer now who is responding the DeFreitas publication. So that's why the responsibility really falls on Wistar to be sure they're right and to get that information out in public, because the taxpayer now is heavily invested."

Chicago Illinois

Chicago's McCormick Place convention center was the largest such enterprise in the nation, its 1.6 million square feet divided between two airplane hangar–sized halls straddling Lake Shore Drive, a ten-minute taxi ride from the Loop. During the first week of October more than 9,000 scientists swarmed into McCormick Place to listen to presentations by their colleagues on subjects as diverse as the effect of tetanus immunizations on patients suffering from AIDS and the usefulness of topical sunscreens in preventing cold sores, a study that happened to be written by, among others, the NIH's Stephen Straus. One hundred and sixteen reporters and approximately fifteen hundred pharmaceutical company representatives were monitoring the Thirty-first Annual Interscience Conference on Antimicrobial Agents and Chemotherapy. During their breaks, scientists roamed through the brightly lit exhibition court where salespeople from mega-firms like Searle, Pfizer Roerig, Lilly, Ortho-McNeil, Burroughs Wellcome, Bristol-Myers Squibb, and Hoechst stood in welcoming poses at booths. A steady line of scientists awaiting complimentary coffee snaked around Abbott Labs' towering copper espresso machine.

Less than three weeks earlier and months after the official deadline, HEM Pharmaceuticals president William Carter had asked the committee on presentations for an eleventh-hour consideration of his paper on Ampligen therapy in CFS. In an exception granted to only a dozen other late submissions among the 2,200 presentations already scheduled, the committee added the HEM study to the agenda.

On the eve of Carter's presentation, HEM investors, scientific consultants, potential backers, Maryann Charlap, and Carter himself sat down to a lavish dinner in a Chicago restaurant. Spirits were high. In less than three days the Food and Drug Administration would be forced to meet its thirty-day deadline to rule on the company's application for an expanded trial. In a matter of just three days, then, a governmental green light might breathe new life into a foundering company. Financial backers at the table knew little about the disease itself; in many cases, their appreciation for the phenomenon was limited to what they had read in the lay press. They knew only that a trial had been conducted with good results. To allay their curiosity, Carter had invited Dan Peterson and Paul Cheney to the dinner.

Carter asked the former Nevada partners to describe the epidemic disease in detail.

The doctors quickly realized that their audience was especially interested in hearing anecdotes about specific patients who had experienced dramatic improvement on Ampligen. Carter drew Dan Peterson out about Patient 00, Nancy Kaiser, who had been in a wheelchair for nearly a decade and who was barely able to write her own name prior to treatment with Ampligen. Now Kaiser was close to 50 IQ points smarter, and on her best days the former golf fanatic could play nine holes.

Carter, Cheney recalled later, "also asked us to comment about various issues around the disease: what do we think it is, how do we think it's transmitted, do we think it's new or old, what are holes in the brain—that kind of thing. There was a *lot* of commentary about the brain lesions."

The malady's possible retroviral etiology was another point of fascination for Carter's guests that evening. "Oh, yes, they were interested," Cheney commented. "They were *very* concerned. Their attitude was 'This is incredible!' The other major issue of the evening," Cheney continued, "was 'Be careful about exceeding the gag order.'"

Since September 3, when HEM submitted its application to the Food and Drug Administration for approval of expanded clinical trials, the company had been instructed by the FDA to confine all public commentary to the scientific data in the company's abstract. Carter warned Cheney and Peterson in particular, who he knew would be sought out by reporters, to avoid making claims that the drug was "safe and efficacious"—the sole standards by which the drug agency was required to rule on Ampligen—in ways that might be perceived as advertisement.

Privately Cheney had significant reservations about the drug and was increasingly uneasy in the face of HEM officials' excitement over the success of the trials. The Charlotte clinician believed there were important questions about the long-term use of the drug that had yet to be addressed. In low doses, Ampligen stimulated the immune system; in higher doses, it down-regulated an overactive immune system. What if, Cheney postulated, a patient was prescribed Ampligen at a high dose in order to down-regulate immune system activity, thus reducing toxic levels of cytokines such as interleukins, but was later taken off the drug. Would the patient's immune system be rendered inoperative?

"I really think this drug *could* make you worse," Cheney ruminated. "That doesn't mean the drug's not effective. And it doesn't mean that the drug's not good. It's just that there are some pitfalls in its use that we damn well better know about."

Cheney's theoretical musings seemed well founded, given the testimonials of patients who had been abruptly cut off from their Ampligen lifeline at the trial's end. More than a few sufferers reported that they felt worse in the weeks following the trial than they had felt at any time in their years of illness.

On the morning of October 1 several hundred scientists attended virology session number 46 in an auditorium on Lake Michigan's shore. William Carter, who would describe the Ampligen trial, was the morning session's final presenter. Eyeing the diminutive, frail-seeming Carter as he stepped to the lectern were Stephen Straus and Steven Jacobson, the government neuroimmunologist who had helped Straus test a handful of patient blood samples for HTLV1 and HTLV2 after the Wistar announcement a year before. Larry Corey, the herpes expert from the University of Washington who had published two studies promoting CFS as a psychiatric disorder, studied the wraithlike Carter as well. Carter commenced his rapid-fire reading of the HEM study results with a statement that likely did little to help him with this crowd: "The topic that we're going to discuss today," he began, "is built on the pioneering observations of Dr. Dan Peterson and Dr. Paul Cheney, who are in the audience today."

Carter had less than twelve minutes to present the voluminous findings. His delivery was brusque and matter-of-fact as he started by describing the demographics of the study subjects: their average age was "about forty," most of them had been sick for four to six years; nearly all were being cared for either by spouses or by professional custodial caregivers. Carter then described patients' physical condition upon entering the trial: "At baseline, the two groups [placebo and treatment] were severely debilitated," according to two standardized measurements of morbidity, the Activities Daily Living test and the Karnofsky Performance Status. Approximately eight to twelve weeks had passed before patients receiving Ampligen began to diverge from the placebo group in their Activities of Daily Living scores. By twelve to sixteen weeks, the Ampligen patients' Karnofsky scores also began to diverge to a statistically significant degree. Placebo patients demonstrated zero improvements. "There's less than one chance in a thousand that this would have occurred by chance alone," Carter said.

Even more significantly, perhaps, those patients who received the drug did not experience "physiologic deterioration," Carter said, adding, "which . . . was seen in the placebo group."*

Carter then said, "I should mention, by the way, that eight percent of the patients [four people] in the placebo group attempted suicide during the six-month observation interval, but there were no attempted suicides reported in the drug-treated arm."

Patients on the drug improved on tests of cognitive ability, Carter continued, but placebo patients demonstrated no statistically significant intellectual improvement.

Before the trials, Carter added, 85 percent of all the patients had elevated levels of human herpesvirus 6, as demonstrated by monoclonal antibody tests. Levels of the virus's activity are "known to be reduced" among Ampligen recipients, Carter said.

Carter concluded with the comment that, although the drug was "not without side effects . . . in no instances, to date, were any of these side effects sufficient to discontinue therapy in patients."

* The history of the placebo group during the six months of the trial was at least as revealing as that of the patients on Ampligen. Over six months, placebo recipients, as a group, experienced an *accelerated* rate of hospitalization, compared to a diminished rate in the drug-treated group. On treadmill tests, which every patient undertook at frequent intervals during the six months of the trial, placebo recipients deteriorated significantly in terms of their degree of oxygen consumption and endurance, whereas Ampligen patients improved significantly.

In the question session afterward, Straus, Jacobson, and Corey dominated the floor. Straus introduced himself to Carter with the collegiate "Straus, Bethesda." In an Edwardian show of civility, he commended Carter for "speeding these data to us." The comment generated a frisson of amusement in the audience, given its cynical subtext. "You showed a lot of data, Dr. Carter," Straus said, getting down to business. "There are several questions. One is that the rate of hospitalizations that you seem to see indicated in this study is surprisingly high for this population. I'm wondering what that's due to and how representative this population is for the kind of patients that many of us see with chronic fatigue. But in addition, you commented on side effects of the Ampligen treatment not sufficient to terminate therapy. But what about sufficient to unblind therapy?"

Straus's line of questioning indicated he was suspicious that patients' good responses had been generated by a placebo effect—that is, an awareness that they were getting the drug. His question ignored the fact that the HEM trial's scientists had focused not upon patients' own sense of well-being—as Straus did in his 1986 acyclovir trial—but upon objective laboratory data such as viral activity, cytokine levels, white blood cell ratios, oxygen uptake, and so on, to measure improvement. In addition, many patients who actually *were* receiving placebo got even sicker, suggesting that the normal placebo effect noted in most double-blind trials was almost entirely missing in this particular trial.*

Carter's unruffled elucidation of these issues silenced Straus for the time being. But his NIH colleague, Steven Jacobson, stood to pursue Straus's original question about the remarkable degree of debilitation exhibited by patients in the study before starting therapy. "I was really surprised by the low Karnofsky performance of these patients," Jacobson said. "I mean, it a little bit strains credulity . . . to have patients who were that sick and were able to comply and perform all the studies— just even coming back for follow-up, biweekly I.V. infusions on an outpatient basis—"

"Well, virtually all of these individuals have a custodial caregiver who brings them to the unit," Carter responded. "As Dr. Straus mentioned," he added, "we are not representing here that this is the typical CFS patient. This appears to be the far end of the spectrum of the disease."

Larry Corey stood to dispute Carter at some length about the study's finding that 85 percent of patients had elevated levels of human herpesvirus 6. Corey insisted that "at least in our hands, it's been very difficult to find active viral replication of HHV6."

"Our results agree with those of Anthony Komaroff and Dan Peterson that were published in the June 6 issue of *Lancet*," Carter told Corey. "And in fact we've looked at several hundred individuals, and it looks like the incidence of virus reactivation is not isolated to a specific geographic region of the country. It's in your part of the country, it's in the Southwest, the Northwest, et cetera."

Immediately after the presentation a conference press aide announced that, due to the status of the drug at the Food and Drug Administration, HEM would not be

---

* On the other hand, a few patients receiving the placebo reported improvement. In fact, remarkably, two placebo recipients joined the lawsuit against HEM, so certain were they that they had been receiving the drug.

holding a press conference, nor would Carter be answering questions from the press. Even so, Carter was surrounded by reporters within moments of stepping down from the lectern. The scientist remained mute as he advanced down the center aisle of the auditorium toward his waiting colleagues, a throng of bristling journalists at his elbows. Bill Jenks, HEM's Manhattan-based public relations officer, stepped into the crowd of correspondents from CBS, *Medical World News,* and other publications and struggled to explain why Carter would be unable to talk to them. Eventually the reporters dispersed.

David Strayer, HEM's principal scientific adviser who had been at Nancy Kaiser's side in Incline Village when she became the first CFS patient to receive Ampligen, had stood quietly at the back of the large room throughout Carter's talk. At its conclusion, he was approached by a clinician from southern Florida who reported that his practice was inundated with CFS sufferers and asked if some of his most severely stricken patients might be included in the next Ampligen trial. Strayer explained that the drug's future was in the hands of the FDA.

For the moment, Strayer added, Ampligen's potential as a CFS therapy occupied a high priority inside the Philadelphia company, but the FDA would determine whether the company would continue to afford the disease such high status. (HEM was also planning to continue testing Ampligen in AIDS, in hepatitis B, in renal and lung cancer, and in severe burn patients.) In addition, Strayer indicated, the fate of patients who had received the drug in the clinical trials and now were seeking continued infusions of the drug, whether by pressure from civil courts or from Congress, rested with the drug agency, not HEM. "We could not justify continuing everybody on the drug without some evidence that the drug was efficacious," Strayer said. "We're still waiting for guidance from the FDA on that."

The *Chicago Tribune* published the Associated Press's story about the drug trial under the benighted headline "Viral Drug Helps Fight Yuppie Flu."

Ron Winslow, writing in the *Wall Street Journal,* quoted an unnamed FDA source whose comments hinted at what the agency's action would be the following day. "It's too early to claim that Ampligen is a dramatic treatment for chronic fatigue syndrome," the agency spokesman said. "The product has significant side effects that would have to be considered against any claimed benefits." Winslow quoted Anthony Komaroff, too, who told the reporter, "This isn't a medicine that acts on the psyche. It acts on the body."

On the eve of the FDA's response to HEM, Paul Cheney and Dan Peterson, independent of one another, were gloomy about the drug's prospects. "There's not a chance the Food and Drug Administration is going to approve this drug," Peterson said over dinner the night of Carter's presentation. "How can they approve a drug for a disease the NIH says doesn't exist?"

Cheney predicted the agency would "probably delay approval pending toxicity issues, but it's just a way to delay. They don't have the guts to kill it, because the patients will kill them. But they don't have the guts to approve it, because Straus will kill them."

30

Creative Accounting

On October 4 the FDA, citing its concerns about "serious and potentially life-threatening reactions that were observed during the study," denied for the time being HEM's request for expanded Ampligen trials in CFS sufferers. The agency put the request on "clinical hold," awaiting HEM's response to criticisms and questions raised by David Kessler, the commissioner of food and drugs, in a private letter to attorney John Rapoza, HEM's vice president of regulatory affairs.

The "life-threatening reactions" cited by Kessler were "acute hepatic [liver] toxicity, severe abdominal pain, and irregular heartbeat." All three symptoms had occurred in one patient in Incline Village. Dan Peterson had insisted that she be taken out of the study. In the four-week period that the woman, Cynthia Modica-Gaines, was Ampligen-free, she suffered a severe relapse of CFS and pleaded to be allowed to continue the trial. Peterson returned her to the study, but at half dose. She suffered no further ill effects. A patient in Houston had passed a gallstone while on the drug. Neither reaction was as toxic as, say, the kidney failure suffered by some patients in Stephen Straus's acyclovir trial who had not received enough fluids.

In an FDA talk paper, offered as a reference source by agency public affairs people to reporters and the public, the agency also blamed the rejection on "numerous deficiencies in the application." "The data provided do not allow us to make an independent assessment of the results," Kessler wrote attorney Rapoza. "Please provide a complete listing of all outcome measures for each of the patients."

Perhaps the most damning point Kessler made in his letter had to do with adverse reactions to Ampligen, although Kessler's emphasis seemed to be less on the adverse reactions themselves than on HEM's failure to report them to the drug agency. If HEM had deliberately withheld such reports, the drug agency might well have construed the action as obstructive or as an attempt to mislead. HEM's spokespeople responded with the comment that fever, muscle pain, and flu-like symptoms were so much a part of the illness itself that it was difficult to differentiate between Ampligen-induced symptoms and CFS-induced symptoms. Undoubtedly the most striking aspect of Kessler's letter was its unintended highlighting of the government's misreading of the disease. FDA staff seemed to harbor only the vaguest notion of just how disabling the disease could be and of the degree of physical suffering it imposed. In the agency's talk paper on the subject, Kessler pointed out that CFS sufferers eager for government approval of Ampligen must understand that the "significant side effects associated with Ampligen" needed to be "weighed against any claimed benefit before the drug could be approved for widespread use." Kessler apparently did not know that CFS victims suffering from a globally disabling disease would hardly regard flu symptoms as "significant side effects" when weighed against the benefits of a drug that might restore their ability to function. In the world of CFS everything was relative; as Paul Cheney said, "What has to be weighed here is the toxicity of the drug versus the toxicity of the disease."

Patient activists, not surprisingly, were bitterly disappointed by Kessler's action and viewed it with extreme cynicism. "To approve Ampligen would be the single most powerful blow for the credibility of this disease," said Marc Iverson, the CFIDS Association's president. "This was not a decision based on science. It was politics." In a newsletter published later that fall, the CFIDS Association's executive director, Kimberly Kenney, wrote, "We suspect that this is a delay tactic employed by the FDA to prevent the approval of an antiviral drug by one government agency for an illness that another, namely the NIH, still considers to be simply depression by another name." She added that FDA approval would have been an "unnerving prospect for the thousands of government officials, clinicians, and medical school academics who stand by Stephen Straus's psychoneurotic theory." The patient association's mistrust went even further. Was the FDA's action, Kenney asked, a deliberate delaying tactic meant to give Straus and other government scientists time to "advance their science and offer public statements acknowledging that CFIDS is indeed an organic illness, allowing NIH and other institutions to save face?"

HEM's official posture was one of nonchalance. A company spokesman described the Kessler letter as "routine" and said HEM would be able to resolve the agency's concerns about side effects in a matter of weeks. Dan Peterson reported, however, that William Carter had called him soon after receiving Kessler's letter and that "he was very depressed. . . . There was significant congressional pressure, apparently, but the FDA snubbed Congress. They would rather have congressional anger than NIH anger."

Suspicion ran high that the long arm of Stephen Straus had been at work in the FDA's decision to halt further Ampligen trials. Although HEM's David Strayer said the drug agency had not revealed to HEM officials the identities of its scientific advisers on the study, both Cheney and Peterson were under the impression that Straus had been the FDA's primary adviser in its ruling. Certainly Straus had been present during HEM's meetings with federal health officials the year before.

In an ironic turn of events, HEM vice president and attorney John Rapoza used Kessler's letter about Ampligen's safety as ammunition against the Nevada patients who were suing the company for additional infusions of the drug. On November 20, Rapoza mailed portions of Kessler's letter to James Beasley, the Reno lawyer representing the Nevada patients, along with an affidavit.

For the moment only the six patients who still remained in Dan Peterson's original Nevada pilot study—Nancy Kaiser, Marylou Guiss, Andy Antonucci, Billee Reed, Gerald Crum, Joyce Reynolds, and Candace Gleed—were allowed to stay on the drug, as were the seventeen patients who had persuaded Reno judge Edward Reed to order HEM to give them Ampligen for at least one additional year. Half of the original fifteen pilot study patients—Nancy Taylor, Tom Miller, John Trussler, Amy Long, Ellen Mears, and Gloria Baker—had chosen to go off the drug by 1990. A few made that decision because they did not feel significantly better on Ampligen. For the rest, however, money was the issue. Most, having been disabled for some years, were living at subsistence level; the cost of paying for housing in Incline Village, while maintaining their homes out of state, simply was too great. Thus, after three years of clinical trials and several million dollars invested, only twenty-four CFS patients, out of a potential pool of hundreds of thousands or more, would be allowed access to the drug during that year.

Centers for Disease Control, Atlanta, Georgia

Tom Folks and Walid Heneine had tried for two months, without success, to recover the sensitivity they had achieved in mid-June. As a result, on October 10 a think tank–style group of molecular biologists within the Division of Viral and Rickettsial Diseases convened to examine the problem. Heneine walked his colleagues through the steps and missteps of his multiple attempts to reproduce De-Freitas's work. Ultimately the agency's microbiologists suggested to Folks that he stop testing the Atlanta epi-aid study specimens until he solved the sensitivity problem. The committee proposed to Heneine and Folks that they continue to experiment with the amplification conditions and "master mix cocktail"—the primers—until they could achieve "consistent sensitivity" equal to the Wistar test. The microbiologists, in addition, told Folks that, with respect to airflow, his retrovirus laboratory was set up poorly for PCR experiments. Because of the airflow problem, there existed a possibility of contamination of specimens and cell cultures by airborne pathogens.

"The epi-aid study is dead," Walter Gunn said on October 16. "Tom Folks hasn't been able to get sensitivity up again, so they've stopped."

Frustratingly, division chief Brian Mahy's gag order prohibited Gunn from describing to DeFreitas with any clarity the problems in Folks's lab, nor could he even hint at his own increasingly tenuous hold on his job, a situation that could be blamed, in part, on his advocacy on her behalf. He could do little more than entreat her to continue the collaboration.

But there were other pressures. As the specter of the agency's failure to confirm the Wistar data loomed larger, administrators in Gunn's division began to talk about publishing the results, either as a report in the *Morbidity and Mortality Weekly Review* or as a full-blown paper in a medical journal like the *Annals of Internal Medicine* or the *New England Journal of Medicine,* forums where the agency's conclusions could be read by an enormous body of clinicians likely to have CFS sufferers in their practices. Gunn knew such a paper would make a laughingstock of DeFreitas and her institution. More tragically, it would wreak additional suffering among patients by seeming to support Stephen Straus's theories. Gunn's passion on the subject ran so high that he warned Larry Schonberger that he would interfere with the publication of any reports or papers on the subject.

"I will *not* let a report be issued saying they've done the study and that they couldn't confirm Elaine's work," Gunn said. "It would not be fair. The only way I would let Schonberger do that is if he said, 'We tried, and we failed, but we did not follow DeFreitas's protocol.' But the *real* report, the one that should be issued, is: 'We've got a problem in our labs.' " Gunn had tried to impress upon Schonberger what he believed was the inadequacy of the agency's efforts to duplicate the Wistar study: "I told him the CDC has *never* done the work properly," Gunn recalled. "What really bothers me is that they've already frozen the stuff two or three times! Even if they do get the sensitivity back, the experiment probably won't work because they've frozen and thawed the DNA so many times!"

Gunn's confrontational stance was taking its toll. "The stress of this is just overwhelming," he confessed. After a conversation with Schonberger on the subject, Gunn measured his heart rate. It was 104; a normal resting heart rate is 60.

U.S. Congress, Washington, D.C.

By 1991, victims of a myriad of incurable, often devastating ailments had uncovered a stark truth about the nation's health agencies: political pressure was the water that drove the federal research wheel. Anyone who doubted that proposition needed only to look to history for confirmation. Twenty years earlier there had existed patient advocacy associations for sixteen diseases. In 1991, however, national patient organizations represented more than eighty diseases; a majority of these groups had fund-raising arms to support congressional lobbying efforts.

On October 16 several members of the CFIDS Action Campaign for the United States (CACTUS), a group that included patient support group leaders from Massachusetts, Washington, D.C., and California, gathered in the offices of the Sheridan Group on Capitol Hill for a lesson in congressional networking. Lobbyist Tom Sheridan, who had been hired by the CFIDS Association and CACTUS to represent chronic fatigue syndrome in Washington, and his associate Brent McCaleb spent a day teaching lobbying skills to the CACTUS members.

The federal response to AIDS, around which an unprecedented advocacy movement had mushroomed by the mid-1980s, was proof that lobbying worked. In 1990 more federal research dollars were being spent on AIDS than on any other disease except all cancers combined, even though AIDS failed to rank in even the top ten causes of death in the United States.*

The next morning, Paul Cheney joined the group, which then split into teams of two and fanned out into the marbled halls of the Senate and House office build-

---

* One investigative report that year by *Minneapolis Tribune* reporter Lou Kilzer laid bare the fundamentals of government spending on AIDS: "On a per-patient basis, no other major disease comes close. For each AIDS death reported in the United States in 1990, the government spent $53,745 in research and education. That's more than fifteen times the $3,241 spent per cancer death and about 58 times the $922 per death parceled out to researchers fighting heart disease."

ings. Sheridan's soldiers met with legislative staff members whose bosses sat on health appropriations subcommittees.

After 5:00 P.M., a small group that included Cheney, Sheridan, CACTUS president Joan Iten-Sutherland, and Oklahoman Ed Taylor made their way by cab to the White House to see Hanns Kutner, the domestic policy adviser on health and social issues to President Bush.

Afterward, Cheney recalled the interview in disheartened tones: "Kutner said he would orchestrate some kind of communication between the White House and the secretary of health's office, but that he did not want to dictate or redirect health policy, which is code for saying, 'We don't want to rock the boat unless we feel a political wind is blowing.' "

Although Cheney refrained from saying so, others in the room told Kutner categorically that Straus should be removed from the study of chronic fatigue syndrome at the NIH.

Kutner, in response, merely reiterated his view that the White House could not intervene. "I told them the entire policy posture between our office and the National Institutes of Health is hands-off," Kutner recalled later. "James Mason's office is much more in a position to consider this issue on its scientific merits than certainly our office is." Mason, the assistant secretary of health, had headed the CDC during the agency's Tahoe investigation.

Throughout the day, Tom Sheridan checked periodically on the fate of the Health and Human Services appropriations bill for fiscal year 1992, then in a House-Senate conference committee. As frequently happened, the House and Senate had passed different versions of the bill. The House had proposed its biggest sum yet—$2.8 million—for Centers for Disease Control research on CFS. The Senate, in contrast, proposed a federal investment of $2 million, a sum nearly identical to the previous year's appropriation.

According to Joan Sutherland, the steel-willed president of CACTUS, legislative aides in every office they visited that day promised their members support for the House's $800,000 increase in research funds. "By midafternoon," Sutherland said, "we learned that we had made the first cut. But the deliberations were continuing when we left Washington."

On October 29, Sutherland and the other CACTUS members were delighted when Tom Sheridan called their California headquarters with news that the full $2.8 million had survived the conference committee's budget trimming; the entire sum was going to the CDC.

Language in the 1992 appropriations bill from the House was specific about how the agency was to spend its nearly $3 million. The contested $800,000 was earmarked for expansion of the agency's surveillance to new cities. But the agency was also asked to include children in the surveillance, to "provide prompt team reaction to CFS outbreaks, . . . to conduct a national CFS prevalence survey to provide national prevalence estimates of CFS in the general population ages 12–65," and to implement Walter Gunn's proposal to measure the disease in health professions.

By early 1994, the CDC had undertaken two of Congress's requests: the four-city surveillance system was expanded to include teenagers; and that same year, the agency investigated two purported cluster outbreaks of CFS, one in twin office towers in Sacramento, California, where state employees had filed a petition about poor air quality, the other in two small towns in Huron County, Michigan. Neither investigation resulted in a conclusion that CFS clusters actually had occurred.* In 1995, after their four-county surveillance data was contradicted by the findings of several independent epidemiologists, agency staff brought the costly project to a quiet end.

HEM Pharmaceuticals, Philadelphia, Pennsylvania

In spite of the Food and Drug Administration's clinical hold on further trials of Ampligen, and despite the company's own grim financial outlook, HEM was striving to expand its investigation into Ampligen's usefulness in the treatment of chronic fatigue syndrome. On October 17 the company held a scientific advisory board meeting at its Philadelphia headquarters. Several CFS investigators, including Anthony Komaroff, Elaine DeFreitas, Paul Cheney, Dan Peterson, John Martin, C. V. Herst, and Nancy Klimas, were invited to participate.

DeFreitas described the meeting as "very upbeat." The Wistar scientist was dismayed by Martin, however. She complained that, once again, his proof for a novel recombinant virus seemed thin indeed. "I think he's on a self-destruct mission," she noted, "and I think he's going to take a lot of people down with him. . . . At first I thought he was just being coy because he had some commercial deal going, but he was asked dozens and dozens of questions by everyone in the room, as was I, and I don't remember [Martin offering] one straight answer."

William Carter questioned Martin at length, saying at one point that the FDA wanted to see "etiological studies," studies which demonstrated that Ampligen suppressed the pathogen causing the disease. "I don't think we're there yet," Carter eventually told Martin.

HEM's medical adviser David Strayer invited DeFreitas to collaborate with him on a study of one CFS sufferer—the twenty-one-year-old daughter of a mem-

---

* Agency staff compared the number of people with a "CFS-like illness" in the twin towers, where seventeen of a total of two thousand employees had been diagnosed with CFS by their doctors, with rates of CFS in a comparable office building in Sacramento. Although the agency determined that there were more people with a "CFS-like illness" in the twin towers than in the "control" building—twenty-one versus eleven—the agency reported that the difference was not "statistically significant." Therefore, by the agency's logic, no cluster had occurred. Kimberly Kenney, executive director of the CFIDS Association in Charlotte, was dissatisfied. The agency had "failed to include employees who had left their jobs due to illness," she complained. Indeed, in a report issued about the research ("Investigation of Chronic Fatigue among Employees in Two State Office Buildings, Sacramento, California, Summary of Survey Findings"), the agency stated that although "questionnaires were also provided to some former . . . employees, these questionnaires were not included in the data analysis."

In Michigan, the agency had mailed questionnaires to residents of four small towns, or three thousand households, in Huron County. A local doctor administering to residents of two towns had called the state's epidemiologists out of a concern that a CFS outbreak was occurring. "Basically, there was just as much fatiguing illness in the two towns we used as controls as there were in the two towns the [local] doctor was concerned about," noted the agency's John Stewart afterward. By mid-1995, the agency had yet to release any official report about the Michigan investigation.

ber of the Wistar board of directors. Irrespective of the turbulent events of the past several months, the young woman had been able to obtain Ampligen under the FDA's compassionate care clause and was slated to begin treatment with the drug in one week. Along with an eighty-four-year-old professor emeritus from the University of Pennsylvania who was also suffering from the disease, the young woman had the highest blood concentrations of retrovirus gene fragments that DeFreitas had yet seen. Strayer wanted DeFreitas to monitor viral levels in the woman while she was on the drug.*

Over the next several months, HEM's revised application to the FDA would be turned down and all remaining patients would be removed from the drug. By the end of 1993, no CFS sufferers in the United States, including Nancy Kaiser, the Albuquerque housewife who had been Patient 00, was receiving Ampligen. HEM, in addition, was a reported $33 million in the red and nearing dissolution. Stocks of Ampligen were virtually depleted.

Centers for Disease Control, Atlanta, Georgia

Congress had awarded the Centers for Disease Control $2.1 million for the fiscal year just ended for the purposes of investigating the prevalence and the cause of CFS. The agency had spent the money, but its accomplishments seemed thin indeed. For twelve months Abt Associates in Cambridge, Massachusetts, had kept the agency's four-city surveillance project afloat; through Gunn's efforts a new plan was in place to include teenagers in the next year's surveillance. Walid Heneine and others in Building 15 had struggled to reproduce the Wistar finding, without definitive results; Heneine had begged off traveling to Wistar to learn DeFreitas's techniques firsthand. Gunn's division had launched a case-control study, then aborted it when logistical problems arose, with the result that twenty-two specimens were partially analyzed then set aside. Agency scientists failed to produce any scientific findings about the disease in fiscal year 1991, nor did they publish any scientific papers on it. In violation of a congressional mandate, they failed to investigate any cluster outbreaks until 1994, although several were reported to the agency's epidemiologists, nor did administrators exhibit any inclination toward launching national surveillance, thus ignoring yet another congressional mandate. In short, seven years after the Tahoe outbreak, the number of people suffering from CFS in the United States continued to be a mystery, as was the disease's rate of spread and the mode or modes of transmission.

Financial records from that period suggest administrators were employing unorthodox accounting practices to justify depletion of the CFS fund:

- The Division of Viral and Rickettsial Diseases charged $162,954 in employees' salaries to the CFS project in 1991. Included in that sum was 80 percent of Gary Holmes's salary, or $26,788. Holmes was not employed

---

* In the first pilot study of Ampligen in AIDS, concentrations of HIV in the blood dropped in concert with the prolonged administration of Ampligen (William A. Carter et al., "Clinical, Immunological, and Virological Effects of Ampligen, a Mismatched Double Stranded RNA, in Patients with AIDS or AIDS-Related Complex," *Lancet* 1, no. 8545 [June 6, 1987]: 1286–92).

at the CDC in 1991, however; he worked his last day at the agency on December 7, 1990.

- The same division reported that seven employees had worked on the CFS project in 1991, committing anywhere from 10 percent to 90 percent of their time to the effort. On examination, however, several percentages appeared to have been exaggerated. For example, Susan Good was a "flu coordinator" whose task was to talk to people who called the agency about flu, and yet 20 percent of her salary, $7,780, was charged off to the CFS investigation. Leone Schmeltz, a former secretary to Walter Gunn, had refused to work on any agency effort related to CFS, according to Gunn, and had become a flu surveillance officer within Gunn's division that year; nevertheless, 20 percent of her salary, $5,028 was charged to the CFS investigation. Howard Gary was a statistician in the viral diseases division. "I don't think Gary did more than a few days' work on CFS in 1991—at *most*," Walter Gunn commented. Yet 10 percent of Gary's salary, or $4,929, was charged to the CFS project. Larry Schonberger's contribution, also measured at 20 percent, cost the project $17,158.
- Although agency director William Roper had reported to Congress that twelve full-time employees, or their equivalent, were working on the project that year, the division charged with the investigation claimed just 3.2 FTEs. That figure was achieved by adding together the percentage commitments of seven employees.

Other investigators at the agency were also dipping into the CFS money. Scientists in the enterovirus section may have made the most lavish use of the fund. British researchers, of course, had advanced enteroviruses as a possible cause of the disease. As a result, Gunn's case-control study included a proposal that all patient and control specimens be tested for enterovirus. As noted, however, because the case-control study was aborted early in 1991, just twenty-two specimens were collected and analyzed. Scientists in the enterovirus section could have analyzed, at most, twenty-two blood samples that year. Yet, incredibly, the enterovirus section charged the CFS fund a whopping $320,774.92 in 1991. Some, but not all, of the money was accounted for in agency documents.

- Four scientists in the enterovirus section, including the section chief Mark Pallansch, charged ten percent of their annual salaries, or $28,433, to the fund.
- The enterovirus section charged another $40,000 for supplies and equipment, and $5,000 for travel.

There remained $247,331 unaccounted for. A close reading of the enterovirus scientists' summary of their scientific objectives for the project suggests that the researchers were using CFS money to develop sophisticated new ways of detecting enterovirus in human specimens. This might have been a worthy goal, but it was hardly directly related to the CFS epidemic.

"One of their favorite ruses is that they're 'developing tests that they will use eventually in the case-control study,' " Walter Gunn explained. "Like Bill Reeves [chief of the Viral Exanthems and Herpesvirus Branch] will work on developing a test for HHV-six. He can charge that to chronic fatigue syndrome. Or 'building up their lab capability'—that's another favorite generic excuse, except that if you look for papers out of that particular lab that were published at that time, there are no papers."

Indeed, Philip Pellet, a microbiologist in William Reeves's Viral Exanthems and Herpesvirus Branch, was principal investigator for an ambitious plan to develop highly sensitive assays—specifically, polymerase chain reaction—for three human herpesviruses, the proposed budget for which was to be $215,000. The money would come from the CFS fund, of course. Pellet's rationale for the undertaking, according to official agency budget documents, was as follows: 'The herpesviruses, EBV, CMV [cytomegalovirus], and HHV6 have been suggested as possible etiologic agents for chronic fatigue syndrome. . . " Yet, in a series of interviews during the late 1980s, few at the agency were more passionate in their insistence than Pellet and his associate Jodi Black that HHV6 or any other herpesvirus were unlikely to cause CFS.

- Finally, by November of 1991, the agency had also charged the CFS fund $19,446 for employee travel costs, even though Gunn was the only employee who traveled with any frequency for the project, and he estimated his travel expenses as under $7,000.

In September of 1991 Larry Schonberger was quizzed about his division's activities in CFS. Having turned down several requests for a formal interview, Schonberger was encountered in the agency's cafeteria one afternoon as he sat down, a plate of steaming cod on the tray in front of him.

Asked why his agency had failed to investigate a cluster of CFS for six years, Schonberger replied simply, "This is not how I wanted to spend my lunch," and lapsed into silence.

He was asked a second time: by congressional mandate, the CDC had been told to investigate clusters—why hadn't that been done?

A long pause ensued, during which Schonberger grimaced and pushed his folded forearms out in a defensive posture, as if to deflect the inquiry. "May I ask what clusters you are talking about?" he said eventually. "Is there something I'm missing?"

According to agency documents and his own staff, he was told, medical professionals and citizens had been reporting clusters to the agency every year for several years.

"We—" he responded, but stopped. "Um . . ." he said after a while, then stopped. "If we could find a *true* cluster, we would jump on it and investigate it."

He was reminded that his division's surveillance system was identifying bona fide CFS patients in four cities. Why couldn't the same technology be applied to cluster outbreaks?

"What's a cluster to one person isn't a cluster to another," Schonberger responded after another lengthy pause. "Look," he continued, "it's no secret that we are having trouble with this one. We've let people up and down the line at the CDC and other agencies know. There's no simple answer to this problem."

Had Congress given the agency enough money to crack the problem?

For the first time, Schonberger responded unhesitatingly: "Don't ask me about money. I don't know anything about it."

Was that year's appropriation of $2.8 million going to CFS exclusively? he was asked.

Whatever the source of his emotion, it was powerful. As his face turned tomato-red, the artless Schonberger insisted, "I don't know anything about the money. Don't ask me about the money!"

U.S. House of Representatives, Washington, D.C.

On October 30 the chairman of the Human Resources and Intergovernmental Re-lations Subcommittee of the Committee on Government Operations, New York congressman Ted Weiss, sent Assistant Secretary of Health James Mason a letter informing Mason that the subcommittee was conducting a full review of "the fed-eral response to chronic fatigue immune dysfunction syndrome (CFIDS). This condition has been on the agenda of the Public Health Service for many years, in-cluding research into its epidemiology, etiology, pathogenesis, manifestations and treatment," Weiss wrote.

Weiss's subcommittee, unlike the House and Senate appropriations subcommit-tees, which had set the CFS funding levels, was a true oversight committee with a history of aggressive investigation into activities inside the federal health agen-cies.* Not surprisingly, many patient advocates who were familiar with the Weiss subcommittee muscle hoped the congressman might someday be persuaded to turn his penetrating gaze on the CFS epidemic and the Public Health Service's missed opportunities. Jane Perlmutter, a New York State patient support-group leader, was among many constituents who attempted to interest him or his staff in the epi-demic. Perlmutter's letters, according to Patricia Flemming, the congressman's as-sistant on the subcommittee, resulted in Weiss's October 30 letter to Mason.

"CFS was something that Ted had wanted to look into for a while," Flemming recalled later. She suggested that Stephen Straus, in particular, might come under the congressman's scrutiny. "We had some indication that the person in charge of research at the National Institute of Allergy and Infectious Diseases might have had some feeling that this was not an important disease—that it was psychogenic in nature."

Soon after Weiss's inquiry was mailed to Mason, however, Flemming and Weiss were overwhelmed with work relating to AIDS and were unable to turn their attention to CFS. Less than a year later, in September 1992, Ted Weiss died of a heart attack, and the matter of a full-scale congressional investigation into the activities of the federal health agencies in the realm of CFS receded into the gray zone of lost or forgotten issues on Capitol Hill.

---

* Under Weiss's chairmanship, the subcommittee had completed hundreds of investigations of Public Health Service activities and issued as many reports to document its investigations. The committee's best-known oversight projects included the Food and Drug Administration's program to monitor ani-mal residues in food; the slow pace of the development of drugs to treat AIDS; failures in the CDC's AIDS prevention program; scientific fraud among federal research grant recipients; the government's monitoring of breast implant data; dioxin in drinking water; and the resurgence of tuberculosis.

National Institute of Allergy and Infectious Diseases, Bethesda, Maryland

Stephen Straus's agency met its congressionally mandated September 30 deadline to award money to independent researchers. On November 12 NIAID announced in a press release that it had awarded grants to establish three "cooperative research centers" for the study of CFS. Two of the researchers were well-known investigators in the field: Anthony Komaroff and James Jones, both of whom had previously won grants to study the disease. A third, Benjamin Natelson, a neurologist and a professor of neuroscience at the New Jersey Medical School, was a newcomer to the CFS grant application process, but not to the disease. "I had never published on CFS," Natelson admitted later, "but I had a *ton* of preliminary data." Beginning in 1989 the doctor had decided to limit his practice to "[P]atients—people who fall between the cracks of establishment medicine. It's a very tiny practice," he added, "but it has been *filled* with CFS patients since then." In a conversation, it was easy to see why Natelson had impressed the NIH. "We are splitters rather than lumpers," he said of himself and his collaborators. "Stratify—that's our middle name." He viewed the disease not as a cohesive entity but rather as "subsets of illnesses, possibly including fibromyalgia, mitral valve prolapse syndrome (a heart disturbance that caused fatigue and palpitations), and CFS.*

Komaroff, Jones, Natelson, and their institutions would share $1.2 million. Each center would receive an average of $400,000 for the first year of what were to be four-year projects. After overhead and administration costs, those sums would be closer to $200,000.

One member of the independent panel selected by the government to review the grants hailed the agency's action as a breakthrough in the troubled CFS field. "Three out of five grants got funded. That's *amazing* in this day and age," the panel member said, pointing out that the NIH in recent years had been funding just 10 percent of all grant proposals submitted to them. "This is an incredibly high percentage for chronic fatigue syndrome grants. The NIH is making up for lost time."

At least one scientist who had come innocently to the CFS grant process that season was left resentful and puzzled, however. Michael Tarter, a biostatistics professor at the University of California at Berkeley, had spent two months writing a two-hundred-page proposal. Tarter, a twenty-five-year veteran of the Department of Biomedical and Environmental Health Sciences at Berkeley, envisioned developing baseline information about the disease, something that had never been undertaken in the field. He proposed setting up statistical models for evaluating both the clinical and epidemiological parameters of the disease. The scientist, who had received more than thirty NIH and Environmental Protection Agency grants dur-

---

* If success could be measured by the acquisition of federal dollars, Natelson went on to be quite successful in the CFS field. The data he produced turned out to be less than groundbreaking, however. In 1994 Natelson announced that his team had discovered that CFS patients experienced intellectual or cognitive abnormalities, and that, when compared to healthy people, CFS sufferers exhibited a reduced capacity for exercise, i.e., exercise made CFS patients tired.

ing his long career, was doing nearly identical research in the field of AIDS. Using the same tools, he had been able to demonstrate, for instance, that survival patterns for AIDS varied radically according to sex and race. If implemented, Tarter's plan likely would have advanced proof of the brain and immune system aberrations in the disease and would have revealed patterns of transmission and other critical epidemiological information. In addition, his methods would have established computerized standards for assessing these patterns in different populations.

The government's panel attacked every aspect of the proposal, however.

"The whole experience was amazing, to tell you the truth," Tarter said several months later. "I don't think the people in Washington dealt with us fairly." His score was the worst he had ever received on a federal grant application. "Biostaticians supposedly occupy the most objective of all scientific niches, and if any disease ever needed the objective parameters that biostatistics could provide, it's this disease," he continued. "I'm absolutely sure there is a great deal of politics in this disease. And I wouldn't be surprised if politics had entered into the killing of our grant."

Tarter's suspicions seemed credible, considering the identity of his primary clinical collaborator: Dan Peterson of Incline Village, Nevada. Berkeley neuropsychologist Sheila Bastien, who had revealed the disease to be a bona fide brain syndrome in 1986 and who by 1991 had evaluated more than three thousand patients, was also named on the proposal.

Tarter clearly believed his recent endeavor had been a profound waste of time and one he had no intention of repeating: "I think this was a fiasco. It would take a *lot* of inducement to get me or anyone else I know at Berkeley to apply for a CFS grant in the future."

Centers for Disease Control, Atlanta, Georgia

Gunn would later describe himself as "totally frustrated" by the pace of research in the retrovirology lab. Tom Folks's work had been stalled since midsummer by his inability to regain a sensitivity equal to Elaine DeFreitas's. Unknown to Gunn, however, Folks was facing bigger problems in his laboratory. Over a cocktail at a party one Saturday evening in mid-November, Folks had told Larry Schonberger about the most remarkable development in the retrovirology lab since the effort to duplicate DeFreitas's work began: contamination appeared to be occurring among the CFS specimens and controls. The first incident had occurred early in September. One of the Atlanta CFS co-cultures—a culture in which an uninfected human blood line had been laced with white blood cells from a CFS sufferer—looked "strange." Folks had the co-culture sent to the agency's electron microscopy center for analysis. To his amazement, the electron microscope results indicated that the culture was infected with an HTLV-like retrovirus. The virus was budding from cells in the co-culture. The lab chief immediately sent the control sample to the agency's electron microscopist for an analysis; the control sample turned out to be infected with the mystery virus as well. Folks began sending more and more of the CFS cultures and their controls for electron microscopy analysis, with similar results each time.

Folks had already been warned by other agency microbiologists after their study of the retrovirology lab's airflow system that contamination was a danger. Nevertheless, the question remained: where had the virus come from? There were two obvious possibilities: the mystery virus had been in CFS tissue samples from which Folks had created the co-cultures, and a lab tech had accidentally contaminated the control cultures with material from the infected ones by forgetting to change pipettes; or the cell line Folks had used to create his cultures was itself contaminated.

To make co-cultures, Folks used a human cell line, patented at the NIH, called A3.01. While on staff at the National Institute of Allergy and Infectious Diseases, Folks had worked with the cell line, which was known to be highly receptive to retroviruses. Folks, in fact, had discovered its utility in HIV research and had created additional cell lines from it as well. Now he began to wonder if A3.01 itself had been contaminated in Bethesda before it was shipped to him. He asked Cynthia Goldsmith, an electron microscopy expert at the agency, to test the main A3.01 cell line to see if it, too, was contaminated.

Meanwhile, Folks began to wonder if the so-far unidentified retrovirus had come from the spinal fluid of a CFS patient who had participated in the Ampligen trial in Charlotte. Because of the severity of her illness, Paul Cheney had suggested to the patient's neurologist that he send a sample of her spinal fluid to Folks. Folks had kept the culture made from this spinal fluid in Black Diamonds, the same lab where the Atlanta epi-aid cultures were kept.

"We were worried that maybe we had infected the other cultures from this woman's spinal fluid," Folks recalled later.

Indeed, electron microscopy revealed that the cell culture from the Ampligen trial patient was infected. But the control sample for this culture turned out to be positive, as well. The mystery deepened when Folks and his staff checked the control cell line, A3.01, in a second lab. They learned that the A3.01 line was contaminated with the same pathogen that was flourishing in Black Diamonds.

Folks felt both excitement and dread. Perhaps the severely ill woman's spinal fluid held the key to the disease; perhaps it harbored the retrovirus Elaine DeFreitas was suggesting lay at the heart of the disease. But if that was true, then it was a highly infectious agent, possibly able to travel through the air, or aerosolize, from lab to lab. And if the virus could aerosolize, the only defense against it was a rubber suit.

On November 20, Gunn submitted another version of the case-control study protocol to the CFS steering committee. It was his eighth such proposal since May. The committee decided to put off its decision until after the New Year. Six years had passed since the submission of the original proposal, and the agency had yet to conduct a case-control study of CFS.

HEM Pharmaceuticals, Philadelphia, Pennsylvania

During the first week in December the Food and Drug Administration turned down HEM Pharmaceuticals' second, revised application for permission to begin expanded clinical trials of Ampligen in CFS. With the chances of approval for additional clinical trials seeming virtually dead in the United States, HEM officials began to discuss approaching the Canadian government about an expanded clinical trial in that country.

Centers for Disease Control, Atlanta, Georgia

On December 2, electron microscopist Cynthia Goldsmith left a note on Walter Gunn's desk: "Just wanted to let you know that I looked at a sample of A3.01 that [a lab tech] was working with out in the main lab, and it does have the same virus."

Goldsmith's note confirmed Folks and Gunn's worst fears. None of the CFS specimens had been prepared or analyzed in the main lab; Folks's lab techs handled CFS samples in Black Diamonds, a much smaller laboratory. Seemingly, it would have been physically impossible for the cell line in the main lab to have been contaminated by any CFS specimens. Two interesting possibilities remained, however: either the main cell line had arrived at the agency from the NIH in a contaminated state, or the lab tech who worked with the CFS specimens in Black Diamonds had carried the virus into the main lab on her clothing or—worst-case scenario—on her breath, which would mean that she herself had become infected and that the bug was transmitted by inhaling airborne particles of virus.

Folks assured Gunn he was working to establish whether the cell line had been contaminated at the NIH or in his own labs. Remarkably, Folks added, the mysterious virus had contaminated experiments all over his laboratory.

In a matter of days Folks established that the A3.01 line at the NIH was free of contamination, which meant that somehow the cell line had become contaminated in the Atlanta retrovirology labs.

Gunn was increasingly suspicious that the new virus was the same bug Elaine DeFreitas and John Martin had been investigating.

"The most likely source of the contamination is the CFS patients," Gunn said. He raised the possibility that one of the Building 15 lab technicians had been exposed to the disease outside the agency and was carrying the virus. "Right now," he said, "no one knows *what's* going on, except that we have contamination in the epi-aid specimens."

By December 9, Walid Heneine and Tom Folks at last had been able to recover the sensitivity required to find the virus in amounts of no more than one viral copy per cell. Nevertheless, Gunn doubted the agency's ability to succeed with the Wistar project using the epi-aid specimens gathered in August. "By now," he said, "the samples have been frozen and thawed a number of times. And they may be contaminated." Folks, in contrast, believed it would be possible to perform the test. Gunn encouraged him with a collegiate "Go for it!" After running ten to fifteen samples, some of which were from healthy controls, some of which were from cases, however, it became apparent that something was wrong. A disproportionate number of samples were positive. "It looks like we've gained sensitivity but lost specificity," Walter Gunn observed.

Although he had originally told his associates he would retire in June, Gunn more recently had decided to leave before the New Year. In his final two weeks at the agency, he turned his attention to calling the twenty-four local CFS sufferers who had been enrolled in the epi-aid study five months before. He asked them to come into the agency one more time to provide blood specimens. Gunn planned to send Elaine DeFreitas fresh whole blood from these patients, and he wanted to be certain the blood had never been frozen. (If Elaine DeFreitas could tell the difference between patients and healthy controls among the Atlanta patients, it wouldn't matter whether Tom Folks's staff ever achieved parity with DeFreitas, Gunn reasoned.) Above all, Gunn wanted to be certain the blood was free of contamination. Each patient blood sample was collected in the afternoon; the following morning, a control specimen was taken from a healthy agency employee; the samples were sent together the same day to Philadelphia.

Before sending the blood to Wistar, Gunn divided the samples in half, saving half for the agency. Walid Heneine said he wanted to test the new blood with his newly sensitized test. Now, however, when he ran the assay on ten specimens, all ten were negative. Perhaps he had dialed up the sensitivity of the PCR to such a degree that he had now lost specificity entirely.

According to Walter Gunn, Larry Schonberger struggled to persuade Tom Folks to publish Heneine's latest results in the *Morbidity and Mortality Weekly Report*. Gunn stepped into the fray. "I told Tom Folks and Walid and Larry that if they did that, I would go public with the fact that there had been serious contamination, that serum was frozen and thawed several times, that Elaine DeFreitas's protocol was not followed, that the data were flawed, and that I could prove it."

With Gunn's declaration, the move toward publishing Heneine's results in the agency's weekly bulletin of infectious disease trends lost momentum.

Paradoxically, Gunn privately expressed optimism about the agency's future in the search for the agent. If Tom Folks and his associates had actually discovered a new human retrovirus in their lab, they would be able to create cell cultures stocked with growing virus. Soon, Gunn imagined, they would develop probes and primers for it, with which they would be able to test CFS blood. "At a minimum," he said, "there's a new retrovirus. Maybe it's not related to CFS. But I said to Folks, 'What patients' serum have you had up here that have immunological and neurological problems?' "

There was only one answer: it was Gunn's CFS serum.

Wistar Institute, Philadelphia, Pennsylvania

In mid-December, DeFreitas was thrust back into her painful struggle with the retrovirologists at the CDC. Early that month Walter Gunn had called to ask if she would run her retrovirus assay on the agency's twenty-four Atlanta cases and approximately twice as many controls. If DeFreitas could prove to the agency that she could differentiate between the controls and the cases, Gunn reasoned, her case would be made, irrespective of the agency retrovirologists' failure to replicate her original study. DeFreitas agreed to the test but balked when Gunn called her back to tell her that the agency staff had neglected to extract the DNA from the samples they were planning to send her. "We're right back in the same vicious circle," DeFreitas said. "I told them it would take too long for me to extract the DNA. *They* should extract it. We don't have the money," she said.

Like other scientists at Wistar, DeFreitas had been put on notice by Giovanni Rovera, the Wistar's new director: every Wistar lab had to be self-sufficient by 1992. "He's telling me I have to balance my budget by January or fire half my staff," DeFreitas said at the time. "Wistar, in the last year, has absorbed about $100,000 for the CFIDS project. The leukemia project is the only federal money I have. I would be out on the streets selling pencils if I didn't have that." DeFreitas had no idea where she would find the money or the manpower to pursue the investigation Gunn was proposing to her now. More painfully, it was work she had done long ago and was trying desperately to move beyond.

Centers for Disease Control, Atlanta, Georgia

On December 28 Walter Gunn resigned from the federal agency that had been his home for fourteen years. In a lengthy letter to Elaine DeFreitas some months later in which he freely recounted the tumultuous history of the agency's effort to replicate her work, Gunn wrote that he left the agency because he was "convinced that a fair replication of your study was not possible at CDC" and that he wished to pursue the matter of retroviral infection in the disease as an independent investigator. But on closer examination, Gunn's reasons for leaving cut deeper than his colleagues' ambivalently executed retroviral research. They reached back to Gunn's earliest suspicions that money appropriated for CFS research was being used to stock laboratories with extra supplies and equipment and to enrich pet research projects wholly unrelated to the epidemic disease. (As it was, division head Brian Mahy's use of money earmarked for CFS research had been so questionable that Gunn believed the British-born scientist was destined someday to face a congressional inquiry on the matter. "I'll be seeing Brian Mahy across the table in Washington," Gunn said darkly soon after his departure.) His reasons for leaving the CDC encompassed, too, the cavalier responses of his superiors when he voiced his suspicions, and the constraints they placed on him in an effort to punish and silence him. At bottom, it was Gunn's challenge of his superiors' peculiar accounting habits that forced his hand. If he attempted to stay at the CDC until June, Gunn feared, he would be fired.

"I was on a real collision course. I could see where things were going," he said privately upon resigning. "I don't want to undercut the CDC's ability to go forward with this, nor do I want to hurt the CDC as an institution. This is an aberration. Otherwise, it's a great institution. I'm not even sure if what they did is illegal. I just didn't like it, and I put my career on the line."

The public posture Gunn struck bore little resemblance to the truth; as far as patient organizations were aware, Gunn was pleased with the agency's progress in the disease and had opted for early retirement, thus clearing the way for a wide variety of experts with backgrounds more steeped in medicine than his to assume responsibility for the investigation. It was a posture Gunn adopted under duress; he needed his pension. The agency, for its part, worked overtime to exert spin control over news of the sudden departure of its principal CFS investigator.

One week before leaving, Gunn arranged a conference call between the agency and the Charlotte-based CFIDS Association's president and executive director, Marc Iverson and Kim Kenney, to alert the patient organization to his departure. "I told Mahy it was an important call," he explained. "I said it was critical that [the CDC] have a good relationship with Marc Iverson's organization and with the others." With his superiors breathing over his shoulder, Gunn read from a prepared script that had been carefully worked over by Mahy. In it, Gunn said he was leaving because the project required "the leadership of an experienced medical epidemiologist, assisted by a highly trained staff of immunologists, virologists, infectious disease specialists, and epidemiologists. I am a psychologist with cross-training in epidemiology, and I have taken this project as far as I can with the training I have had. It is time that I step down to make room for someone with training more appropriate to the task. . . . CDC is currently searching for a new principal investigator with medical training to take over my duties in relation to CFS research."

Larry Schonberger had balked when Gunn proposed to say in his script that the agency's surveillance study had generated evidence that CFS was an organic, or medical, disease and not a psychiatric condition. "Larry said, 'You can't say that!' " Gunn recalled later. Gunn ignored his soon-to-be former boss and kept the sentence in his script.

Gunn's reading of a prepared statement was a stilted performance that by its very nature undermined its intent: to convey the agency's goodwill toward patient advocates and its commitment to unraveling the disease.

CFIDS Association president Marc Iverson was unimpressed. "Something else came through loud and clear between the lines," he said afterward. "We asked if they were going to put news of Gunn's resignation out in a press release. They were stunned. Then Dr. Reeves said, 'The CDC should be the focus—*not* the individual.' I then paid tribute to how much Gunn had done to help this disease. Their response was 'This is not about an individual. It's a team effort. The *CDC* is committed to investigating this disease.' "

Gunn had taken his colleagues on their word when they assured him they would find a full-time replacement for him. He had recommended that they recruit a CFS expert from the outside, "a Komaroff or a Nelson Gantz to come in for two years and take over." (Gantz was an infectious disease specialist at the University of Massachusetts with clinical experience and a stated research interest in the disease.) Privately, he commented, "This project has such a bad reputation at CDC, with all these people laughing at it for so long, that it's possible that nobody with good skills will want to jeopardize their career at the agency by taking it on. I also think someone from the outside would be able to push harder. Gary Holmes, as an EIS officer, was here at their pleasure. They could sign a paper, and he's gone! Someone who is here for a two-year stint from the outside, they're not going to mess around with, because he would be able to report that to people outside the agency." But even the recruitment of an outside scientist would be little more than cosmetic if a major restructuring of responsibilities failed to occur within the agency, according to Gunn. Years of hilarity, ridicule, and corrupted science had contaminated virtually everyone who had been involved in the discovery process: "The only way the CFS investigation will be run well at CDC is when it's out of the purview of the Division of Viral Diseases, and even out from under the Center for Infectious Diseases. This disease needs its own program at the agency, just like AIDS."

Gunn's departure was a calamity for CFS victims, his resignation testament to the agency's continued negligence in the realm of the disease, as well as Congress's failure to regulate the agency. When Gunn left, agency officials announced that William Reeves, the Viral Exanthems and Herpesvirus Branch chief, would be assuming the post of principal investigator on the project on an interim basis. In fact, agency staff never searched for a new principal investigator; when Reeves absorbed Gunn's title into his own, the agency in effect eliminated the position of CFS principal investigator, although Reeves continued to carry the title well into 1995. Significantly, Reeves had been, Gunn said, one of his "greatest antagonists" on the CFS steering committee.

1992
THE
DISAPPEARED

The physician needs a clear head and a kind heart; his work is arduous and complex, requiring the exercise of the very highest faculties of the mind, while constantly appealing to the emotions and finer feelings.

—Sir William Osler, *Counsels and Ideals*

31

Subculture of Invalidism

Harvard Medical School, Boston, Massachusetts

Seven and a half years had passed since a wealthy Houstonite summering in Incline Village, Nevada, brought her complaint of paralyzing weakness to a young internist named Dan Peterson. The doctor's children, toddlers when the epidemic in northern Nevada began, were nearly through grade school. Paul Cheney's children, grade-schoolers at the start of the outbreak, were now in college. None of the children could remember a time when chronic fatigue syndrome had been anything but a nearly palpable presence in their households and the dominating passion of their fathers' lives. In spite of the tumultuous publicity the Nevada outbreak had garnered in the middle 1980s, its three hundred victims were, by 1992, seemingly invisible, their experience banished into forgotten history. The import of the Tahoe epidemic itself had slipped into the haze as well; Gary Holmes and Jon Kaplan's cursory investigation had submerged the outbreak's urgent lessons in a miasma of doubt and confusion.

A handful of investigators had been unable to forget the events of 1984 and 1985 in the mountain resort town, however. On January 15 their version of events, the scrupulously examined Tahoe manuscript, was published at last in the *Annals of Internal Medicine*.[1] The paper was the most exhaustive and medically sophisticated study of the disease ever undertaken. Two hundred fifty-nine patients who had sought care in the Alder Street clinic for long-term, disabling illness were studied using techniques ranging from magnetic resonance imaging of the brain to polymerase chain reaction tests for human herpesvirus 6 DNA. The paper's value was more closely tied to its conclusion than to its scope, however. The authors characterized the disease as a "chronic, immunologically mediated inflammatory process of the central nervous system." Thus, eight years after the first known case in Incline Village, the truth about the disease was laid bare for the scientific community: chronic fatigue syndrome was a disease of the brain.

The seventeen names at the top of the paper were a compendium of the scientific history of the Tahoe epidemic. They included controversial figures such as the NIH's Robert Gallo and Gallo's associate Zaki Salahuddin, in whose laboratory blood samples from Tahoe were tested for human herpesvirus 6. CDC retrovirology chief Tom Folks, who, while at the National Institute of Allergy and

Infectious Diseases in 1986, had tested—with negative results—fourteen Tahoe samples for reverse transcriptase, an enzyme associated with retroviral activity in cells, was named too. University of Nevada microbiologist Berch Henry, who directed the PCR experiments on more than one hundred blood samples, was named, as was Reno neuroradiologist Royce Biddle, who had read hundreds of magnetic resonance imaging brain scans of CFS sufferers from northern Nevada. Biddle's Harvard counterpart, radiologist Ferenc Jolesz, was another author. Susan Wormsley, the flow cytometrist who in 1986 had provided an electron micrograph of an unidentified virus budding from the B-cells of Pam Butters, a diagnostic laboratory supervisor in Incline Village, was listed as well.

Anthony Komaroff's name appeared last, as was standard in the case of senior researchers who functioned as the facilitators and coordinators of research. To the surprise of many, however, Komaroff positioned his former research fellow Dedra Buchwald as first author, the place of honor in scientific articles, usually reserved for the scientist who contributed the most. Paul Cheney's name came next; Dan Peterson's was third. For Cheney, who had been the innovator behind most of the scientific avenues explored by the Tahoe collaborators, from brain imaging to the search for a retrovirus, Buchwald's ascension to first author aroused a bitterness he struggled to control in conversation. "I have a letter from Komaroff that states I will be the first author on the Tahoe study," the doctor said. Indeed, in 1991, Komaroff had sent a letter to all of the authors notifying them of Cheney's top position on the paper. There had been no quibbling: Cheney's driving curiosity, intellectual creativity, and scientific contributions were known to all involved. Buchwald's contributions had included extracting medical charts over a period of four days in 1986 in the Peterson-Cheney Alder Street clinic during her Harvard fellowship. She had, in addition, located a group of healthy control subjects willing to undergo brain scans, an achievement that had advanced the paper's fortunes considerably. Nevertheless, her role in the discovery process at Tahoe hardly approached that of either Cheney or his partner, Dan Peterson.*

For Anthony Komaroff, the manuscript's publication was a personal triumph. Although he had performed none of the bench work, his commitment to orchestrating the research and pushing the study along its tortuous course toward publication had been nearly obsessive. Without his devotion to the project, the reality of the Tahoe epidemic likely would have remained buried forever. His Nevada collaborators on occasion had criticized Komaroff as an opportunist who merely coordinated research without actually performing any himself, but there was something to be said for his particular administrative faculty: Komaroff and no one else, after all, had piloted the complicated project to fruition. "Given the biopolitical nightmare that paper had to go through," Paul Cheney noted soon af-

---

* When he was asked why he had elevated Buchwald to first place, Komaroff confirmed that he had indeed named Cheney first on the first two versions of the manuscript. However, the first such version was rejected by the *New England Journal,* the second by *Lancet.* By the time the manuscript was accepted by the *Annals* in 1991, Komaroff said, "the manuscript had been entirely rewritten, and many new substudies conducted and analyzed. . . . Paul Cheney was not involved in any of this." Nevertheless, Komaroff agreed, along with Buchwald and Cheney, to name *both* doctors as first authors, as in "Dedra Buchwald and Paul Cheney"—a departure from convention which the *Annals* editors categorically ignored.

ter the paper's publication, "it wouldn't have happened without Komaroff. In the end, the paper needed a politician as well as a scientist." The passion with which the Harvard doctor pursued publication of the paper was proportional to the degree to which the disease jeopardized his academic career; it was vital for Komaroff to prove to his peers in medicine that the malady to which he had devoted so much of his time and skill was real. Dan Peterson, who had watched from his rural retreat in Nevada as Komaroff struggled for years in Boston to bring the Tahoe research into the mainstream, commented, "He's tried—I think he's tried harder than you would ever know—because it's his reputation on the line."

Komaroff had submitted the original manuscript to the *New England Journal of Medicine* in 1988. The journal's reviewers rejected it, complaining that Cheney and Peterson had failed to collect laboratory and clinical data in a systematic fashion. Komaroff had argued that to expect clinicians in the midst of an outbreak of a severe and mysterious disease to engage in a scientifically pure system of data collection was asking the impossible. The journal's reviewers had complained, too, about the absence of healthy controls with whom to compare the magnetic resonance imaging brain scans of epidemic patients. Radiology experts at Harvard had assured Komaroff and his collaborators that the brain lesions in the patient group were abnormal, but the journal's reviewers had insisted upon controls nonetheless. It had taken Komaroff two years to find a suitable group of healthy controls willing to undergo the protracted and claustrophobic procedure. In the meantime, the *Lancet,* too, declined to publish the paper pending healthy MRI controls. After a two-year hiatus, Komaroff had submitted the paper to the *New England Journal* once more. Komaroff found the editor's criticisms that time wholly insupportable, and he withdrew the manuscript. Next he sent it to the *Annals,* whose editors turned the manuscript over to four independent reviewers. In the following eighteen months, the study underwent two separate, grueling revisions; each revision was twice sent to two reviewers.

"Let me put it this way," Komaroff said on the subject of his second and final revision. "My response to the criticisms of the article were much longer than the article itself. It took me a *month* to write that letter. But, although I cursed it at the time, I was delighted in the end. The review made the article much stronger." In the course of responding to critics, he had been able to "greatly expand the discussion of the CFS field" in an unusually long discussion section that accompanied the study in the *Annals.* "I was able to refer to all of the work in the field, and I took the liberty to cover the work of a *lot* of people, including Nancy Klimas, Jay Levy, and others. Now, there has *never* been a discussion of this field in a major journal. It's part of a big fabric," Komaroff continued. "I wanted to open that fabric to the world, and the *Annals* editors let me do it! I expected them to call back and say, 'We simply don't have room,' but that phone call never came."

As generous as the journal's editors had been, they exhibited extreme caution in the matter of the article's title, in which the disease was called a chronic illness characterized by fatigue, neurologic and immunologic disorders, and active human herpesvirus type 6 infection" rather than "chronic fatigue syndrome," the malady's government-sanctioned name. By doing so they avoided any suggestion that brain lesions, immunologic abnormalities, and reactivation of normally latent herpesviruses were unique to most cases. By implying the syndrome at issue was an obscure phenomenon seen exclusively in northern Nevada, the editors undermined the paper's achievement, which was to synthesize an extraordinary wealth of new information about a pandemic disease.

Science writers were not confused by the journal's hairsplitting; they recognized the paper for what it was: a research article on chronic fatigue syndrome. Reporting on the study in the *Boston Globe,* journalist Richard Knox began: "The largest in-depth study of people with chronic fatigue syndrome has established that the great majority have brain damage and evidence of active infection by a common virus. The long-awaited report strongly supports the view of some doctors and thousands of patients that the disorder often has physical causes. . . . Reflecting the medical establishment's skepticism toward the syndrome, the study was rejected by medical journals until enough data accumulated to show undeniable evidence of viral, immune system and brain effects."

New York Times medical reporter Lawrence Altman wrote two stories on the study in as many days, both of them referring to the disease under study as "chronic fatigue syndrome." He led his first report, "The largest study yet of chronic fatigue syndrome has found evidence of inflammation in the brains of patients, the first documentation of a neurological abnormality connected with the mysterious ailment."

Ron Winslow's story in the *Wall Street Journal* was headlined "Chronic Fatigue Study Points to Herpes Virus," a reference to the high proportion of patients—70 percent—who exhibited evidence of active replication of the normally latent human herpesvirus 6. The *Annals* paper, Winslow wrote, "adds to mounting evidence that an immune system dysfunction underlies the condition."

Nevertheless, despite its documentation of an extraordinary peril, the study failed to attract anywhere near the notice won by the Kaplan and Holmes 1987 study of the same population. It is possible that the size and complexity of the Tahoe manuscript precluded snap judgments and in effect camouflaged its importance.

Komaroff had enrolled in the study approximately 85 percent of the people who were diagnosed with the disease by Paul Cheney or Dan Peterson from 1984 through 1987. Most of them lived in the rustic communities along the California-Nevada state line near Lake Tahoe; seventy-six were residents of large urban centers, frequently Los Angeles or San Francisco, who had sought help from Peterson and Cheney during the same years. The study subjects' mean age was 38.8 years, almost 70 percent were women, and 40 percent were college graduates. Choosing his words carefully, Komaroff noted that, although the "non-Tahoe group" of patients could hardly be said to represent an epidemic, the Tahoe group might well have represented an epidemic because "most of these patients became ill within a two-year period and many had close contacts who became ill." The disease appeared to be contagious, he continued: "Enough cases occurred among family members, co-workers, and other close contacts to suggest the possibility of an infectious agent transmissible by casual contact." Specifically, Komaroff revealed that "several groups of patients who had frequent close contact became ill within several months of each other: ten of thirty-one teachers at one local high school [at least one student from the same school was similarly affected, but this student chose not to participate in the study]; five of twenty-eight teachers at another local high school; three students and one teacher at a third high school; and eleven employees at a casino. The spouses or sexual contacts of six patients were similarly affected, and there were eight instances in which at least one parent and one child both had the illness."

NIH theorists who had worked to promote the notion that the epidemic disease in Tahoe in the middle 1980s was distinct from the disease affecting other people around the nation sporadically could find little justification for their hypothesis in this study. "Clinical and laboratory findings in the 'clustered' patients did not differ from those of the larger patient group," Komaroff wrote. "Patients in the non-Tahoe group were more frequently shut-in and had a slightly higher frequency of headaches, adenopathy, arthralgias, paresthesias, and rashes, but generally the two groups were similar. In most patients, the chronic debilitating illness was of sudden onset, beginning with a 'flu-like' syndrome; 29 percent of the patients were regularly bedridden or shut-in. The symptoms were chronic and experienced on a nearly daily basis in the months and years after the typically sudden onset of the illness."

Komaroff also found little difference between patients who had fallen ill in the epidemic years and those few who had fallen ill before 1984: "No statistically significant differences were found when patients who experienced the onset of illness before 1984 were compared with those who had a later onset of illness."

Interestingly, Komaroff added, there emerged "no statistically significant differences" between sufferers who fell ill abruptly with what seemed initially to be flu-like symptoms and "the few patients who experienced a more insidious onset."*

Patients from the Tahoe epidemic and those from the larger cities shared another worrisome commonality: "Altogether, 55 percent of the patients in the Tahoe group and 51 percent of the non-Tahoe group stated that a close contact was similarly affected."

Komaroff proposed that despite the presence of brain lesions in 21 percent of apparently healthy subjects, the appearance of such lesions in nearly 80 percent of the Tahoe sufferers suggested they were "experiencing a genuine but as yet undefined pathologic process." In addition, some patients had deeper and larger white matter lesions than any healthy controls, lesions more typical of severely afflicted multiple sclerosis sufferers. Finally, in some patients there existed clear correlations between the position of the lesions in the brain and clinical symptoms. "A relation was seen between the anatomic area affected and the clinical presentation," Komaroff wrote. "One patient with ataxia had [lesions] involving the cerebellum. Seven patients with visual symptoms had [lesions] involving the occipital cortex [the brain's vision center], and one patient with paresis [numbness] had a [lesion]

---

* Komaroff's finding again contradicted a commonly held notion among federal scientists that there were "Tahoe types," whose disease began literally overnight, and "non-Tahoe types," whose illness began insidiously over a long period of time. The National Cancer Institute's Paul Levine and his colleagues had hypothesized that "non-Tahoe types" were more likely to be psychologically ill.

involving the contralateral internal capsule. In several cases, MRI studies were repeated, and the scans showed that areas of [lesions] persisted even after symptoms resolved."

Even if the publication of the Tahoe manuscript failed to generate widespread interest among the lay press and public, its purport—that CFS was an infectious disease of the brain—was hardly lost on the scientists at the Centers for Disease Control, particularly those whose credibility it threatened. Komaroff's study, after all, utterly destroyed the validity of the agency's own Tahoe study. The Division of Viral and Rickettsial Diseases staff, who had held an iron grip on the agency's CFS investigation for almost nine years, reacted angrily to Komaroff's paper. Within days of the study's appearance, William Reeves, the division's herpes chief who had assumed Walter Gunn's title of CFS principal investigator, epidemiologist Jon Kaplan, and others began to write their reply. Over the next several weeks, the group produced several versions of a letter attacking Komaroff's paper, which they planned to send to the *Annals.* According to one agency scientist, the letters were so wrathful that at least eight versions were prepared until the team arrived at a document their superiors considered "civilized" enough to send to the *Annals* letter department.

By late March faxes of the agency's letter to the journal and Anthony Komaroff's labored response were circulating among the Tahoe manuscript authors. "It's not pretty," was Dan Peterson's comment after reading the documents. "They are suggesting we're trying to legitimize an hysterical disease."

Paul Cheney, in Charlotte, remarked, "The other shoe has fallen. . . . We obviously have an enemy in Bill Reeves. This letter suggests he is not receptive to valid research on this disease and that he cannot be trusted to run the agency's program."

In a letter subsequently published, on August 15, in the *Annals,* the CDC's scientists attacked Komaroff and his collaborators for their choice of controls and accused them of mismatching controls with patients.[2] Reeves and his coauthors spread their net further, however, lambasting nearly every facet of the study and ending with a categorical dismissal not only of the research but also of the disease the Tahoe authors had described: "Although the term 'chronic fatigue syndrome' is not used in the article title, the first two paragraphs of the discussion implicate this syndrome as the condition affecting their patients. Because the chronic fatigue syndrome has no known cause or specific treatment and it exists in a highly charged medical, social, and political atmosphere, new potential causes and treatments are accepted by many as gospel before scientific confirmation. Accordingly, published studies on this syndrome must be as precise as possible. We conclude that the disease Buchwald and co-workers described is not the chronic fatigue syndrome or any other clinical entity."

Charlotte, North Carolina

On January 2, Charles Lapp, an associate clinical professor at Duke University, joined Paul Cheney's clinic as a full-time partner. Lapp's decision meant that patients needed to wait just two months rather than six or seven for their first appointments. So far, Cheney had personally evaluated 1,200 CFS patients since his move to North Carolina.

National Institute of Allergy and Infectious Diseases, Bethesda, Maryland

February 3 marked the third meeting of the Chronic Fatigue Syndrome Inter-agency Coordinating Committee (CFSICC), of which CFS grant administrator Ann Schleuderberg was chairwoman. Like the second meeting of this impressive-sounding group, which had taken place five months earlier, it consisted of a con-ference call among the five members. The handful of people who had played a role in the committee's formation the year before—Walter Gunn and Minnesota governor Rudy Perpich were the prime movers—had envisioned it as a consor-tium of scientists from the CDC, the NIH, and other health agencies that would promote communication between Atlanta and Bethesda while functioning as a high-level task force devising complementary schemes to eradicate the disease and to coordinate the assault. In reality, the CFSICC had evolved under Schleu-derberg's leadership into a toothless organization of middle-level scientists and bureaucrats whose biannual kaffeeklatsches revealed them to be committed to maintaining the status quo.

The CFSICC's evolution—for the sole purpose of pacifying a distraught con-stituency—was among the most graphic demonstrations of the manner in which the bias of federal scientists and their bureaucratic machinations compounded to erase the epidemic from public view. In February 1990, late in his tenure as gov-ernor of Minnesota, Rudy Perpich had traveled to Washington to plead with James Mason, then assistant secretary of health, for improved communications between the CDC and the NIH on the matter of the new disease. He also complained to Mason about the slow pace of research. In May 1990, realizing nothing had been done, Perpich wrote to Mason.

"I again ask that you quickly act to increase . . . research activities related to CFS," he said. "I and others have long called on the Congress to provide funding for the CDC for [CFS research], and the Congress has responded. I ask the CDC to urgently carry this work forward."

In June 1990, Mason assigned his deputy, Audrey Manley, to organize a meet-ing among CDC and NIH officials "to look at this issue and to identify the ways the two agencies can better coordinate this effort." Eventually the matter filtered down to Fred Murphy of the Center for Infectious Diseases in Atlanta, then fur-ther down to Brian Mahy, director of the Division of Viral and Rickettsial Dis-eases, and finally to epidemiology activity chief Larry Schonberger, who dropped the problem in Walter Gunn's lap.

Gunn approached his assignment with an ardor not shared by his co-workers. He suggested that a task force "provide oversight in regard to the appropriateness and quality of research" inside the health agencies—a suggestion that made his colleagues especially nervous. "The CDC didn't want *any* scrutiny of where the money was going," Gunn remembered later. "That was the *last* thing they wanted." By the time a planning meeting was held on November 14, 1990, enthusiasm for the interagency coordinating committee was all but dead among Gunn's superiors. The NIH's Ann Schleuderberg was named chairperson.

Schleuderberg convened the first meeting of the CFSICC five months later in Bethesda, immediately following her agency's March 19, 1992, workshop on the disease—the one during which participants were prohibited from discussing etiology. Records of that first meeting revealed that the participants spent much of their time congratulating themselves on the success of the workshop. Eight months later, on October 7, the CFSICC held its second meeting—by teleconference. Murphin Williams of the Food and Drug Administration informed the committee that HEM Pharmaceuticals' application for an expanded clinical trial of Ampligen had been denied; the *Wall Street Journal* had reported the same news three days earlier. Ann Schleuderberg relayed her agency's decision to fund Anthony Komaroff, James Jones, and Ben Natelson—more stale news. Then, according to Gunn's minutes of the proceedings, "it was agreed that Dr. Schleuderberg would continue as CFSICC chairperson for another term and that the committee will be convened by teleconference each quarter, the time and date of the next conference to be announced at a later time." The phone call had lasted sixty-nine minutes.

Gunn had left the CDC by the time the next teleconference occurred in February 1991. In a memo to members before the call, Schleuderberg defined the committee's future scope: "The consensus so far is that an agency-by-agency report of current activities continues to be the most useful approach."

And in her January 1992 report to Congress about activities related to CFS inside her agency, Schleuderberg boasted that the committee's existence was yet more evidence of the government's "steadfast and growing commitment to the advancement of CFS research."

University of Toronto, Ontario, Canada

A firmly held belief that CFS was a psychiatric, or even imaginary, illness pervaded prestigious American universities and medical centers like Stanford, UCLA, and the Mayo Clinic well into the 1990s. In such institutions a few powerful department heads or widely published professors were able to command the spotlight and drive their theory home in the lay press and elsewhere (also, incidentally, chilling free expression on the matter in their own universities, where less influential faculty members, fearful of derision or even loss of employment, kept their contrary thoughts to themselves). The phenomenon was hardly confined to the United States. At the University of Toronto a handful of university staff had fashioned a revisionist view of the Canadian CFS epidemic as an example of mass delusion.

Irving Salit, head of the university's infectious disease department and chief of infectious diseases at Toronto Hospitals, led the charge with his often stated faith in the disease's psychiatric basis.[3] In 1992, for instance, Salit was invited to address the annual meeting of the Institute of Underwriters, held in Toronto, on the subject. The institute included many of the most senior insurance industry executives in North America. Ottawa CFS expert Byron Hyde, who was invited to address the group and who heard Salit's speech, later described it as "a *Saturday Night Live* stand-up comedy routine with CFS patients as the brunt of the joke."

Salit was not the only philosopher of CFS to emerge from Toronto University. In 1992, Edward Shorter, a history professor, published a book on the subject, *From Paralysis to Fatigue.*[4] In the context of a fiercely destructive epidemic of, by then, seven years' duration, Shorter's book loomed as the most truculent assault ever on the legitimacy of the disease. Shorter portrayed the spread of CFS as a wanton, even conspiratorial "subculture of invalidism" populated by lonely single women seeking attention and the unscrupulous medical charlatans who attended them. He blamed the rise of this "psychic epidemic" on two villains: the popular media, which were spreading "a plague of illness attribution" among a "hypersuggestible" citizenry, and a loss of "medical authority." The long-standing primacy of doctors in the culture was eroding, Shorter complained, with the result that patients were less willing to believe doctors who brushed off their symptoms as fanciful.

The historian's research citations bore the mark of a polemicist whose argument depends on the omission of an entire body of data that is contrary to his conclusion. His sole acknowledgment that patients demonstrated objective physical abnormalities, for instance, came in the following comments: "Needless to say, psychiatrists are unwelcome in the subculture of chronic fatigue. . . . Behind this fear of psychiatry is the horror that one's symptoms will be seen as 'imaginary.' . . . Thus patients welcome the occasional blood abnormalities that turn up in their testing."

Predictably, Shorter invoked the research of NIH scientist Stephen Straus to buttress his argument. Straus, Shorter wrote, was "a distinguished internist" who became "an object of vilification" when he introduced his psychoneurotic theory. Thoroughly enmeshed in a worldview wherein the medical profession stood unassailable, Shorter was blind to his own and to Straus's vilification of CFS sufferers.*

Lay readers greeted Shorter's argument with ambivalence. Writing in the *New York Times* on December 10, 1991, book reviewer Michiko Kakutani took exception to Shorter's pugnacity, noting that, in his arguments against CFS, he "abandons the dispassionate tone of historical inquiry that gave the earlier chapters of his book such an authoritative air. Instead of judiciously presenting both sides of the issue, he becomes increasingly dogmatic, eager to persuade the reader of the correctness of his own position. As a result, *From Paralysis to Fatigue* feels like an odd hodgepodge of a book; part medical history, part hypothesis, part diatribe."

Anthony Komaroff also criticized Shorter's theories, in the May 1993 *Harvard Mental Health Letter* of the Harvard Medical School. Adjectives such as "fallacious," "disingenuous," "misinformed," and "ludicrous" peppered Komaroff's text, which culminated in this sentence: "In my judgment, no serious scientist,

---

* With its politicized science and forsaken victims, the CFS epidemic was ripe for Shorter's exploitation. It was inconceivable, however, that in 1992 Shorter could have found a publisher for a similarly mean-spirited book about multiple sclerosis, lupus, or AIDS—all disorders that medical experts had once characterized as dependent upon the victim's emotional state.

whether historian or physician, can examine the available evidence and confidently assert that CFS is merely a state of mind."[5]

National Cancer Institute, Bethesda, Maryland

As a result of monitoring diseases suffered by AIDS victims, cancer researchers had become aware of a stunning worldwide rise in non-Hodgkin's lymphoma—the cancer that in 1994 would end the lives of Dr. Lewis Thomas and Jacqueline Onassis. Statisticians studying the problem realized the increase had begun as long ago as the 1950s. Since 1950, the disease's attack rate in the United States, in particular, had tripled.[6] The reasons for the phenomenon were unknown, but many scientists felt that a transmissible agent, probably a virus, might play a role. That January, cancer epidemiologist Paul Levine was preparing a manuscript for publication on the troubling matter, then under study at the National Cancer Institute. Levine's particular focus was the seemingly large number of non-Hodgkin's lymphomas among CFS suffers and their relatives in the Incline Village, Nevada, practice of Dan Peterson. Levine had presented the material three months earlier to his colleagues in Bethesda. "But," he said, "now that it's coming to writing it down, we're really being *very* careful about the conclusions. . . . We need to show the kinds of serious analyses that go into a conclusion of making an association between chronic fatigue syndrome and cancer." Nevertheless, Levine admitted, "There's a blip—there's definitely a blip—and we are figuring out how to put that blip into perspective. We want to be sure that whatever is said is phrased properly.

"This study was just done as a first look, just to counter what I thought was inappropriate reporting of data," he added in a reference to Seymour Grufferman's cancer data. "It may be that CFS predisposes people to cancer, but Grufferman's data can't show that. Cheney and Peterson may turn out to be right, but we don't think the anecdotal reports are solidly based."

National Institute of Allergy and Infectious Diseases, Bethesda, Maryland

Although the Food and Drug Administration had crushed hopes for an expanded clinical trial of Ampligen in the United States anytime soon, patient support organizations took heart when they learned that the agency that frequently advised FDA administrators on drug approval issues, the National Institute of Allergy and Infectious Diseases, had requested a presentation on the drug by its inventor, HEM Pharmaceuticals. It turned out that Stephen Straus had asked the company for the briefing, which occurred on February 10. Straus apparently expected one or two HEM officials to make the presentation. Instead, Ampligen co-inventor William Carter, the firm's chief executive, invited David Strayer, HEM's medical adviser; Robert Suhadolnik, the Temple University molecular biologist who was studying Ampligen's effect in CFS and AIDS sufferers; Miami immunologist Nancy Klimas; and Paul Cheney to accompany him. On the agency side, Straus, his research nurse Janet Dale, National Cancer Institute epidemiologist Paul Levine, herpes expert Dharam Ablashi, and Warren Strober, an immunologist from Straus's institute, were present. Ann Schleuderberg dropped in for a portion of the discussion, then left. In all, approximately thirty-five people were gathered in a small classroom on the eleventh floor of the Warren Magnuson Clinical Center.

Cheney noted that Straus seemed surprised and annoyed that the HEM group was so large. The government scientist made it clear he wanted the presentation limited to twenty-five minutes. David Strayer, who had managed all of the company's clinical trials, was slated to speak for twenty minutes, followed by a five-minute talk by Nancy Klimas. The meeting ended abruptly when Straus completed his interrogation of Strayer and Klimas, the only participants he questioned.

France

On February 13, *Le Nouvel Observateur,* the French newsmagazine, published a ten-page cover story on CFS, headlined, "La Fatigue, Une Vraie Maladie" (Fatigue—A Real Disease"). Was a virus or retrovirus responsible for the fatigue that seemed to be affecting greater numbers of the French populace, or was it merely a *maladie des yuppies*? the magazine's editors asked. "Across the Atlantic, researchers are asking: is CFS caused by a retrovirus? Meanwhile, the charlatans prosper," a French journalist wrote.

The magazine, in addition, described Elaine DeFreitas's Kyoto presentation and published the Center for Disease Control's definition of the disease.

Chiron, San Francisco

Six months earlier, scientists from Chiron, a biotechnology firm in Emoryville, California, a small town adjacent to Berkeley, had called Elaine DeFreitas to ask if she would be willing to enter into a confidential collaboration. Chiron was among the top three biotechnology firms in the world, with revenues then of $250 million. Chiron staff explained that they wanted to study her technology with an eye toward developing a commercial diagnostic test kit for CFS.

"We have business development people at Wistar who are open to *any* technology that's generated here," DeFreitas said later. The Wistar scientist had gamely entered into the collaboration with the understanding that it was secret—that neither side could discuss the process with outsiders.

Not long into the collaboration, Chiron's scientists told DeFreitas they were having trouble reproducing her work. The company's scientists were using a technique called "Southern blot" by which to visualize bands of protein from the virus. DeFreitas and her lab associate, Hiroshi Terunuma, sent a highly detailed written explanation of their protocol to Chiron. Still, the scientists said, they could not reproduce the experiment. In turn, DeFreitas asked Terunuma to go to Emoryville and shepherd a second effort. Terunuma spent a week in Chiron's laboratories.

"The data went from zero correlation to eighty-seven percent correlation," DeFreitas recalled. When she called a sample positive, Chiron did, too—87 percent of the time; the percentage held steady for negative samples as well. "In essence, they were seeing what we were seeing as soon as they started doing it Terry's way."

The development boosted morale in DeFreitas's lab and gave the scientist a measure of confidence that her collaboration with the CDC had begun to erode. "I felt [that] if Chiron could do it, I don't *care* what CDC says, and neither did Chiron. Because sooner or later, once Chiron began manufacturing a test kit for the retrovirus, CDC would *have* to come around."

During the initial six months, while Chiron scientists had been working to reproduce the finding, DeFreitas had moved forward and now had live virus growing in cultures. Chiron told DeFreitas they would like samples of her live virus; in addition, company executives were sufficiently impressed by the finding's commercial potential that they asked DeFreitas to extend the secret arrangement another six months.

Soon afterward, early in February, DeFreitas was shocked to discover from Jay Levy that Chiron had violated the confidentiality clause of their contract. Without alerting anyone at Wistar, Chiron executives had invited Stephen Straus, Anthony Komaroff, Jay Levy, and Gary Holmes to its headquarters to discuss DeFreitas's finding and the retroviral etiology theory in general. As Levy described the scene to DeFreitas, Komaroff was characteristically neutral on the subject; Levy told Chiron that more data was required, including isolation of the agent itself. Straus, on the other hand, "did nothing but ridicule it," DeFreitas reported.

DeFreitas was angered by Chiron's violation of the secrecy agreement. In addition, she noticed that, after the company's conference with Straus, "the whole feeling of the interaction changed. They got gun-shy about pursuing the collaboration. Apparently CDC didn't bother them—but Straus did."

When DeFreitas realized what had happened, she was reluctant to send samples of her virus to the firm, especially after spending six grueling months nurturing the cultures. For one thing there wasn't very much virus to go around; she was especially unenthusiastic about sharing the precious commodity with scientists whose commitment to the project had grown suddenly cold.

DeFreitas called the project manager at Chiron, Michael Richman. "I said, 'Look, if we're going to spend six months growing this virus, I'm not going to send it to you to give it a halfhearted effort. *We'll* keep it,' " DeFreitas said. "[Chiron] basically said 'Fine.' "

Some years afterward, project manager Richman, who is today head of business development for the firm, confessed regret that Chiron executives had decided to involve outsiders in the field without alerting DeFreitas or inviting her to be part of the deliberations. "I personally think she should have been here," he said. He explained that there had been "a lack of technical results" that led executives at the company to question the legitimacy of the finding. Richman added that Chiron had asked Levy, Straus, Holmes, and Komaroff to sign confidentiality agreements regarding their Emoryville conclave; when Levy and possibly others violated those agreements, Richman said, "we were surprised and we took some action on that."

Asked about DeFreitas's accusations that Straus's denigration of her work had queered the Chiron-Wistar interaction, Richman said, "I think she may be right.

We were investing a lot of money and time in this—eight or nine months—and when you bring in experts in the field who are negative about the prospects for success—But," he continued after a moment, "I don't think it was just Stephen Straus. He gave one perspective."

Wistar Institute, Philadelphia, Pennsylvania

Elaine DeFreitas had sent her grant proposal to the National Institute of Allergy and Infectious Diseases on February 1. She had been encouraged to do so by lobbyist Tom Sheridan, who had received assurances from members of Senator Ted Kennedy's staff that the tide would soon turn at the Bethesda agency and that CFS grant proposals would be processed on an "expedited basis," just as AIDS grants had been for several years.

Her proposal, DeFreitas said, was "very conservative." She had avoided claims of causation; she simply wanted the time and resources to pin down the nature of her discovery. "We have to identify this thing—give it a name," DeFreitas said. "Even if it turns out that this virus is nothing, we need to find out."

Her grant proposal included the names of her clinical collaborators, David Bell and Paul Cheney, in spite of Ann Schleuderberg's warning of a year before that the federal agency considered neither clinician bona fide and that any grant proposal containing their names would flounder. "She may well be one hundred percent right," DeFreitas commented, "but Paul Cheney and David Bell are my clinical collaborators. The virus is in their patients. It's like Willie Sutton—when they asked him why he robbed banks, he said, 'Because that's where the money is.' "

DeFreitas had been forced to fire two of her staff early in 1992 because of a shortage of funding for her CFS research. One of them was Brendan Hilliard, the postdoc who had been working at her side since the earliest phase of her CFS research. "Thanks for isolating a new virus—you're fired" was how DeFreitas characterized the painful act of firing Hilliard. "I've got two and one-half people working on this now," she added.

With Koprowski's departure from the Wistar, DeFreitas found herself more vulnerable than ever. "I don't have the leeway I had with Koprowski. . . . He would come up with contingency funds, but that is finished."

Several months earlier, Elaine DeFreitas had halted the sequencing process in her laboratory. "We had to make some really hard decisions," the scientist said, "because we weren't getting enough genetic material from our polymerase chain reaction. . . . We finally decided we were going to have to grow something to get enough, so everybody turned their attention to that."

DeFreitas had discovered just five human cell lines in which her virus would thrive. Into these she mixed white blood cells from patients with CFS. "From sample to sample, it looks identical," she said. "It's like following a shadow."

Her next step, DeFreitas said, would be to load the gene sequences into her lab's computer in an effort to identify the pathogen. She needed to complete that phase of the work within six months, in time for the meeting of the committee that would determine the fate of her grant proposal. In her proposal, DeFreitas had promised she would be far enough along by the time the grant committee met that she would be close to identifying the virus. Should she be unable to provide the information, she said, "we'll be dead in the water."

DeFreitas reported she was still working with blood samples that Walter Gunn had sent her from the CDC patients and that she was unable to report definitive results. "I don't know if it's a technical problem or if the timing of taking the samples was too early," she said. "We don't know when this virus is in the blood. I *do* know we've gotten our best signals from people four years into their illness."

DeFreitas was feeling the pressure of a watching, waiting scientific world, one that was not universally friendly. She had been invited by the Ciba Foundation, an independent academic institution funded by the giant, Switzerland-based pharmaceutical firm Ciba-Geigy, to present her work at a CFS conference the foundation was holding at its London headquarters in May. As always, the conference, the foundation's 173d, was being limited to just twenty-five participants. "We like very small, closed meetings focusing on topics where there have been interesting developments," the foundation's deputy director, Gregory Bock, explained later. "I had been following this field for several years and my intention was to bring together the most prominent people in the field." Other invitees included Stephen Straus; Peter Manu, the clinician from the University of Connecticut who maintained that CFS was a psychiatric problem; and Peter Behan, the University of Glasgow neurologist who had cast DeFreitas as a fraud during his visit to the United States the previous September. Remarkably, Ciba officials had asked Toronto University history professor and pop author Edward Shorter, whose recent book had ridiculed the disease and its sufferers, to moderate the conference (Bock later defended his choice, insisting, "He's a perfectly respectable medical historian.")

DeFreitas discussed the invitation with her Boston collaborator, David Bell, who had become the scientist's confidant in the turmoil of recent months. "It sounds like a turkey shoot—and you're the turkey," Bell told her when she described the guest list.

On February 19, DeFreitas presented a scientific grand rounds on her work at Philadelphia's Jefferson University. The mother of a CFS patient who had been in the audience approached her afterward. "She said something very disturbing," DeFreitas recalled. "She said, 'You're like Joan of Arc.' I said, 'Do you remember what happened to Joan of Arc?' "

Centers for Disease Control, Atlanta, Georgia

On February 20 retrovirology chief Tom Folks reported he had low expectations of ever confirming Elaine DeFreitas's work. Folks had never been able to repeat his first success of July 1991; instead, he and Heneine had consistently found signals for the retrovirus in both controls and patients, suggesting to them that the Wistar retrovirus was endogenous and therefore incapable of causing disease. During a lengthy conversation on the subject, Folks evinced neither joy nor righteousness; instead, he sounded depressed and, on occasion, angry. He had little doubt that an infectious pathogen was at the heart of the disease; in fact, he suspected a retrovirus. But he resented the time and effort he had been forced to expend looking for the DeFreitas pathogen. Since 1986, when Anthony Komaroff had asked him to evaluate a handful of Tahoe blood samples for reverse transcriptase, Folks had always been coolheaded about the disease in contrast to his agency colleagues. CFS had never been a topic of hilarity for him, nor did he, even now, disparage its gravity. Even so, he forecast an imminent career meltdown for DeFreitas and perhaps for her former boss, Hilary Koprowski. He cited his own lab's inability to reproduce the Wistar's retroviral finding in CFS, which was coming on the heels of a similar failure by researchers to confirm the team's retrovirus finding in multiple sclerosis. "This one will wipe them out," Folks predicted.

Folks, in addition, suggested that DeFreitas would be vilified by patients. Victims of the disease would turn on her when they learned they had been duped, whether out of incompetence or venality, about the cause of their disease, he said. "Chronic fatigue syndrome is a bigger disease than multiple sclerosis," he said. "A greater number of people are devastated for a longer period of time. And when you tangle with people who are so devastated . . . it's going to be difficult for her to bounce back from that."

Folks said that his lab had been performing their test for retrovirus using the Wistar primers on sixty blood samples, some of them from controls, others from patients who had been evaluated by the agency as "class one." These were presumed CFS sufferers without evidence of psychiatric symptoms, including depression, and without any abnormal laboratory tests. They were, in other words, an unusual group; finding CFS sufferers who weren't seriously depressed was difficult indeed. Agency scientists believed the class one patients were probably the "purest" for research purposes, since they could never be confused with psychiatric patients. To many people who were familiar with the disease, however, class one patients were an anomaly.

Naturally, patient samples were mixed in with control samples and secretly coded in such a way that Folks and his staff were unaware of health status. Folks estimated that one-third to one-fourth of the sixty samples were true CFS patients.

"We have *very* few positives," Folks reported. "Two or three people. If we're hitting the patients, then so be it. But I don't see even a third lighting up with our marker. It may be that the CFS patients that we're seeing have a window when they're expressing the agent, and we've missed that window. Maybe our case definition is wrong, but I don't think so. Now, there are no absolutes in this business. Maybe Elaine DeFreitas was getting blood at a different time in patients' illnesses. Clearly, Cheney's patients may have been at a different point in their illness than the Atlanta patients." In addition, Folks said, "We're only looking at a frequency of one in 150,000 cells in peripheral blood. If the virus is in one cell in a million, we would have to run it one in ten times."

As they wound down their efforts, Folks waited for the results of DeFreitas's analysis of the Atlanta samples sent to her by Walter Gunn on December 12. Folks had given DeFreitas a March 1 deadline to complete her study. If she managed to define which samples came from controls and which came from patients, Folks said, "Walid Heneine and I will travel to her lab. You have my word on that." Until that moment, however, Folks had no intention of accepting DeFreitas's invitation to come to her lab so that she could demonstrate how she performed her experiments. Folks defended his refusal on grounds that he was saving taxpayers' money. "Every time someone makes a discovery, am I supposed to take taxpayers' money and go charging off to their labs?" he asked. "We can't run to their lab—we just can't do it. I can't take people in my lab away from other important health issues just because someone makes a claim."

Folks and his colleagues were confident enough of the integrity of their efforts that they were gearing up to write a paper on their retrovirus investigation for the scientific literature. Folks wanted to broadcast his results to as wide an audience as possible, one in which clinicians as well as bench researchers were well represented. "We're thinking about the *New England Journal of Medicine, JAMA,* or *Lancet,*" he said.

Folks's own increasing distrust of DeFreitas was evident. "I could tell you four groups who've tried to confirm this and failed," he commented. On questioning, he listed Robert Gallo's lab at the NIH, neurologist Peter Behan's lab at the University of Glasgow, Jay Levy at the University of California, and his own lab. The reason for their failure to confirm, Folks added, "was the sixty-four-dollar question. There's the obvious—that she's making it up. But I don't believe that. I believe she's really finding this. But there could be mistakes. Maybe she found it once and couldn't find it again. Maybe she got away with that, and now her back is against the wall.

"Let's step back," he continued. "Here's a person who has isolated the etiology of chronic fatigue syndrome. Can you imagine the monetary value of that? Can you imagine the personal satisfaction? If that were me, I would take that into another lab—I would be *jumping* to get it confirmed. Now, we've been willing to sign affidavits—we've been willing to sign our souls to the devil to help her confirm it. Yet she chooses not to do that. She could come to our lab. She could send her materials to me. The government works for everyone; we would sacrifice our *publications* to help her confirm it! You tell *me* why she won't send that material to me! Or why she won't come to our lab! If I were [DeFreitas], I would go to some world-class retrovirus lab and let them help me prove the validity. But she's chosen to sequester herself in her lab. Her track record is good. Why she would put that in jeopardy, I don't know.

"I supported her for a year," Folks continued. "We are the closest at being able to produce her work," he added in a reference to the sensitivity his lab had achieved, "and we *still* can't identify her markers. . . . It's a very embarrassing situation at this point if she's wrong, and it becomes an ethical issue if she kept getting windows where she saw the marker, but not all the time. She's basically taken a year of the government's money to work on her technique."

Once the DeFreitas discovery "had been put to rest," as he phrased it, "I'm going to be somewhat depressed," Folks said. "One, we've spent all this time, and two, chronic fatigue syndrome has taken a setback. We really need a marker for this disease. The only good thing about this is it will tell you not to pursue this particular marker. Although," he added, "we will probably always use the DeFreitas primer, now that we've got it working."

In fact, Folks suggested, he was hardly giving up on the retrovirus search. "Everything has been put on hold because of this," he said, "but once this has been answered, you'll see a lot of things take off in our lab. My own personal bias," he added, "is that it *is* a virus like a retrovirus, because a retrovirus is chronic and it's latent and it's slow. That's how retroviruses work. And this is a slow, debilitating disease. It probably has a latent phase, it probably hides, and that's exactly what a retrovirus does. The only thing that *doesn't* fit a retroviral etiology is the epidemiology of the disease," Folks continued in a reference to the apparent casual transmission of CFS. "But we've only got two human retroviruses so far—AIDS and leukemia—and maybe there are other ways of transmitting other retroviruses."

Throughout the course of his conversation, Folks made no reference to the contamination in his laboratories, a mystery that had yet to be solved.

Ali Kahn, the new Epidemic Intelligence Service officer hired to handle the CFS epi-aid investigation, had completed his evaluation of the "exposure histories" among the patients and healthy controls enrolled in the study. Kahn had been looking for exposures to infectious agents among these patients to see if their illness could be explained by past exposure to known pathogens. After extensive questioning of all the patients, Kahn had found just two similarities among patients' histories that distinguished them from healthy controls: CFS sufferers had a wider acquaintanceship with other victims of the disease, and they used over-the-counter medications, particularly painkillers, with greater frequency. They failed to demonstrate any higher exposure to known infectious pathogens than normal people.

The finding could not have pleased Kahn's boss, Larry Schonberger, who held that the disease was a grab bag of common infections and psychiatric disorders. Even more annoyingly, the finding suggested that the disease was infectious.

Medical College of Wisconsin, Milwaukee

Although his demand for secrecy continued, virologist Sidney Grossberg relayed to his patrons at the CFIDS Association in Charlotte that his progress during the past year had been exceedingly good.

"He's made strides," Marc Iverson said that spring. "He's now got the retrovirus in eight patients. He recently sent us an electron micrograph of it; it looks like Elaine DeFreitas's micrograph. He's very slow, very conservative, and very tight-lipped," Iverson continued. "When he gets published, it will be in the *New England Journal of Medicine*. But maybe not for five or ten years. He does *not* want to have happen to him what has happened to Elaine DeFreitas and John Martin. He's the turtle; Martin and DeFreitas are the hares."

Nevertheless, unlike a number of other researchers in the field, Grossberg had skipped a step in the learning curve: having been completely ignorant of the disease when patient JH first described her symptoms to him in January of 1989, he had never experienced a phase of skepticism or disbelief. "I'm convinced this is *really* a *true* illness," he would say later, a distinctly emotional tone entering his voice. Thus convinced, the scientist was increasingly aghast at the politics that were now threatening to swamp his efforts, most particularly in the realm of financial support. Indeed, some years later, Grossberg would describe his struggle to secure funding as "painful" and "very difficult." Likely, it had been hard for the distinguished scientist to appeal to a fledgling patient organization for money, but "CFIDS money," as Elaine DeFreitas called it, had been the only cash available to scientists searching for viral etiologies in the disease for some time.

Fairly or not, the scientist blamed DeFreitas for some portion of his pain.

"It is profoundly unfortunate that she chose to go public with this after the meeting in Japan," he commented. "It raised the level of suspicion among scientists who review grant applications at the NIH. . . . That's why I've been so careful to avoid any sort of public disclosure."

Grossberg had applied for funding from the National Institute of Allergy and Infectious Diseases. Remarkably, his grant had been approved by the institution and was awaiting funding. And when the government makes such a decision, that scientist's success enters the public domain.

News of Grossberg's grant approval and likely funding struck Elaine DeFreitas with predictable force. After a three-and-a-half-year investment with immeasurable personal costs, she had seen federal support for retrovirus investigation go to a member of the scientific old boy network. DeFreitas, in contrast, continued to struggle against a tide of prejudice, most of it stemming from her choice of clinical collaborators—Paul Cheney and David Bell.

"If Grossberg gets funded and I don't," DeFreitas said defiantly, "I'm going to pitch a fit. I'll be goddamned if, after all this time, some guy from Dubuque is going to find this!"

Grossberg had been making inroads at the CDC in Atlanta, too. Tom Folks reported later that spring that he and Grossberg were having conversations about Grossberg's findings. By summer, in fact, Grossberg had begun sharing his data with Folks.

Vancouver, British Columbia, Canada

In the months since the Food and Drug Administration placed all further testing of Ampligen in CFS on clinical hold, the drug's manufacturer, HEM Pharmaceuticals, had hardly been idle. The company's directors were searching for new markets in Canada, continental Europe, and the British Isles in which to complete the next phase of their clinical trials. HEM had already submitted a proposal to launch an Ampligen trial in Canada to the Canadian Ministry of Health. In the early spring, they took their act on the road. On March 8, David Strayer and Robert Suhadolnik, who had played a major role in the company's AIDS and CFS trials, presented the results of the firm's recent clinical trial in ninety-two American CFS sufferers to a meeting of Canadian scientists in British Columbia.

In the meantime, officials at the Food and Drug Administration had transferred HEM's application for additional clinical trials of Ampligen in CFS sufferers from the Division of Biologics to the Division of Antiviral Drugs, where approval was reportedly even more difficult to come by.

Wistar Institute, Philadelphia, Pennsylvania

In early March, Elaine DeFreitas's problems were amplified when Tom Folks informed her that she had failed to differentiate between patients and controls among the class one blood specimens Walter Gunn had sent her on December 12.

DeFreitas had found just three positives among the twenty-three samples; worse, the samples DeFreitas called positive were all from healthy controls. She had found one marginal positive; that specimen had come from a CFS sufferer. All the rest of DeFreitas's samples—she had been sent eleven cases and twelve controls, according to Walter Gunn—were negative for her retrovirus marker.

Much later, Folks would say, "We were ready to stay with her if she had found positives to be negatives. But she found negatives to be positive. That ruined her. It broke her back. She lost all credibility with that."

In conversation that spring, DeFreitas was unapologetic about the results. The samples had taken a long time to process, she said, because it took ten to twelve days to perform the experiment according to her protocol. "*Theirs* take three days," she noted in a reference to the experiments being performed by Walid Heneine and Tom Folks in Atlanta. More important, the Wistar scientist had been plagued by a technical problem, discovered only near the end of the tedious work with the twenty-three samples. "We found out we had been using truncated primers. They were bad primers which we were getting from the core facility at Wistar," she said.

DeFreitas had wanted to perform the experiments again with good primers even before she had completed the experiment. She had explained her problem to Folks, but she recalled that he was unsympathetic. "They were *demanding* the re-sults," she said. Reluctantly DeFreitas persisted. She released her results to Folks "with a caveat. I said the primers were probably no good."

Afterward, and independently of her collaboration with the government, De-Freitas decided to run her assays a second time on the specimens, this time using better printers. After seven weeks, she had completed the work. Even with im-proved materials, however, DeFreitas remained unable to distinguish between healthy people and people suffering from CFS. Frustrated, she tried the experi-ment again, and then again. Each time the patients were negative. "We've redone it now multiple times," she reported later. "And in fact there are *still* no patients positive. I don't know what that means. Are the government's exclusionary crite-ria excluding the very patients we want?"

DeFreitas's specimens, of course, had come from class ones, people lacking ev-idence of either depression or abnormal lab tests. "Walter Gunn says they would exclude everyone who had preexisting or even current psyche problems," DeFre-itas said. "So they were cutting *all* the cognitive people out of group one. Those kinds of patients were being *systematically* excluded from the epi-aid study."

DeFreitas knew that the patient specimens being sent to her by Paul Cheney and David Bell came from people who were extremely ill, all of whom demon-strated intellectual and emotional enervation.

"I would like to look at people in the other categories. Those eleven [CDC] pa-tients went through so many layers of exclusion! This data is so difficult to inter-pret without having gotten a random sampling from groups one, two, three, and four. Our theory is that the retrovirus hides out in the central nervous system, so you won't always find it.

"We ran those specimens once, and they were negative," DeFreitas continued in a reference to her experiment with the class one patient samples. "We then ran them again—multiple times—and they were *still* negative. And Tom Folks said,

'There you are—the chronic fatigue syndrome patients are negative!' And I said, 'No! This is *only* class one patients. This is the class that's been excluded for having *any* abnormal test. This could really tell us something! Maybe the positive patients will be in group two or three or four.

"I *begged* them to do class two, three, and four patients. And they wouldn't send them to me," DeFreitas continued. "And that's when I realized *they don't want to know!* They're so delighted that these eleven patients were negative!"

Whether DeFreitas's idea—to test patients from all four categories in the government's surveillance study—was a reasonable one was uncertain. Certainly most pathogens were known to wax and wane in their hosts at varying points during any infectious disease. Anthony Komaroff, who had been a member of the government's physicians panel to review cases reported into the surveillance system, was queried on the matter. He said, "There is no right answer here." Yet, he continued, "If I had looked for an association between a novel infectious agent and group one CFS patients, and did not find it, I would probably not pursue the matter further . . . particularly if the testing was labor-intensive and expensive and the [CDC] technicians were thereby tied up and unable to study other important problems [such as hantavirus or Ebola virus]. Given that resources are finite, I think I would not have recommended applying the assay to the group two to four patients." Certainly Larry Schonberger and others at the agency felt that way. Eager to cut bait and publish the results of their epi-aid investigation begun the previous summer, they rejected DeFreitas's proposal.

The Wistar scientist was quick to note what she viewed as the agency's hypocrisy: "When Tom Folks did his test last July on [David] Bell's Lyndonville patients and *all* of Bell's patients were positive and four out of five of the CDC's Atlanta patients were positive and *none* of the controls were positive," she said, "they wouldn't publish that, because they said that's just *one* experiment." Now, after one experiment in which the patients were negative for the marker, the agency was pushing for publication of the results.

DeFreitas was devastated by the CDC's aggressive stance. Prior to publishing her paper on the retroviral marker in 1990, she had performed her experiments repeatedly, each time searching for clues that her assays were affording false positives. She held off publication for more than a year, in fact, looking for evidence of the virus by several different methods, to be certain of her finding. "Their basis is just *glaring*," DeFreitas complained. "If it's positive, it shouldn't be considered for publication. If it's negative, you use it."

As the full weight of the agency's decisions settled upon her, she felt defeated. "I realized that I had been used so that Bill Reeves could get up in front of Congressman John Porter and say, "We're collaborating with Elaine DeFreitas—*that's* what we're spending our money on.' "

To compound her anguish that spring, she received word from Wistar director Giovanni Rovera that, in DeFreitas's words, he no longer wanted the institute associated with CFS. "He advised me strongly to get out of CFS," she said. Some years later DeFreitas would recall that "Rovera never really made it his business to understand the science of this. It wasn't important enough to him to ever sit me down and ask me what was going on. The only thing that he was interested in was getting commercial money for Wistar." The crash of the Chiron collaboration no doubt fueled Rovera's decision at least as much as the CDC's impugning of De-Freitas's abilities and the integrity of her research.

DeFreitas was unsurprised by Rovera's move. Years earlier, she had waded into the swamp of the disease with Wistar chief Hilary Koprowski's blessing, but Koprowski's departure eight months before had left her without advocates within her institution. Now, with the government's virologists threatening to publish a paper negating her discovery, University of Miami immunologist Nancy Klimas extended her hand to DeFreitas. Klimas suggested DeFreitas move to Miami and establish her own laboratory within the university's immunology department in order to continue her work on CFS.

Sarasota, Florida

As government hostility to their work escalated that spring, fence-mending as well as a subtle emotional bonding was occurring among the competitive, if tiny, cadre of scientists searching for the pathogen at the heart of the disease. On the weekend of March 14 and 15, the sprawling Sarasota Marriott was the site of yet another weekend medical conference on CFS, the eighth since 1987. Present were the "usual spear-carriers and singers," according to Walter Gunn. He meant himself, Paul Cheney, Elaine DeFreitas, Anthony Komaroff, John Martin, Byron Hyde, Nancy Klimas, David Bell, and other investigators who by then were well known to each other and to members of patient organizations. Although retired from government service, Gunn had by no means lost interest in the disease. He had established a consulting firm, headquartered in his basement home office in an Atlanta suburb; from Lilburn, Georgia, he intended to continue the work he had begun at the Centers for Disease Control. He hoped not only to function as a facilitator of research, but also to establish a professional society for doctors and scientists interested in the disease.

Little that was said at the lectern in Sarasota was newsworthy, with the exception of Elaine DeFreitas's update on her work at Wistar. During a twenty-five-minute presentation to an audience of five hundred, 80 percent of whom were patients, she revealed that she had cultured, weighed, and measured her virus. It was definitely an RNA virus, she said, adding that it was just as definitely a novel virus. In addition, she had tested more than thirty samples of umbilical cord blood of newborns, which was highly unlikely to be infected with any pathogen, known or unknown; the cord blood was uniformly negative for her virus, suggesting that it could not have been an endogenous agent. The viral particles were lighter and smaller than either HTLV1 or HTLV2 particles, DeFreitas told her audience. She suspected her bug was neither spuma nor lenti nor onco—the three known families of retroviruses. Instead, she believed it might constitute a new branch of retrovirology altogether. In fact, when studied under the electron microscope, she said, the virus most resembled in size, shape, and morphology an animal retrovirus, the simian D virus. DeFreitas had discovered, in addition, a protein band that she suspected might be a precursor to a diagnostic test: the band appeared only in people who were symptomatic for CFS. She had submitted all of this data in manuscript form to the *Proceedings of the National Academy of Sciences,* the journal that had published her original retroviral findings in the disease the year before. The title of her article was "Non-C-type Retrovirus in Children." As he had her first paper, Hilary Koprowski, a member of the National Academy of Sciences, sponsored the paper's publication in the organization's journal.

DeFreitas and Martin were seen huddled in conversation during the weekend, a scene that would have been unthinkable one year before. DeFreitas, Martin, Paul Cheney, and David Bell took their Saturday evening meal together in another demonstration of revived solidarity. The peppery Brooklyn native, the self-righteous Australian, the cerebral grandson of Georgia sharecroppers, and the patrician, Harvard-educated Rhode Islander were an unlikely foursome, and the circumstances that inspired their need for fellowship were at least as remarkable. If enmities had existed among members of this group in the past, it was increasingly apparent to them that the fire-breathing dragon just outside the door was the greater foe. There emerged particular empathy for DeFreitas. Even Cheney appeared to have recovered his affection for the scientist from the prestigious institute who had taken his concerns seriously while the federal agencies dismissed him. As a result of her collaboration with him, she was about to be publicly discredited by the government's disease detectives. At weekend's end, Cheney was seen enfolding the bone-thin DeFreitas in a comradely hug.

Gunn, noting the newfound solidarity among the embattled research fraternity, seized the opportunity to propose a collaborative study to DeFreitas and Martin to counter the CDC's study. Gunn had been impressed that when Folks and his team most closely followed DeFreitas's protocol for handling blood specimens, they had found the Lyndonville children's samples positive for the DeFreitas marker. On the strength of that observation, Gunn proposed to Martin and DeFreitas that they collaborate in a study of Lyndonville children. David Bell agreed to select the patients and controls from the little upstate New York village. Bell would send the blood to Gunn to be secretly coded, after which Gunn would send the coded samples to DeFreitas and Martin. Independently, the two scientists would perform their own assays for retroviral infection in these specimens.

Gunn had a second motive: the government's dismissal of Martin's data had left unanswered for too long the question of whether Martin and DeFreitas were indeed working with the same or different pathogens. A concordance of results, Gunn knew, would go a long way toward proving that the virus growing in cell cultures in Philadelphia was kin to the bug growing in John Martin's Los Angeles lab. "At the very least, we'll be able to find out if they've got the same agent," Gunn said.

A year earlier, such a collaboration would have been unimaginable to either Martin or DeFreitas. With the storm clouds gathering, however, they welcomed Gunn's suggestion.

Some days later, in a phone conversation, Gunn described his plan to Tom Folks.

Atlanta, Georgia

Given his former role as principal investigator, Walter Gunn was slated to be the first author on any journal articles relating to surveillance, viral markers, or the epi-aid and case-control studies. For months, however, he had been reminding his former CDC colleagues that he would forbid the use of his name on any paper refuting Elaine DeFreitas's study and that he would counter any such paper with a public dissemination of his carefully compiled record of the agency's star-crossed effort to replicate to the Wistar protocol.

In early April, Ali Kahn, the new Epidemic Intelligence Service officer in Larry Schonberger's section, told Gunn that the agency's paper on the Atlanta epi-aid study was already written. Two versions existed, Kahn said—one with their Wistar test results, one without them. Kahn's superiors were debating which version of the paper to publish and whether to publish it quickly, without peer review, in the *Morbidity and Mortality Weekly Report.*

"They're going to say the CDC got specimens from thirty patients and thirty controls and conducted the following tests—and the tests were all negative, including tests for retroviruses. If they include DeFreitas's data, they'll say they weren't able to confirm DeFreitas's finding," Gunn said. "I told CDC, 'You guys weren't willing to publish her one positive—why are you willing to publish her one negative?' If they're foolish enough to go ahead with it, I will say they didn't follow her protocol."

Larry Schonberger called Gunn at home to discuss the matter.

"I told him, if the CDC results are positive, I'll be on the paper," Gunn said. "If the results are negative, I don't want to be on it."

By that spring, government virologist Tom Folks had identified the retrovirus that had first contaminated his laboratory when he began receiving blood samples from CFS sufferers.

"We thought maybe it had been derived from CFS patients," Folks responded when asked about the contamination. "But it turned out to be a fairly common monkey virus. When we cloned it and sequenced it, it turned out to be gibbon ape leukemia virus. We did a fairly low-key investigation," he added. "Within six months, we knew."

Folks confessed he had failed to ascertain the origins of the contamination, except to prove that it had occurred somewhere in a CDC lab. "Where it got introduced into the lab, we don't know," he said. "These things happen even with the best technical people. A pipette may have started the contamination. But we know it's not related to CFS—that's the main point."

He strove to underplay the event. "I think maybe there was a week's worth of excitement," Folks said. "Maybe a month. These things happen. These things may have happened to Elaine."

32

The Greatest Underestimate
of All Time

Wistar Institute, Philadelphia, Pennsylvania

On March 24 scientists from the Centers for Disease Control arranged a teleconference among themselves, Elaine DeFreitas, and David Bell to propose yet another retrovirus study. Agency investigators seemed to be making a last-ditch effort to establish definitively—or to crush definitively—the validity of DeFreitas's original finding, even as they were readying their paper refuting it.

Schonberger and Folks's new proposal resembled the study Walter Gunn had proposed to DeFreitas in Sarasota, with one exception: the agency had no intention of involving John Martin; the collaboration was to be between Wistar and the CDC. This time, Tom Folks and Larry Schonberger explained, agency staff would get blood samples from the same nine Lyndonville, New York, children DeFreitas had called positive in her 1990 paper. Each of these samples would then be divided in half and interspersed with specimens from healthy controls. A secret code known only to Epidemic Intelligence Service officer Ali Kahn would be established. Kahn would send DeFreitas half of the blood. She would undertake to reproduce her original experiment for the umpteenth time, differentiating between the Lyndonville children and healthy controls. The retrovirologists at the CDC would attempt to do the same, using DeFreitas's primers.

DeFreitas and Bell listened carefully as Folks and Schonberger described the study. The agency investigators promised to send the Wistar scientist a written protocol, and DeFreitas delayed giving her answer until she received the document. Bell and DeFreitas felt squeamish about attempting another collaboration with the agency. But if the government scientists could be counted on to follow through with the work as DeFreitas insisted it must be done, there remained a tantalizing chance of success. The Wistar scientist called Walter Gunn and described the new proposal to him.

Gunn was unsentimental about the motives of his former colleagues. "I advised her that it was a trap," he said later. Gunn suggested strongly to DeFreitas that she ask for a third, independent molecular biologist to be included in the collaboration. The agency, he pointed out, had devised the study in a manner that allowed them to undermine her once again. "I said it would only be the CDC doing the testing, and they don't know how to do the test, so it will definitely come out negative. Then they could wrap this whole thing up."

Gunn suspected the agency had proposed the study to circumvent the possibility that DeFreitas would raise the matter of the patients' selection criteria in a public forum. After all, she could hardly gripe that the patients in question weren't well selected if they were the same patients she had called positive for retroviral fragments in her 1990 paper. If Gunn was correct, then, the latest proposal was less a scientific inquiry than an offensive weapon in the agency's growing armament against the Wistar scientist. If the CDC opened the collaboration to a third scientist, however, its "sure thing" might be less certain.

DeFreitas, as a result, countered the agency's proposal with a request that a third investigator be brought into the collaboration; she asked that some of the blood be sent to C. V. Herst, the molecular biologist at Oncore Analytics in Houston. Folks and Schonberger rejected DeFreitas's request on the grounds that Oncore Analytics was a commercial lab.

Finally, when DeFreitas read a draft of the protocol devised by Folks and Schonberger, any possibility of a continued collaboration faded entirely. In DeFreitas's view, the government's new proposal was as high-handed and unfair as any she had seen.

Most glaringly, the agency insisted that on all publications stemming from the collaborative study, the disease that had afflicted Bell's patients would be called "idiopathic chronic fatiguing illness in Lyndonville, New York." Clearly the government sought to avoid an association between the contagious, incurable viral disease and the benign-sounding "chronic fatigue syndrome." Folks and Schonberger justified their nomenclature to DeFreitas with the argument that Bell had diagnosed the Lyndonville children before the agency's definition of CFS was published, an argument she found absurd. In addition, she recognized it as a tool by which the government could manipulate her own claim that the retroviral marker was specific for CFS; the agency's name transformed the meaning and scale of her discovery from macro to micro.

In a long written response to the agency regarding its protocol, a letter DeFreitas later described as "asbestos-gloved," the scientist fairly spat her objection: "By analogy, this reasoning would suggest that no one ever suffered from multiple sclerosis or lupus before the symptoms of these syndromes were published."

DeFreitas also seized upon another disparity in the government's plan. Folks and Schonberger, no doubt weary of DeFreitas's criticism of their methods, had inserted into their protocol the caveat that "the specifics of the techniques used to detect these [retroviral] sequences [would be revealed] at their discretion." In other words, Folks's team would not be obliged to tell DeFreitas or anyone else how they had achieved their results, leaving DeFreitas and others without a means of assessing the validity of the government's assays.

"I find it interesting," DeFreitas wrote, "that now, after I have supplied Dr. Tom Folks at CDC with all the written protocols for our methods . . . that we used in our original published study, plus all the details of our viral isolation studies yet to be published, the CDC has now decided, as stated in this protocol on p. 9, that the specifics of the technique used to detect these sequences [will be revealed] at their discretion. Since I have revealed all my techniques, only CDC's techniques would be in question, yet they have no obligation to discuss the differences between our and CDC's experimental protocols.

"On the same topic," she added, "Dr. Folks has told me that this procedure can be completed in three days, while ours requires six to ten days. Clearly he is not using the same procedure we are."

In their protocol, Folks and Schonberger had further dictated that all polymerase chain reaction experiments had to be completed in four weeks; the results had to be sent to Atlanta four weeks after receipt of blood specimens. The protocol decreed that agency staff would break the code "after written reports from both laboratories are received or at four weeks, whichever comes first."

DeFreitas commented: "This deadline would allow Dr. Folks, using a three-day assay, considerably more opportunity to replicate his results than my lab, using our published six- to ten-day assay."

DeFreitas also questioned the timing of the agency's recent overture to her, coming as it did just as the agency's investigators were readying their paper refuting her own 1990 report in the *Proceedings of the National Academy of Sciences,* and in spite of the fact that Folks had discovered a possibly novel retrovirus of his own by accident (Gunn had apprised DeFreitas of the contamination occurring in Folks's laboratories).

The Wistar scientist ended with an angry declaration of independence from the agency: "My only conclusion from these series of interactions with CDC is that despite our continued efforts at communication and collaboration on the potential involvement of a retrovirus in chronic fatigue syndrome, CDC's position will continue to undermine a fair assessment of the topic. The short-range effects of this attitude will unfortunately be borne by those afflicted with the illness, but I believe the longer-range consequences will be CDC's to bear. Therefore, my laboratory will not be collaborating with CDC on this protocol."

DeFreitas sent copies of her letter to Bell and Paul Cheney as well as to CFIDS Association president Marc Iverson, Anthony Komaroff, Tulsa philanthropist Ed Taylor, Walter Gunn, and members of the National CFS Advisory Council.

Privately she said, "It is inconceivable to me that [the CDC] could be considering publishing a study refuting my work when they themselves are growing a retrovirus. Folks told me that because they haven't characterized it they can't write about it," an explanation that failed to mollify her.

Upon receipt of DeFreitas's tie-severing letter, Folks and Schonberger called David Bell in Boston, hoping he might influence DeFreitas in their favor. Bell, however, barely entertained the government scientists' overture. "Elaine's letter," Bell told them, "is self-explanatory."

On April 15, two days after receiving a fax of DeFreitas's letter, Folks, Schonberger, and Ali Kahn sent another letter to DeFreitas in which they regretted "several important misunderstandings." The agency scientists went on to ask that DeFreitas reconsider her decision to withdraw. "Confirming the association you reported could lead to public health measures to prevent and treat this devastating illness and," they wrote, "stimulate our obtaining new resources and personnel to expedite our studies."

DeFreitas, bitter and distrustful, was unmoved by their appeal. "I'm as disappointed about it as I can be," she said later. "I really thought that the rumors about CDC having a bias against this disease—and that's what I thought they were: rumors—were unfounded. I felt that these people were epidemiologists and virologists and that they would want to know as much as *we* wanted to know, that they would have the same curiosity. But I really have to say now that that's the case—the agency is biased. It took a long time for the world to fall on me, but when I read that protocol, it was right there. They were stacking all the cards in favor of negative data.

"I know for a fact that if I had had a crystal ball in 1988 and could have seen even a few of the events to come, I would have run for the hills," DeFreitas continued. "But I'm still curious. *We* are still curious. We want to get some answers. And we are so close—that's what's fueling us."

Washington, D.C.

The bias that DeFreitas observed at the CDC was reflected in the ranks of many doctors who, seven years after the Tahoe outbreak, continued to be ill equipped, intellectually and emotionally, to cope with the rising phenomenon of CFS in their clinics. A 1992 survey conducted by clinical psychologist Leonard Jason of DePaul University suggested that close to 40 percent of CFS patients eventually dropped out of mainstream medicine altogether. Brutalized by their reception in doctors' examining rooms, they ceased consulting doctors, preferring instead to wait out their disease away from the medical profession's unhelpful counsel.

Wells Goodrich, a clinical professor of psychiatry at Georgetown University, was increasingly disturbed by what he viewed as doctors' abdication of their professional duty to CFS sufferers. Goodrich's wife, also a psychiatrist, had become severely ill with CFS in 1988. As his wife consulted doctor after doctor in the Washington region, Goodrich was troubled by clinicians' callous responses to her devastating medical problems. She, meanwhile, slid deeper into disability. The couple turned to purveyors of alternative therapies like acupuncture and megavitamins; the therapies failed to effect a cure, but they were dispensed with a degree of humanity and compassion, Goodrich said, that eased his wife's psychic pain considerably. The experience, he recalled later, "broadened my view of medicine." In addition, he admitted, the experience left him angry.

On May 3, Goodrich felt compelled to speak out on the subject in a forum of his peers: the annual meeting of the American Academy of Psychoanalysis, the more liberal of two national organizations devoted to psychoanalysis. Goodrich had entered medicine in the late 1940s as a researcher at the NIH and had watched as the ascendancy of medical technology displaced the humanistic clinical values of William Osler's era. "Thirty or forty years ago," he said, "most physicians assumed that if a patient was in pain, something should be done to try to understand at least part of the pathophysiology. Some . . . supportive interventions were expected of the physician, however incomplete his understanding of the patient's disease happened to be. Unfortunately, this viewpoint is no longer common." When confronted by patients who could offer little evidence for their dilemma besides their subjective experience, doctors became defensive and adopted "avoidance" behaviors, treating their CFS patients with "neglect or even contempt," Goodrich noted.

There was an obvious precedent for the mistreatment of CFS sufferers, he continued. "We know that the stage of medical confusion for AIDS lasted five years," he said, "from 1978 to 1983, by which time both the National Institutes of Health and the Centers for Disease Control had acknowledged its existence." Prior to 1983, however, AIDS victims suffered from the same negligence to which CFS patients were now subjected. Goodrich cited the experience of a pediatrician who in 1979 presented to the Bronx Medical Society a series of seventy infants born to drug-addicted mothers. "He concluded these infants suffered from AIDS," Goodrich said. "He was laughed off the medical society podium, since the doctors who listened to his presentation were then in the process of trying to accept that AIDS was a disease of male homosexuals.

"Now there are twice as many chronic fatigue–immune deficiency syndrome patients in the world as there are AIDS patients," Goodrich added. "Unlike AIDS, only a few [CFS] patients die. When they do die, it is of suicide, overwhelming infection, or cancer secondary to immune deficiency. A case can be made that CFS is a worse disease than AIDS, at least for the fifty percent of cases that are severe, since these patients' lives are totally disrupted by pain, mental confusion, physical weakness, and other manifestations of central nervous system inflammation. Such patients often envy AIDS patients who can anticipate eventual relief of symptoms through death."

Goodrich was worried he might be pelted with rotten tomatoes after his speech, but he was, as he phrased it, "showered with lilies" instead. During the course of his presentation, the audience more than doubled in size; when he ended, he was surrounded by fellow psychiatrists who confessed that they either suffered from the disease themselves or had spouses or other close relatives who did. Several other psychiatrists complained that they had struggled to find suitable medical doctors for their CFS patients, but had been stymied by the dearth of clinicians willing to help such patients. "It was remarkable," Goodrich recalled afterward.

In addition, although he had published more than fifty research papers during his long career, none of his previous papers had generated as many requests for reprints or as much general interest as did his May 3 speech to his professional association.

Atlanta, Georgia

Since the Sarasota meeting, Gunn's plan to engage David Bell and Elaine DeFreitas in a study of Lyndonville children had become more elaborate. He had expanded the study to include a group of adult CFS sufferers who were patients in the clinical practice of Susan Levine in New York City. An internal medicine and immunology specialist, Levine had become interested in the disease in 1987 during her residency at Sloan Kettering Memorial Cancer Center in New York. She began seeing victims in her private practice in 1988; by 1995 two thousand patients in Levine's practice were CFS sufferers. Gunn had invited C. V. Herst in Houston to test specimens for the retroviral marker, too. If all went according to plan, then, blood samples from adult sufferers in Manhattan and adolescent sufferers in Lyndonville would be tested for evidence of retrovirus infection in Wistar's laboratories in Philadelphia, Herst's in Houston, and Martin's in Los Angeles.

The CFIDS Association of Charlotte, supported entirely by contributions from patients and wealthy philanthropists, would foot the bill for the study. "We have to pay for the original research," CFIDS Association head Marc Iverson complained. "Then we have to pay for the research to *confirm* the original research."

Wistar Institute, Philadelphia, Pennsylvania

On April 30, Elaine DeFreitas informed the scientists at the CDC that she and David Bell had chosen to perform their own blinded study "with Dr. Walter Gunn as principal investigator." She then invited the agency to join the new study: "If CDC would like to participate . . . the samples can be divided into four aliquots with one going to Dr. Folks's lab." She asked the agency to advise her or Gunn of its decision, "since sample collection will begin in early June 1992."

Centers for Disease Control, Atlanta, Georgia

Tom Folks, Larry Schonberger, and Ali Kahn responded to DeFreitas's letter on May 8. Decorously, Folks and his colleagues turned down DeFreitas's invitation to join the new study being orchestrated by their vexatious former colleague, Walter Gunn. During a conversation the week before, Tom Folks had reported that publication of the paper refuting DeFreitas was "imminent." Moreover, he expected someone from the agency's CFS working group to present their findings at the Ciba Foundation conference on the disease in London during the week of May 11.

Once DeFreitas's findings had been dispensed with, Folks said, his lab would aggressively pursue the retroviral theory of the disease. But he cautioned that the search for the cause of CFS was "going to take years."

"When did we first recognize AIDS as a clinical entity?" he asked rhetorically. "It was '81. The etiology wasn't recognized until '84. It took a long time—and that was an *easy* one! There were clear markers—CD-four cells dropped; the end point was death. You don't have that with these patients. The fact that people are finding little hints of a virus here and there is great, but you don't want to chase a falsehood or an artifact. The investigation of this disease is at the early, formative stage."

U.S. Senate, Washington, D.C.

Lobbyist Tom Sheridan had asked his staff to determine what should have been a simple number: the amount of money being spent on CFS research each year at the National Institute of Allergy and Infectious Diseases. He needed the figure for a report he was writing on the federal government's response to the CFS epidemic, which he planned to release in October at a medical conference on the disease in Albany, New York. Considering the matter routine, Sheridan sent a staff member, Kristin O'Connell, to Bethesda to speak to Stephen Straus, who was, after all, the head of the Laboratory of Clinical Medicine at NIAID and the self-acknowledged chief of CFS research at his institute. Straus agreed to see O'Connell, but upon her arrival he asked her who was funding the Sheridan Group's lobbying efforts. When she named the CFIDS Association of Charlotte, Straus announced he would provide no information about money expenditures at the National Institutes of Health until the patient organization offered him an apology for its newsletter's coverage of his research, as well as a written promise never to criticize him again.

When O'Connell returned to the Sheridan Group's offices on T Street and told Sheridan what Straus had said, Sheridan thought she was joking. When she persuaded him that she had reported Straus's words accurately, Sheridan decided to call Straus himself.

The government scientist was no less adamant with the lobbyist. "Straus said the information would not be available," Sheridan said later. "He said, and I *quote,* 'I require a letter of apology.' "

Faced with Straus's recalcitrance, Sheridan decided to respond in kind. "I said, 'You can tell me or you can tell the U.S. Congress *why* you wouldn't tell me,' " Sheridan recalled. "And I told him I would quote his remarks in our description of NIH activities in our report in Albany."

Straus terminated his conversation with the lobbyist without capitulating, but the scientist then called Ann Schleuderberg, the CFS grant administrator in his institute. Sheridan soon heard from Schleuderberg, who struggled to make light of Straus's behavior, dismissing it as the predictably emotional reaction of a redhead.

"Schleuderberg is a very well trained bureaucrat," Sheridan said. "She understood this was a problem, that this was not going to be good politically. I told her, 'If [Straus] wants to play that game, I will play hardball.' "

Sheridan later mused, "I don't want to ruin this man's career, but he's got to understand that he's a public employee and is accountable to the public. He is obviously a very resistant, angry, personally offended, and personally possessed person. In science, there's no room for that."

Schleuderberg headed off Sheridan's threat with a promise to submit the financial information her colleague had refused to provide. In time, she told Sheridan that the intramural CFS research effort at the National Institute of Allergy and Infectious Diseases, being orchestrated by principal investigator Straus, cost $946,225 in 1991.

Sheridan's education in the politics of CFS did not end with the Straus incident. He was becoming increasingly aware, as well, that accounting practices employed by government scientists who claimed to be researching the disease were nebulous at best. In preparation for his report in Albany, for instance, Sheridan had dispatched Kristin O'Connell to Atlanta to inquire into the CDC's expenditures on the disease. While staff at the Atlanta agency addressed the matter with considerably more grace than had Straus, "the information left something to be desired," Sheridan reported. "The actual dollar figure they report is higher than the activity around the disease [would indicate]." When Sheridan tallied up the numbers submitted to him by the CDC and NIH, he found the federal government claimed to have spent, altogether, $6 million in 1991 to investigate CFS. "We can add up only about four million dollars' worth of project work," Sheridan commented that fall. "What happened to the two million?" he continued. "This is thirty-three percent of publicly claimed CFIDS expenditures. What happened to that money?"

Sheridan had been a lobbyist for AIDS organizations for seven years. He was used to focusing his efforts on one primary goal for his clients: acquiring more money for research. As a result of his experiences of the past year, however, Sheridan now realized that CFS presented a more complicated dynamic. Appropriating money in ever-larger sums to the CDC and the NIH was probably not going to help victims if the research effort was spearheaded by the same scientists who had been controlling the government's investigation for the last decade. Years of struggle by patient activists, for instance, had forced the CDC to launch a surveillance system; but overwhelming bias among the scientists who designed the system ensured that the true magnitude of the epidemic was unlikely to be revealed, in spite of multimillion-dollar expenditures. Straus's work, which cost taxpayers about three-quarters of a million dollars every year, had served only to propagate the view throughout mainstream medicine that the disease was a psychological disorder. In short, the small sums patients had been able to pry out of Congress for the health agencies had been used by those agencies primarily to perpetuate misconceptions about the disease.

"This situation is actually . . . unique," Sheridan admitted in a conversation that fall. "I have told my clients: 'I can go to the Congress and get more money for the National Institutes of Health and the Centers for Disease Control. But before we ask Congress for money, let's get an infrastructure in government that is *helpful* to you rather than hurtful. There is no point in asking the government to spend money that will ultimately harm your goals. Your advocacy efforts have to be smartly done, and that may mean reforming institutions that are not working *before* you give them money.' "

Sheridan had added CFS to his firm's portfolio, he said, because he had been impressed with the dedication and intelligence of the patient activists he met. The politics surrounding the disease, in addition, were familiar to him. "I've fought these battles before," he said. Nothing had prepared Sheridan for the degree of opposition he was encountering on CFS, however. He remarked on the fact that, while the Food and Drug Administration deliberated over HEM Pharmaceuticals' application for expanded clinical trials, doctors had been lobbying agency officials, demanding that the government prevent CFS patients from obtaining Ampligen. "I'm always surprised by the level of antagonism the opposition demonstrates," Sheridan said, "but I've never seen *that* level of vitriol, not even in AIDS," the lobbyist said.

Ciba Foundation, London, England

Gregory Bock, deputy director of the Ciba Foundation and organizer of the foundation's conference on CFS, had struggled to keep the meeting exclusive. Bock allowed just twenty-five people to attend the week-long gathering, which began on May 11 in Ciba headquarters at 41 Portland Place in London. Bock had appointed the NIH's Stephen Straus co-chairman of the event, along with Harvard psychiatrist Arthur Kleinman, who, like Straus, had written a paper on depression in the disease.[1]

Moderating the conference was Toronto history professor Edward Shorter, whose recent book had called the disease a sham. Invited to place chronic fatigue in historical perspective, Shorter inaugurated the meeting by portraying CFS as a contemporary manifestation of the "hysterical" diseases afflicting women in every century, supporting his argument with slides of centuries-old illustrations.

Walter Gunn, in London to describe the CDC's surveillance data, was sickened by Shorter's contribution. "He showed pictures of naked women with their limbs twisted in paralysis. If I had been a woman, I would have walked out," Gunn said, adding, "It was all opinion. He has no data. His take is that the epidemic is due to press publicity."

The symposium's membership was top-heavy with psychiatrists. "It was very tedious listening to all the bullshit," Gunn commented later with uncharacteristic abandon. "I said that if we listened to the psychiatrists, we'd still be treating lupus with psychotherapy," he added. "Occasionally people would get up and present evidence to show that it's an organic disease. What seemed to be coming up was that maybe there's something organic about mental illness."

When it became clear Elaine DeFreitas would not attend the Ciba Foundation's 173d symposium, the CDC's Tom Folks was asked to fill the vacuum. Folks, afforded less than five days' notice, recalled that he went from the plane directly to the Ciba Foundation's stage in London to read his paper.*

Gunn listened intently as the agency retrovirologist described his team's efforts to replicate the Wistar finding.[2] Folks said he had not only failed to find evidence of the retroviral fragments DeFreitas had described two years earlier, but he had also searched without success for regions of bovine leukemia virus, simian retroviruses, types one and two, simian T-cell leukemia virus, and human spuma virus.

"The lack of a positive signal from patients and controls using these primers and probes does not rule out completely their presence either as a primary etiology or [as] co-factors," Folks said. "It merely indicates that we could not locate the signal. However, it does imply that, if present, the frequency must be extremely low."

Judiciously, Folks qualified his report, suggesting that it hardly exculpated the role of retrovirus in CFS patients. "Our inability to identify CFS patients from controls using these retroviral markers could possibly be due to a difference in study populations," he said. "Second, the retroviral primers we used still leaves open the possibility for another known or unidentified retrovirus as the etiology using other primers. And lastly, if the retrovirus is only transiently present in [white blood cells] or resides primarily in other tissues, then absence of a retroviral signal in our study would not preclude the presence of a retrovirus."

But Folks did not hesitate to point out that five groups had by then tried and failed to replicate the Wistar finding.

When Folks was finished speaking, Gunn challenged him: "I mentioned the autoradiograph that had all of David Bell's Lyndonville patients positive on DeFreitas's marker as well as four out of six Atlanta patients. Folks responded that the finding had been due to contamination."

---

* Much later, Folks commented, "I got off the plane, walked on the stage, and presented the data, and it's been downhill for retroviruses and CFS ever since."

Gunn sensed that DeFreitas's standing was all but crushed by Folks's report. "She's destroyed in the eyes of everyone there. Straus, Folks, and others there concluded that DeFreitas is *done*," Gunn said.

Privately, Gunn was becoming concerned about the consequences of his study to determine if DeFreitas, John Martin, and C. V. Herst were working with the same pathogen. What if the results indicated that the DeFreitas finding was an anomaly that could not be repeated? After investing so heavily in the Wistar work in particular and the retroviral theory in general, would the large patient organization be willing to admit defeat and change the direction of its research funding?

"Science writes itself," Gunn said. "Eventually it will all be sorted out. But what if she's *not* right? What if it turns out that she and Martin and Herst can't differentiate cases from controls? What if there is no retrovirus? What then?"

And though he did not give voice to his thoughts, Gunn had to have been thinking about the implications for his own credibility should the new study produce negative results.

Washington, D.C.

Spring in the capital brought with it the usual round of testimony by federal health agency officials to Senate and House appropriations subcommittees and the by now ritual equivocations to Congress about the state of CFS research inside those agencies. CDC director William Roper's written testimony in response to questions by Congressman John Porter of the House Appropriations Subcommittee on Labor, Health and Human Services, submitted to the committee in May, was no exception.

"Dr. Roper, how many Americans suffer from CFS?" Porter asked.

"A preliminary estimate based on our ongoing surveillance system," Roper responded, "is that approximately ten thousand persons over age eighteen in the United States meet the CDC case definition of chronic fatigue syndrome."

Roper had not written the CFS testimony; its authors were high-ranking members of the agency's CFS working group—"sneering committee" members, as Walter Gunn had once dubbed the obstreperous group.

Ten thousand people was less than half of the membership of the Charlotte-based CFIDS Association, approximately half of the membership of a Kansas City–based national patient organization, and slightly less than half of the past membership of the defunct Portland-based patient organization. Ten thousand people was, in addition, half the number of people suffering from the disease who wrote to the CFIDS Association *in a typical month.* Just three months earlier, on March 5, the Charlotte group had received 15,000 calls about the disease after its toll-free telephone number was momentarily flashed on the TV screen at the conclusion of a Christian Broadcasting Network report on the disease.

Roper's prevalence estimate, in addition, was equivalent to the number of telephone calls from CFS sufferers to his agency in a typical five-month period. It approximated, too, the number of patients in the combined clinical practices of a handful of the most prominent CFS experts, doctors such as Paul Cheney, Dan Peterson, Jay Goldstein, Carol Jessop, Mark Loveless, and Susan Levine—none of whom, except Dan Peterson, had been afforded the opportunity to refer patients into the agency's surveillance system. Of the approximately sixty CFS patients Peterson referred to the agency from his practice, the doctor said, "seven or eight made it through the gauntlet" as government-approved CFS sufferers.

Walter Gunn estimated that more than 75 percent of CFS patients referred into the system were eventually eliminated by the agency through one means or another. When the retired investigator learned of Roper's estimate he commented cheerfully: "Totally incorrect. It's only off by a factor of ten. Nobody's perfect!"

Paul Cheney, who had been following the government's head count, was privately dismissive of the data. "It may be the greatest underestimate of all time," he said. "It means that, certainly, I have all the cases in the state of North Carolina in my practice. I spoke to a support group in Monroe, Louisiana, recently. Four hundred patients came to that support group. There were people being pushed into the auditorium in wheelchairs. Now, the disease is there, in a small town, by the hundreds if not the thousands. And there may be a *thousand* times that amount with subclinical illness."

Porter veered into money matters as well, his questions harder-hitting than in past years, a reflection of the growing involvement of patient advocates and lobbyists in the appropriations process. Porter wondered why the agency's budget justification for the year just past failed to include references to any of the congressional directives regarding use of the money. Included in these directives were a "prompt team reaction to CFS outbreaks which may occur," "conducting a national CFS prevalence survey to provide national prevalence estimates of CFS in the general population," and "conducting a survey of CFS in health professionals."

"Why does the budget justification omit reference to these important items?" Porter asked.

"Our current chronic fatigue syndrome program addresses all suggestions," Roper said, for the second year in a row violating the law against lying to Congress. "We provide prompt team reactions to possible CFS outbreaks." He added, "As detailed in previous responses, the request for a national prevalence survey is premature. . . . At present there is no reason to expand beyond the current sites."

Porter pressed Roper on the issue of cluster outbreaks, asking him to describe the agency's efforts and to tell the committee whether those efforts were adequate. The query pressed the hapless authors of Roper's testimony to the wall, since there was nothing to describe. Apparently gambling that legislators and patient organizations were too dim to notice, Roper touted the Atlanta epi-aid study—an efficient way to acquire blood from local CFS sufferers in the agency's effort to replicate or repudiate the Wistar finding—as a response to a cluster outbreak. He also noted that the agency had been "contacted regarding a possible outbreak on the Pacific coast." What Roper did not say was that the person doing the contacting had been none other than the assistant secretary for health and Roper's predecessor, James Mason, who had called out of concern for the young Mormon missionaries who reportedly had contracted the disease in California. Nor did he tell Porter that the CDC had chosen not to investigate this outbreak.

When Porter sought details of how the 1991 appropriation of nearly $3 million had been spent, the agency head responded with a vague "estimated budget breakdown," which claimed that $30,000 had been spent on travel related to the disease. The agency also claimed $1 million worth of charges to laboratory supplies and equipment, a sum Gunn later scoffed at. "They ran tests on twenty patients that year," he said.

Herpes branch chief and now CFS principal investigator William Reeves also testified before Porter's committee about his branch's research into the disease. As Elaine DeFreitas had predicted, Reeves touted the agency's collaboration with her before Congress, going on at some length about the government's labors and its commitment to finding the cause of the disease. DeFreitas, when she read Reeves's testimony, was particularly incensed that Reeves had made his self-aggrandizing presentation to Congress while his colleague, Tom Folks, was busy in London discrediting her work.

Porter questioned Bethesda officials on the same subject that spring. When he asked Anthony Fauci, director of the National Institute of Allergy and Infectious Diseases, if the agency needed more money to fund extramural grants, however, Fauci said that his institute did not, because "the pool of experienced investigators in the CFS field remains small. We are trying to attract new researchers by stimulating interest through workshops, publications, and program announcements. As the number of investigators increases," Fauci added, "the availability of resources will become more important."

Porter then asked Fauci if the institute needed more money for its intramural investigations.

"We have expanded our intramural program to a level that we feel is appropriate, given the state of the science and staff commitments in this area," Fauci assured Roper, in effect turning down Porter's offer of additional money.

Chicago, Illinois

CDC director William Roper's underestimate of the number of Americans afflicted with chronic fatigue syndrome was less than surprising given the nature of the government's surveillance system. Relying on doctors to report cases of a disease, as the government had done to obtain its prevalence data in CFS, was such an unreliable method of measuring prevalence that health departments rarely employed it. Fran Taylor, for example, infectious diseases chief for the city of San Francisco, noted in 1988 that designating a disease a "reportable disease"—that is, one that doctors were required to report to the local health department—rarely produced statistics reflective of the true number of cases. "These ordinances are very poorly complied with by physicians," she said. "Only those doctors who have a particular interest in the disease report, and sometimes even *they* don't."

The CDC's Larry Schonberger, an experienced epidemiologist who had studied at the Johns Hopkins School of Public Health, the nation's premier training ground for epidemiologists, surely knew the drawbacks to doctor-based surveillance programs when he conceived the agency's CFS surveillance plan. More particularly, he had to have known how poorly a disease like CFS would fare in such a study; after all, most doctors had been taught to believe that CFS did not exist, and few were competent to diagnose it. In committing the government to doctor-based surveillance, Schonberger had selectively ignored a second means of measuring the prevalence of a disease, a method that epidemiologists universally recognized as the more accurate system: turning directly to the population itself. D. A. Henderson, investigating the Punta Gorda epidemic in 1959, used this method, literally going from door to door in the little Florida town with a team of epidemiologists to unearth cases; in this fashion, Henderson had found many more cases than had been diagnosed by local doctors.

During his final two years at the Atlanta agency, Walter Gunn had repeatedly asked that his agency undertake a population-based method of surveillance. He proposed, for instance, that the agency perform a random telephone survey of several thousand American households, looking for people suffering from the sign-symptom complex of the disease as defined by the agency's own diagnostic criteria. Citizens whose responses suggested a possible case, Gunn had suggested, could be investigated further. There was nothing unconventional about Gunn's proposal. Random-digit dialing, as the practice was known, was a standard tool of modern epidemiology; in addition, he was proposing to use the agency's own Physicians Review Committee to arbitrate suspected cases. Yet Schonberger, disregarding the annual directive of Congress to use money appropriated to the agency for national prevalence studies, had repeatedly vetoed Gunn's idea.

By 1992, however, researchers had emerged in the private sector who believed that ascertaining true prevalence rates in the American population was both crucial and within the means of contemporary epidemiology. Leonard Jason, a clinical psychologist at DePaul University in Chicago, was at the center of a collaborative group of epidemiologists, statisticians, and doctors at Northern Illinois University, the University of Illinois Medical Center, and DePaul who were attempting to measure the prevalence of CFS by eliminating doctor-intermediaries. Jason himself had fallen ill with the disease in 1989 at the age of forty. An investigator who had served on grant review panels for the National Institute of Mental Health in Bethesda and been the recipient of $3 million in federal research grants, Jason was leveled and took a leave of absence from DePaul. When he returned in a state of partial recovery eighteen months later, he was stirred by the idea of attempting a population-based prevalence study.

Like Walter Gunn, Jason and his collaborators were especially cognizant of the seeming high number of cases of CFS among nurses and doctors. They were aware, too, of the early literature on "epidemic neuromyasthenia," which revealed that medical workers, especially hospital employees in close contact with patients, exhibited the highest rates of the disease during community outbreaks.* Jason's team decided to perform a preliminary prevalence study among nurses. They obtained a random sampling of 3,400 nurses' names and addresses from the Illinois Nurses Association and the American Holistic Nurses Association. Forty-three percent of these nurses returned a questionnaire mailed to them by Jason and

---

* Although he did not report a clear-cut cluster, retired surgeon Thomas English of Asheville, North Carolina, lobbied the CDC's William Reeves that year about the contagion issue, without success. "There are a number of people around me who fell ill," English recalled later. "We cut our fingers in the operating room all the time. It's why I've stopped practicing—there is no way I'm going to risk putting someone else through what I've been through. I wrote to the damn CDC," English continued. "I tried to talk to them about this, but all they would say is, 'We can't investigate unless the state invites us.' Yet, I know a [CFS sufferer] who has a letter from Bill Reeves advising her not to give blood."

his collaborators. Of those 1,474 nurses, 202 checked a box indicating they had suffered extreme, debilitating fatigue for six months or more. Subsequent questioning revealed that at least 70 of them appeared to have bona fide CFS by the government's own definition.

Jason's research produced sharply higher prevalence rates than the Atlanta agency's: 680 cases per 100,000 people, in contrast to the CDC's average of 3.5 cases for every 100,000 people in the nation. And although Jason conceded that the prevalence data among nurses might not be pertinent to the population at large, he suggested that the data had intrinsic value for all interested researchers. "If rates of CFS-related symptoms among nurses are as high as the study suggests, then nurses might be a high-risk group," Jason said. "Future studies might be focused on identifying possible etiological agents."

Jason and his collaborators were eager to expand their prevalence studies beyond nurses to the Chicago community at large, using random-digit telephone dialing. They would be unable to proceed without money, however. That spring they sent a grant proposal to Ann Schleuderberg at the National Institute of Allergy and Infectious Diseases.

"If it gets funded," Jason said, "it will be the first community-based prevalence study that will not rely on physicians as intermediaries but will go directly to individuals."

Incline Village, Nevada

Dan Peterson's despair over the state of medical progress on CFS continued that summer. "I don't think this is getting better," he said in June. "I think it's going backward. Everybody selectively ignores evidence, like sky-high cytokines, brain lesions. I just sent one of my patients to UCSF. She had *huge* brain lesions. She saw a world-famous neurologist there. She came away with a psyche diagnosis."

For Peterson, the failure of mainstream medicine to grasp the severity of the problem after so many years was almost incredible. This lack of resolution struck Peterson as surreal. "It reminds me of those [Ingmar] Bergman flicks that just end—you're left sitting there in the dark," he said.

Prospects for the legalization of Ampligen had faded as well, Peterson believed. "We're never going to see Ampligen as a commercially available drug," Peterson continued. "Never. [FDA head] David Kessler is a tough cookie. He won't let Ampligen sneak by. HEM will run out of money, and that will be the end of it."

Centers for Disease Control, Atlanta, Georgia

On June 10, Brian Mahy, director of the agency's viral diseases division, wrote Giovanni Rovera, the new director of the Wistar Institute. "During the past year, we have committed considerable resources" to the Wistar replication effort, Mahy advised Rovera. Deftly, Mahy described the ill-fated collaboration in terms that left DeFreitas looking manipulative and recalcitrant. Agency scientists, meanwhile, emerged as paragons of reason. Much later, DeFreitas characterized the letter as "basically a veiled attempt to put me in political jeopardy at my institution," adding, "This was my *collaborator!*"

Mahy also advised Rovera that his agency was "preparing a peer-reviewed scientific article on the results of our attempts to detect HTLV2-like sequences and retroviral risk factors in CFS patients. We would like to include Dr. DeFreitas as an author, but if she disagrees, we intend to omit her part of the study from the manuscript. I hope that this would meet with your approval."

Mahy enclosed, "in confidence," a draft of Tom Folks's Ciba Foundation presentation one month earlier.

Sebastopol, California

The patient lobbying organization CACTUS, established the year before, folded in June due to lack of money. Executive director Joan Iten-Sutherland sent a letter to the group's organizing committee enumerating the CACTUS assets on June 17: a cash balance of $2,000, a fax machine, a mailing list, and a wooden shelving unit. "I am in the process of determining whether we have any outstanding obligation to the IRS or the state of California," Iten-Sutherland wrote. Should there be any money left over, Iten-Sutherland promised to send it to the Massachusetts CFIDS Association "to be placed in a fund for PWC [people with CFS] advocacy in Washington." With Iten-Sutherland's letter, the sole patient-staffed lobbying organization for CFS sufferers dissolved, leaving the Tom Sheridan Group, paid for by the Charlotte-based patient association, the only CFS lobbyist in the capital.

Ottawa, Ontario

During the first week of July the Canadian Department of Health and Welfare granted HEM Pharmaceuticals permission to undertake an expanded clinical trial of Ampligen among two hundred Canadians with CFS. The study was identical to the proposal rejected by the U.S. Food and Drug Administration the previous October. As promised, two hundred Canadian patients, or their insurance companies, would be required to pay for the drug and its administration, a cost estimated by some to be $50,000 over the course of the six-month study. Patients would be selected from ten sites across Canada. According to Temple University's Robert Suhadolnik, who had been a HEM collaborator on the firm's AIDS and CFS trials, the Canadian government had committed more than $10 million to the trial, so enthusiastic were Canadian health officials about Ampligen's promise in CFS.

HEM officials, in addition, submitted the data from their 1991 clinical trial in the United States to the *New England Journal of Medicine.*

Canada's ruling was good news for CFS sufferers; the bad news was that HEM Pharmaceuticals was crashing financially. Whether or not the company could stay afloat long enough to carry off an ambitious multi-site clinical trial in Canada remained to be seen. Outsiders were puzzled, however: if the Canadian government and its own CFS patients were footing the bill, why was HEM balking? For the moment the project was in limbo, mysteriously so, and HEM officials weren't talking.

Wistar Institute, Philadelphia, Pennsylvania

By July it was official: Elaine DeFreitas was moving to Florida. She had been awarded a tenured associate professorship at the university. She would take with her all of her laboratory equipment, which had been purchased with funds from NIH grants to study multiple sclerosis and acute T-cell leukemia, and most of her laboratory staff. There were potential complications, however: Miami had granted her lab team non-paid status, which meant DeFreitas would need to support them with grant money. So far, however, the CFIDS Association was providing just $12,000 a month to DeFreitas—as well as $8,000 a month to John Martin and $8,000 a month to Sidney Grossberg, making the Charlotte-based patient organization the only source of funding in the United States to investigate the etiology of the disease.*

That month her grant proposal to the National Institutes of Allergy and Infectious Diseases, which sought government funds to support her research, was turned down.

Early in July, CDC retrovirologist Tom Folks sent Elaine DeFreitas the agency's manuscript describing his lab's unsuccessful efforts to replicate her work. It was the seventh and presumably final draft of the paper, though it remained in an unfinished state. Folks alerted DeFreitas that the manuscript was bound for the *Annals of Internal Medicine.* He asked her permission to add to the article her name and the results of her evaluation of eleven class one Atlanta patients.

DeFreitas found much to criticize in the agency's report, but she was especially incensed by the government's failure to describe its four-tiered system of classifying patients, nor did it describe the selection criteria for the group one patients who were the study subjects. "They don't even say that there could be different phases or stages of the disease," DeFreitas complained. "Stage one *could* be a stage where the virus can't be found in the blood. And, perhaps serendipitously, David [Bell] and Paul [Cheney] tend to send me group four patients."

In the days following her receipt of the agency's draft, DeFreitas was in communication with Walter Gunn. When he read the draft to be submitted to the *Annals,* Gunn's worst expectations were confirmed. "They lied in that article," Gunn said.

And as he had threatened to do, Gunn sat down and wrote a description of government efforts to replicate DeFreitas's discovery. He put the information in the form of a letter to DeFreitas, beginning, "Since the CDC is about to publish their recent study of retroviruses in chronic fatigue syndrome patients, I thought you should know the facts pertaining to their study as observed by me while I was working at CDC as principal investigator for chronic fatigue syndrome studies."

Gunn revealed every detail of the agency scientists' endeavors, unveiling the history for DeFreitas, much of it for the first time. His story poured out over four single-spaced typed pages. It began with the agency's failure to properly prepare the blood specimens, then proceeded to the early positive results of the Lyn-

---

*Paul Cheney had intervened on DeFreitas's behalf and convinced the philanthropy to reinstate her monthly stipend.

donville children. Gunn went on to describe Walid Heneine's departure for a two-week Beirut vacation, a move that had resulted in the freezing of specimens, and then he told of the discovery of a mysterious retrovirus in Folks's lab. He concluded: "Convinced that a fair replication of your study was not possible at CDC, I retired on December 28, 1991, and have been pursuing the evaluation of a retroviral etiology of chronic fatigue syndrome from my own consulting firm."

"She needs this information to defend herself," Gunn said soon after faxing the document to DeFreitas.

"We've discussed what to do," DeFreitas reported, after talking to Gunn. "My game plan is as follows: I wrote a letter to the *Annals* editor. It takes the paper point by point, from a scientific perspective. I said the paper was an inadequate, narrow report that asks more questions than it answers. If they decide to publish the government's paper after reading my letter, then I want them to publish my letter."

With Gunn's blessing, DeFreitas planned to send his letter along with her own to the *Annals* editors. The two braced themselves for the likelihood that their dispute with the CDC would emerge in the popular media if the *Annals* published their letters. DeFreitas, however, hoped that the *Annals* would choose to avoid publication on the subject altogether out of a sense of decorum. The battle raging between the Wistar scientist and the Atlanta agency, complicated further by the apparent defection of a former government scientist, obviously surpassed the bounds of a standard scientific dispute.

In Charlotte, Paul Cheney was dismayed by the CDC's aggressive move. He pointed out that Tom Folks had recently invited Sidney Grossberg, the Wisconsin researcher, to Atlanta to present his retroviral findings in CFS to agency scientists. "To imply that there is *no* evidence for a retrovirus when there is evidence in *three* labs!" Cheney said. "It's the most disingenuous thing. I think Tom Folks's claim goes beyond the fact that he could not replicate the finding with the Wistar probes. He's claiming no other retrovirus by any other mechanism—at the same time that they have a novel retrovirus in their lab. It's almost reckless."

DeFreitas's concern that the agency's group one patients, while bona fide CFS sufferers, might be in a phase of their disease when the virus was difficult or impossible to find struck Cheney as eminently reasonable. He too wondered why the agency was unwilling to investigate any of the other three groups of patients for the virus.

"Something that's become increasingly obvious to David, Elaine, and me is that when patients are improved, or feeling better, we see the biggest signals on PCR [polymerase chain reaction]," Cheney said. "Some of the strongest signals in the early cases came from patients who were less sick than others. Two years later, some patients who had been the sickest improved, and they went from testing negative to testing positive." In the earliest days of his collaboration with DeFreitas, Cheney said, the two were puzzled by the phenomenon. "The first thing we wondered was how can these patients be so sick but negative? What came later, what completed the circle, was that the people who were negative when they were most sick developed an incredibly strong signal as they became better." The volatility of the results among patients in different phases of their disease was hardly exclusive to CFS, Cheney continued. In people infected with HIV, the pathogen was easily recovered at the earliest stages of infection and much later, usually years later, when the patient became terminally ill. In between those two stages, the virus was harder to detect. Viruses causing the common cold were hardest to find just before the cold sufferer recovered.

There was no doubt in Cheney's mind that Elaine DeFreitas had found what she said she had found. He was equally certain that the government scientists had failed to find the Wistar marker out of impatience and ambivalence.

"At the National CFS Advisory Council meeting in Atlanta in September Elaine was very detailed about certain aspects of her procedure," Cheney recalled. "She said she had made a matrix of variables in order to optimize the experiment. And only when it was optimized could she distinguish between the cases and controls. The DNA extraction that she uses is a laborious test that Tom Folks doesn't even do. The magnesium concentrates are extremely important, too. But the thing that's really important is that she found that when she ran the PCR procedure at high stringency, if she kept dropping the temperature, [the primers] would bind to human genes, so *everybody's* result would be positive. But she found there was a window where [the primers] would bind to HTLV, and only the patients would show up positive, not healthy people. The magic window—it comes down to the temperature of the PCR."

Much later, when DeFreitas had been unblinded to the machinations of the agency's investigation, she sought to explain Heneine's negative results. "Tom Folks was so horrified about the low sensitivity that he started to play around with the PCR conditions, and that's where it started to go wrong. He made the stringency so high that the PCR couldn't pick up anything but HTLV-two, and *that's* where he lost the Lyndonville signal."

Some years later, responding to DeFreitas's criticism, Folks said, "That's a good question—why we started mucking around with the primers and probes after we got results the first time. But when we started attempting to repeat it, everything began to turn up low-level positive. Her probe would jump on endogenous material."

In time, both Cheney and DeFreitas would insist the agency's push to publicly repudiate DeFreitas's work was beneath the professionalism of the government's Tom Folks. It had been far too early in the game to dismiss DeFreitas's finding, the two claimed; much additional work needed to be undertaken before making claims about the virus's existence in patients or its relationship to disease. Not long after the agency's move to publish their negative study, Folks was asked why he felt such urgency to do so when there remained so much suggestive evidence for retrovirus infection in the disease. "I feel it's my public responsibility," he said. "Congress told us, 'Here's some money to see if this is real.' And when you invest that level of money, you report it. Also, keep in mind that I have scientists who have invested their careers in their research. I can't tell them that this can't be published. They have to have something to show for their time."

With the passage of years, Folks's answer to the same question changed. In mid-1995, two and a half years after his lab's negative study had appeared in the *Annals of Internal Medicine,* the scientist was more reflective. "If Elaine hadn't been thrown into the limelight the way she had been, it would have made a difference in the way we went after it," he admitted. "Basic science is slow and methodical—you don't rush. But, at the public health level, it can get very scary."

He also revealed that the decision to end the investigation and publish the negative findings had not come from him but from "the second floor" of Building 1, where the CDC's top administrators spend their days. "This was not my decision," Folks said. "This was a CDC decision, as in, 'That's it—we've done it, guys and gals.' [Walter] Dowdle called me," he added. "I didn't have any choice."

It had been Dowdle, then, the agency's second in command, who had defined for Folks the Wistar project's end.

U.S. District Court, Washington, D.C.

On July 8, Prem Sarin, a top administrator and scientist in the Tumor Cell Biology Laboratory of Robert Gallo, was convicted of embezzling $25,000 meant for AIDS research and of lying on government documents to hide his crime.

Sarin was the first federal scientist in Bethesda to whom Paul Cheney had sent blood samples from the Tahoe epidemic. Cheney had asked Sarin to examine the blood for evidence of retroviral infection, but Sarin had studied it for human herpesvirus 6 instead, a discovery that had launched the Gallo laboratory on an investigation of the role of the newly discovered herpesvirus in CFS.

33

HIV-Negative AIDS

Eighth International Conference on AIDS,
Amsterdam, Netherlands

For a decade, two pandemic diseases had been moving through the world's population like a pair of graceless mute beasts on some fantastic migration. Over time, one had become the most public of maladies, its very name—AIDS—an international symbol of death recognized in every language and by every government. The other went by a thousand names—AIDS minor, the Tahoe malady, Lyndonville disease—few of them meaningful to anyone but the sufferers and the clinicians who ministered to them. The first disease sent its victims to the grave; the second suspended them in a twilight between living and dying.

Although there was one clear, indisputable distinction between the two maladies, regions of the borderline between them were increasingly blurred. As imaging technology and biological assays were revealing, the diseases shared a number of brain and immune system abnormalities, most prominently brain lesions and corresponding cognitive deficits, chronic activation of normally latent herpesviruses, and—possibly—infection with a retrovirus. In the summer of 1992 the borderline grew even more ragged.

On July 23, the fourth day of the Eighth International Conference on AIDS, news from a small press conference in Irvine, California, diverted attention from the hundreds of formal papers being presented in Amsterdam. Sudhir Gupta, a University of California immunologist, reported he had isolated particles of a previously unknown retrovirus from an ailing sixty-six-year-old woman, her symptomless daughter, and six other patients. Investigators and the lay press gathered in Holland were riveted by Gupta's announcement that the older woman suffered from an "AIDS-like" condition wherein a component of her immune system, a subset of T-cells called CD4 cells, were severely depleted. In addition, she had suffered a bout of *Pneumocystis carinii* pneumonia, a so-called opportunistic infection that afflicted many AIDS patients whose CD4 cells were depleted. Her thirty-eight-year-old daughter was without symptoms, but on careful analysis she appeared to be experiencing a mild abnormality of the immune system sometimes seen in the earliest, symptomless stages of AIDS.

Taken in isolation, Gupta's announcement might have been dismissed as unimportant. However, as many of the scientists meeting in Amsterdam were aware, other researchers had reported isolated findings of retrovirus particles in HIV-negative patients with AIDS-like symptoms. In the spring, in fact, the CDC had issued a request that all such cases be reported without delay. Gupta's findings were the first to hold up to peer review. His article describing his discovery was scheduled for publication in the *Proceedings of the National Academy of Sciences* in August; complying with the government's request, the *PNAS* editors had released Gupta's paper in July. Gupta's university followed suit with a news conference. If Gupta's discovery was borne out in further studies, it would indicate that yet another retrovirus capable of harming the human immune system was at large—one for which the world's blood banks weren't screening.

Organizers of the Amsterdam meeting immediately convened a three-person panel of experts to respond to the Gupta finding, which had electrified the assembled researchers and press. One of the three experts, co-chairwoman of the National AIDS Commission June Osborne, counseled calm. "The public should not be unduly frightened by a very preliminary report," Osborne said.

Max Essex, a Harvard AIDS researcher, expressed skepticism bordering on ennui. "I'm not overwhelmed by it," he commented after reading the paper. "I'd place the odds at five to ten percent that this might lead to something."

David Ho, director of the Aaron Diamond AIDS Research Center in New York City, was similarly dismissive. "There is absolutely no proof of an association" between the syndrome described by Gupta in his paper and the virus he had isolated, Ho said. Nevertheless, Ho himself had presented a paper at the Amsterdam conference describing his discovery of reverse transcriptase, an enzyme manufactured by retroviruses when they reproduce themselves, in eleven patients with an AIDS-like syndrome who were negative for HIV.[1]

Both Ho and Essex raised the specter of laboratory contamination in the matter of Gupta's findings. Microbes such as Gupta described, they said, were notorious laboratory contaminants and could easily have come from an animal cell line. They also pointed out that such viruses had been described in the literature for more than twenty-five years, but that no link to human disease had been established.

In spite of the cool response of Essex, Osborne, and Ho, Gupta's *PNAS* paper eclipsed virtually all other scientific news at the conference, dominating print and broadcast reports for several days. The editors of the *New York Times* deemed Gupta's paper and the explosion it detonated worthy of a cautionary editorial on July 23, the same day that *Times* medical writer Lawrence Altman filed his story on the subject. "AIDS Puzzle: No Cause for Panic," the editors intoned. Even so, the *Times* recommended that patients considering elective surgery bank their own blood. The newspaper also had harsh words for scientists who kept their discoveries secret prior to publication in scientific journals, and it scolded the CDC, whose scientists reportedly had been sluggish on the conundrum of non–HIV positive AIDS.

The inquiry will not be helped by the disgraceful behavior of some scientists. A few key researchers, apparently eager to gain credit as the discoverers of a new AIDS virus, have not been sharing their data or insights with health officials until their findings are published in scientific journals. And the Centers for Disease Control, normally quick to sound a health alarm, has foolishly been sitting on some early case reports while awaiting the unavailable data.

There is no time to lose in getting to the bottom of this mystery. All scientists with relevant data have an obligation to report their cases to the CDC immediately, and the CDC has an obligation to speed its investigation.

Months before Gupta's press conference, early in the spring, Tom Spira and Bonnie Jones of the CDC's Division of AIDS/HIV had reported on six cases of non–HIV positive AIDS. Doctors had referred the cases to the agency over a two-year period. Jones and Spira's report, which they presented at a small scientific conference in Colorado, contained a brief summary. "HIV may not be the only infectious cause" of immunodeficiency, they stated. Their abstract failed to receive wide circulation among researchers who were studying the worrisome problem of patients with AIDS-like symptoms who tested negative for HIV, and the agency's involvement in the matter seemed to end there.

Just days after the Amsterdam conference, however, researchers and the lay press subjected the CDC and its scientists to a rare condemnation for their failure to respond to the emerging threat. The censure began in Amsterdam and was graphically described by *Times* writer Lawrence Altman, himself a former Epidemic Intelligence Service officer, three days after the conference ended:

> [T]he criticism shouted by participants at the AIDS meeting here was astonishing. It started after Dr. Jeffrey Laurence of Cornell University Medical School in New York City not only reported five cases of an AIDS-like illness but also said he had tantalizing clues suggesting that a new virus might be among them.
>
> Dr. James Curran, the CDC's leading AIDS expert, followed, adding the agency's six cases. He asked aloud whether the CDC should have published them earlier in its widely read weekly report [the *Morbidity and Mortality Weekly Report*], and he also put out a call for doctors to report additional cases. Participants shouted "Yes!" because earlier reporting could have speeded up the recognition and investigation of the problem.
>
> Then a number of European and American scientists stepped forward to report even more cases. The number was small, about two dozen. But the CDC's embarrassment was now huge because the agency had lost control over the dissemination of new information in the field of AIDS.

Altman accused the agency of overlooking "two fundamental principles of public health," which he defined as "swiftly investigating mysterious cases of an illness to determine their cause, and rapidly communicating with the public and scientists to allay alarm about the perceived threat." Here Altman revealed a bias perhaps instilled by his government background. Few things were more alarming to citizens than a perception that the government was trying to "allay alarm" before its scientists had fully grasped the nature of the threat. Given the plethora of unanswered questions raised by the non–HIV positive AIDS cases, any assurances by the government that the public had nothing to fear were premature.

Nevertheless, when the press asked U.S. government officials in Amsterdam about the safety of the blood supply, they received standard assurances that blood banks were capable of excluding any donor with AIDS risk factors. Only one agency official acknowledged the obvious contradiction in such an assurance: James Curran admitted that the risk factors for the new syndrome were unknown. (In fact, as would become apparent in the coming weeks as doctors reported additional cases, few victims of the new syndrome shared the same risk factors that AIDS patients exhibited.) At that point, other agency officials switched their argument: they told the press the blood supply was safe because there were still so few cases of the new syndrome, perhaps no more than thirty. Too many reporters present could recall a period in the early 1980s when federal scientists had dismissed the fear that the few known cases of AIDS would blossom into a pandemic.

When the agency officials were reminded of the early dismissal of the AIDS epidemic, Curran suggested the analogy was misguided. Cases of the new syndrome, he said, were not restricted to any particular region of the country, nor did they seem to be clustered in time, unlike the early AIDS cases. "It's easy to slip into this AIDS mentality because we are talking about it at an AIDS conference and we have AIDS researchers doing the work," Curran said. "This is not AIDS caused by something else."

Curran's words may have been prophetic. Certainly, many CFS researchers were thinking the same thing.

Sudhir Gupta characterized his microbe as an intracisternal retrovirus. "Intracisternal" was another name for foamy, or spuma, retroviruses. Gupta's collaborator, the scientist who had actually performed the laboratory isolation of the virus, was Zaki Salahuddin. The former AIDS researcher had established a lab for himself at the University of Southern California and had been collaborating with Gupta on the emerging puzzle of non–HIV positive AIDS. Like Elaine DeFreitas, Gupta and Salahuddin next needed to clone their new virus and sequence its genetic code in order to fully identify it, a project that could take months or even years.

Not surprisingly, many in the CFS field were gripped by Gupta's report. They wondered whether Gupta's mother-and-daughter subjects were, in fact, CFS sufferers, and whether Salahuddin's latest viral discovery was merely a reprise of Elaine DeFreitas's finding, or perhaps John Martin's. Martin, who was chief of pathology at Salahuddin's university, was a friend of Salahuddin and had discussed his work with the exiled scientist; in fact, the two had called upon the same electron microscopist at the university to help them visualize their respective viruses. Even so, little effort had been expended toward answering questions the CFS research community would have liked answered. In a conversation soon after the Amsterdam conference, Salahuddin admitted that Gupta's and Martin's pathogens looked virtually identical, but he pointed out that most herpesviruses looked alike under an electron microscope, too. When Salahuddin was asked point-blank whether the syndrome being called "non–HIV positive AIDS" might actually be misdiagnosed CFS, he commented, "It's a fair statement, but I'm not a prophet. Time and money [are] required for this. Right now I'm just trying to firm up the virus."

Salahuddin confirmed that he and Gupta, who had a cohort of CFS patients in his clinical practice and who had presented papers on the immunology of CFS at medical conferences on the disease, had discussed the possibility that CFS and non–HIV positive AIDS were the same disease. Gupta, according to Salahuddin, "feels strongly that his two patients in *PNAS* don't have CFS. . . . But *I* don't have a definition of chronic fatigue syndrome. And I don't know two doctors who agree on the definition of chronic fatigue syndrome. It's a nest of hornets!"

It was apparent, too, that the question was unlikely to be resolved anytime soon. Salahuddin had already received a call from Anthony Komaroff, who had asked Salahuddin to test some of the CFS patients in Komaroff's New England practice for the latest retrovirus.

"He's a prince," Salahuddin said of the Harvard researcher, who had written a letter in praise of Salahuddin's scientific talent to the prosecutor at Salahuddin's felony trial in 1989, "but I do not have NIH money. I told Komaroff, 'Look—I love you, but I don't have funds.' "

Charlotte, North Carolina

Paul Cheney was hardly surprised by the news from Amsterdam, and he could well understand the confusion. For years he had observed that some CFS patients met the government's defining criteria for AIDS on every count except infection with human immunodeficiency virus. Early in August, stimulated by the coverage of Gupta's *PNAS* paper, Cheney consulted his computerized database. "I have four patients in this practice who would meet AIDS criteria. Two have CD-four counts below two hundred," the doctor said, referring to the immune system T-cell subset that, when depleted to 200 or less, qualified a person for an AIDS diagnosis by the CDC's latest definition of the disease. In healthy people, CD4 counts were thought to hover somewhere between 800 and 1,200 per cubic millimeter of blood. "Fifteen percent of my patients have CD-four counts below five hundred," he added. It was hardly unheard of, Cheney continued, to diagnose the kinds of opportunistic infections that torment AIDS victims—maladies like thrush, candida, and pneumonia—in CFS sufferers.

His patients with strikingly low T-cell counts and opportunistic infections resembled patients with CFS in all other respects, he said. Their disease had begun as a clear viral syndrome, one that Cheney liked to describe as mono-like, and had evolved, over a period of months and years, just as unmistakably, to a debilitating neurological disease. In addition, unlike AIDS sufferers, who had long periods of remission, sometimes lasting for years, during which they felt well and were able to function, Cheney's CFS patients never felt well. Finally, unlike seriously ill AIDS patients, they had not died. "They're not evolving like HIV. They're evolving like CFIDS," Cheney said.

New York City

New York Native publisher Charles Ortleb viewed with bemusement news of the sudden attention being paid to people who lacked evidence of HIV infection but were suffering from a chronic AIDS-like illness. Ortleb, who for years had conceptualized AIDS patients as a subset of a far vaster epidemic of immune dysfunction affecting the entire population and caused by the casual spread of human herpesvirus 6, felt vindicated, though hardly appeased. In his editorial of August 10, he took issue with the government's position that, because just thirty cases had been reported so far, the syndrome was exceedingly rare. "Actually, the number of cases is not small," Ortleb wrote. "Last week, when Dr. Anthony Fauci of the National Institute of Allergy and Infectious Diseases asked that all cases of HIV-negative AIDS be reported to him, we did our civic duty.

"We reported thirteen million American cases.

"That's one estimate of the number of cases of chronic fatigue and immune dysfunction, a condition that research (if anyone bothers to read it) suggests is essentially HIV-negative AIDS."

National Institute of Allergy and Infectious Diseases, Bethesda, Maryland

The August 15 edition of the *Annals of Internal Medicine* carried a double-barreled blast at chronic fatigue syndrome from the CDC and the National Institute of Allergy and Infectious Diseases. The first, in the letters section, was William Reeves's angry response to the Tahoe manuscript.[2] The second blast came in the form of a report by Ann Schleuderberg, Stephen Straus, and other participants in the NIAID conference the previous March.[3]

Schleuderberg et al. wrote that CFS was "not a homogeneous abnormality," nor was there any "single pathogenic mechanism" among cases. (Such an argument, of course, obviated a public health campaign to control or eliminate the disease.) They offered absolutely no data to support such comments. In addition, they wrote that "no currently existing laboratory tests can be used to confirm the diagnosis of CFS" and that "diagnostic testing in patients with suspected CFS should be done solely to exclude other diagnoses." In addition, they sought to widen the CDC definition to include people with psychiatric disorders, excluding only those with symptoms of schizophrenia, "psychotic depression," manic-depression, and drug abuse. In their final paragraph, Schleuderberg et al. posed this question: "What kinds of research are needed to advance our understanding of CFS?" Because "no convincing evidence exists as yet for a single pathogenic mechanism," they continued, future research should proceed along a "broad range" of disciplines, including psychology and psychiatry. Nowhere in their seven-page report did they endorse additional research into the actual cause—or, as they would prefer, "causes"—of the disease.

They also noted that "no objective physical measure of disability exists." That was because patients with CFS scored so low on any known disability measurement that investigators were forced into "extending the scale(s)," as Philip Peterson of Minneapolis did when CFS sufferers scored on average 16 out of a possible

100 on the Medical Outcome Survey (MOS). With 100 as "best health," such low scores had never before been recorded on the MOS. CFS patients exhibited a significantly greater degree of morbidity than even heart attack sufferers.

"The validity and reliability of such adjustments are unknown," Schleuderberg and her colleagues wrote.

Centers for Disease Control, Atlanta, Georgia

Stories of a second AIDS-like condition and its association with a new retrovirus stayed in the news through the summer, though the tenor of the coverage was beginning to change. On August 2, *New York Times* medical writer Lawrence Altman, reporting from Paris, revealed that Luc Montaigner, the scientist who discovered HIV, had said "there is no evidence of such an association."

On August 15, federal scientists convened a meeting in Atlanta to discuss the emerging health threat of non–HIV positive AIDS. In the three weeks since Sudhir Gupta's paper on his isolation of a new intracisternal retrovirus in a handful of cases, the number of reported cases had risen from approximately thirty to fifty. Nobel prize winners, members of the National Academy of Sciences, CDC's AIDS administrators, and Anthony Fauci, head of the National Institute of Allergy and Infectious Diseases, formed a panel to query scientists Gupta, David Ho of the Aaron Diamond AIDS Center in New York, and Jeffrey Laurence, a Cornell University Medical College cancer and AIDS specialist and associate professor of medicine, each of whom had been studying cases of the syndrome and discovered evidence of retroviral infection in patients. Reporters were admitted to the meeting, a decision that made a number of scientists uncomfortable, Lawrence Altman noted in his report of the meeting. The government's decision to admit the lay press had come reluctantly. "If we didn't have the meeting," Anthony Fauci told Altman, "we would be accused of having a cover-up."

Martha Rogers, a CDC scientist, reported on some of the characteristics of the thirty patients whose cases were under study by the agency. Interestingly, although 96 percent of AIDS sufferers had exhibited risk factors for their disease, such as illicit drug use, fewer than half of the thirty cases did. In addition, most AIDS patients die within two years of developing an AIDS-defining illness such as *Pneumocystis carinii* pneumonia, but the non–HIV positive patients who had suffered such illnesses had survived and remained symptom-free for as long as seven years afterward. Demographic differences among the two groups were perhaps the most striking of all. Thirty percent of the new cases were female; only 11 percent of U.S. AIDS patients were female. Eighty-four percent of the new cases were white, compared to 53 percent for AIDS patients. Finally, 27 percent of the new cases were at least fifty years old; among AIDS victims, just 10 percent were over fifty.

New York City

On August 18, *New York Newsday* reported that at least two of David Ho's seventeen non-HIV AIDS cases had been originally diagnosed with CFS. When queried on the matter some time later, Ho insisted the CFS diagnosis had been made in error.

Charlotte, North Carolina

In mid-August the government diplomatically renamed non-HIV AIDS, calling it "idiopathic CD4 T-lymphocytopenia." The name denoted a dramatic loss of the T-cell subset known as CD4 cells, which until recently had been considered a diagnostic hallmark of AIDS. The new name was immediately shortened by scientists and the press to "ICL." One month earlier, in July, the CDC had instituted a formal surveillance program for ICL, asking infectious disease specialists and other clinicians to report all cases of the syndrome to the agency. They defined the malady in the following manner: the patient must be HIV-negative and score less than 300 in two or more consecutive tests for CD4 cells. The patient's subjective symptoms played no role in the definition, and indeed a few of the ICL patients who had been reported to the agency felt fine.

In Charlotte, Paul Cheney had a number of ICL patients in his CFS practice, none of whom felt remotely well. He had sent blood from one of them to De-Freitas, who reported that the ICL case was "one of the *most* positive people on our assay." Early in September, Cheney decided to analyze—with the aid of a powerful computer and his sizable patient database—the extent of the ICL phenomenon among his CFS patients, with the intent of reporting his findings to the CDC. After extensive analysis, Cheney called the agency's Tom Spira, a scientist in the agency's AIDS/HIV Division, who had been assigned to the ICL investigation. Cheney had limited his focus to the 873 CFS patients who had entered his practice since 1989.

"We put a good deal of analysis into this," Cheney said afterward. "We went through our database and found eighteen people who had CD-four counts below three hundred. Three of these patients had CD-four counts of below two hundred. We also found four additional people who had AIDS-defining opportunistic infections, just one of whom was among the eighteen." The government required that at least two CD4 count tests be performed consecutively before a legitimate diagnosis of ICL could be made. "Of the eighteen," Cheney said, "only seven had been done more than once. Only one was *consistently* below three hundred. We've not had *anyone* consistently below two hundred."

Spira told Cheney that, in fact, very few ICL patients had consistent CD4 values below 300 when they were followed over long periods of time.

"The other thing we did was give Spira a distribution of CD-fours on all 1,350 of our CFS population," Cheney continued. "We basically had a histogram in which we displayed the CD-four counts of 1,350 people. The X axis was the CD-four count value, and the Y axis was the number of people. You end up with a curve with tails. Superimposed on that were the controls, of which we had about ninety. So you could see, if there was a shift, what the shift was."

Included in the data Cheney forwarded to Spira were the results of forty different tests, most of which had been performed on all patients. "We sent the flow cytometry results of lymphocyte types and subtypes, including T-cells, subpopulations of T-cells, and sub-*sub*populations of T-cells; B-cells and subpopulations of B-cells; and the natural killer cell data," the doctor added. "The chronic fatigue syndrome patients have both lower and higher CD-four counts than normals," Cheney said. "This scatter is relatively characteristic in our patients."

In addition to the data from his computer, Cheney also filled out ICL case report forms sent to him by the agency and returned them to Spira. The forms were modeled after the agency's AIDS case report forms, with which most doctors were already familiar.

In the midst of preparing his data for Spira in Atlanta, Cheney had also been telephoned by Jeffrey Laurence, the Cornell Medical Center researcher. Laurence had been among the first AIDS specialists to report cases of non–HIV positive AIDS, and like Sudhir Gupta, he had found suggestions of retrovirus infection among these cases.[4] He asked Cheney to send blood specimens from his ICL cases to Cornell.

"They have several probes against putative lentiviruses [a class of retrovirus] that they want to test against our patients," Cheney said. He complied with Laurence's request, but as he described the inquiry from the New York lab, Cheney sounded almost bored.

He had recently spent some time in Idaho with his son, who was enrolled in college there. Away from his clinic, in quiet moments, the doctor found himself viewing the current spasm of interest in the chronic disease he had been investigating since 1984 with something approaching detachment. "I was walking in the mountains," Cheney said. "I was at twelve thousand feet. And I thought, We've already *done* this! We've been doing this for some time."

New York City

On September 7, *Newsweek* published an article called "AIDS or Chronic Fatigue?" Aside from *New York Native* publisher Charles Ortleb, who for years had insisted that AIDS and CFS were not merely related but the same disease, *Newsweek*'s science editor Geoffrey Cowley was the only journalist who, prompted by the phenomenon of HIV-negative AIDS, ventured to describe the ways in which the two conditions overlapped and to suggest that scientists explore the relationship between them. Cowley profiled a CFS sufferer, a forty-eight-year-old woman from Stevensville, Michigan, who, Cowley wrote, "can also count herself among sufferers of the 'AIDS-like illness' that public health officials are now scrambling to investigate." The woman had lost most of her CD4 cells, putting her well into the ICL category. "So far," Cowley wrote, "the search has produced few answers. But as more cases come to light, it's becoming clear that the newly defined syndrome has as much in common with CFS as it does with AIDS."

Cowley noted that both Paul Cheney and Anthony Komaroff had a number of ICL cases in their CFS practices in Charlotte and Boston, and that both planned to report their cases to the CDC. "In the wake of the recent furor over ICL, Cheney amassed CD4 counts for 873 patients he's seen since 1989," Cowley wrote. "Twenty of them had dropped below the crucial 300 mark, and nearly four times that number had dipped below 500 (anything below 800 is abnormal). Dr. Anthony Komaroff, a CFS specialist at Boston's Brigham and Women's Hospital, says similar percentages of his patients have suffered CD4 depletion. . . . Between them, they could substantially boost the tally."*

Cowley's speculation, perhaps predictably, was met with a blast from *Science* weeks later. Writer Joe Palca suggested Cowley's work was irresponsible. The National Cancer Institute's Paul Levine also dismissed the Cowley story. "Cowley tried to link two groups of problems in a way that is totally arbitrary," Levine complained. "We don't even know yet if low T-cell counts are clinically significant. The feeling at the NIH is that HIV-negative AIDS is not one illness—and that it may even be a genetic disorder. So I think [the controversy over ICL and CFS] is a distraction. There's enough confusion about chronic fatigue syndrome as it is."

Harvard Medical School, Boston, Massachusetts

Walter Gunn had spent much of the previous spring and summer orchestrating an ambitious study to compare the ability of Elaine DeFreitas, John Martin, and C. V. Herst to differentiate between CFS patients and healthy controls using their respective tests. Should there be agreement among the three, or even among two of the three, their scientific credibility would be enormously enhanced. Gunn, too, had an interest in the outcome. He had, after all, staked his own credibility on what he believed was the legitimacy of DeFreitas's discovery, even giving up his job in the process. With this new effort, he had created for himself an opportunity to prove his old government colleagues wrong and to undercut their impending publication.

A month earlier, on June 23, Gunn had gone to tiny Lyndonville on the shore of Lake Ontario where, with David Bell's aid, he had collected samples from fifteen children in whose blood Elaine DeFreitas had found her retroviral marker. Ten of the children had been included in her original *PNAS* paper; another five, originally selected as healthy controls, had changed from negative to positive in subsequent tests by DeFreitas and, in addition, had developed severe CFS in the two years since the paper was published. Since Bell had closed his Lyndonville practice early in 1991, there existed no medical office in town. Jean Pollard, whose daughters had suffered from the disease since 1985, offered her commodious kitchen with its wood-burning oven to Gunn and Bell for their blood draws on the fifteen cases, most of whom were either entering or well into adolescence, as well as healthy controls chosen by Bell.

In early May, Gunn had traveled to New Jersey, where he arranged for a phlebotomist to draw blood from seventy-three CFS sufferers and healthy controls. Susan Levine, the Manhattan CFS specialist, had selected the patients and controls from her own practice. Levine's patients had all been called positive by C. V. Herst in previous tests.

In June, Paul Cheney gave Gunn specimens from what the doctor described as "ten *good* CFS cases" and ten controls.

---

* Unlike Cheney, although Komaroff discussed the incidence of ICL among CFS patients in his Boston clinic with the government's Spira, the Harvard doctor never sent Spira any formal documentation of the phenomenon.

As he obtained them, Gunn divided the Lyndonville, Charlotte, and Manhattan blood specimens into three portions and sent them in thermal containers to Martin, Herst, and DeFreitas.

At 11:00 A.M. on Saturday, September 19, Gunn and two collaborators, David Bell and Anthony Komaroff, gathered in Komaroff's offices to break the codes. Participating in an eight-way conference call were Ann Schleuderberg in Bethesda, who had learned of the study from Gunn and asked to be included in the code-breaking, and David Patterson, the Charlotte-based CFIDS Association's controller, whose foundation had paid for the study; Marc Iverson was too ill that day to join the call. Elaine DeFreitas, who had moved herself and her staff to Miami in July, had been unable to complete her portion of the study; personnel shortages, equipment shipping delays, Hurricane Andrew, and ensuing power outages, she told Gunn, had conspired to stifle progress, but she was listening from Miami. John Martin and C. V. Herst, who had completed their respective tests, were on the line in Los Angeles and Houston, as was Susan Levine in New York. "I basically wanted *everyone* there when I broke the code," Gunn said later.

For those who had been involved in the study, the results couldn't have been more devastating. It wasn't simply that neither Martin nor Herst seemed able to separate patients from controls using their tests, it was the apparent extraordinary *degree* of error their tests evinced. In most instances, the investigators had found as many—and in some cases *more*—healthy controls positive as they found patients negative. "They might as well have thrown darts," Patterson said afterward.

Breaking the code took nearly thirty minutes. An enduring, painful silence followed the reading of the results. Finally Susan Levine ventured a comment that was no doubt at the forefront of everyone's thoughts. "It looks like these tests cannot adequately differentiate between cases and controls," she said.

CFIDS Association controller Patterson noted that, after the codes were broken, "Most of these people didn't have much to say. No one hypothesized as to why the results had come up so skewed. . . . It puts us in a very awkward situation. We have to go before our scientific advisory board with these results and explain them."

The code-breaking seemed to be a watershed for Walter Gunn. Interviewed soon afterward, he was volatile, careening from regret to defensiveness. "One would have to conclude that there is no indication that these two labs could tell patients from controls," he said. "I'm sure they're growing a virus by the gallon, I'm sure they're sequencing it and doing all the things they're saying they're doing, but I'm not seeing any association between their virus and the illness. One possibility is that whatever they're testing for has no association with CFS. Perhaps the specimens were damaged in shipment—except that if the virus had died, there wouldn't have been so many positives."

Although DeFreitas's results remained unknown, Gunn nevertheless seemed to cast blame on her. "Maybe it's the hurricane, maybe it's the move from Wistar," he said, "but Elaine DeFreitas is disappointing a lot of people. I might still be at CDC if I hadn't defended her so staunchly." A few minutes later he blurted, "When I think about how I fought to protect Elaine at the CDC! The people at CDC are probably laughing up their sleeves."

But then Gunn abruptly pointed out the limits of the study: "All this shows is that using polymerase chain reaction to look for HTLV2-like segments does not distinguish patients with this disease."

And he suggested that what needed to be done next was a bigger study involving the same researchers but larger numbers of patients and controls; perhaps as many as three hundred samples should be collected and dispersed to Martin, Herst, and DeFreitas.

Gunn advised Patterson that he "should not be thinking about defending the researchers," however. "What's the best thing for the *patient*?" Gunn said rhetorically. "I encourage you to write a letter to the National CFS Advisory Council asking for their advice. *They* could advise you to do a more intensive study with two hundred or three hundred samples. Let's give this council something to do!"

Privately Gunn said, "The CFIDS Association is spending over $300,000 a year on this stuff. They need expert advice."

University of Southern California, Los Angeles

On September 28, John Martin reported to the scientific advisory board of the CFIDS Association that he and his lab had "achieved a major goal of essentially cloning the entire viral genome" of the virus he had discovered a year and a half before. Nevertheless, Martin remained unable to identify the type of virus or to explain what he described as "the characteristic foamy cell cytopathic effect seen in tissue culture," because he had cloned only a portion of the virus, albeit the most important part. Before he could publish his finding, he needed to clone the complete genetic sequence of the virus, which required the virus to be broken up into its smallest genetic units, or base pairs. That process was so time-consuming that Martin had asked for the aid of United States Biochemical Corporation, a commercial firm that offered custom viral sequencing for academic and industrial clients. The cost was estimated at $27,000 to $34,000.

Martin devoted another portion of his report to his poor results in the Gunn study. Before undertaking the study that summer, Martin said, he had identified CFS patients by putting blood specimens into cell cultures, obtaining viral isolates, studying the isolates under an electron microscope for cytopathic effect, and confirming the result by "repeated serial passage" of the infected cells into more cell cultures. His method was labor-intensive, however, and he used a simpler culture method for the study. "[T]he cultures were not passaged to confirm that the cytopathic effect was due to a transmissible agent, and no other confirmatory test was tried," he explained. Martin's lab had called half of the healthy controls positive and half of the CFS patients negative.

"These disappointing findings are being carefully evaluated so that we may improve our culture techniques," Martin wrote. "In particular, we have resumed our previous practice of testing for the transmissibility of all cytopathic effect to secondary cultures."

Martin's standing with the CFIDS Association board was beginning to crumble under the weight of Walter Gunn's influence. Said David Patterson, the organization's controller, "We have some theories about Martin. We think he's either a genius who has not only found the cause of CFIDS but perhaps several other diseases, or else he may possibly have something, but he's too scattered to bring his finding to fruition, or—third option—he's found something that's completely unrelated to the disease."

One anomaly that troubled the organization's scientific advisory board, Patterson continued, was the fact that Martin's electron micrograph of his virus revealed it to be nearly five times bigger than the viruses that Elaine DeFreitas and Sidney Grossberg were studying. In the spring, Grossberg had sent the CFIDS Association an electron micrograph of his presumed retrovirus, which appeared to be about five thousand base pairs long, a size considered typical of retroviruses. Grossberg's picture resembled in size the virus in DeFreitas's electron micrograph. Martin's virus, on the other hand, appeared to be of a size more suggestive of a herpesvirus than a retrovirus.

In the meantime, as a result of Gunn's persuasion, Martin's funding had been severed.

Geneva, Switzerland

On September 29 the World Health Organization concluded a two-day session on the new syndrome of idiopathic CD4 T-lymphocytopenia, or ICL, at its headquarters in Geneva. The international agency's meeting was closed to reporters, but Michael Merson, its AIDS chief, told journalists afterward that the World Health Organization believed the new syndrome to be rare. "We don't have a new epidemic on our hands," Merson said. "It does not look like a major problem, and we have no definitive evidence that there is a new virus causing immunosuppression."

Countries that had reported cases to the World Health Organization included the United States, Australia, Denmark, England, France, Ivory Coast, New Zealand, Russia, Rwanda, Spain, Switzerland, and Thailand. The United States had reported forty such cases, but Merson was unable to offer a worldwide tally because researchers were still filling out forms and trying to determine possible overlap in reported cases.

CIFDS Association president Marc Iverson, who had been disabled for fourteen years and was an ICL case himself, noted the World Health Organization's apparent dismissal of the syndrome with rueful bitterness. "I understand WHO swept it away," he said. "A two-day meeting in Geneva—that's how we got swept away."

National Cancer Institute, Bethesda, Maryland

Months before, cancer epidemiologist Paul Levine had said he was trying to find a way to "phrase properly" the "blip" of non-Hodgkin's lymphoma cases Dan Peterson and Paul Cheney had reported in Nevada during the epidemic years of 1984 to 1986. With the publication of his article on the subject that month, it seemed he had found a way.[5] In evaluating the state's cancer registry, Levine reported he had been unable to find a statistically significant rise in cases of non-Hodgkin's lymphoma statewide. Levine's analysis, however, failed to take into account the fact that outbreaks of CFS may not respect county and state lines. A great many of the CFS epidemic patients who sought help in Incline Village, Nevada, were Californians, even though they may have lived just four miles away. In addition, Levine had not compared rates of non-Hodgkin's lymphoma from county to county inside Nevada. An honest researcher, Levine noted these weak points in his abstract and promised that "additional studies are in progress analyzing the data at the county level."

As of 1995, the government's cancer researcher had failed to undertake any further investigations into the seemingly high rate of non-Hodgkin's lymphoma cases in the northerly region of Lake Tahoe. That same year, Levine, the only federal cancer researcher who had felt compelled to investigate the relationship between CFS and cancer, retired from the National Cancer Institute.

Centers for Disease Control, Atlanta, Georgia

On October 3 the CDC leaked its preliminary surveillance data to reporter Kim Painter, who had been following the CFS story for *USA Today*. The following day the agency's Division of Viral and Rickettsial Diseases was sending Howard Gary, chief of biometrics activity at the agency, to an Albany, New York, medical conference to report the surveillance results. "At most, we're talking about sixty thousand cases" nationwide, John Stewart, chief of the clinical virology section at the agency, told Painter. According to the government's estimate, there were five to eleven CFS sufferers for every 100,000 people in the four cities under surveillance—Atlanta, Reno, Wichita, and Grand Rapids.

Marc Iverson was disappointed by the government's first release of surveillance data. "The government is saying there are sixty thousand people with chronic fatigue syndrome in the country," he said. "But there are one thousand people with this disease in the Greensboro, South Carolina, support group alone. Hell, if this is what we're working so hard to get congressional funding for," added the former banker, "let's use the money to pay off the national deficit instead—or pay interest on the deficit."

Albany, New York

Those who had begun to suspect Elaine DeFreitas of hiding from her critics were disabused of that notion when she attended the Albany conference, an event that attracted seven hundred people, 80 percent of them patients, on the first weekend in October. The public spaces inside the Albany Marriott teemed with doctors and sufferers; regional support group officials had made certain the hotel staff stocked the hotel's main floors with extra chairs and sofas for debilitated patients unable to walk from the conference halls to their rooms without resting along the way. Representatives from patient support organizations as far away as England, Denmark, Norway, and Australia were in attendance. *New York Native* publisher Charles Ortleb did not attend, and he forbade Neenyah Ostrom, his CFS beat reporter, to attend, so fearful was he of contagion.

DeFreitas was about to receive a triple-barreled blast from the CDC, the University of Glasgow's Peter Behan, and Walter Gunn, who would report the poor results of his recent study. Not surprisingly, DeFreitas was less than calm. On Saturday night, the eve of the conference's virology meeting, she sat in the hotel's chrome-and-glass bar with her friend and counselor, pediatrician David Bell. Lighting fresh cigarettes as soon as they finished their old ones, the two conferred on ways in which DeFreitas might answer Scottish virologist John Gow and, most particularly, Walid Heneine of the CDC, from the conference floor, since she herself had not been invited to present her data.

Bell advised her to take the high road. "Don't even respond," he said.

DeFreitas took her own counsel the next day, however. She sat through the presentations by Gow, Gunn, and finally her old adversary, Heneine, who was listed as the first author on the agency's *Annals* paper refuting her findings.[6] When Heneine had finished, the National Cancer Institute's Dharam Ablashi, the herpesvirus expert who was moderating the session, seized on the data to suggest that CFS was something other than a retroviral infection. "I think it is very important that here are three negative studies presented by three different groups," he commented. He noted that, in addition, "in the beginning when this Lake Tahoe epidemic was identified, a number of samples were sent to the Gallo lab. They were tested and were found to be negative [for retrovirus]."

When Ablashi had finished, DeFreitas, speaking from a microphone placed in the aisle for health professionals in the audience who wished to ask questions, began with a point of logic she obviously believed capsulized the conflict. She pointed out that even though John Gow in Scotland and the scientists in Atlanta claimed to have followed her protocol, their results were diametrical. "Dr. Gow reported that *all* patients and *all* controls in his assay were positive, whereas *all* patients and *all* controls in Dr. Folks's and Walid Heneine's assays were negative," DeFreitas said. "Clearly that means they were not doing the same assay, and if they were not doing the same assay as each other, they were not doing the same assay as we are. And I think that if one is going to stand up and confirm or repeat another scientist, one has, at minimum, a responsibility to do that assay the way the original investigator did it."

DeFreitas continued, saying that she had generously offered both groups her protocol and primers before her original *PNAS* article was published. In addition, she had invited Heneine, Tom Folks, and "anybody else in his laboratory to the Wistar Institute to do the assays side by side with us, using CDC samples and samples from Lyndonville and Dr. Cheney's office." Mystifyingly, she said, her invitation was turned aside. "And when that offer was rejected," she continued, "we offered to pay our own way to go to Atlanta, to stand side by side with Dr. Heneine and Dr. Folks and do this assay with the same reagents, the same materials, and settle this once and for all. *That* offer was rejected.

"I do not think that this was a valid attempt to reproduce our data. I think what they've succeeded in doing, rather than improving their sensitivity, was actually *decreasing* their sensitivity."

DeFreitas took up Ablashi's comment that retrovirus infection in the Tahoe specimens sent to the Gallo lab in 1986 had been definitively ruled out by government scientists. "The samples that were sent from Dr. Cheney's to Dr. Robert Gallo, I know from personal conversations with Dr. Gallo, were tested for HTLV-one antibody *only*," she said. "We reported in *PNAS* [that] all antibody to HTLV-one, specifically, was negative."

Ablashi shot back, "I tested those samples for HTLV-two antibody myself! I also got samples from Dr. Tony Komaroff, which he sent me about seventy samples, only two of them I found positive." Ablashi thundered on: "Now a question I want to raise is, were tests presented by Dr. Gunn done with the probe *you* provided, and were they done according to *your* protocol?"

"Let me speak to Dr. Gunn's study separately, because one important point was left out of Dr. Gunn's excellent presentation. And that is that *our* data is not in yet," DeFreitas replied. "We received the coded samples from Lyndonville as well, but because of my move from the Wistar Institute to the University of Miami, which began in July, was interrupted by [Hurricane] Andrew, and still goes on--I still have equipment sitting on loading docks to be moved into the university—we were not able to complete the study. The code for Lyndonville has *not* been broken for us, and as soon as those experiments are run, they will be provided to Dr. Gunn and Dr. Komaroff, and the code will be broken. And then we will see if *we* can detect patients from controls in our own assay, using our own level of sensitivity and specificity. So that's the point."

She made a second point about C. V. Herst's results: "I won't take words out of C.V.'s mouth, but [his] test—while I think [it is] an excellent and interesting test, and a quick test for a commercial laboratory, and an inexpensive test, which is very important for a commercial laboratory—is *not* the same test that we use. It is analogous to, but not identical to, the test we use."

Ablashi again butted heads with DeFreitas. "I want to make a comment to the general public," he said testily, clearly addressing the CFS sufferers present. "These are only research tools; they are *not* diagnostic tests."

Ablashi had at last tripped DeFreitas's flash point; her aplomb evaporated. "Does that imply," she began in a style that was both deliberate and contemptuous, "that Dr. Herst cannot do PCR as well as Dr. Walid Heneine?"

Her slight against Heneine silenced Ablashi. It had an altogether different and unexpected impact upon the audience, however. At first, there were only surprised murmurs and a few gasps as the depth of her hostility registered. Then there was tentative applause in support of DeFreitas—applause that soon escalated into an explosion of noise. The audience whooped and cheered and whistled their approval with the fervor of a Metropolitan Opera audience after a bravura performance. A wall of sound bore down on the scientists on the dais and enveloped DeFreitas, pale and almost painfully thin, standing alone before the microphone. For an interminable period, it seemed that the private rage and despair of every patient in the hall had been unleashed in a demonstration of solidarity against the government's scientific establishment. Tom Folks, who had predicted the patient community would turn its anger on DeFreitas when his agency's inability to confirm her finding was announced, had sorely underestimated that community's growing sense of betrayal by their government and the underdog loyalty DeFreitas inspired.

When the demonstration ended at last, Heneine took the microphone to respond to DeFreitas's barb. "Dr. DeFreitas and our lab at CDC, we have had a long history of interaction," he began. "And everything that she said about this interaction is true. Before publication, she let us know about her primers and everything, and we, all the time, have been in good faith interacting with her. Now, when we come to the specifics—this is very important here, where sentiments and feelings are different from facts—as far as running the tests, we have been in contact with her and the people in her lab to make sure that the test we are running in our lab has the same sensitivity and the same ability to detect this fragment she reported in her article.

"You have seen the results, and these are the facts," he concluded, "and we stand by them, and we will let the medical literature to be the final judge of this."

Before a new interchange could begin, Jay Levy reprimanded the audience for its unruly behavior. "This is not a popularity contest," he said. "It is not decided in this forum who's right and who's wrong. It will be decided by the scientific community and the clinicians and others when the data is put into a publication. This is a privilege to have this information presented, and I'm sure Elaine and C.V. and the others should be pleased that people are trying to confirm them, and they may have different results. The debate is very helpful, but let's not have the applause."

To DeFreitas's surprise, Paul Levine, the epidemiologist from the National Cancer Institute, then spoke in her support, cautioning that final judgment about her work was premature. "The point is," Levine said, "until Dr. DeFreitas finishes her studies, the question is still open." He challenged his colleague Ablashi, noting that Ablashi, too, had used tests for HTLV2 on Tahoe samples but that, as DeFreitas had made clear, "she doesn't *have* HTLV-two."

"I can just say," Levine added, "that Dr. Grufferman and I sent Dr. DeFreitas coded samples from the Tahoe epidemic a *long* time ago and she's finally tested them, and we know that there are positives and there are negatives." (Levine had gone to Nevada earlier in the year to obtain blood specimens from patients he considered classic cases in Incline Village and Yerington for analysis by DeFreitas. He had sent the specimens to the Wistar in the spring. Privately, he confirmed that "Some were positive.")

After Levine's remarks, Ablashi ended the session, calling it a success.

Afterward, DeFreitas, to her embarrassment, was embraced by a patient, a young man with a ponytail. "Elaine," he told her, "kick ass and take names!"

Walter Gunn's view of DeFreitas's behavior in Albany was gently disparaging. "Two-thirds of the audience were patients and were unable to judge the scientific issues, but she hurt herself," Gunn observed. "She was emotional. She felt attacked and was counterattacking, but she would have been better off not responding." His old colleagues at the Centers for Disease Control, Gunn continued, were eager to put the DeFreitas controversy to rest, he continued. "They're very anxious to finish her off. They've been angry since the beginning. They were angry when her paper was published in *PNAS*! I don't doubt for a minute that Elaine DeFreitas has a virus," he added, "but is it related to CFS? Same thing with John

Martin: I'm sure it's not a vat of clams—I'm sure he's got something there. But is it unique to the disease?"

Certainly Gunn's former government associates saw his role in the Wistar controversy as the retired investigator's Waterloo. Tom Folks, who did not attend the Albany conference, commented, "I think Walt Gunn's a very dejected man who was hoodwinked by Dr. DeFreitas and others into believing this marker was real. It's an especially sad situation for chronic fatigue syndrome sufferers who have put a lot of faith in her."

Seymour Grufferman of the University of Pittsburgh had been invited to Albany to speak about the challenges the disease presented to epidemiological investigation. He had listened with a sharply critical ear to the CDC prevalence data as it was presented by biostatistician Howard Gary and witnessed the fireworks in the virology session, and was disappointed in the agency's performance. He had hoped the Atlanta scientists, who had been silent on the subject of the epidemic disease since 1988 when they published their definition, would emerge as strong investigators. At least, he had hoped, they might be less biased than those at the NIH.

"When I saw the kind of sloppy analysis they had performed on the surveillance data, I started getting the idea," Grufferman said. "It was so amateurish—it was garbage. It just reminded me of a government being forced to do something to placate the rumbling masses. So they do something, but in a sloppy, belated way."

Walid Heneine's report on the agency's effort to replicate the Wistar finding struck Grufferman as a "whitewash." "Heneine did not have the appearance of a dispassionate scientist. He seemed to take great relish in stepping all over DeFreitas," Grufferman said. "It's very bothersome to me. This is the problem of not having independent research grants—the NIH and the CDC wind up doing all the research.

"You get the feeling from the government bureaucrats that this is a disease that's in people's heads, and if they wait long enough, it will go away. We're not going to move forward in this way. We're really not making progress at all! It's a time warp. There needs to be a case-control study and a population-based surveillance study by people who approach the disease as an infectious disease. The virology really needs to be sorted out, too. But, with the priority given this by the government, that's never going to happen.

"I do think it's a real disease, but we don't have good researchers tackling it. We have Anthony Komaroff and Dedra Buchwald, who staked this out early but are really not contributing any new insights—there's no creative science there. And then we have the virologists, who are being crapped on, and they just sort of drop in and out. There's poor Elaine, with all of her black clouds all over her, although I really have to hand it to Elaine—she's got balls. Then you have the patients, who remain desperate for help. You could hear them in the hallways exchanging quack remedies," Grufferman added. "And the quack M.D.'s were there offering to write prescriptions—'Ten more drops of this, five more drops of that.' It was a carnival."

DeFreitas, the subject of so much speculation by scientists and patients alike, returned to Miami feeling triumphant but exhausted. She was ill—extremely ill, in fact. Her throat felt as if it had been burned with acid; her head felt swathed in cotton. She told herself she had been struck by a bad case of flu; it had been drafty in the hotel, she reasoned; she had been tired even before she left for the stressful event. Underneath such thoughts, fear festered.

"You can imagine what was going through my mind, having been in such close quarters with so many patients," she confessed. "I took a whole week's worth of acyclovir."

In three weeks her symptoms subsided.

At the Albany conference research psychologist Leonard Jason presented his preliminary data on the extent of the disease among Chicago nurses. His estimate of 680 afflicted nurses per 100,000 nurses stood in stark contrast to the prevalence data offered by the Centers for Disease Control. Many in the audience, in fact, were aghast. Walter Gunn, who heard Jason speak, was not.

"When I was at the Centers for Disease Control, we were getting one thousand to three thousand calls a month from people who thought they had this disease," Gunn recalled. "Roughly twenty-five percent were nurses—a lot of them, interestingly, pediatric nurses. I consider this disease to be a real problem for the health care industry."

Two weeks later Jason and his collaborators learned that their $1.5 million research proposal to pursue his investigation of CFS prevalence among both nurses and the general population of Chicago and surrounding suburbs had been turned down by the National Institute of Allergy and Infectious Diseases. A special ad hoc study section assembled by grant administrator Ann Schleuderberg told Jason and his collaborators their proposal was unfeasible.

"They threw the Centers for Disease Control's prevalence rates at us. They said, 'You can't do this study because there are too few people who are sick—five or six per hundred thousand, according to the CDC—and you'll have to call millions of people to pick up cases of the disease in a community-based surveillance.' Of course," Jason added, "we don't believe those rates."

In the previous months, Jason had sought financial support for his work from more than thirty private foundations. He had been turned down by all of them. "The lack of interest in this disease around the country is mind-boggling," he said.

HEM Pharmaceuticals, Philadelphia, Pennsylvania

In the first week of December the Food and Drug Administration refused HEM Pharmaceuticals' second request to begin expanded clinical trials of Ampligen in CFS victims in the United States. (The company's clinical trial in Canada, however, had been approved by the Canadian health agency.) The decision came two months after Jean Hardy, a CFS sufferer in Charlotte and a patient of Paul Cheney's, committed suicide.

Hardy, a once beautiful, lively woman who had been bedridden for several years, was the subject of a CNN story on the disease six months before her death. "If only I knew what I had done to get this disease!" she had told the interviewer as she lay on her bed, her arm over her eyes to deflect the glare of the camera-man's lights. Hardy's hopes had been raised by results of the Ampligen trials the previous fall. In September, however, it was apparent to her that approval for Ampligen, if it came at all, was years away. That month, in fact, HEM officials had begun negotiations to withdraw the drug from even the handful of patients in the original Nevada study—people like Albuquerque resident Nancy Kaiser and former Truckee, California, English teacher Janice Kennedy, who were receiving Ampligen through the FDA's compassionate care clause. Overwhelmed by disap-pointment and the prospect of additional years of suffering, Hardy took her life.

Charlotte, North Carolina

At the end of the year, Paul Cheney performed a search on Medline, the largest of the medical literature computer search services. "In the last six months alone," Cheney reported, "there have been one hundred twenty-eight articles about CFS in the literature."

National Institute of Allergy and Infectious Diseases, Bethesda, Maryland

The National Institute of Allergy and Infectious Diseases agreed to support Wis-consin scientist Sidney Grossberg in his investigation of retroviral infection in CFS. Grossberg was awarded $166,079 for this purpose.* At least the government agency could claim—truthfully now—that it was funding research into the cause of the disease, however meagerly. Grossberg was in fact the first scientist to be funded by the government to explore a viral etiology for the disease. CDC virol-ogist Tom Folks was among the scientists who encouraged the Bethesda institute to fund Grossberg.

There were other hints that the government was moving slightly left of center on the retrovirus issue. When Walter Gunn asked Ann Schleuderberg to review his paper on his study of the previous summer, the NIAID official advised Gunn to avoid stating categorically that his investigation ruled out retroviral infection in the disease. Anthony Komaroff, too, had suggested to Gunn that he add a sentence near the end of his report pointing out that the results of the study "don't mean that a retrovirus couldn't exist in this disease," Gunn said. Komaroff, although pub-licly a proponent of the multiple-cause, or multifactorial, theory of the disease, and a NIAID contractor, had sent blood specimens to Grossberg for evaluation that fall.

Centers for Disease Control, Atlanta, Georgia

Tom Folks reported during the winter of 1992 that he had "some very interesting leads" on retroviral infection in the disease. "Other investigators have called me

---

* The grant was to last three years. In 1994 Grossberg was awarded another $158,030; his 1995 fund-ing was estimated by NIAID officials to be $162,000.

from other areas," he said vaguely. "One national,* one international.† They're sending me materials. We've already had some pieces of sequences that we've been able to find that may suggest some retrovirus homology. If we can clone these sequences, maybe we can get a marker."

He insisted there was enough news from his lab on the retroviral front that he had developments to report at the beginning of each week's meeting of the newly named CFS Group, the former sneering committee, headed by William Reeves. He insisted his research into a retroviral etiology would continue, in spite of the Wistar project's bad end.

By the end of 1992 at least four labs were actively investigating the CFS retrovirus theory in the United States. And although DeFreitas had been the first to publish on the subject, she still ran the risk of being outpaced. If a retrovirus caused CFS, the Nobel prize awaited the first scientist to establish the connection beyond all doubt.

As Paul Cheney described the competition, "The person who publishes the definitive positive study will get all the marbles."

---

* Folks's national contact was Wisconsin scientist Sidney Grossberg. Commenting much later on Grossberg's evidence for retrovirus activity in CFS patients, Folks remembered, "There were hints of retroviral sequences—without a doubt. The problem is that we were not really able to distinguish whether it was exogenous or endogenous." An endogenous retrovirus, of course, is one carried in the human genome over the course of millennia; presumably endogenous material does not cause harm. Not surprisingly, Folks's collaboration with Grossberg came to an end. "It's clear [Grossberg] has something unique," Folks said, "but whether it's CFS-related or not I don't know."

† Folks's international contact turned out to be microbiologist Michael Holmes, a researcher at the University of Otago medical school in Dunedin, New Zealand, who had found suggestions of retroviral infection in CFS patients as long ago as 1986. In 1992, Folks put the New Zealander in touch with the CDC's CFS Group. Although Folks had no explanation for it, Holmes eventually decided to forgo any collaboration with the American agency.

1993

TALKING
THE TALK

Never springing, Minerva-like, to full stature at
once, truth may suffer all the hazards incident to
generation and gestation. Much of history is a
record of the mishaps of truth which have struggled
to the birth, only to die or else to wither in premature decay.

—Sir William Osler, *An Alabama Student
and Other Biographical Essays*

34

A Failed Initiative

Department of Veterans Affairs, Washington, D.C.

Between the fall of 1990 and February 1991 half a million American military personnel were sent abroad to wage a war against Iraq in the Persian Gulf. Conditions
were rugged. Soldiers lived in close quarters in warehouses and tents. They ate
food prepared in military mess units and, not infrequently, sampled the cuisine of
local vendors; diarrhea was a hazard common to either fare. Camp stove heaters,
which used diesel fuel, warmed tents at night but exuded pungent smoke and
gases that made sleeping difficult. In the course of their duties, a great many Gulf
War conscripts were exposed to vapors from myriad fuel oils, pesticides, and, to a
lesser degree, paint. At war's end, some of the soldiers were exposed to smoke
and fumes from the oil well fires burning out of control on the Kuwaiti desert, an
aftermath of Iraqi bombing raids. The large number of reservists who served in
the Gulf had been forced to abandon their civilian lives on short notice, leaving
jobs and families behind; at least one-fifth reported that they worried virtually
around the clock about being killed or wounded. All of them, no doubt, were victims of stress during their deployment in the war.

One would have expected the rigors of Desert Storm to exact a toll on its participants. Indeed, even before the war was officially over, officials in the Department
of Veterans Affairs had begun worrying about potential health implications for military personnel serving in the Gulf. "Anyone watching the oil fire in Kuwait had to
wonder what kind of problems that would cause," the assistant chief of health for
the veterans department, Susan Mather, told *New York Times* reporter Philip Hilts,
on November 23, 1993. With those extraordinary infernos in mind, months before
most troops began to be sent home from the region, Dr. Mather had looked into the
toxic health effects of the fires and other possible Gulf War health hazards.

As she and others in her department had expected, Mather began hearing about
sick Gulf veterans within months after their return to the United States. The only
problem was, the veterans' complaints departed from the anticipated scenario.
Their symptoms, observed over time, failed to suggest that veterans were suffering from smoke inhalation, chemical exposure, or any known infectious disease.
Military experts found the stories Gulf veterans told about their physical decline
utterly mysterious, in fact.

The army's first investigation into veterans' complaints was requested by the Office of the Surgeon General on March 30, 1992, fourteen months after the war's end. That inquiry, headed by a team of six doctors and epidemiologists from Walter Reed Army Institute of Research, focused on a group of Gulf War veterans living in Indiana, members of the 123rd Army Reserve Command at Fort Benjamin Harrison in Lafayette. None had served in combat. Once in the Gulf, they were split by companies and battalions and deployed throughout the region. In all, 1,200 reservists from the 123rd ARCOM had been sent to the Gulf. A majority of them transported supplies; some drove trucks carrying latrines and water; others used forklifts to move supplies from warehouses to trucks; some refueled supply trucks. When the war ended, several were employed scrubbing military vehicles with steam hoses and degreasers in preparation for the equipment's return to the United States.

In some cases, their symptoms began in the Gulf—fatigue and, frequently, upper respiratory ailments that failed to resolve. Between May and August of 1991, when the majority of them were sent home, the complaints grew more serious. By April of the following year, 125 of them, or 10 percent, claimed to be suffering from a multitude of ailments. Symptoms ran the gamut from hair loss to headaches, joint pain to diarrhea, with two constant, unifying symptoms: varying degrees of exhaustion and a peculiar intellectual cloudiness marked by short-term memory loss and poor concentration.

Over the course of two days in April, seventy-nine ailing Indiana reservists reported to the team from Walter Reed, which had set up a small clinic in the base military hospital. The army's thirty-page account of the investigation, which became available to the public on June 15, 1992, reflected an earnest effort to uncover the etiology of the veterans' problems. Doctors examined the reservists, studied their medical records, interviewed them, and administered questionnaires to eke out clues to their psychological state. In addition, they tested reservists for Lyme disease, brucellosis, enteric parasites, and hypothyroidism. Importantly, using records of troop deployments, they studied, and ruled out, potential chemical and radiation exposure the seventy-nine veterans could have suffered in the Gulf. (The army's camp stoves had been used all over the world with no ill effects to soldiers; the Kuwaiti oil fires had deposited their most dangerous fumes in the upper atmosphere, beyond the reach of earthbound soldiers; so far it appeared there had been virtually no chemical warfare in the Gulf; radiation hazards had been minimal.) Most persuasively, the report stated, "there were very few exposures common to the entire group. Reported symptoms did not correspond with known effects of those exposures."

As inconclusive as their investigation had been, the costliness and the public nature of the effort required that the medical team draw some conclusion. With little else to pin the problem on, the army team resorted to offering stress as an explanation for the wave of illness among the 123rd ACROM reservists. "There is at present no objective evidence to suggest an outbreak of any disease in 123rd ARCOM," they wrote. "Post-deployment adjustment to civilian life," they added, was always a stressful event, and stress was a "plausible etiology for many of the symptoms reported, especially sleep disturbances, depression, forgetfulness, and cognitive difficulties."

In testimony before the Senate Veteran Affairs Committee that year, Steve Robertson, a Gulf veteran and American Legion lobbyist, commented, "The only stress I'm experiencing now is the failure of the Department of Defense to accept this problem."

When Robertson was first evaluated for his medical problems, a military doctor had suggested that he see a psychiatrist. The psychiatrist then told Robertson his symptoms were a manifestation of anger at being deployed in the Gulf. Robertson's tour of duty had ended in the spring of 1991. Some time later he described living conditions in the Gulf as "probably one of the most unsanitary places I've ever been in my life." Robertson said army latrines and showers were infested with insects. He shared a tent with fourteen people. "You had about two feet on either side of your cot," he recalled. Soon after his return to the United States, Robertson developed a severe cough, aching joints, extreme fatigue, and diarrhea. The cough and diarrhea eventually dissipated over a period of two years; fatigue and joint pain were still prominent symptoms two years later.

Interestingly, the Walter Reed doctors considered chronic fatigue syndrome as an explanation for the veterans' ills but ultimately rejected it. The government's CFS case definition required a daily reduction in activity of 50 percent or more and the exclusion of all other chronic clinical conditions. Although some sick veterans fit this description, not all of them did. "We feel that the chronic fatigue syndrome may apply to very few of the soldiers, if any," the Walter Reed doctors wrote.

Irrespective of the army's investigation and the assignment of veterans' symptoms to a probable cause, namely stress, the problem refused to go away. In fact, as the months rolled on, it was apparent to all that the problem was not confined to Indiana. Gulf War veterans from many states and regions of the nation were demanding attention from the Veterans Affairs Department, claiming disability as a result of their participation in Desert Shield and Desert Storm. The symptoms of the great majority of these veterans were identical to the amalgam of complaints described by Indiana reserves. Sensitive to charges that the "Gulf War syndrome" had the potential to become another Agent Orange debacle in which the military would be accused of covering up or ignoring a service-related health crisis among veterans, the military's experts continued to mine the mystifying outbreak with their epidemiologic arsenal.

In the fall of 1992, under pressure from veterans' associations, the Veterans Administration established a Persian Gulf registry. Gulf veterans who were ill, or worried about falling ill as a result of their service in the Gulf, were invited to add their names to the registry. By early 1994, thirteen thousand veterans had signed up.

░

Infectious diseases have stalked the participants of war for most of history, causing more fatalities than the warring factions imposed upon each other. In the nineteenth century, typhus, malaria, cholera, dysentery, and typhoid fever were known throughout medicine as "camp diseases" because of their persistence within troop encampments throughout the world. When their mode of transmission was understood and measures were taken to combat transmission of these diseases at the turn of the century, their incidence waned.

By the 1980s, most military medical experts and civilian doctors enjoyed a comfortable certitude that infectious disease had been conquered, both on the battlefield and in civilian life. Many of those familiar with CFS were less sanguine. As early as May 12, 1987, the disabled cardiologist Jake Lindsay had written to Surgeon General C. Everett Koop predicting that chronic fatigue syndrome might soon emerge as a major health crisis for the American military. Lindsay cautioned the surgeon general: "I have already been told of the occurrence of total disability due to CEBV recently requiring some soldiers to leave the service. The CEBV epidemic could have a disastrous effect on our armed services, much more dangerous than AIDS, due to its ability to rapidly spread like the common cold. Since it can be spread as quickly as it recently did in Lake Tahoe . . . it could disable entire bases, as well as leave a large number of personnel permanently disabled, at great expense."

Lindsay urged Koop to appoint senior investigators at both the CDC and the NIH who would devote their full attention to investigating the disease. "Power similar to that of the general in wartime should be given these senior officials," Lindsay wrote. "This would help ensure full and rapid cooperation between competing labs and scientists working on these problems."

Koop never spoke publicly about CFS during his tenure as surgeon general, although by 1989 his wife was rumored to be bedridden with the affliction. By 1988, however, the military's infectious disease chiefs had been curious enough about the subject to seek Stephen Straus's expertise. Captain Kenneth Wagner, head of the infectious diseases and HIV program for the Department of the Navy, and Colonel Edmund Tramont, Wagner's army corollary at Walter Reed, invited Straus to a meeting of the Tri-Service Infectious Diseases Society at Homestead Air Force Base in Miami on March 10.

Tramont, in a conversation at Walter Reed on April 20, 1988, was asked if CFS was a problem in the American military. "Not really," he responded, then amended his comment to suggest that there was no more of the disease in the military than in the general population. "We see people who were much, much, much better a few years ago; then they got sick and they just never returned," Tramont said. "It happens. It's real." Nevertheless, Tramont, who retired from the military in 1992, did not view the disease as a catastrophic illness, and certainly not as a discrete, infectious one. He cast his lot, instead, with the "yuppie burnout" theorists, suggesting that society, in recent decades, was perhaps asking too much of its members, particularly women, leading to a degree of fatigue and stress that likely had not existed in earlier decades.

In 1991, in his capacity as CFS research chief at the CDC, Walter Gunn began hearing from members of the military who suffered from the disease. Many of them complained that the armed forces were discriminating against them with respect to disability support for the condition. "I got a call from a female army lieutenant who was having problems getting disability," Gunn said. "They were trying to give her thirty percent disability. She said she knew people in the navy who had been retired with this disease at a sixty percent disability." Nearly a decade before, Gunn, a formal naval officer, had called a friend in the office of the undersecretary of the army and suggested that he focus on AIDS as a potential health issue for the military. "Now," Gunn mused, "I think they should be thinking about chronic fatigue syndrome."

Dorothy Knight seconded his view. Soon after she was hired to respond to the agency's voluminous mail and calls from CFS sufferers, the perspicacious Knight concluded that the malady her callers described was the same disease afflicting military personnel and their families at the Fort Stewart military base in Hinesville, Georgia, where Knight had been secretary to the branch chief of pharmacy services in the base hospital.

If small outbreaks of CFS—either recognized or unrecognized—occurred on U.S. military bases before the war, it was not unreasonable to imagine that conditions in the Gulf War theater might have hastened the rate of spread, resulting in a more conspicuous attack rate. The history of CFS—indeed, the history of most casually transmitted infectious diseases—suggested that institutional settings, or any setting where groups of people lived in close contact, enhanced opportunities for outbreaks to occur.

National Academy of Sciences, Washington, D.C.

Late in 1992 a committee of distinguished scientists from the National Academy of Sciences published a book that inadvertently explained how an epidemic of such proportions could have remained submerged throughout its first decade. *Emerging Infections: Microbial Threats to Health in the United States* described in stark language the virtual inability of the U.S. public health establishment to detect and aggressively pursue epidemics of new infectious diseases. As things stood now, its authors insisted, there existed no mechanism by which either the CDC or the NIH could recognize the emergence of new diseases. Experts in the fields of epidemiology, microbiology, and public health, the authors wasted little effort on subtleties. "[T]he United States has no comprehensive national system for detecting outbreaks of infectious disease (except for food- and waterborne diseases)," they wrote. "Outbreaks of any disease that is not on CDC's current list of notifiable illnesses may go undetected or may be detected only after an outbreak is well under way."[1]

By 1990, fifty-three diseases were federally ordained as reportable to the CDC. They included Hansen's disease (leprosy), gonorrhea, syphilis, rabies, Lyme disease, polio, plague, mumps, and botulism. (Each state also had its own rules regarding notifiable diseases, rules that often either expanded or duplicated the federal agency's list.) But surveillance even for reportable diseases in the United States "was a passive process," the authors wrote, in that doctors and hospitals were expected to report cases to the state authorities who, in turn, would report them to the CDC. And this system had flaws; for one thing, doctors' reporting practices were notoriously lax.

Discussing remedial strategies, the report's authors suggested two methods: the establishment of a hot line to CDC epidemiologists that doctors could use to report "unusual syndromes," and "using electronic patient data collected by insurance companies to assist in infectious disease surveillance."*

Above all else, the authors portrayed national surveillance as "the key to recognizing new or emerging infectious diseases." Its importance "to the detection and control of emerging microbial threats cannot be overemphasized," they continued. "Poor surveillance leaves policymakers and medical and public health professionals with no basis for developing and implementing policies to control the spread of infectious diseases." In addition to measuring the magnitude of the problem, they said, surveillance enabled scientists to "help describe the natural history of the disease, identify factors responsible for [its] emergence, facilitate laboratory and epidemiological research, and assess the success of specific intervention efforts." (The committee noted that it was impossible to know whether the impact of AIDS might have been "limited had there been an effective global infectious disease surveillance system in place in the late 1960s or early 1970s.") At any rate, they added, "without such a system in place we would have little chance for early detection of emerging diseases in the future."

National surveillance remained nonexistent in the CFS field, although the U.S. Congress had for seven years been pressing the agency responsible for such surveillance. Politicians were intuitively aware of the critical importance of having prevalence data, as were patient advocates, but the epidemiologists at the Atlanta agency, while accepting taxpayer dollars earmarked for the purpose, had steadfastly failed to comply. The career of epidemiologist Walter Gunn, who alone had pressed for national surveillance, had ended prematurely, so out of step was he with his agency's policy on the matter. "Walter was rather biased,") one agency scientist commented shortly after Gunn's departure.

As powerful as national surveillance would be, however, it could not be relied upon as the nation's sole method of documenting new epidemics, according to the report. A "full clinical documentation of unsolved cases, with a system for archiving sera and pathological specimens," would be required as well. Congress and patients had, of course, asked repeatedly for the establishment of a central archive where tissue specimens from CFS cases might be collected, yet neither the Atlanta nor the Bethesda agency had displayed a willingness to establish such an archive. The report, in addition, listed a series of "clinical circumstances that require high-priority surveillance efforts." On that list were cases of unexplained encephalitis—precisely the clinical dilemma University of

---

* The first suggestion sounded reasonable, except that doctors and patients had been reporting CFS cases to the agency at the rate of 2,000 to 3,000 a month in recent years, without effecting a change in agency policy. The second suggestion, if issues of patient confidentiality could be solved, might have aided in tracking the disease. After all, by 1987 the major health insurers had received enough claims for CFS that they had classified the disease as a preexisting condition serious enough to deny insurance to new applicants, even though the federal health agencies had maintained it was psychological in origin.

Southern California pathologist John Martin had brought to the government's attention in 1991.*

As for CFS becoming a notifiable disease someday, Centers for Disease Control staff brushed off the suggestion as unrealistic. "CFS will never be a notifiable disease," insisted agency medical epidemiologist Keiji Fukuda, "because it's too controversial. Some doctors don't even believe in it. Why ask for something that's never going to happen?"

Fukuda seemed to have temporarily forgotten that his agency had based its entire surveillance program on doctors' referrals.

Emerging Infections had its genesis three years earlier at a conference sponsored by New York's Rockefeller University and the National Institute of Allergy and Infectious Diseases. Although the agenda had been viruses, many participants broached another topic: complacency on the part of the scientific and medical communities, policital leaders, and the public toward the threat of new infectious diseases. During the conference, a committee was formed to prepare a report that would serve as a call to arms. Microbiologist Joshua Lederberg, a Nobel prize winner and former president of Rockefeller University, was named co-chairman of the committee.

Ironically, one of the committee members was the father of William Reeves, the CDC scientist who had absorbed Walter Gunn's job. The senior William Reeves was a professor emeritus of epidemiology at the School of Public Health at U.C. Berkeley and the recipient of numerous awards for distinguished service in the public health arena. Alexis Shelokov, the epidemiologist who had investigated the outbreak of epidemic neuromyasthenia in 1953 at the Chestnut Hill Hospital in Bethesda, was another author and committee member. With D. A. Henderson, Shelokov had written papers on epidemic neuromyasthenia which appeared in the *New England Journal of Medicine*.

In the book's introduction, Lederberg noted that, far from having conquered infectious diseases, as many seemed to think, the world had never been in greater danger from epidemics of pathogen-borne new diseases. The threat "may even intensify in coming years," Lederberg added.† In addition, he wrote, the next epidemic was likely to come from a previously unknown microbe: "It is this committee's considered opinion that the next major infectious agent to emerge as a threat to health in the United States may, like HIV, be a pathogen that has not

* Martin had even reported isolating a previously unknown virus from the spinal fluids of such cases. Still, the agency refused his invitation to send a team to L.A. to examine the encephalitis cases and to note firsthand the laboratory evidence for his claims.

Martin had been stunned and angered by the agency staff's cavalier dismissal of his concerns. The pathologist had blamed the government scientists' refusal to investigate on the fact that he had tentatively linked the encephalitis cases to the CFS epidemic.

† The outbreak of rat-borne pneumonic plague in parts of India in the fall of 1994, after severe floods left garbage and sewage strewn across the land, was evidence enough that even the oldest diseases had yet to be defeated. The 1995 Ebola outbreak in Zaire was an even more recent reminder of humanity's vulnerability.

been previously recognized." No matter where the pathogens come from, however, Lederberg added, "we can be confident that new diseases will emerge." How could he be so certain? "Jet spread," made possible by modern transportation systems; genetic alterations in disease-causing microbes; human population growth; and invasion of "new ecological settings," he insisted, all "favor exposure to new pathogens and more efficient transmission" of old microbes.

World Health Organization, Geneva, Switzerland

By early 1993, chronic fatigue syndrome appeared in the World Health Organization's tenth revision of its International Statistical Classification of Diseases and Related Health Problems. On page 494 of the volume, known as the ICD-10, the disease was given a designation, or code, G93.3, and named postviral fatigue syndrome, benign myalgic encephalomyelitis.

The World Health Organization's classification system limited all diseases in the G90 to G99 category to disorders of the central nervous system; G93 diseases, in particular, were disorders of the brain.

Milwaukee, Wisconsin

On January 2, 1993, Sidney Grossberg of the Medical College of Wisconsin began receiving money from the National Institute of Allergy and Infectious Diseases to investigate the role of human JHK virus in chronic fatigue syndrome. Over the next three years, he would receive nearly a half million dollars in support of his effort.* Grossberg was slated to receive blood samples from CFS sufferers and healthy controls from NIAID's Stephen Straus and from the Centers for Disease Control. Privately, however, he confessed to staff at the CFIDS Association that he had little faith in the Atlanta agency scientists' ability to identify cases of the disease. After government retrovirologist Tom Folks reported that "we were really not able to distinguish whether [Grossberg's virus] was endogenous or exogenous" or "whether it was related to CFS," Grossberg, like DeFreitas before him, decided to pursue his research without further government collaboration.

National Institute of Allergy and Infectious Diseases, Bethesda, Maryland

By early 1993 it appeared that Stephen Straus, long a promoter of the view that CFS was a potential psychiatric disease, was now engaged in a game of scientific catch-up. In the January issue of the *Journal of Clinical Immunology,* Straus's research group reported finding immune aberrations in CFS patients.[2] On February 5 the NIH touted the findings in a press release as if they were a breakthrough, even though scores of scientists around the world had been finding immune aberrations in CFS sufferers for years. Asked if there was anything new about Straus's

---

* In addition, the CFIDS Association was providing the scientist with an additional $106,000 a year, bringing Grossberg's total funds closer to $1 million.

findings, Boston's Anthony Komaroff was characteristically diplomatic. "The work was consistent with what others have reported," he said.

Food and Drug Administration, Rockville, Maryland

On February 18 executives from HEM Pharmaceuticals and its consulting scientists met with FDA officials. In what oncologist David Strayer, HEM's medical adviser, described as an "educational" session, the company sought to explain the clinical and biological manifestations of the disease to the government scientists. Listening were officials from the FDA's Antiviral Drug Advisory Committee.

Perhaps the biggest hurdle HEM needed to overcome was the FDA's stated concern about the side effects of Ampligen. In clinical trials in other diseases such as AIDS and cancer, Ampligen had been shown to be remarkably nontoxic. "Adverse events" that worried the FDA included fever, chills, rashes, myalgias [muscle aches], arthralgias [joint aches], palpitations, and sleep disturbance—all aspects of CFS itself. In a report to HEM board members in 1991, William Carter, HEM's president and a co-inventor of Ampligen, had noted, "New data . . . indicate conclusively that the 'side effect' profile is directly attributable to an elevated lymphokine, such as IL-1, and not [to] Ampligen. Independent physicians have corroborated our conclusion that the 'side effect' profile is simply manifestations of the underlying disorder itself."

Indeed, in the paper about the clinical trial, published early in 1994, HEM scientists calculated that the "total number of adverse events reported by patients receiving [Ampligen] was virtually identical to that reported by patients receiving placebo."[3] There were no statistically significant differences in adverse events between the two groups, in fact, except that patients on placebo reported more insomnia.

FDA scientists were stymied on another matter as well. What would be considered "end points" for successful therapy for the disease? If Ampligen was not a cure, then how could improvement be measured, and what degree of improvement might be expected? In an effort to answer these questions, Carson City, Nevada, resident Gerald Crum, a former electronics technician and software programmer, testified at the February meeting about his own experience with Ampligen. After falling ill in 1985, he had suffered three years of progressive deterioration, a condition that included frequent seizures and short-term memory loss. His IQ, formerly 130, fell to 85. "When I went for walks in my neighborhood," Crum told the FDA panel, "I couldn't find my way home." Crum had been part of the early pilot study in Nevada in 1989. After three months on Ampligen, his IQ was measured at 120, his seizures became far less frequent, and he could do complex math again. Crum pointed out that, although he wasn't recovered, he had "regained a measure of quality to my life which I thought I would never experience again."

In 1990, Crum voluntarily withdrew from the drug to see if its good effects could be sustained. "Within six weeks," he recalled, "I began experiencing seizures, several per week, and I lost the cognitive ability I had regained. In short, I regressed to the same seriously ill condition I was in prior to receiving Ampligen." Four months later he was started on Ampligen once more and was still receiving the infusions. Crum said he was now in the best shape he had been in since contracting the disease. In addition, he said, he had never experienced "toxicity or severe side effects from this drug." His experience, Crum testified, demonstrated that "CFS is treatable and that the most severe symptoms can be stopped from advancing." It also demonstrated that treatment was required for sustained periods of up to years, even perhaps for the duration of the patient's life. "I urge immediate compassionate access to the drug for the most severe cases of CFS," Crum said. "I also urge fast-track licensing of the drug to make it available to the vast population suffering from CFS."

Paul Cheney also testified before the FDA scientists. As he had done nearly ten years before with two Epidemic Intelligence Service officers from the Centers for Disease Control, he tried to convey the profundity of the medical and social impact of the disease. At best, Cheney told FDA officials, the disease was a "prolonged postviral syndrome" from which people recovered or improved within one to five years. At worst, he said, "it is a nightmare of increasing disability with both physical and neurocognitive components." In the last six months alone, he continued, five of his clinic's patients had died, "two by suicide and three by intercurrent infections. All were in a progressive, debilitated state." Immunologically, the doctor added, many of his clinic's 1,200 patients had remarkably reduced levels of T-cell subsets. Four patients had developed "AIDS-defining" opportunistic infections. "Most have abnormal neurologic examinations," Cheney continued. "Half have abnormal MRI scans, eighty percent have abnormal SPECT scans, ninety-five percent have abnormal cognitive evoked EEG brain maps.

"We regularly admit [patients] to the hospital," Cheney continued. "The most common admitting diagnoses are acute and chronic encephalopathy, uncontrolled head pain, and debilitating fatigue with inability to care for self." One of his patients, he said, had been hospitalized for five months and was awaiting nursing home placement; she was thirty-seven. The doctor called the disease "a disaster, from an economic standpoint." Four-fifths of the patients evaluated at his clinic were unable to attend school or work: "Most are already on or will shortly be on some sort of disability plan, public or private. In a recent survey of twenty consecutive patients at our clinic, the average dollar figure spent on medical care before coming to our clinic was $15,000, with a range of from $2,500 to $50,000. Most patients had seen more than ten physicians."

Cheney also described the manner in which his practice had become tied to litigation by CFS sufferers. "We are frequently depositioned for disability and other types of litigation," he explained. "Many cases involve divorce as we witness the disintegration of the family unit. We have seen litigation against schools to force homebound teaching of impaired children with CFS. The medical–legal aspects of our practice steadily grow as this disease eats at the fabric of our communities."

According to David Strayer, the medical oncologist who was in charge of the pharmaceutical firm's AIDS and CFS clinical trials, FDA officials seemed to accept HEM's explanation for the "adverse events" noted in the CFS trial. In fact, it was increasingly apparent to all that the drug agency now looked favorably on the prospect of a second round of expanded trials in the disease. Just one problem remained: by all reports, HEM Pharmaceuticals was poised on the brink of insolvency.

Centers for Disease Control, Atlanta, Georgia

The retroviral theory of the disease took a serious battering in the medical press as 1993 began, chiefly as a result of the Atlanta agency's failed efforts to replicate Elaine DeFreitas's finding. First, the Ciba Foundation published the paper Tom Folks had read at the foundation's 1992 London symposium, in which he described his laboratory's inability to reproduce the Wistar immunologist's work.[4] In February, the lead article in the *Annals of Internal Medicine* reprised the Ciba paper: scientists in Atlanta had tried and failed to find HTLV2-like gene fragments in patients suffering from chronic fatigue syndrome.[5]

In March, the CDC's *Morbidity and Mortality Weekly Report* carried news of the failure of John Martin and C. V. Herst to differentiate between patients and controls using their respective tests for retroviral infection.[6] The article noted that Walter Gunn's experiment was the first "controlled, blinded trial to examine the ability of these retroviral tests . . . to distinguish CFS case-patients from controls." The study's findings "do not support the hypothesized association between infection with retroviruses and CFS and are consistent with findings from other studies assessing evidence of retroviral infection."

The response to the CDC study on the part of activists in the CFS field was strong and swift. Ottawa clinician Byron Hyde, an irrepressible critic of the agency since its publication of what Hyde believed were criminally faulty diagnostic criteria for the disease in 1988, took umbrage in his advocacy newsletter, the *Nightingale*, which reached 12,000 Canadian and American CFS sufferers.

"How Reliable is the CDC?" Hyde thundered in a banner headline. "First . . . the CDC published incorrect physical diagnostic criteria for CFS," he continued in his article. "Now the CDC, in a non–peer review announcement [the *MMWR*], states that there is no apparent basis to the Cheney-Bell-DeFreitas retrovirus. This is not a scientific approach worthy of a federally funded organization, but appears more like state terrorism." Hyde suggested that the agency's zealous report might make it harder for DeFreitas to publish her work in a peer-reviewed journal "where this fascinating research would face proper scientific scrutiny." He accused the agency of being determined to bury "potentially important scientific information," adding, "If the CDC were truly interested in scientific truth, a more reasonable approach would have been to assist the DeFreitas group with adequate funding. This, of course, was not done."

It was amid this atmosphere that Hilary Koprowski decided that it would be wise to subject Elaine DeFreitas's paper, "Non-C-type Retrovirus in Children," to a formal review before publishing the article in the *Proceedings of the National Academy of Sciences*. As an academy member, Koprowski had the right to request the publication of articles in *PNAS* without formal peer review. The privilege afforded academy members the opportunity to see papers published that they deemed important without the long lead times imposed by a formal review; Sudhir Gupta's article about the discovery of an apparently novel virus in non–HIV positive AIDS sufferers had been such a paper. Now, though he continued to support DeFreitas's work, Koprowski sensed the glut of refutations against her had rendered impolitic the use of his academy privilege. Far better for DeFreitas, he reasoned, if the article were peer reviewed by scientists outside the academy, even if only for the sake of appearance. Fully confident the article could stand up to any scrutiny, Koprowski requested an independent review.

David Bell, who was following the fate of the paper with special interest since the three children described in it had been his patients for years, recalled that the first reviewers were reasonable in their criticisms. Primarily, they expressed concern about the potential for contamination. In order to satisfy them, DeFreitas performed the experiments again, checking for the contaminants that had worried the reviewers; she included her negative findings in her new draft. That paper was then sent to two more reviewers. It was then, according to Bell, that the process began to go haywire.

"The next two reviewers' comments were totally off base," Bell recalled later. "The reviewers contradicted each other, and their criticisms were irrelevant. At that point, I remember thinking, We're now getting away from science and into the politics of the disease."

DeFreitas was unable to satisfy the new reviewers—one of whom Bell strongly suspected was Stephen Straus—and *PNAS* rejected the article pending her ability to do so.

American Medical Association, Chicago, Illinois

For years federal health agencies had fostered a view that CFS was grossly over-diagnosed and that most cases were probably better-known chronic diseases that doctors had failed to recognize, such as lupus, multiple sclerosis, or, most popularly, garden-variety depression. Yet, in focusing on what else CFS might be, the government stubbornly ignored mounting evidence for what it was. Moreover, in the world outside the NIH's ivy-covered brick buildings, those who looked in a systematic way had discovered that very few people bearing the CFS diagnosis were suffering from any other known illness.

Lyme disease was high among the maladies commonly assumed to be CFS-masqueraders that had falsely inflated the magnitude of the CFS epidemic. The tick-borne bacterial disease theoretically lent itself to cure by antibiotics. In many cases, however, the "cure" failed, and victims of Lyme disease suffered a debilitating course of illness, frequently neurological in nature, that defied treatment, sometimes lasting for years. Five years earlier, pediatrician David Bell had privately advanced a precocious notion about the Lyme phenomenon: perhaps, Bell mused, chronic antibiotic-resistant Lyme cases were actually misdiagnosed CFS. Bell was not speaking out of ignorance; his wife, Karen, an infectious disease specialist, had diagnosed the first case of Lyme disease in western Massachusetts several years before, and Bell himself was well versed in Lyme's signs and symptoms.

On April 14 the *Journal of the American Medical Association* published a paper that supported Bell's radical inversion of the government's theory.[7] The article suggested not only that more than half (57 percent) of Lyme disease diagnoses were made wholly in error but also that the disease most commonly mistaken for Lyme was actually CFS. Moreover, 20 percent of patients who had originally had Lyme had rapidly developed another disease, most commonly CFS, "soon after objective manifestations of Lyme disease."

Many misdiagnosed Lyme disease cases were also found to be suffering from fibromyalgia, a condition similar enough to CFS that some fibromyalgia and CFS experts believed the two were either the same or closely related diseases.*

The *JAMA* researchers, who were rheumatology and immunology experts at Tufts and a neurologist at Harvard's Brigham and Women's Hospital, had evaluated the cases of 788 people referred as Lyme disease sufferers to the Lyme disease clinic at the New England Medical Center in Boston during the previous four and a half years. "The greatest diagnostic problem demonstrated in this study was distinguishing Lyme [disease] . . . from chronic fatigue syndrome or fibromyalgia," they wrote. Lyme arthritis typically caused swelling of knees; neurological side effects of Lyme were "subtle memory deficits" and numbness in hands and feet. "These symptoms . . . improve gradually over a period of months following intravenous antibiotic therapy. In contrast," the authors continued, "chronic fatigue syndrome or fibromyalgia, which may be variants of the same disorder, tend to produce more generalized and disabling symptoms. They include marked fatigue, severe headache, widespread musculoskeletal pain . . . difficulty with concentration and sleep disturbance . . . [the] illness is not cured with antibiotic therapy. . . .

"In our experience," the authors added, "Lyme disease has become an overdiagnosed and overtreated illness."

HEM Pharmaceuticals, Philadelphia, Pennsylvania

By the summer of 1993, HEM Pharmaceuticals had, by reports, crashed financially. Although Food and Drug Administration officials gave every indication that they would now allow expanded trials of Ampligen in chronic fatigue syndrome patients, HEM had no money to go forward with an expanded trial. Company officials remained silent on the problem, but one rumor put the company's deficit at $33 million. Efforts were under way to raise money from private investors, but there was little enthusiasm among company officials for raising money by taking the firm public; 1993 had turned out to be a disastrous year for biotechnology stocks.

As HEM's fortunes plummeted, so would those of CFS and AIDS sufferers receiving the drug under the compassionate care clause. Soon Ampligen stocks would be depleted.

* There were subtle differences between the two: in one comparison, for instance, fibromyalgia patients had less severe intellectual impairments than patients with CFS (Curt Sandman, "Is There a Chronic Fatigue Syndrome Dementia?", paper presented at Chronic Fatigue Syndrome and Fibromyalgia: Pathogenesis and Treatment, First International Conference, Los Angeles, Cal., Feb. 16–18, 1990). In addition, fibromyalgia patients had several consistent pressure-sensitive pain regions throughout the body; although CFS sufferers experienced muscular pain, regions of pain were not necessarily consistent from patient to patient.

CFIDS Association, Charlotte, North Carolina

Since hiring professional lobbyist Tom Sheridan to help them negotiate the corridors of Congress, executives at the large Charlotte-based patient organization were growing more focused in their oversight of the CDC and NIH. And, as he was being paid to do, Sheridan was thinking strategically. Increasingly, it was apparent to him that the effort to rehabilitate these agencies from within was not working. In particular, lobbying for more money in the hope that they would use that money to advance the discovery process was clearly a failed initiative. Money was not the problem; the people in charge of the research programs were the problem. Money could do many things, but it could not expunge scientific bias. Sheridan knew that the CFS Interagency Coordinating Committee (CFSICC), as constituted, was a bureaucratic fraud, a committee on letterhead only. If it could be broadened to include powerful health officials, however, it might just be the tool with which patient advocates could pry loose better science from Atlanta and Bethesda. If, for instance, the CFSICC chairperson was the assistant secretary of health, he could ride herd on the handful of ineffectual scientists and bureaucrats currently on the tiny panel. After all, the assistant secretary was chief of the Public Health Service, which included the NIH, the CDC, and the FDA, and he was the second most powerful health official in the nation after Donna Shalala, the secretary of health and human services.

Sheridan had worked with the appropriate congressional committees the previous fall to include language in the new NIH Reauthorization Act that would give his idea the force of law. On June 10, 1993, President Clinton signed the act, which ordered that the CFSICC be chaired by the assistant secretary of health. The act further required that the committee's first meeting in its reconstituted form be held no later than December 15, 1993.

That the recent Clinton appointee to the post happened to be Philip Lee, a medical doctor and former chairman of the San Francisco Health Commission, was the first piece of good fortune CFS victims could claim since the ascendancy of Walter Gunn at the CDC three years before. In contrast to Gunn, however, Lee, who represented the authority of a cabinet member, had real power. He was, in addition, sophisticated in the realm of medical politics, having served as assistant secretary of health in the Johnson administration. In addition, as city health commissioner, Lee had followed the CFS epidemic in San Francisco and had demonstrated his support of patient advocacy groups there.

Like many doctors and scientists who had a proven interest in the disease, the new assistant secretary had a personal stake in the disease as well: a close friend suffered from CFS. Lee had been witness to the onset of his friend's ordeal, which he originally had suspected might be hepatitis; he had watched with dismay as the malady developed into a chronic condition.

Finally, one of Lee's closest friends happened to be Alexis Shelokov, the epidemiologist who had investigated outbreaks of epidemic neuromyasthenia during the 1950s and co-authored papers in the *New England Journal of Medicine* on the topic. Over the years, Shelokov's ideas and observations about the disease had left a deep impression on Lee. During a private meeting in 1992 in San Francisco with several CFS experts, including Paul Cheney, Nancy Klimas, Jay Levy, John Martin, and other local health officials, Lee had said, "I have a strong interest in the policy process and how one might move an illness like this onto the policy agenda. . . . We're almost reaching the point where there is a critical mass of scientific information that can help to move this fairly quickly. And my own view would be that one focus for this effort has to be identifying some people in the executive branch who can have a significant influence on the process." He also said, in talking about James Mason, who was then assistant secretary of health, "If he changed his position on this issue, it could make an enormous difference." Now Lee himself had Mason's job and the attendant political clout.

On August 4 the CFIDS Association's executive director, Kimberly Kenney, wrote a letter of protest to Lee about the most recent report to Congress from the CFS Interagency Coordinating Committee. She recounted no fewer than eighteen outright misstatements of fact and a number of grossly exaggerated assertions in the committee's report about its achievements. She ended by asking Lee to assume his rightful post as chairman of the committee. Lee responded to Kenney a month later. Without committing himself to the chairmanship, he told her that he had met with the CFSICC "to review their activities." He expressed his support of the committee.

Centers for Disease Control, Atlanta, Georgia

By the fall of 1993, the CDC had revised its original estimate of the prevalence of the disease to a figure that was even smaller than the previous year's estimate of 10,000 cases. In the draft of a publication prepared for distribution to the public and to doctors, the agency's epidemiologists wrote that, based on their four-county surveillance study, now three years old, there were between 3,000 and 10,000 people in the United States with chronic fatigue syndrome. The agency planned to circulate the figures in their new booklet, "The Facts about Chronic Fatigue Syndrome."

The agency's statistics, which suggested there were 3.5 CFS victims for every 100,000 people, induced a slack-jawed incredulity among CFS experts outside the government.

"It's a gross undercount, because they insist on using doctor referrals," said Paul Cheney, "when in fact doctors either aren't reporting cases to the CDC case monitors, or they don't believe in the illness." Cheney noted that there were approximately one million people in the five-county region surrounding Charlotte. "At three per hundred thousand, there should be thirty cases in all of Charlotte. But I have three hundred patients from Charlotte in my clinic, and I would say we are seeing only about ten percent of the cases in Charlotte, because I tend to see only the sickest patients. I would say [the CDC epidemiologists] are off by one or two orders of magnitude."

In the final draft of the booklet, the sentence that claimed a mere 3,000 to 10,000 people in the United States suffered from the disease was removed.*

---

* In May 1995, the Centers for Disease Control's William Reeves participated in a congressional briefing on CFS. In the eight months between August 1994 and April 1995, Reeves said, 100,000 copies of "The Facts About Chronic Fatigue Syndrome" were sent in response to public inquiries. In the month of April 1995 alone, the agency mailed another 7,000 copies of a second edition of the booklet.

The CDC's booklet, targeted at doctors and laypeople alike, aimed to answer "the most frequently asked questions about CFS and to clarify areas that are often misunderstood." But *New York Native* reporter Neenyah Ostrom noted after seeing the draft that "it appears to be intended to show that essentially no facts have been established about CFS." The agency determinedly denied scientific findings already established by experienced investigators on matters of immunology, contagion, prevalence, and cancer risks, she wrote. The booklet, Ostrom concluded, "does not describe the chronic fatigue syndrome that exists in the peer-reviewed medical literature." Ostrom's newspaper put the story on its front page under the headline "Anatomy of a Cover-Up."

On September 27 the CDC's Division of Viral and Rickettsial Diseases, headed by the British scientist Brian Mahy, convened a two-day meeting in Atlanta to reconsider the government's case definition. In the six years since its publication in the *Annals of Internal Medicine,* the case definition had become one of the most frequently cited articles in the medical literature.* Even so, critics of the "Holmes criteria," as they were often called in homage to Gary Holmes, the lead author on the *Annals* paper, were legion, and included even the authors of the original definition.

By law, the September meeting was open to the public; consequently, a number of patients and the executives of national advocacy organizations attended, and in response to what struck many as arrogance on the part of federal scientists, emotions were quickly frayed. Lobbyist Tom Sheridan noted, "It was clear that the change of administration and the goodwill engendered by the appointment of Phil Lee as assistant secretary of health had yet to translate to Atlanta. [The CDC officials] were far more resistant to a partnership with patient associations than I had ever imagined—the resistance was palpable."

Members of the government panel were culled from the same committee that reviewed all case referrals to the government's surveillance system. They included the NIH's Stephen Straus and Ann Schleuderberg, Gary Holmes (now a practicing infectious disease specialist at Texas A&M University), University of Toronto psychiatrist Susan Abbey, and the CDC's William Reeves.

"They were trying to frame this illness in a medical-social-cultural context," Miami immunologist Nancy Klimas recalled. "But there was no data."

During the meeting, members of the public expressed considerable distress about the composition of the panel, which was decidedly short on CFS clinical expertise. Canadian CFS expert Byron Hyde was the most vociferous, attacking the inclusion of psychiatrist Abbey, saying it was "appalling that such a person should be on this committee." Hyde said Abbey, in a presentation to more than a thousand health insurance executives in Toronto, had made a joke of the disease by displaying a 1987 *Rolling Stone* article on the subject and calling it "the bible of chronic fatigue syndrome patients." Patient advocates present argued for the inclusion of doctors who treated large numbers of CFS sufferers and who had, col-

---

* This is according to the Institute for Scientific Information, a private Philadelphia firm that published the "Science Citation Index" and other reference works for scientific researchers.

lectively, years of active clinical experience with the disease. In a letter to William Reeves mailed shortly after the meeting, CFIDS Association president Marc Iverson demanded that Reeves add David Bell, Nancy Klimas, and Manhattan CFS expert Susan Levine to the committee. Reeves responded that the committee would remain intact for purposes of "efficiency."

This committee had purported to conduct its deliberations in public, but word soon leaked out that the members had planned months in advance to meet behind closed doors on the second day. After threatening to make a formal protest to the assistant secretary of health, Phil Lee, lobbyist Tom Sheridan extricated from the CDC's Keiji Fukuda the time and place of the meeting. Nevertheless, no patients would be allowed to attend.

Dan Peterson, the next day, left the session dismayed. "Straus is a real snake," the doctor said later. "He's the most subtle of the lot. He wants the disease to be renamed 'fatigue.' " Indeed, after more than a decade of intermittent study of 150 people costing millions of dollars, the government's expert now maintained the disease might not really exist as a "discrete entity." In his formal presentation to the committee the day before, Straus had proposed that possibly "no discrete syndromic entity exists, that any case definition would necessarily exclude many affected individuals, and that chronic fatigue merits serious attention unto itself, in whatever context it occurs." Straus, then, would define the disease—and the epidemic—out of existence by embracing all who claimed fatigue under its umbrella.

Eventually, Reeves hoped to submit the new government definition to the *New England Journal of Medicine.* (The journal rejected Reeves's overture.)

Paul Cheney did not attend the meeting. After being on the receiving end of nearly ten years of cynicism, haughtiness, and ad hominem attacks from CDC scientists, Cheney had lost his enthusiasm for the process. Yet again, government scientists rather than clinicians were defining the disease clinically. In spite of Cheney's absence, however, his disembodied presence seemed to suffuse the proceedings, according to Dan Peterson. "It was very odd," Peterson recalled. "Paul wasn't there, but his presence was felt, nonetheless. It seemed as if they were trying to knock him down without ever once mentioning his name." Indeed, by 1993, Paul Cheney's research and observations about the disease were so familiar to those in the field that he had come to symbolize a worldview of the epidemic which the government had struggled for years to suppress: the view that CFS was a transmissible and ravaging disease of the immune system and the brain with profound implications for all of society.

Predictably, patient organizers made a plea to government scientists to incorporate a new name, "chronic fatigue–immune dysfunction syndrome," into a new definition, buttressing their plea with the testimony of immunologist Nancy Klimas. She presented panel members with a handsomely bound book containing nearly fifty scientific articles identifying immunological abnormalities in the disease. "The data exists and is well published," she said later. "My point was that anyone who has looked has found these abnormalities. There is no controversy there. They exist. I said, given that, why not put it in the name?"

Klimas handed the book to William Reeves, who, according to witnesses, accepted it with chilly calm. His only comment to Klimas: "We have a medical library here."

Agency scientists' most remarkable revelation during the conference was that, according to their surveillance data, the average CFS patient in their study was a white woman with an income of at least $50,000. The finding merely served to emphasize what most students of the disease already knew: the government's doctor-based surveillance system had gone terribly askew. Few would dispute that, so far, CFS appeared to be more common in women than men, but there had been absolutely no evidence, until now, to suggest it targeted rich women. The only conclusion to be drawn from such a statistic was that rich women had more money than poor or middle-class women to seek out doctors with the skill and experience to make the CFS diagnosis.

Curiously, it was at this gathering that the agency's own scientists first began to show signs of retreat on the matter of their four-city surveillance and its puny tally. On the first day, in response to a written question from a citizen in the audience—"What can you say is the actual prevalence of CFS in the U.S. population?"—William Reeves responded, "We are trying to get away from just counting up the number of people who have this. I don't think that's the major impact. . . . I can't give you a number." Repeated congressional requests and several million taxpayer dollars since 1988, then, had been of little avail: Reeves, now heading the CFS investigation in Atlanta, had no numbers.

By 1993, University of Nevada researchers, with the support of the Nevada state legislature, had finished the first community-based prevalence study of CFS in Incline Village and neighboring Crystal Bay. Its principal author, epidemiologist Sandra Daugherty, presented an abstract of her study to the government panel meeting on September 27 to redefine the disease. Nearly a decade after the epidemic years of 1984–1985, a portrait emerged of a community ravaged by a contagious disease that was even more widespread than Dan Peterson and Paul Cheney had suspected. Cheney had proposed an attack rate of 1.5 per hundred people for the northern shore of Lake Tahoe. The Reno researchers, however, had discovered that, in Incline Village and Crystal Bay, at least, the seven-year incidence rate was 4.1 percent for the population as a whole. In other words, four of every one hundred people had fallen ill with the disease during the last seven years. The highest incidence of the disease had occurred in Incline Village in 1985 and 1986.

Daugherty, director of the Division of Community Medicine at the University of Nevada School of Medicine, had been the driving force behind the research. Both she and her husband, medical school dean Robert Daugherty, had been dismayed and eventually angered by the government's Tahoe investigation and lack of follow-up. After her husband was brushed off during a meeting with then–CDC chief James Mason in Atlanta in 1988, the Daughertys had successfully appealed to the state legislature for money to perform their own surveillance study.

For every CFS case that turned up in her survey, Daugherty chose a healthy community control, matched to the case by age, sex, and race. This technique provided the means to determine a number of crucial risk factors for the disease, as well as statistics about its natural history and the frequency of certain symptoms. Based on the symptom reports alone, Daugherty and her fellow researchers suggested that cognitive impairment, which they defined as "trouble concentrating, trouble with memory, or confusion," be named a major criterion for diagnosis of the disease. Daugherty found evidence of these disabling symptoms in 100 percent of the patients. As it stood, the government definition had relegated cognitive dysfunction to minor criteria.

The researchers identified a number of risk factors for the disease. These factors, they said, "were found to be associated with CFS and preceded its onset." They included prior histories of infectious mononucleosis, genital herpes, or allergies, and use of birth control pills at the time of CFS onset in premenopausal women. A history of allergies had long been known to predispose people to the disease, and the link with herpes infections had been suspected. The birth control pill connection was new but not dramatic.

Daugherty and her colleagues produced one singular, myth-shattering finding, however: people with lower educational levels and decreased household incomes had been *more* likely to fall ill with the disease than those with higher education levels and higher household incomes. The finding stood in stark contrast to the assessments of Gary Holmes and Jon Kaplan that Incline Village's CFS victims were rich and privileged, definitely "not normal Americans." Daugherty's finding further suggested that a vast uncounted population of CFS sufferers might exist among the nation's lower classes. Certainly many clinicians had suspected for some time that the appellation "yuppie disease" had arisen because it was only the upper middle classes whose education gave them the financial ability and self-confidence to negotiate the nation's health care system to the point of accurate diagnosis. As Paul Cheney had observed in the middle-1980s, "A virus doesn't know whether you're a yuppie." The finding cast further doubt on the government's survey methods, which had relied entirely on doctors to report cases and had resulted in turning up a majority of patients with unusually high incomes.

"We had a lot of people who were very poor—below ten thousand dollars a year," Sandra Daugherty said when queried later about her results. "I wasn't surprised. Practically every illness you can name hits the lower classes harder."

Daugherty had completed her study in two years using approximately $50,000 in state funds.

Social Security Administration, Baltimore, Maryland

Because the Social Security Administration had never officially acknowledged the existence of CFS as a physical disability in its manual, disability awards for the disease—if they were made at all—were typically made under a range of psychiatric categories or for vague-sounding maladies like "organic brain syndrome." On August 26, nine years after the Nevada outbreak, the Social Security Administration sent a Teletype to its branch offices throughout the United States with a code number—688—for chronic fatigue syndrome disability cases. "Effective immediately," the Teletype said, "state agencies will enter code 688 whenever the case involves allegation or diagnosis of CFS."

Assigning a formal code to the disease was a big step for the agency, but according to Barry Eigen, deputy director of the Office of Disability's division of medical and vocational policy, merely having a code did not establish the disease as a physical impairment; it was an epidemiological tool by which to begin to count the number of people who sought disability support by claiming to have CFS. When asked how soon the agency would begin to perform the appropriate statistical analyses that would reveal how many CFS sufferers were seeking disability support, Eigen commented, "It's probably going to be a very long time.

"We don't have a [disability] listing for chronic fatigue syndrome," Eigen continued, "because there's no agreement for what it is and how to establish that someone has it. We can only follow what other scientists and health agencies say—namely the NIH and CDC. *We* have no data. There has to be something we can hang our hat on."

The impetus for establishing a code, Eigen said, had come from within the Social Security Administration—"We wanted to do the right thing"—and because of the agency's representation on the federal interagency committee for CFS, now chaired by Assistant Secretary of Health Phil Lee.

National Institute of Allergy and Infectious Diseases, Bethesda, Maryland

Chronic fatigue syndrome was just one disease under study by the NIH's Stephen Straus. As chief of the Laboratory of Clinical Investigation at NIAID, Straus had also been a co-investigator in a 1993 trial of a drug thought to be helpful in hepatitis B. Given the outcome, it seemed apparent that CFS was not the only disease in which Straus had difficulty assessing the clinical significance of patients' complaints.

On November 15, the *New York Times* called the trial "among the worst catastrophes in the recent history of drug testing." One third of fifteen patients died—deaths Food and Drug Administration chief David Kessler suggested could have been prevented had the investigators viewed their data more critically. "In retrospect," Kessler told *Times* reporter Philip Hilts, "the data were there. There were five deaths here that demanded greater scrutiny."

Straus's involvement in this apparently preventable disaster seemed even more egregious since he had overseen an earlier trial of the drug at the NIH in 1990 in which three people died and five patients developed dangerously high liver enzymes. Straus had collaborated with the University of Washington's Larry Corey on that trial. And there was yet another NIH trial in 1991, during which one death might have resulted from the drug. (A fourth trial was conducted in 1989 at the University of California at San Diego; of twelve patients, one may have died because of the drug.) In these earlier trials, the FDA's Kessler said, as many as five patients may have died from the drug "or its experimental predecessor," but the scientists in charge of those trials had not reported the deaths as drug related because they apparently did not believe the drug had played a role. These scientists "failed to think skeptically about the data they were collecting," Hilts wrote in a paraphrase of Kessler's additional comments. Many of the survivors, some of whom required liver transplants, were expected to sue the government.

Department of Veterans Affairs, Washington, D.C.

On November 16, Veterans Affairs Secretary Jesse Brown announced that his agency would compensate all Gulf War veterans who were able to prove they were suffering from chronic fatigue syndrome as a result of their Persian Gulf service.

Department of Health and Human Services, Washington, D.C.

By federal law, Phil Lee was required to hold a meeting of the newly constituted CFS Interagency Coordinating Committee before mid-December. On November 17 the new assistant secretary of health delivered: thirty-five government scientists and administrators and seven patient advocates were invited to Lee's offices for the committee's first legitimate meeting. For the first time, scientists like the CDC's Brian Mahy and William Reeves were asked to describe in detail and defend their agency's research agendas to the chief of the Public Health Service. Lee listened intently, took notes, and asked pointed questions during the two-hour session.

Afterward, Kim Kenney of the CFIDS Association complained that the committee had yet to "fulfill its mission as defined by Public Law 103-112. There is no CFS action plan, nor are there formal representatives from the CFS or private research communities on the committee." Nevertheless, she was impressed by Lee's familiarity with the current state of CFS research in government labs, and she noted with private enjoyment that scientists Mahy and Reeves seemed unnerved by Lee's demanding inquiry and by his deference to patients and their representatives—a deference that had been sorely lacking in interactions between CDC scientists and patient advocates.

"Now we're waiting to see if he's just talking the talk or if he'll walk the walk," Kenney said.

1994

VIRTUAL MEDICINE

It is not . . . that some people do not know what to
do with truth when it is offered them, but the tragic
fate is to reach, after years of patient search, a condition of mind-blindness, in which the truth is not
recognized, though it stares you in the face.

—Sir William Osler, *Counsels and Ideals*

35

Science by the Rules

Harvard Medical School, Boston, Massachusetts

In 1994 the disease's cause and modes of transmission continued to mystify, but one certainty had emerged: chronic fatigue syndrome, unknown to a previous generation of Americans, was now a common disease. Investigators in private institutions were providing prevalence estimates that surpassed the government's by a hundredfold and more that year. None of these researchers had relied on doctors to report the disease, as had the CDC's Larry Schonberger and his staff. Instead, the independent investigators followed the time-honored epidemiologic tradition of D. A. Henderson in Punta Gorda in 1956 and other like-minded investigators who were in sincere pursuit of disease prevalence: they went directly to the population at risk and searched for cases.

David Bates, a Harvard researcher who was one of Anthony Komaroff's colleagues, analyzed 1,000 consecutive patients coming to a primary care clinic and found that 1 percent of them had CFS, based on the Australian definition of the disease. When Bates used the more exclusive 1988 CDC definition to identify cases, the percentage was slightly less than one-third of that, or 0.3 percent of the population. In a paper on the subject in the *Archives of Internal Medicine,* Bates had estimated there were 300 cases of CFS per 100,000 people.[1] Bates's figures seemed to be a reprise of Dedra Buchwald's finding of the previous year; extrapolating from 4,000 members of a Seattle HMO to the general population, Buchwald had reported an estimate of 98 to 267 people per 100,000.[2]

To lend these figures perspective, it is instructive to recall the polio epidemics of the 1950s, perhaps the last time when—as a result of its easy transmissibility—a potentially devastating infectious disease had posed such a significant threat to the population. In 1953, one of the last important years of the polio outbreak (the first vaccines were introduced in 1955), the incidence of paralytic polio was 20 per 100,000 people.* Based on the Harvard and University of Washington studies, then, CFS—a disease that crippled without paralyzing—was in 1994 somewhere

---

* This is according to the Centers for Disease Control's National Immunization Program, Epidemiology and Surveillance Division.

between five and fifteen times more common than polio at the height of the polio epidemic.*

DePaul University investigator Leonard Jason, who by 1994 had captained two pilot studies measuring CFS rates in Chicago in an effort to obtain federal funding for a wider investigation of prevalence, was impressed by Bates's and Buchwald's numbers. One way to view them, according to Jason, was to restrict the findings to the 190 million people in the nation who were eighteen or older. If 1 percent of American adults had CFS, then nearly 2 million people were suffering. If 0.3 percent had the disease, the number was still impressive: 580,000 people, or slightly more than a half million adults. The more conservative figure suggested that CFS was at least twice as common as multiple sclerosis—and certainly among the most common chronic diseases of this era. By Jason's formula, Buchwald's conservative estimate suggested 190,000 Americans had CFS. Moreover, both Bates's and Buchwald's research included a bias that may have resulted in a significant underestimation of the problem: not everyone with the disease would be found by looking exclusively in medical settings. Jason and his Chicago collaborators had discovered that about 40 percent of CFS sufferers eventually abandoned their effort to seek help within establishment medicine, either because their doctors did not believe they were ill or because they were unable to pay for medical care.

"The bottom line," Jason said, "is that when you have an illness that is this stigmatized by medical professionals, you just can't go about measuring prevalence using physician-based studies. You're going to get biased results."

Based on his own pilot statistics, Jason estimated that at least 200 people per 100,000 in the United States were suffering from bona fide CFS (ten times the 1953 polio rate), a statistic suggesting a half million people had the disease. His data were derived from a random telephone survey of 1,031 Chicagoans. Of these people, 5 percent reported they had suffered severe fatigue for six months or more (a major criterion of the CDC's research definition), but Jason winnowed out just two people among them as bona fide CFS patients. At 200 per 100,000, the national prevalence of the disease among adults would be 387,000. But, Jason noted, because his defining parameters were so rigid, "it could be twice or three times that." The incidence of diagnosed AIDS cases in the United States in 1994 was 30 per 100,000, making CFS—at a minimum—approximately six and a half times as common.

After six years and more than $12 million spent on the disease, the CDC's best official estimate so far, published in the agency booklet, "The Facts about Chronic Fatigue Syndrome," was 2 to 10 people per 100,000.

"If that were true," Jason commented, "[only] four thousand to twenty thousand people in all of the United States would have the disease. . . . Given their

---

* It is similarly instructive to note that, as with most infectious agents, only a small proportion of people who were exposed to the polio agent developed symptoms. Ninety to 95 percent of all polio infections were inapparent, or without symptoms; 4 to 8 percent manifested as a minor illness, without any central nervous system involvement; another 1 to 2 percent were nonparalytic but bore signs of aseptic meningitis. In all, just one tenth to one eighth of 1 percent of all polio infections resulted in paralysis. (From statistics provided by the Centers for Disease Control's National Immunization Program, Epidemiology and Surveillance Division.)

past history," he added, "the Centers for Disease Control should cede the study of the epidemiology of this disease to outside investigators."

As the larger numbers began to filter out in presentations at medical conferences and in the medical literature, staff in Atlanta seemed increasingly willing, even eager, to step back from their own surveillance figures and admit their complicated system had resulted in a gross undercount. Jim Dobbins, an agency demographer and member of the CDC's CFS Research Group, remarked that year, "It seems ludicrous to assume we got them all."

Keiji Fukuda, the medical officer assigned to the disease, acknowledged that "the bias inherent in any doctor-based system is to undercount cases."*

On the strength of the new data filtering out from universities, the CFIDS Association asked Congress for $10 million to support the CDC's surveillance efforts in 1995—with a catch: "The Association encourages the immediate termination . . . of the present [four-city] surveillance study and supports . . . a more effective community-based prevalence study which would allow CDC to collect data on endemic cases and possible cluster outbreaks. The Association also believes CDC should commence a series of studies on possible transmission routes for CFIDS and provide appropriate educational programs." In other words, no more lies.

In early 1994 agency staff revealed that they had in fact halted the original four-city survey and launched a less "passive" form of surveillance in San Francisco, using a random telephone dialing system to survey that city's population. Instead of looking exclusively for CFS, however, the agency again had added a layer of complexity to its surveillance efforts by searching for "chronic fatigue" as well as "chronic fatigue syndrome." Congress had never asked the agency to measure the prevalence of fatigue in urban America.

Nevertheless, agency-watchers found one reason to hope that the CDC might be moving into a more aggressive investigatory mode: Larry Schonberger, who had designed the original surveillance plan in the 1980s and had been, along with Jon Kaplan, among the most cynical of all agency staff on the matter of the disease's existence, was no longer an active participant in the agency's CFS research group.

▨

There was little indication in 1994 that CFS was waning in other parts of the world. A prominent New Zealand researcher reported that an estimated 3,500 people—or 1 percent of New Zealand's population of 3.5 million—suffered from the disease. Gerhard Krueger, a leading German CFS researcher, said that there had been no effort to undertake surveillance in Germany and that the disease was not recognized in most universities and "established teaching institutions," but, he said, "we assume the prevalence is about the same as in the United States—the

---

* On May 12, 1995, designated by patient organizations as International CFIDS/ME Awareness Day, principal investigator William Reeves appeared before interested House and Senate staffs to present the CDC's prevalence estimates. By then Reeves had upped the government prevalence estimate from 2 to 10 per 100,000 Americans over the age of eighteen to 4 to 10 per 100,000.

general estimate is one percent of the population."* Investigators in the Netherlands offered a preliminary estimate based on a doctor-referral surveillance system: from 15,000 to 18,000 people in that country of 15 million suffered from CFS. A Belgian group, representing a country of 10 million, suggested a "crude estimate" of 10,000 to 30,000 victims.[3]

By early 1994 approximately 1,500 patients, most of them Americans, had sought Paul Cheney's expertise in Charlotte, North Carolina. For nearly a decade, Cheney had kept voluminous computerized records on all of his CFS patients dating back to the Nevada epidemic, records that included demographic and medical aspects of each case. Interestingly, 1987 was the year named more often than any other when Cheney asked CFS sufferers when they fell ill. One might have concluded that the national epidemic peaked in the late 1980s, a possibility Cheney allowed. Nevertheless, he noted, "The epidemic is still fairly forceful. There *is* a peak in the late 1980s, but if it took ten years to reach a peak, it could take three times that long to level off. The exponential growth has lessened, but the *numbers* of people getting sick are still high."

National Institutes of Health, Bethesda, Maryland

On January 12, Stephen Straus addressed a "Mind/Body Interactions and Disease" symposium on the subject of chronic fatigue syndrome. The symposium was held under the auspices of the NIH, its stated purpose "to encourage researchers . . . to undertake studies in the burgeoning field of psychoneuroimmunology, the study of the relationship between the brain, the immune system, and the mind." Because Straus avoided CFS medical conferences where patients might be present, his views on the disease, especially of late, were not well known by patient associations.

Mindful of his client, the largest patient organization in the nation, Washington lobbyist Tom Sheridan wrote to Straus asking if the government scientist would share his notes from his presentation.

Straus's response, in full, was as follows: "My presentation on January 12, 1994, was extemporaneous. I have no written outline nor an abstract. Sorry!"

HEM Pharmaceuticals, Philadelphia, Pennsylvania

By 1994, some reports suggested HEM Pharmaceuticals would require at least $80 million to launch new trials and begin manufacturing Ampligen once more. One question puzzling nearly everyone who was following the company's fortunes, however, including its physician-collaborators, was why HEM had failed to pursue its entrée into Canada. "The whole concept of the Canadian trial," said one Canadian official who asked not to be named, "was that the government would pay. It would not cost HEM a penny." Yet, for reasons that were unclear to the

---

* Krueger also said that he knew "offhand" of just ten doctors in all of Germany who "seriously take care of CFS patients—and that's not enough in a country of eighty million."

Canadians, there was no follow-up by HEM. The official could only speculate that "infighting" among HEM executives had somehow derailed the plan.

Beginning in 1994, the last remaining American CFS patients receiving Ampligen under the government's compassionate care clause began to be removed from the drug. Even "Patient 00," Albuquerque housewife Nancy Kaiser, who had been the first CFS sufferer to receive Ampligen in 1990, was forced off the medication. Kaiser told a journalist later, "HEM left us to drown." In addition, all trials of the drug's effectiveness against AIDS ceased.*

Ampligen now had "orphan drug" status at the Food and Drug Administration, a move that had no effect on the availability of the drug but would have given HEM tax credits throughout any future clinical trials. Furthermore, if the drug was approved at the end of the trials, HEM would then have the exclusive right to manufacture Ampligen for seven years. The tax credit boon and all other matters relating to Ampligen, however, remained moot as long as HEM was broke.

"Data from our preliminary trials suggest Ampligen is helpful in both AIDS and CFS," said David Strayer, the oncologist who had supervised clinical trials of Ampligen in both diseases. "But the data is not conclusive. To make it conclusive, we need more trials with more patients."

Ironically, in January the journal *Clinical Infectious Diseases* published the results of HEM's original study of Ampligen in ninety-two CFS patients, which had demonstrated the drug's good results.[4] The *New England Journal of Medicine* had rejected the paper, adhering to its de facto policy of avoiding articles pertaining to CFS. David Strayer wasn't surprised by the famous medical journal's rejection. "They didn't publish anything on Lyme [disease] either, until the agent was found," he noted.

In spite of HEM's public posture of virtual bankruptcy, the firm was quietly moving its research operations to Europe, where it reportedly was easier to achieve government approval of drugs. HEM was collaborating with a Brussels medical team to undertake an open-label pilot study of Ampligen in CFS that year. It was a tiny study—just eleven patients had been enrolled—and the trial lasted for twenty-four weeks, the length of the U.S. trial. The investigators were at the Academic Hospital of the Free University of Brussels.

It seemed apparent from a one-page poster on the study presented at an American CFS scientific conference in Florida in the fall of 1994 that the Belgian protocol for measuring improvement had been modeled on Dan Peterson's pilot trial

---

* In Miami, immunologist Nancy Klimas had been following five AIDS patients on Ampligen for three years as part of a multi-city trial. "My experience with the drug was favorable," she said. "We saw stabilization of CD-four counts." Three other AIDS patients in her care had been receiving the drug under the compassionate care clause. Early that winter, Klimas received a letter from HEM saying that all of her AIDS patients would be removed from the drug unless they could pay for it. None of the patients could afford the drug. "I don't have any patients with AIDS on Ampligen now," Klimas said in late February. Her AIDS patients were considering a class action suit against HEM. In February, when they had been off the drug for two months, Klimas said it was too soon to assess whether the AIDS victims' withdrawal from Ampligen had resulted in deterioration.

in Nevada and the ensuing larger study.* The eight investigators noted that the drug had caused no "major adverse experiences" and summarized, "The preliminary results show that Ampligen is a well tolerated and promising treatment for CFS patients."[5]

There were rumors that a second Ampligen trial was under way among ME patients in Ireland as well, but HEM would not confirm the reports, even to its American collaborators, several of whom were dumbfounded when they learned a trial had occurred in Brussels. When biochemist Robert Suhadolnik, who had collaborated with HEM for a number of years, read the Belgium poster at the Florida conference, he went directly to a telephone and dialed HEM chief William Carter. "I said, 'What the hell is going on?' " Suhadolnik recalled later. The impenetrable Carter was unresponsive. "We were cut out of the loop right there," Suhadolnik added, comprehending by then that Carter had decided to break with his longtime American collaborators and establish fresh, potentially more promising bonds with foreign researchers. (Carter failed to respond to numerous requests for interviews for this book, most recently in mid-1995. HEM receptionists unabashedly reported he was "traveling to raise money.")

"HEM is now using markets outside of the United States," Suhadolnik continued. "Maybe they have a whole new team. But there is no reason the American government could not have approved this drug after that double-blind study. I just don't know where Ampligen fell between the cracks in this country. It's a miracle drug. I know AIDS patients who were being maintained on this drug and died *immediately* when they took them off. Here was a massive, million-dollar investment with good results," Suhadolnik added in reference to the four-city CFS trial. "Why didn't it meet FDA approval? It's just plain crazy." After a moment he added, "The biggest problem that drug has is that it *works*."

Centers for Disease Control, Atlanta, Georgia

Tom Folks and Elaine DeFreitas had neither corresponded nor spoken with each other in nearly a year. The February 1993 publication of Folks's *Annals* paper refuting her finding had ended any semblance of goodwill on either side. According to Folks, the *Annals* article, closely followed by the article in the *Morbidity and Mortality Weekly Report,* which had seemed to further cast doubt on DeFreitas's finding, was "kind of a double whammy on Elaine." He added, "She's sort of not in the picture anymore."

In January, Folks and his colleagues at the Atlanta agency delivered what they felt confident was a triple whammy. For the past year, Folks's lab had been exploring CFS samples for evidence of a myriad of human and animal retroviruses, including bovine, feline, and gibbon ape leukemia viruses and human spuma viruses, with "basically negative results," according to Folks. In February, in the same issue of the same journal in which the Ampligen trials were described, Folks

---

* By mid-1995, a second and much larger double-blind clinical trial was getting under way in Brussels. At least one patient, an American living in Paris who sought entrance into the trial, was told he would be required to pay for the cost of the drug and infusions over a six-month period, a cost set by HEM at $30,000.

reported his results.[6] "Our only disclaimer, at this point," he said later, "is that those viruses could still be there if we looked in the wrong tissue or if they're in such low concentration in the blood that we couldn't find them."

Disclaimer aside, it was apparent Folks and others at the CDC were not only more skeptical than ever about the retroviral theory of the disease, they doubted that a virus was even involved. "It could be microwave radiation," Folks offered flippantly. "It doesn't have to be infection."

Folks was at peace with himself and his agency. "A lot of taxpayer-investigative hours went into trying to find out whether Elaine DeFreitas was right," he said. "I know Elaine can sleep at night now. She would not want to mislead the CFS community. And I can sleep at night knowing that I've done what's right for the taxpayer and the CFS community. In science, negatives are answers, too. They're not the answers you want, but they are answers."

And although the CFS research in Folks's lab had slacked off—"If you pool the percentages of full-time-equivalents who are working on CFS, it's probably down to one or two"—Folks said the investigation spawned by DeFreitas's finding had engendered more retroviral research, including the development of a more sensitive test for retroviruses, which Folks intended to patent. "CFS, in fact, got us into these areas," Folks added, "and it could spin off back into CFS."

"My concern," commented Miami immunologist Nancy Klimas, "is that the people at CDC feel *firmly* that they have disproved an etiology for viruses, and yet they've housed the disease under Bill Reeves's viral section. It's a counterintuitive thing. You have to wonder how they really *feel* about the disease. The *words* coming out speak to a commitment to do the job that Congress has charged them with doing, but . . . then you look at what they're actually doing."

University of Miami, Florida

Since her move to Miami, Elaine DeFreitas had been fighting an uphill battle for professional survival. Hurricane Andrew, which coincided with the move from Philadelphia, had devastated her hopes of a smooth transition from Wistar to academia. Crucial laboratory equipment had sat on loading docks for weeks, then months, as residents of southern Florida struggled to reconstruct the region. In the weeks following the hurricane, there were frequent power outages on the Miami campus. And although she had been able to bring three lab assistants with her, she faced a personnel shortage anyway; there remained too few hands to carry out the ambitious experiments she had planned. She had uprooted three families in addition to her own, and the pressure on her was enormous, compounding the steady pressure to vindicate her discovery. Eventually, she would estimate that the complications of the move had cost her a year.

By January 1994, DeFreitas was burdened by yet another formidable problem: illness. She was suffering from a painful condition called reflex sympathetic dystrophy. RSD is a rare nerve disorder that can occur in people who have undergone extreme physical trauma; although the trauma is over, the nerve damage continues. In DeFreitas's case, the disorder could be traced to her involvement in an automobile accident in 1990 in which she had injured her arm, an injury that had required several seeks of hospitalization. It wasn't until late 1991 that the pain had begun to assert itself in earnest, however. By early 1994, she was increasingly incapacitated by searing pain in an arm, a shoulder, and her neck. Because the condition was rare and poorly understood, most doctors found it difficult to diagnose and treat. As a result, while she struggled to organize her laboratory and captain research, she was simultaneously maneuvering through a maze of specialists' offices in search of relief.

Not surprisingly, whispers began that DeFreitas had contracted chronic fatigue syndrome; after all, she had been working with blood samples from CFS sufferers since 1985. The scientist herself began to wonder, and accepted an offer from Paul Cheney to help pin down the diagnosis. DeFreitas, who was barely able to walk, was hospitalized in Charlotte for a week and seen by Cheney's partner, Charles Lapp; the latter ruled out CFS. Still, the rumors persisted.

DeFreitas returned to Miami, but as time passed, she was increasingly hard-pressed to make it to her lab. Some days she awoke in excruciating pain and was unable to move even her legs. More often than not, she held teleconferences with her staff from her bed or met with them in her living room to discuss experiments. David Bell, who continued to suspect CFS, pleaded with her to come to Harvard for further evaluation. DeFreitas declined; she was in too much pain to handle the trip. By midwinter, the scientist was frequently in a wheelchair, racked by pain so severe her doctors began prescribing morphine.

Not long after her paper on a novel non-C-type retrovirus in three Lyndonville children had been rejected by *PNAS,* she had submitted it to a Canadian medical journal. Now the editors were asking for more data. DeFreitas desperately wanted to comply, but she was too incapacitated to do so.

University of Pittsburgh, Pittsburgh, Pennsylvania

On February 1, 1994, cancer epidemiologist Seymour Grufferman was awarded $1 million from the NIH to pursue his overriding scientific interest: the possibility that some viruses may cause cancer. Specifically, Grufferman won the grant based on his proposal to explore the role of Epstein-Barr virus in the etiology of Hodgkin's disease, a malignancy of the immune system. The government-assembled panel that reviewed Grufferman's grant proposal regarded it so highly that it was ranked in the second percentile. In contrast, his proposals five years before to study issues of cancer incidence and infectiousness in chronic fatigue syndrome had been ranked in the eightieth and ninetieth percentiles by ad hoc review panels organized by grant administrator Ann Schleuderberg.

"Now, what does this show?" Grufferman asked rhetorically soon after his Hodgkin's grant award. "Am I a junky scientist—or is there a bias?"

Although his passion for CFS had not cooled, the epidemiologist had done little research into that disease in the preceding two years. His investigations of the outbreak in the North Carolina Symphony had languished. Blood samples examined under the supervision of National Cancer Institute retrovirologist William Blattner had in some cases demonstrated hints of antibodies to the retroviruses HTLV1 and HTLV2, but Grufferman's collaborator, NCI epidemiologist Paul

Levine, had downplayed the significance of the finding to Grufferman, suggesting it was merely "background noise."*

"That's not science," Grufferman complained, but in truth, there was little apparent impetus on either side to pursue the investigations. For Grufferman, it was a simple matter: he had no funding for CFS research. "This is what happens when you try to do research that doesn't have the backing of mainstream science," he said. "The good investigators eventually get out."

An ambitious scheme devised by Grufferman two years before, for answering the question of whether CFS predisposed its victims or their close contacts to higher rates of cancer, remained in limbo. Grufferman had proposed to send questionnaires to approximately two thousand CFS sufferers from the patient cohorts of several so-called mainstream researchers, like Anthony Komaroff, Stephen Straus, James Jones, and Philip Peterson. He had hoped to undertake the survey with the backing of the National Cancer Institute. Although researchers inside the government cancer institute continued to believe Grufferman's idea was reasonable, there would be no federal money for the project. If the survey was ever launched, Grufferman said, "it [would] be done with private dollars from my university." The National Cancer Institute would not be involved.† "I still do believe there is an association between cancer risk and CFS," he added.

NCI researcher Paul Levine's 1992 investigation into the incidence of certain kinds of cancers in Nevada had led him to the conclusion that "there are clues that there could be an increase in brain tumors statewide. An upward trend in brain cancers was noted." Levine had also studied the incidence in Nevada of non-Hodgkin's lymphoma, the third-fastest-rising form of cancer in the United States, with less certain results. Paul Cheney and Dan Peterson certainly believed non-Hodgkin's lymphoma had increased in tandem with the CFS epidemic in the Tahoe region. "We found an increase in non-Hodgkin's lymphoma," Levine confirmed, "but we couldn't say for sure that it was greater than the general increase around the country." Still, Levine's study had only probed incidences of the cancers statewide. He had yet to tabulate cancer incidences in Washoe and Clark

---

* According to Levine, Sidney Grossberg, the Wisconsin scientist who recently had been funded by the National Institutes of Health to investigate retroviral infection in the disease, "has the only viable study that I know of to suggest retrovirus." He noted that Blattner was only "briefly enthusiastic" about the test results. "The retrovirus theory is moribund," Levine added. "I can't say it's gone over the cliff, but Blattner is not pursuing it, I'm not pursuing it, and the CDC is not pursuing it."

† Indeed, by 1995 it was apparent that the National Cancer Institute was undergoing a major reevaluation of its mission that could reduce its intramural research programs into many infectious diseases, including and most especially AIDS. In an interview that spring, William Blattner, chief of the NCI's viral epidemiology branch within the Division of Cancer Etiology, suggested that the new emphasis on the reduction of AIDS research inside NCI might bleed into any proposed intramural research on CFS as well. Asked if there would be any enthusiasm in the future to pursue chronic fatigue syndrome and its relationship to either cancer or cancer-causing retroviruses within the NCI, Blattner said, "I don't think so. There is a retrenchment under way. It would not be the mandate of the NCI to redirect research into chronic fatigue syndrome unless there was a major cancer component—which has been hard to pin down."

Since the sole intramural effort to discover connections between CFS and cancer had died with the departure of Paul Levine, it seemed clear by early 1995 that this pressing matter simply would not be addressed by the federal government.

counties, the counties where Incline Village and Yerington lay, to see if cancer rates were higher in well-known CFS hot spots, nor had he looked at California counties adjacent to Nevada's Washoe County.

Walter Reed Hospital, Washington, D.C.

By 1994, any number of theories had been advanced about the cause of the illnesses being experienced by Gulf War veterans, their spouses, and in some cases, even their children. These theories included radiation, biological warfare, and chronic fatigue syndrome. In an interview with NBC News on February 22, Major General Ronald Blanck, military spokesman on all matters pertaining to the Gulf War syndrome, insisted he would not be cornered on the matter by theorists but would wait for the military's epidemiological studies to bear fruit, a process that could take years.

Behind the scenes, the chief of infectious diseases for the army, Charles Oster, had come to his own conclusions about the phenomenon. Having carefully evaluated more than two hundred Gulf syndrome cases at Walter Reed, Oster suspected Gulf veterans were suffering from an infectious disease.

"Of course, I'm an infectious disease doc, so that's my bias," Oster said. "But the only thing that could explain this is some chronic infectious agent that has a prolonged incubation period. It's hard for me to imagine that a toxic effect occurred over there, especially since most of them felt fine until they came back. I think there *is* something they picked up in the Gulf," he continued, "and the best candidate is a chronic virus. Having had three years of experience with these people, I'm convinced of that. And we're discovering new viruses every day, so it's perfectly possible."

Oster was highly intrigued by the CFS theory. Certainly the symptoms described by many vets were compatible with CFS's diagnostic criteria, he said, including the neurological aspects. "They do all have memory symptoms, concentration problems, and sleep disturbance," Oster said. But he added that until the illness could be defined by a diagnostic test for the agent, the mystery would continue. In light of this dilemma, Oster had educated himself on the history of the CFS microbe hunt. He was familiar with Elaine DeFreitas's retrovirus claim and he seemed particularly interested in Los Angeles pathologist John Martin's work. The army doctor had hardly been dissuaded by the CDC's negative reports on these findings. In fact, Oster revealed he was orchestrating a research project to search for retrovirus in Gulf War vets, though he declined to name his collaborators or even to say whether they were inside or outside the government's research establishment. Because so little funding was available for CFS research, Oster confessed he was doing [the research] out of my back pocket. . . . I'm not any different from any other researcher in this field," he continued. "We have no money. There is no support for CFS research."

Nonetheless, Oster believed he had an advantage most CFS researchers had yet been able to muster: a politically powerful constituency. "Our guys are pretty well orchestrated," Oster said of the nation's war veterans. "They have strong links to Congress and have a fair amount of political clout." He called his retrovirus research "a fishing expedition," meaning it was in its preliminary stages, but he indicated that veterans' organizations would have the political muscle to redirect major research efforts toward the CFS field if such research proved promising.

"If any of us strike gold in the retrovirus search," he added, "whether it be the army or independent CFS researchers, it will benefit all CFS patients."

Department of Health and Human Services, Washington, D.C.

On March 1 the assistant secretary of health, Philip Lee, convened the second meeting of the CFS Interagency Coordinating Committee. Since the committee's November meeting, Lee had invited four patient advocates to become permanent members of the committee, each of whom would have equal standing to the government participants. Kimberly Kenney, the CFIDS Association executive director, was one of those Lee invited. Lee's move meant that the patient advocates would have the power to directly query government scientists like the CDC's William Reeves, in Lee's presence, about the direction and progress of their research.

"Kim gets to sit there and ask tough questions," lobbyist Tom Sheridan noted. "They *can't* put her down, they *can't* patronize her, because she's not a patient. We'll make sure that these people will no longer get away with the b.s. that they've been getting away with for years now."

Sheridan noted, too, that since the rocky meeting in Atlanta to discuss the case definition the previous September, CDC staff had undergone a change in attitude. "They're not treating these patients like a bunch of misbehaving children anymore. They realize we're informed and monitoring them very carefully."

For each of the last three years, Congress had added from $1 million to $2.2 million to the federal budget for CFS research, Sheridan continued. But he remained concerned with the infrastructure of the federal health agencies, whose administrators seemed unable or unwilling to use the money in a way that effectively advanced the discovery process. Money could do many things, but it could not expunge scientific bias.

"This problem became apparent to us during the first year we became involved with this issue, and our work plan has always been to change the infrastructure," Sheridan said. "This is actually a unique situation. I'm not comfortable going to the Hill asking for money for this disease," he added, as long as that infrastructure remained unchanged. Yet, Phil Lee's chairmanship of the new committee had raised hopes. "The ultimate goal, of course, is to find out what causes this disease and how to cure it," Sheridan said. "And we want the Social Security Administration to stop treating these patients like they're trying to rip off the government. . . . If a superhighway is the best way to get there, we're now on a paved road. We've come off a cow path."

UNUM Corporation, Portland, Maine

Researchers and patients following the progress of the epidemic had frequently suggested that if all of those who were disabled by CFS were actually awarded disability payments from the government, the disease would bankrupt the nation's Social Security fund. This might occur not only because the pool of disabled sufferers was so huge but also because CFS was a chronic illness rather than a fatal one; statistically, one third of the 75 percent of SSA disability recipients who were physically impaired died within five years or less, thus ending the payout.* The Social Security Administration had remained silent on the matter of CFS-related disability throughout the course of the previous decade. In April 1994, however, one of the nation's largest private providers of disability insurance, the UNUM Corporation, issued a press release revealing chronic fatigue syndrome claims to be the fastest-growing sector of their business. According to UNUM, claims for disability caused by CFS had increased 500 percent from 1989 to 1993, a bigger increase than any other category of disability. During that five-year period, UNUM said, CFS-imposed disability had resulted in a 557 percent increase in claims by women; claims for CFS disability had risen 360 percent among men.

Michael Kita, medical adviser to UNUM, called the spread of the disease "impressive to me as both a medical and a sociological phenomenon. It's distressing—startling," he continued. "Doctors like to repair things, and any doctor who has provided care for people with CFS knows how very discouraging it is. . . . There has been a view that this is some form of mass hysteria or overdiagnosis by doctors or depression. It doesn't look that simple anymore. There does appear to be something real happening."

Harvard Medical School, Boston, Massachusetts

The boundary between AIDS and CFS grew even thinner that spring when Anthony Komaroff and several Harvard colleagues reported that the brains of patients with AIDS dementia complex and those with CFS were remarkably similar when viewed by SPECT scan imaging.[7]

SPECT imaging is a computerized method of revealing patterns of blood flow in the brain. Experts on the West Coast had demonstrated as early as 1990 that people with CFS suffered hypoperfusion, or reduced blood flow, to regions of their brains in comparison to normal, healthy people, but Komaroff's paper was the first to compare CFS sufferers with AIDS sufferers.† What was especially significant was that the particular regions of the brain affected, or the nature of the abnormalities, were so similar in AIDS and CFS, suggesting, Komaroff wrote, "a similar origin for the neurologic dysfunction in these conditions." He noted that the blood flow abnormalities in AIDS dementia complex "are believed to be due to direct central nervous system infection with the HIV virus."‡ Komaroff could not point to any particular virus in CFS sufferers to explain their brain damage, especially since brain biopsies on people with CFS were all but unheard of. He

* According to Alan Schafer, director of the Division of Program Information and Special Studies in the Office of Disability, Social Security Administration.

† Komaroff also included clinically depressed and normal people in the study. Interestingly, patients with major depression also had some defects in blood perfusion, though the defects were not as significant as those found in CFS and AIDS sufferers—suggesting an organic basis for their depression and, at the same time, offering an organic basis for the typically severe depression experienced by CFS sufferers. He also noted that abnormal brain perfusion had been revealed by SPECT scan in patients with lupus, cocaine abuse, and dementia caused by stroke.

‡ "Pathologic studies have shown that HIV infection results in a subacute encephalitis characterized by demyelination and the presence of the virus in multinucleated giant cells, as well as in endothelial cells, astrocytes, and neurons distributed throughout the brain," Komaroff wrote.

noted, however, that "the findings in CFS are consistent with the hypothesis that CFS also results from viral infection of neurons [nerve cells], glia [cells that support and bind together nerve tissue], or vasculature [blood vessels]. . . .

"In summary," Komaroff wrote, "this study indicates that SPECT may help in distinguishing patients with CFS from healthy subjects and depressed patients. *SPECT was not useful in separating patients with CFS from patients with AIDS dementia complex,* but that distinction usually can be made with other diagnostic technologies" (italics added).

Centers for Disease Control, Atlanta, Georgia

Curiously, it was an impartial research fellow at the Centers for Disease Control who in 1994 offered documentation for what most CFS sufferers intuitively knew to be true: hardly anyone who had been ill for any significant length of time recovered. Lea Steele had arrived at the agency in 1993, signing on to study chronic fatigue syndrome, which she planned to make the subject of her Ph.D. dissertation. Steele quickly realized that the agency had very little data about the clinical course of the disease, but she noticed that in gathering cases for the four-city surveillance, the agency had kept records of illness duration. Steele decided to analyze these records to seek an answer to the question never before formally posed as a research question: was CFS a disease from which people recovered?

Steele focused her efforts on the agency's 130 class one patients, those considered by CDC staff to be the "purest" cases. These patients had been sick, on average, for 6.4 years when they were recruited into the surveillance program; they had been followed by the government for an average of just under two years. Overall, just 12 percent improved or, said Steele, "substantially recovered," during the two years.

Steele had observed, anecdotally, that there appeared to be two windows of opportunity for recovery: early in the illness, meaning within the first twenty-four months, and then again at between four and five years. "Recovery is *most* likely in the first five years," she said. Those who had been ill more than five to ten years experienced an "improvement" rate of 4 percent. Noted Steele, "The likelihood of recovery was associated with the duration of illness." The longer a patient had been ill, in other words, the less the chance of recovery or even improvement. In addition, no one could be certain the reported recoveries were not in fact temporary remissions.

Steele's analysis wiped out a decade of unsubstantiated assurances in informational pamphlets distributed to the public and the Congress by CDC and NIH staff that the disease lasted for merely "months."

National Institute of Allergy and Infectious Diseases, Bethesda, Maryland

In May, Ann Schleuderberg retired. Since 1987, she had administered the CFS grant program. Many grant hopefuls had viewed Schleuderberg as the bottleneck in the system, and they hoped her successor might prove to be less of an adversary of the disease. When Schleuderberg's immediate boss, John La Montagne, was asked who would succeed her, however, he responded: "We're caught up in the

fact that the government is downsizing. We don't have the ability to bring someone on. The president is determined to reduce the federal work force by 250,000
people. Not that I don't support our president—I *do*."

In other words, Schleuderberg would have no successor.

Federal Court, Reno, Nevada

Late in 1991, when HEM Pharmaceuticals prematurely ended its four-city clinical trial, seventeen Ampligen recipients from Nevada and North Carolina had
filed suit against the company, claiming HEM had made false promises to them
and demanding continued treatment. In response, Judge Edward Reed had issued
a preliminary injunction that required HEM to provide the drug for one year. By
1994, eleven of the seventeen plaintiffs remained in litigation. In July of that year,
Judge Reed ruled in HEM's favor, finding that the company had fulfilled its contract to patients, and the last American patients on Ampligen were cut adrift.

University of Southern California, School of Medicine, Los Angeles

In spite of the CFIDS Association's withdrawal of funds in 1993, pathologist John
Martin had continued to investigate the nature and identity of his viral discovery,
which he felt certain was tied to the CFS epidemic. In August he published a description of the virus in the *American Journal of Pathology*.[8] Martin reported that
he had been able to isolate this virus repeatedly from the blood of a forty-three-
year-old former psychologist, a counselor in the practice of an infectious disease
specialist, with CFS. She was DW, a patient who had fallen ill in 1990 with a sore
throat followed by severe headaches, muscle pain, and fever. Ultimately she was
hospitalized and diagnosed with the vague "possible encephalitis/meningitis."
Because her cerebrospinal fluid appeared to be normal, she was discharged after
seven days, but her illness persisted, eventually evolving into CFS. She was disabled by overwhelming fatigue and developed "impaired cognitive functions, including memory loss and difficulty naming items [dysnomia], intense headaches,
and nonrestorative sleep." By the time Martin's paper appeared, DW had been ill
for nearly four years.

Martin's virus was definitely larger than a classical retrovirus. In size, it more
closely resembled a herpesvirus, and in fact he had discovered partial genetic sequences that were nearly identical to those of the well-known herpesvirus, cytomegalovirus. He had first seen the large viral particles using an electron
microscope in 1991. The virus did not respond to antibodies for cytomegalovirus
or any other known herpesvirus, however. Martin maintained that his virus was
"related to" but was *not* human cytomegalovirus. In addition, unlike most herpesviruses, Martin's virus decimated cells. The cytopathic effect, Martin said,
"can best be summarized by the appearance of foamy cell syncytia."

To be sure there was no contamination, Martin had drawn blood from DW on
eighteen separate occasions over three years. On fifteen of those attempts, he had
been able to infect cultures with the same virus. He had also found the virus in the
woman's spinal fluid.

Martin also reported that he had been able to isolate similar but not identical viruses—which he tentatively termed "stealth viruses"—from a number of patients with "a variety of neurological, psychiatric, and autoimmune diseases, as well as some asymptomatic individuals."

In a conversation some months after his paper was published, Martin stated his certainty that the "stealth" viruses he had at last been afforded an opportunity to describe in the medical literature were the cause of the CFS epidemic. That epidemic, he believed, encompassed a broad range of new illnesses arrayed along a continuum of severity. They included the "atypical" encephalopathies being diagnosed by perplexed neurologists in increasing numbers and mild, subacute brain disease that might either go unnoticed by the sufferer or be attributed to simple fatigue or the natural process of aging. Classic, disabling CFS comprised the vast middle along this continuum.

"No question—this is the cause," Martin said. "The only thing I don't have is a cure," he added. "And just saying 'It's so' doesn't mean much. We have to find a way to inhibit this virus.

"The next challenge," Martin continued, "is to get this finding to the CDC. Not to the research level," he quickly amended, "but to the administrative level."

The pathologist seemed placid about the tumultuous events of the past ten years, during which his own reputation and those of other investigators had been savaged as a result of their research into CFS.

"I think you have to put it into the context of the history of science, and allow for the constancy of human nature. . . . And I don't think a decade is such a long time to spend finding the cause of a disease."

Berkeley, California

Discoveries from the Ampligen trials continued to flow into a vast sea of information accumulating about the disease. Neuropsychologist Sheila Bastien, for instance, had performed the intellectual testing of the nearly one hundred patients enrolled in HEM Pharmaceuticals' Ampligen trials in 1991; Bastien's participation in the study had strengthened her understanding of the damage caused to the intellects of people with CFS. Including the Ampligen patients, she had personally evaluated more than three thousand sufferers from every region of the United States and Canada since her first visit to Incline Village in 1986. By 1994, Bastien was certain that sufferers uniformly were robbed of IQ. "I would say, on average, the IQ loss is fifteen to forty points, conservatively, depending upon how severe the disease is. But there was one social worker in the Ampligen trial whose IQ was one hundred, and after receiving Ampligen her IQ was one hundred fifty-five."

That year, Bastien and Dan Peterson collaborated on a formal study of IQ diminishment in CFS patients.[9] Their subjects were forty people who had undergone repeated IQ testing during the years of their illnesses. Bastien reported that in these forty subjects performance IQ, which measures nonverbal skills like abstract thinking and visual acuity, was significantly reduced. Verbal IQ remained intact. These results were consistent with the pattern of brain impairment Bastien had seen in virtually all of her patients. "What we're finding is that the left temporal lobe, the right parietal lobe, and the left frontal lobe are the three areas with the most damage," she said. "It's like, if the brain was a dartboard, there would be darts everywhere, but the most darts would be concentrated in these three areas."

Several of the brain-imaging experts in southern California had theorized that the brain's limbic system—considered the "seat of emotion" and the center of human instinct, motivation, and mood, including the expression of fear, rage, and pleasure—was damaged in the disease. The limbic system is also important in the establishment of behavior and memory patterns. Since her earliest meetings with CFS patients in 1986, Bastien had become more sophisticated about the psychological impact of the disease upon sufferers, and by 1994 she had begun to synthesize the organic damage with the apparent emotional damage patients experienced. "I think these patients have a lot of emotional stuff that's related to limbic system disturbances," Bastien commented that winter. "They have trouble with decision-making; they're impulsive."

In an earlier article on the subject, Bastien had described in detail the emotional manifestations of the brain damage, symptoms that would be instantly recognizable to anyone suffering from the disease or to people who lived in close contact with them. She wrote that "the patients had trouble making decisions and planning. Many of the patients had a personality change from a previously even-tempered individual to someone easily frustrated, irritable, impulsive, angry, and sometimes verbally out of control."

Bastien routinely asked patients to take the Minnesota Multiphasic Personality Inventory. The test results revealed, she wrote, an "acute psychological disturbance related to their illness. The most prominent features [of this disturbance] are an awareness of somatic and sensory difficulties, marked depression, social withdrawal, anxiety, and pessimism. . . . These patients also had an impulsiveness not part of their premorbid personality. . . . All of the patients met the (DSM-III-R) criteria for dementia."

Bastien required patients to draw a human figure as part of her battery of tests. The figures, sketched with a pencil on paper, were powerful indicators of the emotionally devastating impact of the disease and, in addition, reflected "moderate to severe dysfunction in visual-spatial perception," an organic brain problem, Bastien said. "The quality of the drawings is different from that of dyslexic adults," she added. "Many of the figures look like children's drawings and reflect a regression to an earlier level of functioning."

The sketches, Bastien continued, "often had notable differences between the right and left sides of the body. Many patients' drawings would indicate the side of the body more affected by their illness. Sometimes the figure drawings . . . lean to one side. The eyes in their drawings often lack pupils. These patients frequently drew themselves as sticks, segmented balloons, puppets, or squared-off robots. In summary, most of the organic indicators for these patients are contained in their drawings."

Later that year, Bastien's only child, a son who had suffered from CFS since 1987, committed suicide. Asked for her permission to make her son's illness and subsequent death public, Bastien was momentarily silent. "People need to know," the bereaved psychologist finally said, "that the number one cause of death in this disease is suicide."

Bonaventure Hotel, Fort Lauderdale, Florida

In 1994 Miami immunologist Nancy Klimas commented that although the CDC had seemed to discredit the retrovirus theory, not everyone in academic circles had accepted the government's judgment. Indeed, just when the agency claimed the issues raised by Elaine DeFreitas's work were settled, a New Zealand scientist emerged at a CFS scientific conference in Fort Lauderdale in October to unveil electron microscopy photos of what appeared to be retrovirus particles in cells of New Zealand patients with the disease.

Michael Holmes, a stocky, bearded, chain-smoking man of fifty-two, was a senior lecturer in the department of microbiology at the University of Otago in Dunedin, New Zealand. He had become interested in ME—or "poor man's AIDS," as the New Zealanders who fell ill with the disease sometimes called CFS—in 1984 when a June 13 article in the *New Zealand Medical Journal* described an unusual occurrence of disease in West Otago, a mountainous sheep-herding region of New Zealand's South Island.[10] The cases were centered in Tapanui, a rural inland town of five thousand people.

Tapanui's sole practitioner, Peter Snow, first suspected there might be an outbreak of illness in 1982, the journal reported, "when a number of patients presented with extreme fatigue and a virtual inability to continue with their employment." All but three of the patients were under forty-five. "The majority," the author of the article noted, "were young people and schoolchildren who do not regularly attend their general practitioner." Snow observed that most of them had been ill for four to six weeks when they came to his clinic. The symptoms and unique course of the illness failed to suggest any familiar diagnoses. Indeed, while the end result was the same, the symptoms seemed to vary from patient to patient at onset. "Some of the Tapanui patients said they had had a flu-like illness with a sore throat and generalized muscle aches and pains," the authors reported, "while others complained of severe headaches. All said that after this initial illness they had felt extremely fatigued and had been incapable of a normal day's activity."

Snow recalled several isolated cases of the same unusual illness in the village over the years, usually occurring in the summer. This was the first time, he believed, that a great many cases of the malady had occurred in Tapanui in a short period. Accordingly, the doctor, aided by researchers at the University of Otago Medical School, sought to identify the cause of the outbreak. The investigators ruled out bacteria in Tapanui's water source and poisoning from agricultural chemicals. Next, they searched for viruses in the blood of the afflicted. Their efforts failed to produce evidence of any disease with which they were familiar. In spite of the panoply of complaints, there was a surprising dearth of objective clinical findings.

Snow and his collaborators considered, and dismissed, the notion that the village of Tapanui had fallen victim to mass hysteria. The classic hallmarks of mass hysteria—a preponderance of illness in adolescents and children, a preponderance of female victims, and "benign morbidity" with "rapid remission of symptoms"—were not in evidence. Men and women were afflicted in equal numbers; a year after the outbreak hardly anyone had recovered fully. Instead, on the strength of victims' complaints, researchers concluded the illness was a "definite entity, which has been disabling for those affected." They further argued that "the symptoms are consistent with a viral etiology." Buttressing their theory that "a transmissible agent" lay at the heart of the epidemic, the investigators pointed out that more than half of the patients interviewed had family members and friends who were suffering from the same complaints. Indeed, they suggested, the enigmatic "Tapanui flu" might have spread beyond Tapanui and New Zealand's southern latitudes. "We have no evidence that the disease has been confined to West Otago," they wrote, "and it may be occurring in other rural and urban practices."

In 1986, John Murdoch, a professor at the University of Otago Medical School, asked Holmes to undertake a comparative study of six of Peter Snow's Tapanui patients and six healthy people. Holmes and his colleagues did two studies: they looked for cell death among white blood cells and the presence of viral particles. To his surprise, Holmes discovered reverse transcriptase, the telltale enzyme produced by retrovirus activity, in four out of the six CFS patients at levels 1.5 to 4 times those of controls. "Since each retrovirion has only two molecules of RT [reverse transcriptase]," Holmes wrote later, "this implied that a significant quantity of virus was being produced, especially when the replication rate of this group is normally so slow." In addition, Holmes's electron microscopy views of these cells were suggestive of retroviral infection as well. "In the earliest samples," he wrote, "we found a proportion of . . . cells with convoluted nuclei comparable to those described in the ARC [AIDS-related complex] syndrome. These were not present in controls."

While admitting that his study of six patients—which Holmes had undertaken with the equivalent of $690—was too small to provide anything beyond a suggestion that more research be done, he said, "We would like to propose a retrovirus etiology for CFS based not only on this pilot but on the train of deductive observation which led us to consider it in the first place."

He noted that most of the viruses—Epstein-Barr, enterovirus, and others—that had been red herrings for the cause were "highly persistent or latent organisms which tend to be found in immunologically embarrassed patients. They are not classical opportunists, but they are not far off." Also, when comparing symptoms of patients suffering from poor man's AIDS and AIDS-related complex, Holmes was impressed by the similarity of physical complaints and laboratory signs, especially "Dr. Cheney's report . . . that a lot of interferon is being made," and Australian researcher Andrew Lloyd's observation (also made by Cheney) that the symptoms of CFS and interferon toxicity are virtually identical.

"If the CFS symptoms are due to interferon poisoning," Holmes continued, "they must have a prolonged stimulus . . . a chronic infection. It must also be an intracellular infection, because interferon is induced only by the presence of foreign nucleic acids *inside* a cell. Furthermore, the most powerful interferon inducers are retroviruses. In this scenario, we therefore have a chronic persistent lymphotrophic RNA virus. We also have a plethora of low-grade persistent opportunist epiphenomena, which suggests a degree of immune dysfunction."

After making these observations, Holmes had run out of money to pursue the work further. Two years later, in 1988, his lab was awarded $7,000 by a patients' philanthropy to continue. "We thought we were rich," Holmes recalled. "We took blood from everyone we could lay hands on." Again Holmes found the peculiar "convoluted nuclei" seen in HIV disease. "The virus-like structures were compatible in size and structure with a retrovirus, but it *still* wasn't enough," Holmes said, meaning he was loath to publish his findings until he had been able to do more studies on more patients. "Yet we thought, There's definitely something worth looking at." In 1992, Holmes was able to perform his studies on another twenty CFS sufferers and twenty controls, with similar results. "But by this time," he said, "Elaine DeFreitas had been savaged and thrown to the wolves."

By October 1994, when Holmes made his first trip ever to the United States— the purpose of which was to show his pictures of convoluted nuclei to American CFS researchers—he was exceedingly well versed in the politics of the disease, which were as divisive in New Zealand as elsewhere. "I'm on the hit list because I'm working on this disease," he said. "People who work in this field are considered either black box magicians or charlatans." He was therefore unfazed when, after presenting his photos and describing his work, he suffered a round of particularly condescending criticism from many of the scientists present in Fort Lauderdale.*

The New Zealander's was the only presentation out of nearly sixty that focused on etiology. A sense that looking for one or *any* cause of the disease was a retrograde pursuit pervaded the official proceedings. "To talk about etiologies is to create false hopes," CDC medical epidemiologist Keiji Fukuda—a handsome, voguishly attired young doctor—commented between sessions. "We think it's unlikely that a single agent will be responsible—it's too complicated. It will not be agent X causing disease Y."

🔛

The keynote speaker in Fort Lauderdale was General Ronald Blanck, the military's highest-ranking spokesman on the Gulf War syndrome. At the end of a dinner in the hotel ballroom, the dapper, affable general told the assembled researchers that "our definition for Gulf War syndrome is almost identical to the CDC's definition [of CFS]." After eliminating veterans who turn out to have other diseases, he continued, "what we're going to be left with is a group who I feel have something analogous with CFS." Although as many as 28,000 veterans had signed up with the VA registry, Blanck added, "we're clearly seeing underreporting. We've sent letters out saying, 'You won't be penalized,' but there are people out there hiding their high blood pressure, their diabetes, and their chronic fatigue syndrome."

The military doctor said approximately half of the vets with Gulf War syndrome developed their symptoms on their return from the war theater; the other

* Some time later, David Bell, who attended the conference, noted that criticism of Holmes was limited to his formal presentation. Afterward, Bell recalled, the New Zealander was approached privately by numerous conference participants and congratulated on his work. In point of fact, most of these comments were made to Holmes in the men's room, Bell said. "They would only say these things if it was in the bathroom and there was no recording equipment around."

half reported that their symptoms began in the Gulf. "Most of the people I have seen are totally, substantially disabled and cannot work," he added. "Congressman Buyer of Indiana [a Gulf War veteran] suffers from this and ran for Congress and won, but the spectrum runs all the way to bedridden."*

After his speech that evening, Blanck, clad in his dark green uniform, strolled through the hotel bar, his cap under his arm, and accepted an invitation for a drink from Dan Peterson and Paul Cheney. Over a vintage cognac, Blanck told the clinicians, "*I* think Gulf War syndrome *is* CFS, but if I come right out and say that, it will seem as if we've solved the problem and we can all go home. But we *haven't* solved the problem—we still don't know what chronic fatigue syndrome *is.*" Blanck indicated he hoped to use the military's relatively lavish funding for studying Gulf War syndrome to get to the bottom of the mystery. When he was asked who was providing the military with its primary expertise on chronic fatigue syndrome, Blanck responded, "Steve Straus, of course."

Veterans Administration Medical Center, East Orange, New Jersey

In October the Veterans Administration awarded Benjamin Natelson, a neuroscience professor at the New Jersey Medical School and a 1991 NIH center grant recipient, $2.5 million to study the relationship between chronic fatigue syndrome and Gulf War syndrome. The money would be paid out in $500,000 sums over a five-year period. Natelson's was one of three VA grants to establish what the military was calling "Environmental Hazards Research Centers," but Natelson's group would be the only one of the three with a special focus on chronic fatigue syndrome, both in Gulf War veterans and in civilians.

"When you're in, you're in," Elaine DeFreitas said upon hearing the news. "And he's *really* in."

Natelson attributed his success to a survey he had conducted in the spring of 1993. He had sent questionnaires to eight thousand veterans who had signed the Persian Gulf registry, 85 percent of whom were ill and 15 percent of whom felt well but were concerned they might come down with Gulf War syndrome.† By then, Natelson was aware of the wave of epidemiological data coming from Harvard and elsewhere demonstrating that at least .5 percent of the U.S. population suffered from CFS.

"We feel the rate is higher than that study suggests," Natelson said of the Harvard study. "It's more like one to one and a half percent, perhaps two percent. And when I questioned [the Gulf vets], that group endorsed the complaints of CFS at a lot higher rate than that one-half percent. We were able to suggest that there was a higher incidence of CFS among Gulf War vets than in the civilian population. We got *whole* numbers—in the five-ish range. In fact, we think there has been a mini-epidemic of CFS among Gulf War veterans."

In November, Natelson left New Jersey for the Pasteur Institute in France, where scientists had initially isolated HIV. Natelson was to take a six-month sabbatical at the famous French institute. Rumors abounded that he was in France

---

* Stephen Buyer was elected to represent the Fifth District of Indiana beginning in 1992.
† By mid-1995 the registry had ballooned to approximately 50,000 veterans of the Gulf War, approximately 7 percent of the 700,000 who had been deployed in the Persian Gulf theater.

learning techniques for isolating retroviruses. Instead, Natelson revealed upon his return, he had spent his time in the Pasteur's rabies unit: "I was over there learning about viruses in the brain—viruses that are chronic and smoldering."

University of California Medical School, San Francisco

After five years of effort, virologist Jay Levy was at last awarded a grant from the National Institute of Allergy and Infectious Diseases to study chronic fatigue syndrome. He had asked for $170,000 a year for three years. NIAID reduced the sum to $103,000. As a result, Levy grumbled, he would be unable to pursue the pathogen he continued to believe was at the heart of the disease, but he would continue to investigate the immunological abnormalities in the disease.

Levy's longtime clinician-collaborator, Carol Jessop, who had once been doctor to nearly two thousand CFS sufferers in her Bay Area practice and had introduced Levy to the disease ten years before, would not share in the grant. She had retired that same year from clinical practice to become a hospital administrator.

University of Miami, Florida

By the fall of 1994, Elaine DeFreitas had been totally disabled for nearly one year. In September the University of Miami's medical school dean told her that she would have to close her lab by year's end. DeFreitas had been expecting the call. The NIH had failed to fund her grant proposal, and she had no philanthropic money to pursue her experiments. She gathered her lab associates at her home to deliver the bad news. Whatever the significance of the team's discovery, their work together was finished.

By October, DeFreitas's primary concern was no longer her job or even her career but the precious blood samples she had been collecting since 1985. Lying dormant within the frozen cells of these samples—taken from Lyndonville children, Nevadans, North Carolinians, and dozens of other patients of all ages and in all stages of illness, shipped to her by doctors from all regions of the nation—was her virus. There were, in addition, semen samples from men suffering from the disease and pieces of brain and other organs from Skye Dailor, the teenage suicide, in whose liver and spleen DeFreitas had found retrovirus fragments. Some of the vials held once-pure human and mouse lymphocytes that DeFreitas had infected with cells from patients; in those cases, the virus had flourished for several months in cultures before being frozen. There were, then, several generations or colonies of the virus, some thriving in the source—sufferers' cells—and some inhabiting previously healthy cells that had been infected by patients' cells.

In a manner that perhaps only another scientist might understand, DeFreitas thought of the microbe as her child. She had discovered it, and she had struggled with all her might to keep it alive and to comprehend its place in the world of microorganisms. Stored in narrow polyethylene vials topped with rubber stoppers to keep the tissue from drying out, several of the samples were massed together in a large tank cooled to $-190°F$. by liquid nitrogen. The tank, which DeFreitas had brought with her from Wistar, stood undisturbed in a corner of her now-silent laboratory. The remaining samples were stored in a $-70°F$. freezer, the property of the University of Miami.

DeFreitas's anxiety over the fate of these samples was matched only by the extreme physical pain that now kept her bedridden or wheelchair-bound. She had no money to maintain the nitrogen tank; the samples would be safe from deterioration for only another year. She also needed to find a place to store the samples from the medical school's freezer, and she had no money with which to purchase the equipment. Nearly as worrying was the fact that DeFreitas lacked a trustworthy collaborator to whom she could bequeath her work.

Seated that fall at an antique farm table in the kitchen of her house, a one-story dwelling in a gated, impeccably manicured Fort Lauderdale neighborhood, she commented, "That virus—pretty as a picture—is buried in several vials in my liquid nitrogen tank and will remain alive for a year. After that, it's gone. I don't know whether it causes this disease, but it's alive, and it should be looked at. I've got to send it to someone who will do right by it."

Medical College of Wisconsin, Milwaukee

Sidney Grossberg's progress had been slower than that of either Elaine DeFreitas or John Martin, but he was moving forward nonetheless. By that fall, he had begun the tedious process of cloning his novel retrovirus in an effort to identify its genetic structure. The cloning of the hepatitis B virus had taken four solid years of effort by an entire laboratory staff. Grossberg thought he might be able to complete the cloning process by the end of the year. But then again, he said, it might take another two years. Although Grossberg did not yet have a viral probe or antibody test for the virus, the CIFDS Association had asked him to undertake a case-control study. His CFS samples came from twenty patients under Anthony Komaroff's care in Boston, and twenty healthy people who presumably had not been in close contact with CFS sufferers. Grossberg had promised results by February 1995.

Although the CFIDS Association—as a result of Gunn's persuasion—had ended their support of Elaine DeFreitas when she was unable to differentiate patients from controls in a CDC study, it was more magnanimous with Grossberg, offering him vastly greater margin for error. It was apparent that the patient group, which once had hoped for a quick resolution to the etiology puzzle, was now taking the long view.

"This is obviously too small a sample to be statistically significant," said controller David Patterson. "But we won't stop funding him if the study doesn't work."

By 1994 Grossberg continued to be highly conservative in his comments about his finding, making no claims of causality. Yet, he was readily drawn out about the peculiar nature of his human JHK virus, and his observations were fascinating, particularly in light of the retroviral findings that had come before. Several of DeFreitas's critics, for instance, had suggested that she had found an endogenous retrovirus; Grossberg postulated that his virus could be either exogenous or endogenous, but, if it turned out to be the latter, he offered, "it may be the first endogenous retrovirus found to produce infection." John Martin had for some time been puzzled over his virus's simultaneous qualities of herpesvirus and retrovirus. Said Grossberg, "We may have a genetic recombination of herpes and retrovirus here," and he cited three recent articles in the scientific literature demonstrating an "interaction" between herpes and retrovirus infections in animals. In another study, Grossberg noted, he had collaborated with Yale EBV expert George Miller to prove that "some nucleic acid" of a squirrel monkey retrovirus had "become part of" an Epstein-Barr virus.

After such speculation, however, Grossberg reined himself in and reiterated, "We're unwilling to say whether our virus is causal or whether it's been stimulated, as in HIV disease, as a secondary complication of immune dysfunction."

After a moment, he added, "It's really tough to go this long and *not* have a publication, but we're not going to submit anything for publication until we know exactly what this is and what its relationship is to CFS. And, so far, the molecular clones we've made just don't show up in the gene bank."

For Grossberg, being wrong was vastly more terrifying than any potential glory accrued by being first: "I cherish my good name in science—and I *really* don't want to be wrong on this."

Becton Dickinson and Company, Franklin Lakes, New Jersey

Literally hours before Elaine DeFreitas and her collaborators, Paul Cheney and David Bell, were to present their retrovirus data in Kyoto in 1990, they had been forced to entirely revamp their statistics after Cheney revealed he had diagnosed a nurse in his practice with CFS. For two years the nurse had been used repeatedly by DeFreitas as an "exposed control"—that is, someone who was healthy but had been exposed to people suffering from the disease. Three months before the Kyoto presentation, the nurse had pricked herself accidentally with a syringe she had just used to draw blood from a CFS patient. As the summer of 1990 passed, she became ill. By September she was completely disabled, suffering from all of the symptoms that typify CFS, including neurologic and immunologic aberrations. Throughout most of the previous two years, the nurse had been virus-negative on DeFreitas's tests; after the needle-stick, she had turned virus-positive.

The former nurse had filed a multimillion-dollar lawsuit against the manufacturer of the syringe, Becton Dickinson and Company, the world's largest manufacturer of syringes and among the world's largest purveyors of hospital supplies, including Ace bandages and latex gloves. Cheney's nurse claimed the syringe had malfunctioned, resulting in the needle-stick and the ensuing disability. In preparing for the suit, however, Becton Dickinson was forced to leap beyond the matter of whether or not their product was safe and address the complex issue of the nurse's disease as well as the matter of its transmissibility. Lawyers for the New Jersey–based company took depositions from at least six expert witnesses for the defendant, including a Harvard infectious disease specialist; CFS researcher James Jones, the government grant recipient who for years had maintained that CFS, while serious, was not transmissible; Minneapolis infectious disease specialist Philip Peterson; and Australian Andrew Lloyd. Anthony Komaroff was asked to testify on Becton Dickinson's behalf; he turned the company down.

The plaintiff had just two expert witnesses on her side: Paul Cheney and Elaine DeFreitas. All of the expert witnesses had an opportunity to read one another's depositions. Said DeFreitas, "One infectious disease guy actually said, 'Some viruses are not spread through the blood.' Was he awake in medical school?" She added that Becton Dickinson's experts seemed at times to be "almost vicious. It wasn't just business for them. They were really vitriolic." Cheney's recollection of the testimony of the defendant's witnesses was that Jones, Peterson, and Lloyd were the most adamant in their claim that the disease was not transmissible.*

During the last week of November 1994, Becton Dickinson decided to settle rather than allow the case to be tried before a jury.

"I think Becton Dickinson realized this trial was going to be a three-ring circus," DeFreitas commented upon hearing the news. "They probably figured they were going to have so many reporters at this trial, they caved and said, 'She got it from the needle-stick.' A company like [Becton Dickinson] does not lie down for nothing."

Not surprisingly, Roy Weber, associate general counsel for Becton Dickinson, put a different cast on the firm's decision to settle. "Obviously we weighed the risks of going to a jury against the cost of settling and deemed it prudent to settle," he said. "Now, [the plaintiff] obviously had certain maladies—I think it used to be called melancholia—but we don't believe she got them from the incident she alleged occurred."

Weber denied that the company's directors were afraid of a courtroom circus, or that they would lose their argument that the disease could not be transmitted by a needle-stick.

"The burden of proof is on the plaintiff," Weber said. "*She* had to prove there was evidence it could be transmitted. But there *are* some people who firmly believe this disease is real, that it is transmitted through blood, and that makes it a hard case to litigate if you've got people like that on the jury."

The amount of the nurse's remuneration from Becton Dickinson remained sealed in court documents.

New York City

On November 28 the front page of the business section of the *New York Times* carried a story headlined "New Ailments: Bane of Insurers." Reporter Michael Quint wrote: "Companies that sell disability insurance to individuals are reporting a sharp rise in claims for certain ailments that were little known ten years ago, leaving the insurers with losses of hundreds of millions of dollars. . . . The ailments with by far the biggest increases in claims for the last five years . . . are carpal tunnel syndrome, a nerve disorder that often arises from prolonged use of computer keyboards, and Epstein Barr virus syndrome."†

---

* Queried in 1995, Jones claimed he could not remember whether or not he had participated in a deposition, but he insisted that the lawsuit, itself, was "utter frivolity."

† AIDS was fifth on the list, psychiatric problems were fourth, and back and disk pain were third. Carpal tunnel syndrome was first.

Significantly, Quint observed that among doctors, particularly emergency room doctors and anesthesiologists, disability claims had ballooned to twice the predicted rates in five years. "We are now seeing more and more claims for nervous- or mental-type situations or muscle and soft tissue disorders that are very hard to evaluate," said Stephen B. Center, the executive vice president of UNUM Corporation, the private disability insurer based in Portland, Maine.

A few experts hinted that because of the dramatic rise in such claims, disability insurance might be an outmoded concept that one day simply might become too expensive to offer. Said Eric N. Berg, an insurance company analyst at Bear, Stearns & Company, "In an age of myriad new diseases, the product simply no longer works."

Irvine, California

In 1994, Herman Falsetti, the cardiologist and prominent sports doctor in Irvine who specialized in cyclists and who had diagnosed the outbreak of CFS among the 1984 women's Olympic cycling team, reported that the disease was even more common among athletes now than it had been a decade earlier. Recalling that fear of catching the disease was once rampant among members of the U.S. cycling team, Falsetti said, "It still is, because it's the leading disability affecting professional cyclists. It hit the women in 1986 and 1987 and hit the men later. It is really more prevalent now."

In 1987, Falsetti had estimated that 3 to 5 percent, or almost one of every twenty competitive cyclists, had the disease. He believed the attack rate among elite cyclists had doubled in ten years. "Among athletes, we never even *heard* of this disease ten years ago, and now I would say it affects five to ten percent of professional athletes, especially among the triathletes and in other endurance sports. The training is so much more intense than it used to be, and because athletes press their bodies harder, their immunity is decreased."

Jack Harvey, another sports doctor, agreed. Once the director of the International Bicycle Classic race, Harvey was now the chief doctor for the U.S. Olympic wrestling team. "Wrestlers don't see CFS," he said. "It's not an endurance sport."

National Institute of Allergy and Infectious Diseases, Bethesda, Maryland

Researchers seeking funding for their work agreed: a permanent, or standing, study panel composed of true CFS experts needed to be formed to assess CFS grant proposals. As one investigator said, "We need people who will look at these grants with something less than crossed eyes." Since 1987, when the NIH first expressed an interest in supporting CFS research, grant review panels had been assembled on an ad hoc basis. Traditionally, ad hoc review panels were harsher than standing panels; members of ad hoc panels, typically academics who were unused to working with one another and unlikely to do so again, sought to demonstrate their expertise by engaging in hypercritical evaluations of the grant proposals. More problematically, when applicants reconfigured their grants to appease the most critical members of such panels, they were inevitably faced with a brand-new set of critics upon resubmission. Miami immunologist Nancy Klimas, who had rarely missed a deadline to submit a grant in seven years, complained that year, "Our grants have never been returned to the same study section."

Washington lobbyist Tom Sheridan had attempted to address this dilemma the year before, encouraging Congress to require that the Bethesda agency establish a standing panel for CFS just as it routinely did for other diseases. Congress agreed, and the requirement was passed into law in October 1993 under the NIH Reauthorization Act. The law demanded that the review panel be created within six months of the law's passage. Yet by the end of 1994, fifteen months after the law was signed, the NIH had yet to comply. In fact, in what was perhaps the first overt signal that the CFIDS Association of America might be losing its activist ethos and becoming more malleable as its executives gained wider access to government officials, its lobbyist informed NIH officials that year that the association would no longer press for a standing review panel. Instead, the association agreed to a "standing emphasis panel," which would continue to allow the government to add and subtract reviewers—experts in fields other than CFS—at will. Researchers were unsettled by the compromise.

For some years the CFIDS Association had been viewed as a feisty, challenging group whose leaders were eager to spar with government administrators on behalf of a dues-paying membership of 25,000 CFS patients. Increasingly, there were signs that the executives in Charlotte were far more eager to forge friendly links with government officials than to spar with them—even if it meant compromising the integrity of the organization. The organization's founder, Marc Iverson, once had said he would allow government scientists to peer-review his newsletter when they allowed him to peer-review their scientific papers. Now, editors of the *CFIDS Chronicle,* the organization's primary conduit of communication with its members, were increasingly prone to submit articles containing even mild criticism of federal researchers and policymakers directly to those researchers and policymakers for review prior to publication. Late in 1994 one CFS sufferer, a Ph.D. in philosophy who had been a college instructor before falling ill thirteen years before, proposed an article to the *Chronicle* editors about the "paltry response" of the government to the epidemic. She was told, she said, that her article "might have to be cut, because the CFIDS Association is trying to work with the government." As a result, she declined the opportunity to be a contributor. "My energy is very limited," she explained later, "and I prefer to expend it on something that would remain uncensored."

In the view of at least some of its members, the CFIDS Association was abdicating its adversarial role. Indeed, in a letter to New Yorker James Weir, a disgruntled member of the group's Public Policy Advisory Committee, executive director Kimberly Kenney argued:

> [You] want the Association to discontinue its present style of advocacy and employ "rage" tactics similar to those employed by Act-Up and aggressive activist movements in the breast cancer movement. . . . While I agree that we have a great deal to learn from the successes achieved by AIDS and

breast cancer activists, there are several barriers to the Association adopting an advocacy style that depends so heavily on these strategies. First, CFIDS is not accepted by the general public as a serious, threatening illness, like AIDS and breast cancer are. Second, there are no well-funded public education campaigns to provide a foundation for enlisting the general public in our efforts at this time. Third, rage, while powerful, is a volatile emotion that requires and consumes tremendous amounts of energy (and political capital) to sustain. It is difficult to control and can easily backfire. It erupts spontaneously in response to an incident or crisis and then peaks and subsides quickly. We must use it judiciously.

Kenney advised Weir that in the years to come "the Association will continue to build on [a] moderate, essentially mainstream, approach to advocacy."

Paul Cheney, whose presence in Charlotte had inspired Marc Iverson and others to create the organization eight years before, found a certain irony in the group's newfound compliance with NIH and CDC administrators. "It's an aspect of institutional growth," he commented. "They now see themselves as part of the establishment, and they're adopting the methods of the establishment."

Centers for Disease Control, Atlanta, Georgia

For nearly seven years the definition of the disease drafted by Gary Holmes had reigned supreme. Then, on December 15, 1994, the *Annals of Internal Medicine* published the CDC's revised case definition of chronic fatigue syndrome.[11]

The government's new definition was in some ways better and in other ways even worse than the old one. The "Chinese menu" style of the old definition—which asked that patients meet six of eleven symptom criteria and two of three of the physical criteria, or eight of the eleven symptom criteria—had been abandoned. Now patients needed to meet just four criteria out of a list of eight. In a long-overdue step, the government moved neurological and cognitive problems—"impairment in short-term memory or concentration severe enough to cause substantial reduction in previous levels of occupational, educational, social, or personal activities"—to the top of that list. (Previously, cognitive disabilities had been among the minor symptom criteria.) Other conditions were "sore throat, tender . . . lymph nodes; muscle pain; multijoint pain without swelling or redness; headaches of a new type or pattern or severity; unrefreshing sleep; and postexertional malaise lasting more than twenty-four hours." At least four of these symptoms had to have persisted concurrently for six months or more. There was one more condition to be met: "clinically evaluated, unexplained, persistent, or relapsing chronic fatigue that is of new or definite onset (has not been lifelong); is not the result of ongoing exertion; is not substantially alleviated by rest; and results in substantial reduction in previous levels of occupational, educational, social or personal activities."

The authors proposed a "conceptual framework" for future researchers: "In this framework . . . chronic fatigue syndrome is considered a subset of prolonged fatigue."

For the second time, those who had minimal or no clinical experience with the disease—Anthony Komaroff excepted—were defining it. At least one of the six authors of the new definition, the CDC's James Dobbins, had actually demonstrated a willful desire to *avoid* a clinical acquaintance with the disease. In 1992, he was one of several agency scientists who, during an Atlanta meeting on the disease, had vociferously objected to Paul Cheney's filmed presentation of severely ill CFS patients undergoing neurologic examinations; he had left the room when the film began.

By the government's paradigm, CFS was less a discrete disease than it was merely a state at the extreme end of a continuum of fatigue. Thus, the latest definition served a dual purpose: public demands for efforts to educate or protect the population would again be obviated; fatigue, after all, was not contagious.

Leonard Jason was outspoken in his reaction to the government's new definition. "They fought about this consensus definition for months," he said. "It's a political, not a scientific, event. If these same things were to happen in the AIDS community, it would not be tolerated. . . . I give talks to physicians about this disease. It's 1994, and the majority of doctors still don't believe it's a real disease. The patients think things have changed," Jason added in a reference to the CIFDS Association, "but what's changed is that people don't say these things directly to their faces anymore."

Paul Cheney, mulling the definition and the prime movers behind it, focused on Stephen Straus, who had argued—unsuccessfully—that "chronic fatigue" be named the sole defining element of the disease. In Cheney's view, no doubt tempered by his physicist's education, the government expert had bulldozed the disease into its increasingly well-cemented tomb of confusion and misperception by failing to practice science above "the engineering level."

"*Real* science is leaps of faith that have no logic," Cheney said. "*True* science is *filled* with incongruities. And the better clinicians, trading stories and observations, are not bothered by them—unlike Straus, who becomes dysfunctional. He doesn't know what to do. He can't play a game filled with inconsistencies and incongruities. He plays science by the rules of the day, at the engineering level."

The government's research establishment had pursued a decade-long strategy of avoidance. The fallout from its newest gambit—a second definition as misleading as the first—was likely to ripple through the medical community and academic research centers over time, leaving CFS patients to languish indefinitely in "the night-side of life," as essayist Susan Sontag once described illness. Perhaps the most tangible result of such neglect could be measured in the realm of commerce, where cash rather than medical politics defined priorities. In an interview with journalist Mindi Kitei for *Philadelphia* magazine, published in October, HEM chief William Carter talked about the new direction his company was taking. He told Kitei the Food and Drug Administration had denied fast-track approval for Ampligen therapy, in Kitei's words, "because the scientific community can't even agree on whether [CFS] is actually a disease. For that reason, Carter says, HEM is shifting its focus to cancer and hepatitis."

One can hardly blame the company's investors or Carter. AIDS drugs had been fast-tracked with less supporting data than Carter supplied the government in the wake of HEM's multimillion-dollar four-city CFS clinical trial. In contrast to AIDS, however, CFS—as Carter had learned in a lesson costing millions—remained a medical backwater, a biopolitical morass of huge proportions lying just below the surface of public awareness, from which all but the most stouthearted investigators eventually fled.

EPILOGUE

Knowledge evolves, but in such a way that its pos-
sessors are never in sure possession.

—Sir William Osler, *The Evolution of Modern Medicine*

Gray Hats

Ten years had passed since a crippling disease broke loose in a resort town in the High Sierras. Well into the 1990s, the story of the American epidemic and the people whose lives it destroyed continued to play out in a kind of half-light, unseen and unfelt in most regions of the culture except in the insular realm of clinical medicine, where such patients, by virtue of their numbers and the severity of their illness, were difficult to ignore. Although sufferers seemed to communicate with one another on some curious, uncharted frequency of despair, as a group they inhabited a domain utterly removed from the mainstream. Profoundly debilitated, intellectually compromised, unable to emerge from the "black Jell-O" haze that had claimed them, they dropped from sight. Destitute adults returned to their parents' homes; college students left their campuses, unlikely to complete their education. As the years passed, the society of which they were once a participating member forgot them and moved on. Colleagues were promoted, changed jobs; friends married, had children, moved away; parents aged and died. The ebb and flow of the middle years of life, years during which the majority of patients fell ill, were marked without being experienced. Victims remained anchored in place, longing for redemption, while marriages, careers, incomes, homes, slipped through their fingers. Destitution and suicide flourished.

By the end of 1994 three of the principal players in this drama—Paul Cheney, David Bell, and Elaine DeFreitas—had withdrawn from the public arena as well. Cheney, in particular, was convinced that any further effort on his part to persuade government researchers of the disease's significance or clinical course was pointless. "When in doubt, listen to a thousand patients with an open mind," Cheney had advised a panel of scientists at the Food and Drug Administration early in 1993. "Failing that, then listen to those who have spent countless hours with a thousand patients." The new definition made it abundantly clear that the doctor's observations and research of the last ten years had failed to move the discovery process forward at the highest and most influential levels—the well-financed federal research establishments. He was forty-seven; it was time, Cheney believed, to refocus his efforts.

The doctor's transformation had been gradual. "I'm not sure there was a single point," Cheney recalled late in 1994. "There was a series of events. The attempts by CDC to rewrite the definition without any clinical input . . . Each revision was worse, and the revisions were being driven by the *Annals of Internal Medicine* reviewers, who knew even *less* about the disease. Watching the slide from grace of Elaine and her work. The attacks on her by the Scottish virologist John Gow, and [by] Tom Folks. Then the attacks on John Martin, and his fall from grace."

Cheney had looked on with a kind of stunned dismay as the criticism leveled at his colleagues and collaborators—scientists, funded entirely by patients, struggling to discover the etiology of the disease—had assumed an ad hominem, career-shattering quality.

"Max Planck, a German physicist, said that when you make a paradigm shift that shakes the foundations of established thought, you will not change minds. You're going to have to wait for them to die off," the doctor said. "What I've come to believe is that there is no way in my lifetime that I'm going to change Bill Reeves. He's going to have to die off. . . . I'm looking to other people now, and you won't find them at the CDC or the NIH."

During the two years since the CDC had publicized its failure to replicate De-Freitas's experiments, Cheney's fascination with the trigger—the viral agent that caused the disease—had begun to wane. One of those who had influenced his thinking was Jeffrey Bland, a nutritional biochemist who had been a senior researcher at the Linus Pauling Institute and was the author of several books on nutrition. Bland decried what he described as the "post-Renaissance reductionism of modern medicine," the notion that all diseases can be reduced to a single-point cause—a toxin or a microbe. Some diseases fit the "Western reductionist model," Cheney acknowledged, but most human diseases did not; instead, they fell into a complex matrix of predisposing genetics, environment, and myriad other elements.

"We're all unique," Cheney said. "If you give agent X to ten people, will they all get the same disease? No. HIV is a reductionist model that has failed." Cheney was convinced that the reductionist model ultimately would fail chronic fatigue syndrome sufferers, too.

"The way for me to have made a breakthrough with the CDC would have been to present them with a bug—to define for them a reductionist course. And if Elaine or Michael Holmes or whoever has the bug were to present it to them, the finding would galvanize the agency, but [CFS] would go the way of AIDS," he continued, in a reference to medicine's failure to cure or even dramatically mediate the fatal disease despite the presence of a bug and a multibillion-dollar research effort. "Whatever the mechanism of CFIDS, it becomes *very* complex. Reductionism won't help the patient once the patient is ill. Without a tremendous advance in our ability to kill viruses, we have to start thinking about the *process* of illness."

The process of CFS was like falling dominoes, or the chain reaction of nuclear fission. Once the slide began, Cheney increasingly believed, the instigator was irrelevant to the outcome, which was inevitably a momentous and intricate constellation of "multiple injuries" to the body. "All great avalanches start with something very small," he said. "It is not unlike the theory of chaos in which a butterfly flaps its wings in Japan and starts a hurricane in Florida. It becomes like a snowball going downhill. One doesn't necessarily care what the little pea was that caused all this shit. You can find the pea, but what do you think that is going to do? *Nothing.*

"These patients," Cheney continued after a pause, "are like a ship sitting in the water. And below the waterline the ship is full of holes and they're sinking. You keep plugging holes, but they're still sinking. Sometimes you do exactly the right thing, but you don't know it, because this disease is a *multiple* injury—there are *many* injuries. If I disregulate your immune system, and that disregulates your brain and injures it, and the injured brain now makes hormones that become toxic to you, which further injure you so that your natural killer cells drop and allow the reactivation of viruses you caught in childhood, which further injure you—we now have about seven holes below the waterline. Systems break down, problems beget more problems. There are secondary, tertiary, and 'quartiary' issues. After a while, what is wrong with you is more important than what started the avalanche."

Looking back upon his own and his collaborators' long search for the cause, the doctor noted, "We went through this rising tide of 'science will prevail.' But we need a new way of thinking. This disease is made up of complex networks of interacting systems. One should never give up looking for the bug, because—who knows?—it might exist. But we may never find the bug. And even if we find it we may never be able to do anything about it. Reye's syndrome," he added in a reference to the deadly children's disease that could be triggered by the administration of aspirin during fever, "is caused by chicken pox. But you can't cure Reye's by killing chicken pox. The issue of causality might be important in *preventing* CFS, but it won't help you once you get the disease."*

Along with his philosophical underpinnings, the nature of Cheney's practice in Charlotte was also changing. Once he had drawn patients from all over the United States, Canada, and other foreign countries. Now CFS sufferers from North Carolina and nearby states were claiming most of his attention. "Universities are increasingly starting to set up CFS clinics," the doctor noted. "These clinics are drawing the local patients, and we're turning into more of a regional center. It's becoming rarer and rarer [for us] to see someone from far away."

In addition, unlike those who had sought his expertise in the past, most new patients had been correctly diagnosed with the disease by the time they reached Cheney. What these sufferers needed most from the Charlotte doctor was objective proof that they suffered from a real illness and irrefutable test results demonstrating disability. Most clinicians' understanding of the disease was still too primitive to allow them to provide such documentation for their patients. "Disability issues are a growth aspect of my practice," Cheney said. "These people need a sophisticated defense for disability actions."

---

* Cheney's formidable contributions to the discovery process around any potential retroviral etiology were likely to go unrewarded. Although biotech patent attorney Leslie Misrock agreed that Cheney was a co-inventor along with Elaine DeFreitas, the Wistar Institute's lawyers steadfastly refused to list his name on the patent for the discovery. Now, with the onset of Elaine DeFreitas's illness, scientific progress had stalled and the dispute itself, once so charged, had faded into meaninglessness.

"If no one carries on [De Freitas's] work," Cheney said, "there's no issue. Someone else will just invent around her, and that will be that. But if her work is resurrected in some way, in order to get a clear line of rights, I must ultimately challenge it." Even as he spoke the words, however, it seemed apparent the doctor had lost his passion for the fight.

A Wistar spokeswoman, Dr. Fogg-Johnson, reported in mid-1995 that no patent had been issued. "Whether or not there is one pending, I am not at liberty to say," she added.

In addition to providing such a defense—primarily in the form of multiple imaging technologies demonstrating brain damage and laboratory assays demonstrating immune dysfunction—he and his staff spent more and more time on legal matters related to the seemingly irreversible disintegration of his patients' social and professional lives. Divorce, child custody, employers' refusal to pay out on disability policies, bankruptcy, and even incarceration in psychiatric hospitals were among the crushing issues that compelled CFS sufferers to go to court.

In contrast to other internal medicine specialists, who spend an average of seven minutes with each patient, Cheney typically scheduled only four patients a day. His first patient of the day was always new, and he spent the entire morning taking a history, performing an exam—including a detailed neurological exam—and running tests. His afternoon appointments were repeat visits.

Cheney himself had undergone an upheaval in his private life: he and his wife of nearly twenty years, Jean, had separated that year, their marriage another casualty of the epidemic. Like the unorthodox practitioner in Sinclair Lewis's *Arrowsmith* who moved from a rural clinical practice to a research institution and, finally, to the Vermont woods in order to conduct his own research, Cheney was pondering a move from Charlotte to a small island off the coast of North Carolina. He planned to see new patients in his Charlotte clinic just one day a week; the other four days of the workweek, he said, he would conduct a "virtual clinic," holding telephone consultations with his far-flung patients from his house on the island, and he would continue his reading and studying.

"The movement to a virtual office would allow what's between my ears to be profitable," the doctor said.

Cheney's drift from his once-passionate search for the cause was a remarkable change, given his intimate embroilment with the disease's most famous outbreak a decade before. Another doctor who had been a firsthand witness to a similar event, David Bell, was not ready, emotionally or intellectually, to abandon the quest.

"Paul is very interested in the mechanism of the illness, and he's not so interested in the initiating event anymore. He's now looking at the process, which involves about forty different factors simultaneously," Bell said. "I can see it as a next step for his intellect, although no one will be able to keep up with it. But I want to think about one factor: what was the major hit? Something happened in Lyndonville that made two hundred and thirty people sick."

Nonetheless, Bell, too, was dissociating himself from the political and scientific struggles of the past several years. "I feel very much like Paul," he said. "I'm withdrawing."

His own marriage, like those of his former collaborators, was ending, and by mid-1995, the doctor had chosen to leave his post at Harvard's pediatric clinic to return to Lyndonville, New York. His wife, Karen Bell, would continue to live full-time in Cambridge, working as medical adviser to a Harvard-affiliated HMO. The decision to leave Harvard had crept up on Bell. Throughout 1994, he had worked half the month at Harvard, following the cases of approximately sixty adults and children with CFS as well as children with AIDS; the remaining time he had lived alone in the rambling farmhouse that he and Karen had bought in Lyndonville after their medical training two decades before. While in Lyndonville, Bell worked part-time in the emergency room of the impoverished region's small hospital in Medina. The CFS sufferers he had cared for in his old practice continued to seek him out, but Bell counseled them without charge on his front porch, a sagging screenless structure with a floor of antique wooden planks, a roof supported by four carved Victorian columns, and an unimpeded view of Lake Ontario. "I see people as neighbors," he said at the time. "It's too expensive to carry malpractice insurance."

In his free moments Bell worked on a novel and a nonfiction book about managing the educations of children who suffered from CFS. He was nostalgic about his life and practice before the Lyndonville epidemic that had decimated his own life and the lives of so many of his young patients and their parents. "What an office we had!" he said, his blue eyes merry for a moment. "Even when Mr. Zanke drove through the front wall of the office. He's eighty-five. He said, 'I need an appointment with the doctor to get my license renewed.' People would come in and they had no money, and that was okay. Then they would come in with money and they wouldn't want to pay—and that was okay too."

By mid-1995, however, Bell had decided to revive his Lyndonville practice. "It's caught up with me," he commented. "I'm tired of pretending to be an academic. I haven't learned *anything* about CFS in the last four years. The only way you can do that is to follow someone who's really sick over a long period of time."

He had long ago thrown out an NIH grant proposal to study children with the disease, he said. Given the political history of CFS and his role in it, any further expectation of a grant from the Bethesda institute was, he said, "like me wanting to be an astronaut." A significant portion of Bell's disaffection, like that of his former collaborator, Paul Cheney, stemmed from the almost gleeful dismissal of Elaine DeFreitas and her work by federal researchers. "I've lost my enthusiasm for research," he said. "It went with Elaine." In Bell's view, the CDC and, later, Walter Gunn and the CFIDS Association, had failed to allow DeFreitas the latitude she required to pursue her findings in a supportive, calm environment. "She's scrupulously honest," Bell said when the conversation veered toward the topic of the former Wistar immunologist. "She saw something that she perceived as being real, and she went through a meat grinder. Let's say, just for a moment, that Elaine was spending all of her time on a tissue contaminant," he added. "Let's see what it *is*—there's no reason to be threatened—instead of 'Let's control the damage.' "

Staff at the CDC, Bell conjectured, were likely "horrified by the idea of another human retrovirus." In addition, he said, DeFreitas's precocious discovery had threatened the status quo in Atlanta. "Here was an upstart who was finding something that the CDC couldn't replicate," Bell said. But, he added, "the CDC *still* can't replicate the [natural killer] cell findings! Why is it that about *thirty* other groups have found this, and the CDC can't?"

Interestingly, Bell believed that DeFreitas's former champion, the CFIDS Association, had probably caused her more harm than anyone in the federal research establishment. The nation's largest patient organization, which had supported her research for three years and then withdrawn its support when the government published its inability to reproduce her findings, had abandoned the scientist at a point when she most needed their support, Bell said. "I felt she should have been given some money and then been allowed to do what she could. And a simple double-blind case-control study isn't going to do it in this disease. The CFIDS Association was asking her to do these case-control studies prematurely."

DeFreitas had been unable to perform the study Walter Gunn set up with C. V. Herst at Oncore Analytics in Houston, John Martin at USC and DeFreitas, Bell said, because "Hurricane Andrew destroyed the [University of Miami] campus. She couldn't get it done on time."

At the time, DeFreitas speculated it might be more productive to search for the RNA of the virus rather than the DNA in order to differentiate cases from healthy people. She developed an RNA assay and used it on the samples sent to her by the CDC, but the new test didn't work. "All of a sudden, it gets published that Elaine DeFreitas can't tell cases from controls," Bell recalled. On a final case-control study of just twelve samples, DeFreitas identified five of six patients using her original assay. She had more studies planned to fine-tune the assay, but the CFIDS Association interrupted her work again, demanding that she participate in yet another case-control study.

"The CFIDS Association was patient for three years and then they got impatient. But they were asking for a 1990 Buick in 1964. She's got to do some of the groundwork first, and she's just never had the time to pursue these other studies," Bell said.

The doctor leveled an even more damaging charge at the patient organization's leadership. "Three years ago I came to understand that the CFIDS Association offered [DeFreitas] up," he observed. "They said, 'We need to be on the good side of the CDC and the NIH.' " According to Bell, the leadership had perceived that DeFreitas, no matter how pure her science, needed to be cut adrift in order to build bridges with the government. "Basically there was a certain point at which the politics came up and the money thing came up, and they decided it was time to dump her," Bell said. "I'm stunned that somebody could be hurt so much."

(Marc Iverson, the CFIDS Association's top executive, seemed to tacitly confirm Bell's assessment when, reflecting on his organization's history with De-Freitas, he commented that "if Elaine DeFreitas finds something and *we* funded it, it will never get published. If Sidney Grossberg finds something and [the government] funded it, it will get published in the fucking *New England Journal of Medicine*." Iverson further noted that DeFreitas was currently viewed as too far out of the mainstream for his organization to continue supporting her.)

Ironically, DeFreitas's affiliation with the CFIDS Association, perceived in the early 1990s as an activist organization by federal officials, was in large part what had spun the former Wistar scientist out of the mainstream. "The fact that she was being funded by the CFIDS Association hurt her from getting NIH money. There was *no way* she was going to get funded," Bell said.

The work of countless American scientists is supported in whole or in part by the philanthropic funds of organizations representing patients who are suffering from particular diseases. AIDS, multiple sclerosis, juvenile diabetes, cystic fibrosis, heart disease, cancer, Alzheimer's disease, and other maladies, however, are not mired in high-stakes controversies in which their very existence is debated.

Interferon expert Sidney Grossberg of Wisconsin had sought and been awarded funding from the CFIDS Association to pursue his retroviral experiments. Having watched Elaine DeFreitas crash and burn, however, he had demanded that the organization keep his progress and methods secret. In its quarterly journal, the patient organization made only brief, perfunctory references to Grossberg's work. Using CFIDS Association funds as seed money, Grossberg—one of an elite network of scientists, mostly men—turned to the Bethesda institution for more money and received it.* The CFIDS Association continues to fund Grossberg, but, in contrast to the demands it made upon DeFreitas, the group has requested of him no deadlines, peer-reviewed scientific articles, press appearances, or highly public case-control studies. Marc Iverson, in fact, conceded it might take Grossberg a decade to nail down the identity of his novel retrovirus, a possibility that did not seem to disturb the CFIDS Association chief.

Ultimately, Bell said, it was unfair to expect a poorly funded patient organization to play the role of the National Institutes of Health. "How can you ask a small organization like them to fund basic science?" he asked. The CFIDS Association had merely struggled to fill the void left by the government's neglect.

Tellingly, although the government's CFS expert, Stephen Straus, eagerly sought congressional intervention to halt what he perceived as undue pressure, even harassment, from patients, by mid-1995 he had never testified about chronic fatigue syndrome before members of either house of Congress, leaving it entirely to patients and their advocates to persuade legislators of the need for more research money in the field. His choice suggests that the well-funded government scientist is, at best, indifferent to the fate of scientists outside his institution who wish to be involved in the discovery process and, at worst, hostile to any scientific inquiry not his own.

In 1995, Elaine DeFreitas's medical condition was no better; she remained confined to her house in Fort Lauderdale, attended by her elderly mother. Her ability to pursue the work she had started in the CFS field had faded entirely. DeFreitas believed, in fact, that her scientific career was over.

"I don't know how this virus is going to be classified," she said during a long conversation about her tumultuous history in the disease. "They love to make evolutionary trees for viruses. One of these days someone is going to get their hands on enough of this virus to make it accepted by the scientific community. It's not going to be me, however."

She had closed her lab at the University of Miami and sent most of her blood samples to Paul Cheney's clinic in Charlotte where they could be stored in a −70°F. freezer. DeFreitas had chosen to send tissue samples from human organs, including portions of the teenage suicide Skye Dailor's heart, liver, spleen, and brain to Robert Suhadolnik, the Temple University scientist who had evaluated

---

* When this writer sought Grossberg's successful NIH grant proposal through a Freedom of Information request, Grossberg removed everything but the unrevealing first and last pages of his grant, even though the public is entitled to see successful grant proposals upon request. Only information that might undermine national security is exempted from the Freedom of Information Act.

AIDS and CFS patients enrolled in Ampligen trials for HEM Pharmaceuticals. Suhadolnik could provide long-term storage in a liquid nitrogen tank for the organ samples. Cheney and Suhadolnik agreed to steward the materials until DeFreitas found a trustworthy microbiologist who was willing to take her research to the next level of understanding.

DeFreitas regretted her participation in epidemiological trials with CDC scientists, believing now that the demands made upon her by federal scientists were both unfair and untimely.

"If anyone was powerful enough to go into Gallo's lab in 1981 and say, 'Now we're going to do a double-blind study,' he would have kicked them out of his lab, because he was in the discovery phase," DeFreitas said. "We were trying to code, sequence, and culture. Every time we tried to do publishable science, we were asked to do a double-blind study! The science is done first. Then, when you've got a test—when Gallo says, 'I've got a test for antibodies to HIV; now, CDC, bring me samples from two thousand gay men'—*then* you start work on the epidemiology. But, with two lab people, I was being asked to do *all* these things."

She recalled that Paul Cheney, recognizing the unreasonableness of the demands being made of her, had pleaded with the CFIDS Association's Scientific Advisory Committee members to allow the scientist to drop her collaboration with federal scientists. Unfortunately, the patient organization, her sole source of funding, and Walter Gunn, were ardent in their desire to demonstrate the disease's legitimacy to the government agency and saw DeFreitas's discovery as their most powerful means of persuasion.

"Paul fought Walter Gunn on that issue at every SAC meeting, but he was ignored," DeFreitas recalled. Once Gunn joined the patient organization's advisory group, she added, he "brought the whole CDC attitude into the SAC, which funded me, and began demanding that I focus my efforts on double-blind studies.

"I told Walter to do a Medline search," DeFreitas continued. "I told him to start with Gallo's papers in 1978. I said, 'What you will see is exactly what *we* are doing.' Walter Gunn thought he knew more than Gallo.

"My two Ph.D.'s were going mad," she recalled. "All we had was CFIDS Association money," and yet DeFreitas and her associates were being asked to undertake projects that even a large, well-funded laboratory like Gallo's would not have been expected to undertake at a similar stage of discovery. "It was nonsense," DeFreitas said, "but I couldn't get through to anyone—Marc Iverson, Walter . . ."

Like anyone mourning a terrible loss, DeFreitas focused obsessively on moments in her past that now seemed pivotal—and rued the paths she had chosen. When she returned to her Wistar laboratory several weeks after being hospitalized with injuries she received in a car accident in 1989, for instance, and her lab associate Brendan Hilliard demonstrated to her the evidence for retroviral infection in CFS patients, she recalled that she nearly fainted. "I said, this can't possibly be true, because if it were true, someone like Jay Levy or Gallo would have found this—not me. And I sent them all back into the lab and made them do all the experiments over." The results were the same. "At that point," she continued, "I should have called Bernie Poiesz [the HTLV expert in Syracuse] or Gallo, boxed it all up, and said, '*You* do this.' If the data were right, they would have been believed. If the data were wrong and they believed it and published it anyway, they wouldn't have taken the hit I did because they were already established."

Nor could DeFreitas discount the negative impact of the demands made upon her by the patient organization that had funded her. In hindsight, she now believed the CFIDS Association's insistence that she hold a press conference in San Francisco to announce her discovery before its publication in a scientific journal to be the single most damaging result of her association with the organization. Indeed, the action was destined to bring the full weight of scientific censure upon her. She had agreed to the request because she felt she could not refuse those who had paid for the research. But her initial finding of retroviral gene fragments among patients and people who were in close contact with them was, DeFreitas said, "just a baby step." Once the American press telegraphed the nature of her discovery far and wide, the federal government had no choice but to respond quickly and definitively. That pressure likely contributed to the CDC staff's keen desire to publish their negative study, ignoring DeFreitas's entreaties for time to undertake further experiments.

Wisconsin's Sidney Grossberg, the sole investigator to win federal money to pursue a viral etiology for the disease, cursed DeFreitas's choices. "She created *enormous* pressure," Grossberg complained in 1995. "The Public Health Service had no *choice* but to show whether she was wrong or right," an informal mandate that left everyone else hunting for retroviral etiologies subsumed by dark clouds when the government's verdict became known. "It's made everybody's life harder." Certainly, it is telling that, of the many investigators who tried and failed to replicate the DeFreitas find, only the government's scientists deemed it necessary to publish on the matter, and in no fewer than four journals.

Recently, DeFreitas said, she had had a conversation with Marc Iverson in which he extolled Grossberg's secrecy. Grossberg, Iverson said, did not talk to the press, nor did he attend public meetings on the disease. "This is praised and admired," DeFreitas commented, "when it seems to me that everybody else is being put on the spot. I'm totally confused," she added after a moment. "I thought there were white hats and black hats. There are only gray hats."

Still, she insisted, during those crucial months before and after the presentation of her retrovirus data in Kyoto, Japan, she had not been operating in a vacuum. "Hilary Koprowski, one of the most famous virologists alive, had said, 'It looks good. When are you going to publish?' " Koprowski's confidence made DeFreitas brave. Soon after the Kyoto conference, she had shown her data to Dale MacFarland, a highly respected NIH virologist and friend of Koprowski's. MacFarland, too, had reassured her, telling her the virus looked like HTLV2.

"Even after Japan I was being told that things looked right," DeFreitas noted. "Probably to have remained unscathed I could have handed it off then." After a pause she added, "In retrospect, I say I did the disease a disservice. I might have done the patients a disservice, and I might have done the field a disservice."

In recent months, she continued, she had derived some comfort from a woman whose experience mirrored, in significant ways, her own. Years earlier, DeFreitas had attended a dinner hosted by the Leukemia Society of America during which a young scientist named Sandra Panem was awarded a research grant. At the time, Panem was a postdoctorate fellow working on leukemia viruses at the University of Chicago. "I remember thinking how stunning she was," DeFreitas recalled. "She looked like a young Liz Taylor." DeFreitas had nearly forgotten the striking young scientist whose career had seemed so promising, however, when, during a literature search in the early 1990s, she came across a series of articles written by Panem.

DeFreitas recalled, "She had five or six papers.[1] In each of them, she described a retrovirus in lupus. The retrovirus she had found was almost a hybrid of two monkey viruses. This was a phenomenal discovery. And she was using very basic tools. She did a spectacular job, given the tools. Yet every subsequent paper was in a slightly less prominent journal. Then, abruptly, a wall came down—and from then on, Sandra Panem disappeared."

The first paper Panem published, in fact, appeared in 1976 in the *New England Journal of Medicine,* two years before the Gallo laboratory published its discovery of HTLV.

DeFreitas had been mystified by the apparent vanishing of such an innovative scientist, but she was too caught up in her own struggle to pursue the mystery further. Then, late in 1992, a second group of scientists reported their discovery of a novel retrovirus in lupus sufferers.[2] Reminded once more of Sandra Panem, DeFreitas was suddenly determined to talk to her.

"I finally found her," the scientist recalled. "She's an investment banker in New York."

After explaining her interest in Panem's articles, DeFreitas asked the former scientist, "What happened?"

Panem's reply resonated in DeFreitas's mind for months afterward: "Nobody believed us."

"She became so disillusioned," DeFreitas continued, "that she left science entirely. And suddenly I could see myself twenty years from now, when I'm a high school biology teacher and someone calls and says, 'Hey, they just found a retrovirus in CFS.' And maybe that's how it will happen. And I know how I'll feel—I'll feel great."

Curiously, it was Daniel Peterson, the gifted young diagnostician, as he was remembered by his former colleague, CDC investigator Mary Guinan, who had survived the epidemic with his family and career most intact. "There were some very committed doctors," Peterson said in an oblique reference to Cheney, DeFreitas, and Bell, "who took this cause on as a marriage—at the expense of their real marriages. I never quite gave up everything for this."

Somehow, Peterson had weathered the forces pressuring him to leave Incline Village after the epidemic, just as he had resisted those at the CDC and the NIH who suggested he cease rendering the diagnosis. He had withstood the rage of some of his own patients when HEM ended the ampligen trials prematurely, and he had watched coolly when the company abandoned its principal investigators in the United States and took their drug and research protocol, developed and refined in large part by him, to Europe. For the doctor who had invited the CDC to the famous Tahoe outbreak and inadvertently launched what could well turn out to be among the most shameful chapters in medical history, the epidemic remained a

"Bergman flick" with a last frame, when it came, that left one sitting puzzled and disturbed in the darkness.

"I don't think I ever thought there would be a quick fix for this," Peterson said. "But, to this day, I feel there are probably people more skilled than I who should be seeing these patients—although, who in medicine now wants to do anything out of the ordinary?"

Like that of his former partner in Charlotte, the dynamic of Peterson's practice had changed significantly by 1995. "I do a lot of testimony now," Peterson said. "Third-party referrals." In such cases, his task was to confirm the diagnosis; he was not required to act as a primary physician to the patient, whose needs the doctor now found almost intolerably burdensome, especially given that he, himself, had aged a decade since the epidemic began. "I had much more energy then," he said. The former Vietnam War protester was, in addition, sincerely perplexed by what he viewed as the political passivity of most sufferers. "I'm not sure the momentum is there from the patients. If I had a disease that was totally disabling, I would be *much* more angry and aggressive than most of the patients I know."

In 1994, Stephen Straus continued to be viewed as a chronic fatigue syndrome expert by most in mainstream medicine. On October 23 of that year, Straus was invited to address the American College of Rheumatology, meeting in Minneapolis, on the subject. Over the course of his comments on the pathogenesis of the disease, it was apparent that the government scientist continued to harbor an unmistakable if suppressed contempt for people who suffered from CFS; nor had he retreated from his belief that the malady was, as he told the hundreds of rheumatologists in his audience, "not a single disease entity (but) a mixed bag of entities." He cited, in addition, thirty-year-old medical papers that pinned recovery speed among mononucleosis and influenza victims to "the emotional state of the patient." "If we had been aware of these studies," he said, "some of us might not have tried to reinvent the wheel" by attempting to assign the disease a virological cause, as he himself had done in 1985 when he associated CFS with chronic Epstein-Barr virus infection. And he reiterated his years-long propaganda about the high rate of preexisting psychiatric illness among sufferers. The scientist dispensed with those who would argue the point in a sentence: "The large clinical practices that report in the literature that they don't see a lot of psychiatric diagnoses [among CFS sufferers] can be charged with not using the kinds of techniques that psychiatrists use."

In character, the scientist proceeded to denigrate most research not his own.

"Retroviruses *had* to be considered because this is the era of retroviruses," he said. "In my mind," he added—revealing his failure after more than a decade of study to develop a clinical familiarity with the disease's signs and symptoms— "this doesn't make any sense because . . . retroviral infection . . . include(s) progressive hematologic, immunologic, and neurologic deficits in one mix or another, and those aren't really prominent features of chronic fatigue syndrome." Noting the CDC's failure to replicate DeFreitas's work, Straus said, "Despite the fact that [the retroviral theory] gained a certain cachet, and it made a lot of people very anxious, there's really no good scientific merit to it." He further posited,

"There is no current evidence for chronic infection in CFS. Therefore, broad screening of CFS patients for infections is completely unwarranted. Your patients may demand exotic screenings," he added, "but it's only confusing."

In a few sentences, Straus also dismissed the by-now nearly fifty papers describing immunological aberrations in the disease. "It's fair to say," he said, "that the findings in these studies are not reproducible." He denied the legitimacy of reported neuropsychological abnormalities with the comment "Very little cognitive impairment is actually verified [on careful testing]."

In response to a question from the audience, Straus also attempted to obliterate NeuroSPECT scan data that pointed to functional brain damage in the disease. "Most of these kinds of studies come out of shops with no scientific method," he said, "and have a lot of resonance in certain patient populations because it's a very high-tech, very sophisticated test. And there are practice groups and little mini-institutes . . . around the country who advocate these kinds of things, and our patients bring in this literature saying that so-and-so in San Francisco and so-and-so in Los Angeles and so-and-so in North Carolina showed such and such. And you have to listen . . . but there is no sustained belief that these things are abnormal."

Most remarkably, Straus concluded by blaming patients for at least some part of their dilemma. A significant portion of the symptomatology of the disease, he commented, was a result of "poor sleep hygiene" and failure to exercise: "Patients exacerbate things because they take multiple naps during the day and break up their rest periods and sleep periods. They stay in bed a lot. The diet and medication [with which] they attempt to control some of their other symptoms to keep them alert or awake and functional, in many cases, exacerbates sleep problems."

"To conclude," Straus said, "when we're done thinking about this, this poor miserable patient is still going to end up seeing all of you to understand what it is that all the other specialists he or she has seen over the prior years has failed to diagnose."

The scientist was roundly applauded, with at least one audience member shouting, "Hear, hear!"

On July 19, 1995, Straus responded in writing to a question posed to him through a public affairs officer at the National Institute of Allergy and Infectious Diseases. (He had refused all interview requests since 1987.) "I remain committed to helping resolve the numerous complex problems that chronic fatigue syndrome represents to its many sufferers," Straus wrote, "and foresee active involvement in the field for years to come."

Roll Call

Chronic fatigue syndrome, or myalgic encephalomyelitis, is a disease from which few people recover completely, though many improve over the course of years. Even among those rare few who claim recovery or substantial improvement, the transforming nature of the disease remains manifest; these patients inevitably describe a series of adjustments or realignments of goals and expectations that would have been unthinkable prior to the onset of their illness.

In *The Clinical and Scientific Basis of ME/CFS* (Canada: Nightingale Research Foundation, 1992), Byron Hyde, Sheila Bastien, and Anil Jain describe the phases of the disease in broad strokes. In the "early chronic stage," lasting from one to six years, they write, "the physical and medical aspects start to merge with the psychosocial aspects of the disease. . . . During this period, many patients . . . show a very slow and uneven period of recovery and readaptation to their altered state of central nervous system, muscle, and social function. Recovery should not be confused with adaptation." Any degree of "rehabilitation" in these early years will depend on many things, including the social supports available to the patients—helpful spouses and families in particular—their degree of brain injury, and their intellectual assets and levels of education prior to falling ill.

"Many patients in this stage of illness will not recover sufficiently to enjoy either work or social activities," the authors continue. "[This stage] is marked by major changes in their life pattern. Unstable marriages will become increasingly destablilized, and marriage breakdown and divorce will occur. Money reserves will have been liquidated . . . the social confines of poverty may have set in, and the patients, most of whom will have had life and social expectations set at a higher level, will now see those hopes and expectations destroyed. It is difficult for a physician, in a fifteen-minute visit, to relate to this change. . . . It is the period when students and youths and some adults will be most prone to suicide."

According to these authors, the "late chronic stage"—beginning after the sixth year of illness—is a period about which the least was known medically and socially. Nevertheless, they write: "These patients tend to be forgotten. They have adjusted to their altered abilities. . . . Despite their previous relatively high earning ability, many of these ME/CFS patients will have become poor, long out of the work force, with no appreciable disability insurance. They . . . can become street people. They tend to no longer be recognized as having a post-infectious disease process. . . . It is our opinion that far from ME/CFS simply being a disease of the upper middle class, many of those who fall ill as children, adolescents, and young adults become a significant proportion of the chronic poor" (pp. 25–37).

The following patients (presented in alphabetical order) are all now in the late chronic stage of ME/CFS, having fallen ill during the pandemic years of the middle to late 1980s. Three have died, one by suicide. Most, though not all, report improvement in the form of adaptation, having achieved a degree of forbearance and acceptance.

Darrell Anderson

A former real estate consultant who was fifty-two when he fell ill in 1984, Anderson was featured in a *20/20* piece in 1986. He described the suicidal fantasies he experienced when his family and friends refused to believe he was sick. Nine years later, in 1995, the disease had exacted its social and financial toll: Anderson is estranged from his wife and children and surviving on disability support from the Social Security Administration. "If you can get up one day and take out the trash, and the next day you can't stand up without falling over, your family wonders, 'Is this real or not?'—especially when you're the breadwinner." Anderson says he is "somewhat" physically improved, although he continues to suffer "Alzheimer's-like" intellectual problems. But he adds, "I cannot allow the word 'hopeless' in my vocabulary anymore. I will not allow myself to be degraded by my circumstances."

Nomi Antelman

A CFS victim since 1980, Antelman, who was also interviewed for *20/20,* remains totally disabled. "When CFS made the cover of *Newsweek* in 1990," she says, "I thought, Now I can die happy. I thought things *had* to change. But there's been no real progress. We're where we were five years ago."

Onorio Antonucci

"Andy" Antonucci, a girls' basketball coach and algebra teacher for nearly three decades, was among eight teachers who shared a cramped teachers' lounge two hours a day at Truckee High in 1985, and nearly all of whom acquired the disease in the space of several months. In 1988, after numerous failed attempts to resume teaching, Antonucci, then in his mid-fifties, officially retired and moved to Albuquerque, New Mexico, to be near his mother. He subsists on a reduced California state teachers' retirement pension. The Truckee teachers' 1985 lawsuit against the school district for workers' compensation has so far been unsuccessful. Now sixty-two, Antonucci says, "I've got maybe three or four hours a day in me, as long as it's nothing physical or demanding."

Gloria Baker

Baker, a real estate saleswoman from Riverside, California, had suffered from CFS for a decade when she moved to Incline Village, Nevada, to become one of the original Ampligen recipients in 1989. She chose to go off the drug in 1992. In October 1994 she committed suicide.

Irene and Laurie Baker

Baker, a Truckee High civics teacher, came down with CFS in the spring of 1985. Since 1989 she has been able to work full-time without experiencing major relapses, and she currently claims a 90 percent recovery from the illness. She teaches fifth grade in Truckee. Her teenage daughter, Laurie, who fell ill at roughly the same time, experienced full recovery within a year.

Craig Barshinger

Although he has experienced substantial improvement since falling ill in 1985, Barshinger says he "feels normal" two or three days a year. On those rare days, he adds, "I don't even believe it happened to me." The rest of the time, he continues, "it's like something has snagged in the biochemical knit, like a sweater caught on a thorn, and you want to release the sweater and get on with your life, but you can't." Remembering the early, more severe years of the disease, Barshinger says, makes him "break out in a cold sweat. It's like any life trauma, I suppose—like surviving an airplane crash or a concentration camp." Now thirty-eight, Barshinger sold the company he founded—a firm that made computers to prevent divers from getting the bends on deep dives—eight years ago and moved to Saint John in the U.S. Virgin Islands. He works as a consultant for his former company. "On January 29, 1989, I woke up feeling absolutely normal for the first time," he recalls. "It lasted a week. When [the disease] came back, the severity was gone. Before that, I wasn't sure I wanted to live out a normal life span."

Stephen Beale

An Episcopal priest who fell sick in 1984, Beale abandoned efforts to continue a conventional priesthood in 1994. After suffering a relapse that resulted in ten days of hospitalization, Beale bade his parishioners in Woodland, California, farewell and moved to San Francisco, where he counsels CFS sufferers by telephone and lobbies politicians for research funds. "I've been through hell," he says. "But I'm still a priest. I'm doing priestly things. You could describe me as 'medically retired.'" State chairman of California's Youth for Reagan in his adolescence, Beale also confesses, "I've become a raving liberal."

Sally Bentson (pseudonym)

Along with her mother, Nevada resident Bentson was invited by federal scientists to come to the NIH for study in 1986 when she was twenty-two. Bentson's arm was badly scarred during an anesthesia-free muscle biopsy, performed at Stephen Straus's request. "You become desperate for answers," she says of the experience now. (Straus has yet to provide the test results to her.) Bentson's symptoms have diminished, but at age thirty-one, she continues to suffer fatigue and depression, and in 1994 she experienced a severe relapse that necessitated a three-month leave from her job. Antidepressant medication was helping her cope. "The disease not only lingers in your body," she says, "it lingers in your mind."

Richard Carson

Carson, who fell ill soon after his graduation from college in 1981, remains sick. In 1990, he established the CFIDS Buyers Club, which sells vitamins at low cost to CFS patients and donates half of its profits to research efforts, but he does not participate in the club's day-to-day operation.

Cher

In 1995, a spokeswoman for Cher insisted that the actress is no longer suffering from CFS: "She's well."

Gerald Crum

Crum had been on Ampligen for four and a half years when, in September 1993, he was forced off the drug. Although he testified before the Food and Drug Administration to the good effects of Ampligen, his wife believes her husband had reached a "plateau" on the drug, even though it "saved his life" by halting a progressive dementia. Even without Ampligen, Crum continues to improve in stamina, although, he notes, the improvement comes "at a snail's pace." The former computer programmer lives on disability support from his former employer.

James Dunlap, Jr.

Dunlap, now twenty-three, had just begun eighth grade when he contracted the disease at the start of the epidemic in Yerington, Nevada. He was bedridden throughout his adolescence and was tutored at home until his senior year in high school. With effort, he graduated with his high school class and joined the army. He has no memory of his childhood years prior to the onset of his illness. He also suffers frequent violent tremors, and "continue[s] to get awfully tired," according to his mother. Nevertheless, in 1995 Dunlap was making plans to attend college.

Sonny Dukes

After eleven years, Dukes, once a hard-living motorcycle aficionado, says he has not recovered but has "learned how to accept [the disease] and reconstruct my life around it. . . . I've been through all the stages. If you're going to survive, you've got to sit down and face it, and say this is about as good as it's ever going to get, and hope it doesn't get any worse. At least I'm still here—I'm still alive. I used to hope for a cure," he adds, "but we're not high on government priorities because we don't die. Quality of life doesn't seem to matter much." Dukes says he has married "a good lady" and is leading a reclusive life, taking care of his wife's parents while she works at a drugstore. He cannot hold a job, nor can he ride his bike much. "You don't want to make a mistake on a bike," Dukes says. "There are days when I don't even want to be on it."

Blake Edwards

One of the few Hollywood celebrities to discuss his illness publicly, Edwards first experienced symptoms of CFS in 1983. Over the last decade, he has enjoyed a series of partial remissions. In mid-1995, he was directing a Broadway musical starring his wife, Julie Andrews.

Thomas English

English, a former surgeon, had been ill for ten years by September 1995. Having given up the practice of surgery during the first year of his ordeal, deeming it too dangerous to his patients, he continues to miss his work terribly. "There are days when I would kill to take out an appendix," he says. "Functionally, I'm better than I was at the worst point of the illness, as long as I stay within certain limits."

Gidget Faubion

Called "the little warrior" by her admirers in the middle-1980s, Faubion, now forty-five, ran the national patients' organization in Portland until 1989, when burnout set in. After her departure, the organization dissolved. "The early pioneers had to have tenacity," she says. "It took that to get us on the map. But many of us had to drop out to survive." In the last five years, Faubion says, she has experienced "physical and mental" improvement. Once able to walk only with the support of a cane, she now uses a cane just "ten percent of the time." She works as an independent advocate for the disabled in her Oregon county, focusing on what she describes as the "unique" disabilities suffered by AIDS and CFS patients. "I've concentrated on what we can do to get back into the mainstream." On the matter of her own illness, she says, "There's that twenty percent residual that will always be there, but I'm hopeful."

Candace Gleed

An Ampligen recipient in Dan Peterson's practice for two and a half years, Gleed chose to go off the drug in June 1993. "Ampligen helped, but it became toxic after a while," she says. "In the last six months," she adds, "I've been going downhill." For five years, Gleed had helped educate doctors and nurses who called the Incline Village CFS hot line. When she moved from Reno to Las Vegas in 1995, however, the first board-certified internist she consulted for an infection told her: "CFS doesn't exist." Said the second: "I don't think it's a real disease."

Alan Goldberg

Charlotte resident Goldberg was celebrating his sixtieth birthday when he acquired CFS on a 1985 ski vacation in Incline Village, Nevada. The textile machinery manufacturing executive was forced to retire and remained wholly disabled for five years. With Marc Iverson, he founded the CFIDS Association of America. Now seventy, he says, "I still have problems, but they are not as severe as they once were. I'm able to function."

Cliff Harker

Harker, the Alabama sergeant who inadvertently launched Elaine DeFreitas on her search for the elusive CFS retrovirus, remained ill in 1995. Officially retired from the military in 1992 as a psychiatric disability case, the forty-six-year-old refers to his decade of CFS as "a bumpy ride" and "like looking at the world through a fun house mirror." He adds, "It's a disease of lowered expectations and limitations. If you can find where that limitation point is, you're okay. If you cross it, it comes up and just kicks your butt." In January 1995, Harker experienced three seizures and a mild stroke. Nevertheless, he is working as a receiving clerk, an endeavor that he says does not tax him intellectually or physically. He describes DeFreitas as "a hell of a lady."

William Harvey

Fifty-eight-year-old flight surgeon and pilot Harvey quit flying in 1987 after nearly crashing his small plane during a landing. He did not attempt to fly again until 1992, when he felt sufficiently recovered. "It was a nightmare," he says of his years of severe illness. "I'm still healing." The widespread view of CFS as a psychiatric problem is, he continues, "an optical illusion that just sits here, built into the medical model. When the world flips, and the paradigm changes, it will be because we'll have hard data. But, as doctors, we must try to see reality as it really is." Since writing about his experience in *Aviation, Space and Environmental* magazine, Harvey has been approached by several pilots suffering from CFS, including one of the shuttle astronauts. "We talk about what they should consider doing with their careers, especially if they are flying single-seaters. Inevitably, they must stop. The number of pilots who have [CFS] is pretty damn high," Harvey adds. "We're looking at a *major* problem in aviation, but we just don't know it yet."

Mayhugh Horne

Former Pan Am pilot Horne grounded himself after falling ill in 1985. In 1989 he attempted part-time work at a less intellectually demanding job—selling real estate insurance. Not long afterward, he was involved in a car accident that resulted in additional head injury, destroying his ability to perform gainful employment of any kind. He currently is living on disability payments from the Social Security Administration.

Marc Iverson

Iverson, who became sick in 1979 while a BarclaysAmerica vice president and later founded the CFIDS Association of America, has ceded the day-to-day leadership of the organization to healthy professionals. The forty-two-year-old remains fully disabled.

Martha James (pseudonym)

National Cancer Institute researchers invited James and her daughter, both of whom were stricken during the Yerington, Nevada, epidemic, to come to the NIH in 1986. Nine years later the fifty-five-year-old James continues to suffer cogni-

/

tive difficulties. "Whenever I try to think about a problem," she says, "pretty soon my mind just goes blank. I feel like I've hit a brick wall." Nor can she perform any work with her arms, which continue to be unnaturally weak. "Nobody in Yerington really talks about the epidemic anymore," James adds. "But I think people are still being diagnosed with it. I don't think CFS has gone away."

Sam Josephs (pseudonym)

CFS ended Josephs's dentistry career in June 1985. He was diagnosed by Anthony Komaroff a year later. He lives on disability payments from Social Security and the Veterans Administration. "I'm getting better," the forty-two-year-old says. "I think it's partly because I don't do anything at all, but a lot of it has to do with believing that Jesus will heal you. I've been praying to Jesus to heal me for two years. It has to happen sometime."

Nancy Kaiser

A former golf enthusiast, Kaiser had been ill for nearly ten years and was thought to be in a terminal state when she became the first CFS victim to receive Ampligen in 1989. She experienced dramatic improvement, but she was pulled from the drug in September 1993, and after a two-week grace period she deteriorated rapidly. She is currently confined to a wheelchair or to bed.

Gerald Kennedy

Kennedy, a former drafting teacher, acquired CFS during the Truckee High outbreak of 1985 and was forced into permanent retirement in 1994 at age fifty-five. He receives a partial California state teachers' retirement pension.

Janice Kennedy

Disabled by CFS since February 1985, the former Truckee High English teacher received Ampligen in the 1990 trial. The drug resulted in some improvement, though not enough to allow Kennedy to return to teaching. Now fifty, she is once more housebound and lives on teachers' disability insurance.

Jill Koval

Koval, a member of the U.S. Olympic cycling team, was unable to resume her athletic career after coming down with CFS in mid-1986. Starting in 1988 she experienced gradual improvement. "It wasn't until 1990 that I felt I could live and not worry about it," she says. But she adds, "I'm afraid to ride competitively again because I'm too afraid of getting CFS." Koval manages a personal fitness center in Orange County, California, and occasionally experiences mild symptoms of the disease. "CFS taught me that it's okay not to win—that I don't always have to be number one."

Chris Larson

TWA flight attendant Larson was able to return to work in August 1990 after a five-year medical leave. "I work for three days, rest for four days, then start all over again," she says. Since returning to TWA, she has met other flight attendants who suffer from CFS. "Usually," she says, "I don't tell people I have it, because I'm so misunderstood."

Paul Lavenger

Lavenger, an internal medicine specialist, was disabled by CFS in 1989, two years after his wife acquired the disease. He retired from the practice of medicine after a twenty-five-year career. In 1991 he spoke out publicly about both the epidemic nature of the illness and the federal government's negligence in a lengthy interview in *New York Native*. In April 1995 the doctor died of colon cancer.

Cynthia Modica-Gaines

Modica-Gaines, a former university ballet instructor and performer, was considering suicide before she joined the Nevada Ampligen trial. Having fallen ill at thirty-five, she already had been bedridden for five years. Her sister, who cared for Modica-Gaines during several years of her illness, also acquired the disease, as did a cousin who briefly nursed Modica-Gaines during a period when she was temporarily removed from Ampligen after developing liver problems. The disease, says Modica-Gaines, "is a living death—it's as though you've been kidnapped from your life and locked in your bedroom." When she met Dan Peterson, she recalls, "I could only stare at him like a child in a Keane painting and cry." She received Ampligen for three years. Now, she says, "I'm Lazarus."

Gino Olivieri

The former Rochester, New York, police SWAT team member and Detroit Lions football star, who was featured on the cover of *Newsweek* in 1990, moved to Charlotte that year to participate in the Ampligen trial. He received a placebo, then joined the class action suit against HEM Pharmaceuticals. HEM provided the drug to Olivieri for one year, but the patient recalls that "Ampligen didn't do a thing for me." After the *Newsweek* story, Olivieri received calls from CFS-afflicted policemen in Vancouver, Los Angeles, Seattle, Dallas, and Chicago. He remains housebound and survives on workers' compensation from New York State for job-related injury.

Richard Pearson (pseudonym)

Pearson, the lawyer who was sent by Dan Peterson to the NIH in 1986 for evaluation by Stephen Straus, remains ill nine years later. He is practicing law "half-time," he says. He has remarried and is living in southern California. "On a scale of one to ten, with ten being recovery," Pearson says, "I'm probably a six." He stopped seeing doctors for his condition some years ago. "Have they found the magic bullet?" he inquires.

Howard Penney

Yerington, Nevada, phys ed teacher Penney's near-perfect attendance record began to disintegrate in autumn 1986, one year after the Yerington epidemic began. Over the next four years, he saw seventeen doctors. One doctor diagnosed him with bone cancer, another with lupus, a third with depression; the rest offered no diagnosis at all. Interviewed in 1900, he said, "My life is ruined, my family is ruined, my house is up for sale." In 1995, however, the forty-eight-year-old Penney reported that he is better: "I'm not back to where I want to be, but I'm also ten years older."

Rudy Perpich Jr.

By 1995, Rudy Perpich Jr. had been ill for twelve years. When the disease struck, the son of the Minnesota governor was a twenty-four-year-old second-year law student at Stanford University. His father rallied to his aid, becoming involved in the political process of bringing pressure to bear on federal health agencies, even meeting personally with congressional leaders. The junior Perpich says he now feels "eighty percent better." He works five hours a day as an investment and legal adviser to his father. He is regretful rather than angry that, during the early years of his illness, his doctors advised him to exercise and throw himself into his work. "I drove myself into a furrow," he recalls. As for the politics of the epidemic, he comments, "We got pushed down the rung. I would have preferred to have more attention paid."

Jean, Paul, Hannah, Alison, Libby, and Megan Pollard

The Pollard daughters of Lyndonville, New York, have improved significantly in the six years since their mother, Jean, who was also ill, wrote to Barbara Bush seeking support for research. "They're not cured," Jean says. "They just have great coping skills, and that's what they learned from David Bell. They all have symptoms, but nobody gets bedridden." Their parents, Jean and Paul, are improved, too, though both suffer from short-term memory loss. "We continue to have several new cases of CFS around here," Jean adds.

Joyce Reynolds

A decade after the Nevada epidemic, former bank teller and Truckee resident Joyce Reynolds remains ill. "Sometimes you feel so bad you want to die," Reynolds, now sixty-six, says. An Ampligen recipient for three years under the Food and Drug Administration's compassionate care clause, Reynolds found the drug only mildly helpful. Her two adult sons, believing her to have an imaginary illness, no longer visit.

Sandy Schmidt Fuller

Once an annual participant in the San Francisco marathon, former Incline Village resident Fuller, now fifty-two, was struck by the disease in 1984. "My symptoms began to disappear toward the end of 1988," she says. "There hasn't been anything to bring me back to the doctor since 1989." She adds, "I've had a period of a few years when I wondered if it might come back. I still kind of watch myself." Fuller, who received acyclovir from Dan Peterson, sued Blue Cross/Blue Shield for insurance reimbursement in 1988. The case was settled out of court two years later; Fuller is unable to disclose the sum of money she received, but she reports that she is pleased with the case's resolution. She has remarried and lives in California.

Meghan Shannon

A former respiratory therapist at a San Diego Hospital, Shannon had been severely ill for thirteen years by 1995. When she was reached at a retreat run by nuns in Santa Barbara, she was contemplating suicide. "I will probably not be going home," she said, "not because I'm physically worse, but because I've not been able to find a way to take care of myself without living off other people's generosity and because, in the last few years, the hatred for people with this disease has become so great. I'm forty-five years old. My dreams and hopes are gone. I don't know where else to go, except to the other side, where it's safer."

Susan Simon

Simon, a psychotherapist who had been ill for more than a decade, was killed instantly when a truck collided with her motorized scooter on a New York City street in 1993. A patient in Stephen Straus's NIH cohort and a participant in Straus's acyclovir trial, Simon had talked of suing Straus for malpractice.

Floyd Skloot

Novelist Skloot, ill since December 1988, was a placebo recipient in the 1990 Ampligen study. The former elite-class long-distance racer is bedridden for an average of three days a week, requires a cane to walk, and is able to write for just two hours a day "on a good day." He calls the four-city Ampligen trial "a horror" and says he is working on a fictionalized account of the experience.

Barry Sleight

After ceding his lobbying work to the Sheridan Group, Sleight married a woman who also suffers from CFS and moved from the capital to a small town in Florida. He has since been diagnosed with chronic progressive multiple sclerosis; his wife continues to carry a CFS diagnosis. Sleight's illness began after a case of mono in 1974 when he was in college, but worsened significantly in the middle 1980s, when he was diagnosed with CFS.

Nancy Taylor

Taylor, the wife of a Tulsa entrepreneur and philanthropist, fell ill in 1977 after a blood transfusion, although she was not diagnosed with CFS until 1986. Ampligen, which she received for sixteen weeks in 1989, exacerbated her disease. Her husband, Ed Taylor, who had partially funded the early Nevada trial, was convinced the drug worked in only a small proportion of CFS sufferers and that HEM had toyed with data to cultivate government support for its drug. In 1995, Nancy Taylor remained seriously ill, able to function for only three to four hours every other day. "She is worse, not better," reports her husband, "but that's true of a lot of the ten-year people. Of course, our studies are now telling us that after just five years it's damn near hopeless."

Inga Thompson

By 1995, Olympic cyclist Thompson had suffered from the disease for eleven years, although she reported that her last seriously disabling bout was in 1990. "I still have difficulty with my memory," she says. Somehow, Thompson had managed to race in the 1988 and 1992 Olympics. Training was difficult. "I had to explain to the coaches that I couldn't do the same mileage everyone else could do," she remembers. She retired from the sport after the 1992 games. Now thirty-one, Thompson says the disease prevents her from holding a full-time job. In addition, she must monitor herself carefully to avoid severe relapses. "When I first got sick, I had speech problems," she says. "Now, when I start making up words that don't exist, and have trouble with pronunciation, that's a sign. Another sign is depression."

Paul Thompson (pseudonym)

Computer prodigy Thompson, who fell ill during the Incline Village, Nevada, epidemic of 1984–1985, continues to experience minor symptoms of CFS, but no longer suffers the pronounced cognition problems that originally beset him. "The logic skills are mostly back," Thompson says.

Gore Vidal

Through a spokesman, Vidal reported in 1995 that his 1987 CFS diagnosis had been made in error and that he was no longer ill.

Tracy Watson (pseudonym)

A member of Stephen Straus's patient cohort, former kindergarten teacher Watson has been bedridden or wheelchair-bound since 1986. Beginning that year, she made numerous trips to the NIH, where she underwent four brain scans, two lumbar punctures, an arteriogram, laparoscopy, lymphofluoresis, and numerous other tests for rare diseases. On each visit, she was required to fill out an array of psychological questionnaires. Once a Straus defender, Watson conceded in 1995 that the researcher was erratic in his moods and frightened her.

Romy Zarit

Zarit, ill since March 1986, was never able to resume her career as a flight attendant for PSA; her husband, a minister, acquired the disease one year after Zarit did; the couple recently moved from Los Angeles to Whitefish, Montana, with their two daughters, who remain unafflicted.

Endnotes

1. Clinical Mysteries

1. Richard DuBois et al., "Chronic Mononucleosis Syndrome," *Southern Medical Journal* (Nov. 1984): 1376–82.

2. Gustavo C. Roman and William Sheremata, "Multiple Sclerosis (Not Tropical Spastic Paraparesis) on Key West, Florida," *Lancet* 1 (8543) (May 23, 1987): 1199.

3. James Jones et al., "Evidence for Active Epstein-Barr Virus Infections in Patients with Persistent, Unexplained Illnesses," *Annals of Internal Medicine* 102 (Jan. 1985): 1–7.

4. "Infectious Mononucleosis," NIH Publication, no. 88–142 (May 1986).

5. Stephen E. Straus et al., "Persisting Illness and Fatigue in Adults with Evidence of Epstein-Barr Virus Infection," *Annals of Internal Medicine* 102 (Jan. 1985): 7–16.

2. Raggedy Ann Syndrome

1. William Boly, "Raggedy Ann Town," *Hippocrates* (July/Aug. 1987): 30–40.

2. Hilary Koprowski et al., "Multiple Sclerosis and Human T-cell Lymphotropic Retroviruses," *Nature* 318 (Nov. 14, 1985): 154–60.

3. Foot Soldiers from Atlanta

1. James D. Watson, *The Double Helix* (New York: Atheneum Publishers, 1968).

2. Randy Shilts, *And the Band Played On* (New York: St. Martin's Press, 1987).

3. William Sheremata et al., "Unusual Occurrence on a Tropical Island of Multiple Sclerosis," *Lancet* 2 (1985): 618.

4. W. I. MacDonald and A. M. Halliday, "Diagnosis and Classification of Multiple Sclerosis," *British Medical Bulletin* 33 (1977): 4–8.

5. Robert C. Gallo, "The First Human Retrovirus," *Scientific American* (Dec. 1986): 98.

6. Gallo, p. 88.

7. Gallo, p. 98

4. Rural Disasters

1. Hilary Koprowski et al., "Multiple Sclerosis and Human T-cell Lymphotropic Retroviruses," *Nature* 318 (Nov. 14, 1985): 154–60.

2. Jonathan Trobe, quoted in Robin Marantz Henig, "The Inner Landscape," Body and Mind column, *New York Times Magazine,* April 17, 1988.

5. Folie à Deux?

1. Seymour Grufferman et al., "Burkitt's and Other Non-Hodgkin's Lymphomas in Adults Exposed to a Visitor from Africa," *New England Journal of Medicine* 313 (Dec. 12, 1985): 1525–29.

6. The Prepared Mind

1. C. Alfieri et al., "Lytic, Nontransforming Epstein-Barr Virus from a Patient with Chronic Active EBV Infection," *Canadian Medical Association Journal* 13, no. 10 (Nov. 15, 1984): 1249–52.

2. John Ding-E Young and Zanvil A. Cohn, "How Killer Cells Kill," *Scientific American,* Jan. 1988, p. 38.

3. John L. Sullivan et al., "Deficient Natural Killer Cell Activity in X-linked Proliferative Syndrome," *Science* 210, no. 4469 (1980): 543–45.

7. Not Normal Americans

1. Leslie J. Dorfman, "Lake Tahoe Mystery Disease," *Science* 235, no. 4789 (Feb. 6, 1987): 623.

2. Robert Gottlieb, "*Pneumocystis* Pneumonia—Los Angeles," *Morbidity and Mortality Weekly Report,* June 5, 1981.

3. Byron Hyde, "Three Definitions of Myalgic Encephalomyelitis (ME/CFS) and the History of ME/CFS" (presented at Chronic Fatigue Syndrome and Fibromyalgia: Pathogenesis and Treatment, First International Conference, Los Angeles, Cal., Feb. 16–18, 1990).

4. Denis Wakefield, "Immunological Abnormalities and Immune Therapy in Chronic Fatigue Syndrome" (presented at Chronic Fatigue Syndrome and Fibromyalgia: Pathogenesis and Treatment, First International Conference, Los Angeles, Cal., Feb. 16–18, 1990).

5. Edward Shorter, *From Paralysis to Fatigue* (New York: Free Press, 1992), p. 317.

8. "Dear Sirs, I Am *Sick . . .*"

1. Theodore Van Zelst before the Senate Labor, Health and Human Services Education and Related Agencies Appropriations Subcommittee, 99th Cong., 2d sess., May 1, 1986.

9. Jerry's Poster Kids

1. Syed Zaki Salahuddin et al., "Isolation of a New Virus, HBLV, in Patients with Lymphoproliferative Disorders," *Science* 234 (4776) (Oct. 31, 1987): 596–601.

10. "You Have Been Blackballed"

1. Susan Conant, *Living with Chronic Fatigue: New Strategies for Coping with and Conquering CFS* (Dallas: Taylor Publishing, 1990), p. 24.

11. Antecedent Epidemics

1. Donald A. Henderson and Alexis Shelokov, "Epidemic Neuromyasthenia—Clinical Syndrome?" *New England Journal of Medicine* 260 (Apr. 9, 1959): 757–64; Donald A. Henderson and Alexis Shelokov, "Epidemic Neuromyasthenia—Clinical Syndrome? (Concluded)," *New England Journal of Medicine* 260 (Apr. 16, 1959): 814–18.

2. Berton Roueche, *The Orange Man and Other Narratives of Medical Detection* (New York: Little, Brown and Co., 1971), pp. 95–115.

3. David Poskanzer et al., "Epidemic Neuromyasthenia: Outbreak in Punta Gorda, Florida," *New England Journal of Medicine* 257 (Aug. 22, 1957): 356–64.

4. Alexis Shelokov, "Epidemic Neuromyasthenia, An Outbreak of Poliomyelitis-like Illness in Student Nurses," *New England Journal of Medicine* 257 (Aug. 22, 1957): 345–55.

5. A. G. Gilliam, "Epidemiological Study of Epidemic, Diagnosed as Poliomyelitis, Occurring Among the Personnel of Los Angeles County General Hospital During the Summer of 1934," *Public Health Bulletin* 240 (Washington, D.C.: Government Printing Office, 1938).

6. David Poskanzer, "Epidemic Malaise," *British Medical Journal* 2, no. 5706 (1970): 420–21.

7. Gary P. Holmes et al., "A Cluster of Patients with a Chronic Mononucleosis-like Syndrome: Is Epstein-Barr Virus the Cause?" *Journal of the American Medical Association* 257, no. 17 (May 1, 1987): 2297–302.

8. Dedra Buchwald, John L. Sullivan, and Anthony Komaroff, "Frequency of 'Chronic Active Epstein-Barr Virus Infection' in a General Medicine Practice," *Journal of the American Medical Association* 257, no. 17 (May 1, 1987): 2303–7.

9. David Bell, *The Disease of a Thousand Names* (Lyndonville, N.Y.: Pollard Publications, 1991), 67.

10. T. M. Mukherjee et al., "Abnormal Red-Blood-Cell Morphology in Myalgic Encephalomyelitis," *Lancet* 2 (8554) (Aug. 8, 1987): 328–29.

11. Tadao Aoki et al., "Low Natural Killer Syndrome: Clinical and Immunologic Features," *Natural Immunity and Cell Growth Regulation* 6 (1987): 116–28.

12. Fatigue unto Death

1. Richard S. Tedder et al., "A Novel Lymphotropic Herpesvirus," *Lancet* 2 (8555) (Aug. 15, 1987): 390–92.

2. Paolo Lusso et al., "Diverse Tropism of Human B-Lymphotropic Virus (Human Herpesvirus 6)," *Lancet* 2 (8561) (Sept. 26, 1987): 743.

3. Michael Caligiuri et al., "Phenotypic and Functional Deficiency of Natural Killer Cells in Patients with Chronic Fatigue Syndrome," *Journal of Immunology* 139, no. 10 (Nov. 15, 1987): 3306–13.

4. Igor Grant, J. Hampton Atkinson, John R. Hesselink, Caroline J. Kennedy, Douglas D. Richman, Stephen A. Spector, J. Allen McCutchan, "Evidence for Early Central Nervous System Involvement in the Acquired Immunodeficiency Syndrome (AIDS) and Other Human Immunodeficiency Virus (HIV) Infections; Studies of Neuropsychological Testing and Magnetic Resonance Imaging," *Annals of Internal Medicine* 107 (6) (Dec. 1987): 828–36.

13. Salami Science

1. Galel E. Yousef et al., "Chronic Enterovirus Infection in Patients with Postviral Fatigue Syndrome," *Lancet* 1 (8578) (Jan. 23, 1988): 146–50.

2. William Carter et al., "Clinical, Immunological, Virological Effects of Ampligen, a Mismatched Double-Stranded RNA, in Patients with AIDS or AIDS-Related Complex," *Lancet* 1 (8545) (June 6, 1987): 1286–92.

3. Gary Holmes et al., "Chronic Fatigue Syndrome: A Working Case Definition," *Annals of Internal Medicine* 108 (1988): 387–89.

14. Viral Vicissitudes

1. Stephen Straus, "The Chronic Mononucleosis Syndrome," *Journal of Infectious Diseases* 157 (Mar. 1988): 405–12.

2. James Jones et al., "T-Cell Lymphomas Containing Epstein-Barr Viral DNA in Patients with Chronic Epstein-Barr Virus Infections," *New England Journal of Medicine* 318 (Mar. 24, 1988): 733–41.

3. Stephen Straus, "Allergy and the Chronic Fatigue Syndrome," *Journal of Allergy and Clinical Immunology* 81 (May 1988): 791–95.

4. Peter Manu et al., "The Mental Health of Patients with a Chief Complaint of Chronic Fatigue; A Prospective Evaluation and Follow Up," *Archives of Internal Medicine* 148 (1988): 2213–17.

5. Anthony Komaroff, "The Chronic Fatigue Syndrome," *Annals of Internal Medicine* 110 (5) (March 1, 1989): 407–8.

6. Koichi Yamanishi et al., "Identification of Human Herpes Virus 6 as a Casual Agent for Exanthem Subitem," *Lancet* 1 (8594) (May 14, 1988): 1065–67.

7. Y. Eizuru et al., "Human Herpes Virus 6 in Lymph Nodes," *Lancet* 1 (8628) (Jan. 7, 1989): 40.

8. Anthony Komaroff et al., "A Chronic 'Post-Viral' Fatigue Syndrome with Neurologic Features: Serologic Association with Human Herpes Virus 6 (HIV6)." Abstract presented to the Society of General Internal Medicine, Washington, D.C., April 27–29, 1988.

9. Kurt Kroenke et al., "Chronic Fatigue in Primary Care; Prevalence, Patient Characteristics, and Outcome," *Journal of the American Medical Association* 260, no. 7 (Aug. 19, 1988): 929–34.

15. Return from the Living Dead

1. John C. Murdoch, "Cell-Mediated Immunity in Patients with Myalgic Encephalomyelitis

[ME] Syndrome," *New Zealand Medical Journal* 101 (Aug. 1988): 511–12.

2. Stephen Straus et al., "Acyclovir Treatment of the Chronic Fatigue Syndrome; Lack of Efficacy in a Placebo-Controlled Trial," *New England Journal of Medicine* 319 (Dec. 29, 1988): 1692–98.

16. Black Jell-O

1. Oliver Sacks, *The Man Who Mistook His Wife for a Hat* (New York: HarperCollins, 1987), p. 4

2. Gary Franklin et al., "Cognitive Loss in Multiple Sclerosis, Case Reports and Review of the Literature," *Archives of Neurology* (Feb. 1989): 162–67.

3. E. Premkumar Reddy et al., "Amlification and Molecular Cloning of HTLV-1 Sequences from DNA of Multiple Sclerosis Patients," *Science* 243, no. 4890 (Jan. 1989): 529–33.

4. Marcus J. P. Kruesi et al., "Psychiatric Diagnoses in Patients Who Have Chronic Fatigue Syndrome," *Journal of Clinical Psychiatry* 50, no. 2 (1989): 53–56.

17. The Lie

1. Paul R. Cheney et al., "Interleukin-2 and the Chronic Fatigue Syndrome," *Annals of Internal Medicine* 110 (1989): 321.

2. Steven A. Rosenberg et al., "A Progress Report on the Treatment of 157 with Advanced Cancer Using Lymphokine-Activated Killer Cells and Interleukin-2 or High Dose Interleukin-2 Alone," *New England Journal of Medicine* 316 (Apr. 9, 1987): 889–97; Kirk D. Denicoff et al., "The Neuropsychiatric Effects of Treatment with Interleukin-2 and Lymphokine-Activated Killer Cells," *Annals of Internal Medicine* 107 (1987): 293–300.

3. John L. Trotter et al., "Elevated Serum Interleukin-2 Levels in Chronic Progressive Multiple Sclerosis," *New England Journal of Medicine* 318 (18) (May 5, 1988): 1206.

4. John Dwyer, *The Body at War: The Miracle of the Immune System* (New York: NAL Penguin, 1988).

5. Andrew R. Lloyd et al., "Immunological Abnormalities in the Chronic Fatigue Syndrome," *Medical Journal of Australia* 151, no. 3 (1989): 122–24.

18. Disappearing Fingerprints

1. Carolyn L. Warner et al., "Neurologic Abnormalities in the Chronic Fatigue Syndrome," *Neurology* 39, suppl. 1 (March 1989): 420.

2. *CFIDS Chronicle,* Summer-Fall 1989, p. 166.

19. The Ampligen Effect

1. William T. Harvey, "A Flight Surgeon's Personal View of an Emerging Illness," *Aviation, Space and Environmental Medicine* 60 (Dec. 1989): 1199–1201.

2. Charles Helmick et al., "Multiple Sclerosis in Key West, Florida," *American Journal of Epidemiology* 130, no. 5 (1989): 935–49.

20. The Sneering Committee

1. Floyd Skloot, "Chronic Fatigue Syndrome: How One Victim Copes, Why the Media Trivializes It, Why Some in the Medical Community Dismiss It," *Boston Phoenix,* May 31, 1991.

2. Curt A. Sandman et al., "Memory Deficits Associated with Chronic Fatigue Immune Dysfunction Syndrome," *Biological Psychiatry* 33, no. 8–9 (Apr. 15, 1993): 618–23.

21. Waist Deep in Alligators

1. Molly Haskell, *Love and Other Infectious Diseases, A Memoir* (New York: William Morrow, 1990).

2. Haskell, pp. 9–10.

3. Haskell, p. 274.

4. Nancy Klimas et al., "Immunologic Abnormalities in Chronic Fatigue Syndrome," *Journal of Clinical Microbiology* 28 (June 1990): 1403–10.

5. Deborah Gold et al., "Chronic Fatigue: A Prospective Clinical and Virologic Study," *Journal of the American Medical Association* 264, no. 1 (1990): 48–53.

22. Kyoto

1. Andrew R. Lloyd et al., "Immunological Abnormalities in the Chronic Fatigue Syndrome," *Medical Journal of Australia* 151, no. 3 (1989): 122–24.

2. Ian Hickie et al., "The Psychiatric Status of Patients with the Chronic Fatigue Syndrome, *British Journal of Psychiatry* 156 (1990): 534–40.

3. Andrew R. Lloyd et al., "Prevalence of Chronic Fatigue Syndrome in an Australian Population," *Medical Journal of Australia* 153, no. 9 (Nov. 5, 1990): 522–28.

23. Playing Catch-up

1. Lawrence Altman, "Lymphomas Are on the Rise in the U.S., and No One Knows Why," *New York Times,* May 24, 1994. Altman's source: John O. E. Clark, consultant editor, *The Human Body: A Comprehensive Guide to the Structure and Functions of the Human Body* (New York: Arch Cape Press, 1989).

2. Alejandro Mohar et al., "Non-Hodgkin's Lymphoma and Epstein-Barr Virus: Evidence of Altered Antibody Pattern Prior to Diagnosis." Abstract presented at the 21st annual meeting of the Society for Epidemiologic Research, Vancouver, British Columbia, Canada, June 15–17, 1988.

24. Malfeasance and Nonfeasance

1. Walid Heneine et al., "HTLV-II Endemicity among Guayami Indians in Panama," *New England Journal of Medicine* 324 (Feb. 21, 1991): 565.

25. A Conspiracy of Dunces

1. Donald A. Henderson and Alexis Shelokov, "Epidemic Neuromyasthenia—Clinical Syndrome?" *New England Journal of Medicine* 260 (April 9, 1959): 757–64; Donald A. Henderson and Alexis Shelokov, "Epidemic Neuromyasthenia—Clinical Syndrome? (Concluded)," *New England Journal of Medicine* 260 (April 16, 1959): 814–18.

2. Robin A. Weiss, "Foamy Viruses: A Virus in Search of a Disease," *Nature* 333 (June 9, 1988): 498.

26. Smoke and Mirrors

1. Catherine Macek, "Acquired Immunodeficiency Cause(s) Still Elusive," *Journal of the American Medical Association* 248 (1982): 1243.

2. Susan Sontag, *Illness as Metaphor* (New York: Vintage Books, 1979), p. 60.

3. Robert Gallo, *Virus Hunting, AIDS, Cancer and the Human Retrovirus: A Story of Scientific Discovery* (New York: Basic Books, 1991), p. 148.

4. Elaine DeFreitas et al., "Retroviral Sequences Related to Human T-Lymphotropic Virus Type II in Patients with Chronic Fatigue Immune Dysfunction Syndrome," *Proceedings of the National Academy of Sciences* 88 (Apr. 1991): 2922–26.

5. Mark Scott Smith et al., "Chronic Fatigue in Adolescents," *Pediatrics* 88, no. 2 (Aug. 1991): 195–201.

27. Heartsink

1. Jay A. Goldstein, *Chronic Fatigue Syndromes: The Limbic Hypothesis* (Newport Beach, Calif.: Haworth Press, 1992).

2. Steven F. Josephs et al., "HHV6 Reactivation in Chronic Fatigue Syndrome," *Lancet* 337 (8753) (June 1, 1991): 1346–47.

3. Katrin Bothe et al., "Progressive Encephalopathy and Myopathy in Transgenic Mice Expressing Human Foamy Virus Genes," *Science* 253 (Aug. 2, 1991): 555–57.

28. The "Charly" Syndrome

1. Mindy Kitei, "The AIDS Drug No One Can Have," *Philadelphia,* Oct. 1994, pp. 94–105.

2. Robert J. Suhadolnik et al., "Changes in the 2-5A Synthetase/Rnase L Antiviral Pathway in a Controlled Clinical Trial with Poly(I)-Poly($C_{12}U$) in Chronic Fatigue Syndrome," *In Vivo* 8 (1994): 599–604. "Poly(I)-poly($C_{12}U$)" is the molecular name for Ampligen.

3. Kitei, p. 104.

4. Valerie Fahey, "Waiting in Line at the FDA," *In Health,* September-October 1990, p. 55.

29. The Retrovirus Caper

1. Lauren Krupp et al., "An Overview of Chronic Fatigue Syndrome," *Journal of Clinical Psychiatry* 52 (Oct. 1991): 403–10.

31. Subculture of Invalidism

1. Dedra Buchwald et al., "A Chronic Illness Characterized by Fatigue, Neurologic and Immunologic Disorders, and Active Human Herpesvirus Type 6 Infection," *Annals of Internal Medicine* 116 (Jan. 15, 1992): 103–13.

2. William Reeves et al., "The Chronic Fatigue Syndrome Controversy," *Annals of Internal Medicine* 117 (Aug. 15, 1992): 343.

3. Irving E. Salit, "Sporadic Postinfectious Neuromyasthemia," *Canadian Medical Association Journal* 133 (1985): 659–63.

4. Edward Shorter, *From Paralysis to Fatigue: A History of Psychosomatic Illness in the Modern Era* (New York: Free Press, 1992), pp. 317–18.

5. Anthony Komaroff, "Chronic Fatigue Syndrome: An Alternative View," *The Harvard Mental Health Letter* 9 (May 1993): 4–5.

6. Lawrence K. Altman, "Lymphomas Are on the Rise in the U.S., and No One Knows Why," *New York Times,* May 24, 1994, p. B7.

32. The Greatest Underestimate of All Time

1. Norma C. Ware and Arthur Kleinman, "Depression in Neurasthenia and Chronic Fatigue Syndrome," *Psychiatric Annals* 22 (1992): 202–8.

2. Thomas M. Folks et al., "Investigation of Retroviral Involvement in Chronic Fatigue Syndrome." Presented at Ciba Foundation Symposium #173, London, England, May 13, 1992 (Chichester, England: John Wiley & Sons, 1993), pp. 160–75.

33. HIV-Negative AIDS

1. David Ho et al., "Idiopathic CD4 Lymphocytopenia," *New England Journal of Medicine* 328 (1993): 380–85.

2. William Reeves et al., "The Chronic Fatigue Syndrome Controversy," *Annals of Internal Medicine* 117 (Aug. 15, 1992): 343.

3. Ann Schleuderberg et al., "Chronic Fatigue Syndrome Research; Definition and Medical Outcome Assessment," *Annals of Internal Medicine* 117 (Aug. 15, 1992): 325–31.

4. Jeffrey Laurence et al., "Acquired Immunodeficiency Without Evidence of Human Immunodeficiency Virus Types One and Two," *Lancet* 340 (1992): 273.

5. Paul H. Levine et al., "Does Chronic Fatigue Syndrome Predispose to Non-Hodgkin's Lymphoma?" *Cancer Research* 52, suppl. (Oct. 1, 1992): 5516s–18s.

6. Ali S. Khan et al., "Assessment of a Retrovirus Sequence and Other Possible Risk Factors for the Chronic Fatigue Syndrome in Adults," *Annals of Internal Medicine* 18, no. 4 (1992): 241–45.

34. A Failed Initiative

1. Joshua Lederberg, Robert E. Shope, and Stanley C. Oaks Jr., eds., *Emerging Infections: Microbial Threats to Health in the United States* (Washington, D.C.: National Academy Press, 1992), pp. 2, 3, 136.

2. Stephen E. Straus et al., "Lymphocyte Phenotype and Function in the Chronic Fatigue Syndrome," *Journal of Clinical Immunology* 13, no. 1(1993): 30–40.

3. David R. Strayer et al., "A Controlled Clinical Trial with a Specifically Configured RNA Drug, Poly(I)-Poly($C_{12}U$), in Chronic Fatigue Syndrome," *Clinical Infectious Diseases* 18, Suppl. 1 (Jan. 1994): S88–95.

4. Thomas M. Folks et al., "Investigation of Retroviral Involvement in Chronic Fatigue Syndrome." Presented at Ciba Foundation Symposium #173, London, England, May 13, 1992 (Chichester, England: John Wiley & Sons, 1993), pp. 160–175.

5. Ali S. Khan et al., "Assessment of a Retrovirus Sequence and Other Possible Risk Factors for CFS in Adults," *Annals of Internal Medicine* 118, no. 4 (1993): 241–45.

6. Walter Gunn et al., "Inability of Retroviral Tests to Identify Persons with Chronic Fatigue Syndrome," *Morbidity and Mortality Weekly Report* 42, no. 10 (1993): 183, 189–90.

7. Allen C. Steere et al., "The Overdiagnosis of Lyme Disease," *Journal of the American Medical Association* 269, no. 14 (1993): pp. 1812–16.

35. Science by the Rules

1. David W. Bates et al., "Prevalence of Fatigue and Chronic Fatigue Syndrome in a Primary Care Practice," *Archives of Internal Medicine* 153 (1993): 2759–65.

2. Dedra Buchwald et al., "Chronic Fatigue and the Chronic Fatigue Syndrome: Prevalence in a Pacific Northwest Health Care System," *Annals of Internal Medicine* 123 (July 15, 1995): pp. 81–88.

3. New Zealand CFS incidence estimate by Michael Holmes, senior lecturer, Department of Microbiology, University of Otago, Dunedin, New Zealand (personal communication); Netherlands incidence estimate by J.H.M.M. Vercoulen, Department of Medical Psychology, University Hospital Nijmegen, Nijmegen, The Netherlands (presented at the American Association for Chronic Fatigue Syndrome Research Conference, Fort Lauderdale, Florida, Oct. 7–9, 1994); Belgian incidence estimate by Bernard Fischler, Department of Psychiatry, Academic Hospital of the Free University, Brussels, Belgium (personal communication).

4. David R. Strayer et al., "A Controlled Clinical Trial with a Specifically Configured RNA Drug, Poly(I)-Poly(C$_{12}$U), in Chronic Fatigue Syndrome," *Clinical Infectious Diseases* 18, Suppl. 1 (Jan. 1994): S88–95.

5. Pascale De Becker et al., "Ampligen: Activity in Chronic Fatigue Syndrome." Poster presented at the American Association for Chronic Fatigue Syndrome Research Conference, Oct. 7–9, 1994, Fort Lauderdale, Florida.

6. Tom Folks et al., "Lack of Evidence for Infection with Known Human and Animal Retroviruses in Patients with Chronic Fatigue Syndrome," *Clinical Infectious Diseases* 18, Suppl. 1 (1994): S121.

7. Richard B. Schwartz et al., "SPECT Imaging of the Brain: Comparison of Findings in Patients with Chronic Fatigue Syndrome, AIDS Dementia Complex, and Major Unipolar Depression," *American Journal of Roentgenology* 162 (Apr. 1994): 943–51.

8. W. John Martin et al., "Cytomegalovirus-Related Sequence in an Atypical Cytopathic Virus Repeatedly Isolated from a Patient with Chronic Fatigue Syndrome," *American Journal of Pathology* 145 (Aug. 1994): 140–45.

9. Sheila Bastien and Daniel Peterson, "IQ Abnormalities Associated with Chronic Fatigue Syndrome in Repeated WAIS-R Testing." Paper presented at the American Association for Chronic Fatigue Syndrome Research Conference in Fort Lauderdale, Florida, Oct. 1994.

10. Marion Poore et al., "An Unexplained Illness in West Otago," *The New Zeland Medical Journal* 97, no. 757 (1984): 351–54.

11. Keiji Fukuda et al., "The Chronic Fatigue Syndrome: A Comprehensive Approach to Its Definition and Study," *Annals of Internal Medicine* 121 (Dec. 15, 1994): 953–59.

Epilogue

1. Sandra Panem et al., "C-type Virus Expression in Systemic Lupus Erythematosus," *New England Journal of Medicine* 295 (Aug. 26, 1976): 470–75; Sandra Panem et al., "Viral Immune Complexes in Systemic Lupus Erythematosus: Specificity of C-type Viral Complexes," *Laboratory Investigation* 39(5) (Nov. 1978): 413–20; Sandra Panem et al., "Retrovirus Expression in Normal and Pathogenic Processes of Man," *Federation Proceedings* 38(13) (Dec. 1979): 2674–78; J. T. Reynolds and Sandra Panem, "Characterization of Antibody to C-type Virus Antigens Isolated from Immune Complexes in Kidneys of Patients with Systemic Lupus Erythematosus," *Laboratory Investigation* 44(5) (May 1981): 410–9; Sandra Panem, "HEL-12 Virus: General Considerations [Review]," *Survey of Immunological Research* 2(1) (1983):12–24.

2. S. M. Brooks et al., "The Immune Response to and Expression of Cross-Reactive Retroviral Gag Sequences in Autoimmune Disease," *British Journal of Rheumatology* 31, no. 11 (1992): 735–42.

Index